Heart Physiology
From Cell to Circulation
Fourth Edition

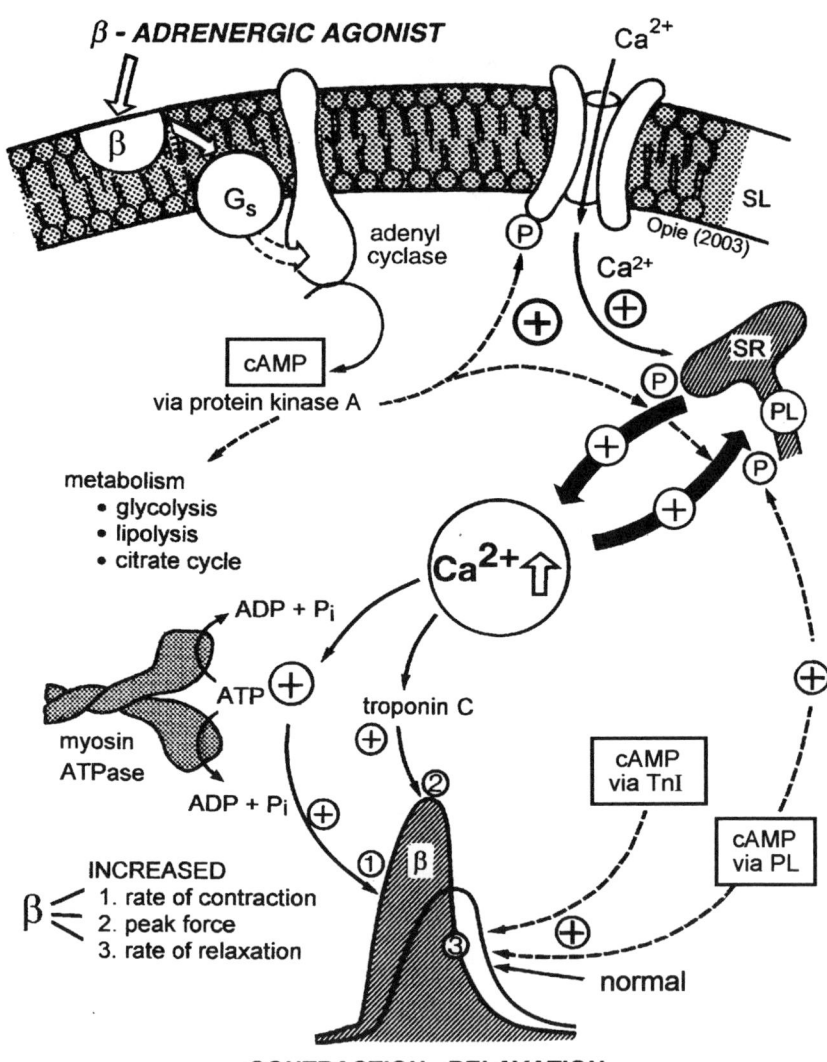

Heart Physiology
From Cell to Circulation
Fourth Edition

Lionel H. Opie, M.D., D.Phil., D.Sc.
*Director, Hatter Institute for Cardiology Research
Cape Heart Centre, Faculty of Health Sciences
Professor of Medicine Emeritus, University of Cape Town
Cape Town, South Africa*

Fellow of the Physiology Society of Southern Africa (2002)

*Visiting Research Fellow (1997), Merton College
Rhodes Scholar (1957–1959), Lincoln College
University of Oxford
Oxford, United Kingdom*

*Visiting Professor (1984–1998), Cardiovascular Division
Stanford University Medical Center
Stanford, California*

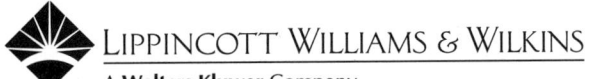

LIPPINCOTT WILLIAMS & WILKINS
A **Wolters Kluwer** Company
Philadelphia • Baltimore • New York • London
Buenos Aires • Hong Kong • Sydney • Tokyo

Acquisitions Editor: Ruth W. Weinberg
Developmental Editor: Joanne Bersin
Production Editor: Frank Aversa
Manufacturing Manager: Ben Rivera
Cover Designer: Christine Jenny
Compositor: Lippincott Williams & Wilkins, Desktop Division
Printer: Maple-Press

© 2004 by LIPPINCOTT WILLIAMS & WILKINS
530 Walnut Street
Philadelphia, PA 19106 USA
LWW.com

Illustrations © 2004 by Lionel H. Opie.

All rights reserved. This book is protected by copyright. No part of this book may be reproduced in any form or by any means, including photocopying, or utilized by any information storage and retrieval system without written permission from the copyright owner, except for brief quotations embodied in critical articles and reviews. Materials appearing in this book prepared by individuals as part of their official duties as U.S. government employees are not covered by the above-mentioned copyright.

Printed in the USA

Library of Congress Cataloging-in-Publication Data

Opie, Lionel H.
  Heart physiology : from cell to circulation / Lionel H. Opie—4th ed.
    p. ; cm.
  Includes bibliographical references and index.
  ISBN 0-7817-4278-1
    1. Heart—Physiology. 2. Heart—Metabolism. 3. Heart cells. I. Title.
    [DNLM: 1. Heart—physiology. 2. Cardiovascular Physiology. 3. Coronary Circulaton—physiology. WG 202 O61h 2004]
  QP111.4.O64 2004
  612.1′7—dc22

2003058870

Care has been taken to confirm the accuracy of the information presented and to describe generally accepted practices. However, the authors and publisher are not responsible for errors or omissions or for any consequences from application of the information in this book and make no warranty, expressed or implied, with respect to the currency, completeness, or accuracy of the contents of the publication. Application of this information in a particular situation remains the professional responsibility of the practitioner.

The authors and publisher have exerted every effort to ensure that drug selection and dosage set forth in this text are in accordance with current recommendations and practice at the time of publication. However, in view of ongoing research, changes in government regulations, and the constant flow of information relating to drug therapy and drug reactions, the reader is urged to check the package insert for each drug for any change in indications and dosage and for added warnings and precautions. This is particularly important when the recommended agent is a new or infrequently employed drug.

Some drugs and medical devices presented in this publication have Food and Drug Administration (FDA) clearance for limited use in restricted research settings. It is the responsibility of the health care provider to ascertain the FDA status of each drug or device planned for use in their clinical practice.

10 9 8 7 6 5 4 3 2 1

To three outstanding teachers
Eugene Braunwald
leader among cardiovascular leaders,
and writer among writers

Arnold M. Katz
an inspiring writer,* teacher, and speaker

William Henry Opie
my late father, who taught me that the search for truth
is the basis of all scientific endeavor

And to my family
I cannot overemphasize my gratitude
for the love and support given to me by my family.
In the words of a Chinese colleague working in Beijing:

I believe the result of work is really the truth, it
takes me all my lifetime; sacrifice the happiness
of my family.

---

* I have read only two books on cardiology virtually from cover to cover. Paul Wood's *Diseases of the Heart and Circulation*, read as a clinical medical student in 1954, and Arnold Katz's *Physiology of the Heart*, when first published in 1977. They both made a profound impression.

Legend to frontispiece

This illustration emphasizes the crucial role of dynamic cell signaling in modern physiology, showing the many steps in the cellular response to β-adrenergic stimulation that lead to the typical stimulation of contraction and relaxation. TnI, troponin I; PL, phospholamban; P, phosphorylation; Gs, G-protein, stimulatory; SR, sarcoplasmic reticulum.

Contents

Contributing Authors ix
Foreword *by Eugene Braunwald* xi
Foreword *by Arnold M. Katz* xiii
From the Introduction to the First Edition *by Richard J. Bing* xv
Preface xvii
Acknowledgments xix

I. Basic Cardiovascular Physiology

1. Introductory Cardiovascular Concepts 3
2. Control of the Circulation 16
3. Heart Cells and Organelles 42

II. Electrophysiology and Electrocardiogram

4. Channels, Pumps, and Exchangers 73
5. Pacemakers, Conduction System, and Electrocardiogram ... 119
   Lionel H. Opie and James M. Downey

III. Calcium and Contraction: Receptors and Signals

6. Excitation-Contraction Coupling and Calcium 159
   Lionel H. Opie and Donald M. Bers
7. Receptors and Signal Transduction 186
8. Myocardial Contraction and Relaxation 221
   Lionel H. Opie and R. John Solaro
9. Signal Systems: Coordinating Life and Death 247
   Lionel H. Opie and Michael M. Sack

IV. The Heart

10. Oxygen Supply: Coronary Flow 279
    Lionel H. Opie and Gerd Heusch

11.	Fuels: Aerobic and Anaerobic Metabolism. . . . . *Lionel H. Opie and Gary D. Lopaschuk*	306
12.	Ventricular Function . . . . *Lionel H. Opie and Mark G. Perlroth*	355
13.	Overload Hypertrophy and Its Molecular Biology	402

V. The Circulation

14.	Blood Pressure and Peripheral Circulation. . . . . *Lionel H. Opie and David J. Paterson*	431
15.	Cardiac Output and Exercise . . . . *Lionel H. Opie and David J. Paterson*	460
16.	Heart Failure: Neurohumoral Responses	485

VI. Pathophysiology

17.	Lack of Blood Flow: Ischemia and Angina . . . . *Lionel H. Opie and Gerd Heusch*	525
18.	Acute Coronary Syndromes: Cell Death	553
19.	Myocardial Reperfusion: Stunning, Hibernation, and Preconditioning. . . . . *Lionel H. Opie and Gerd Heusch*	574
20.	Electricity Out of Control: Arrhythmias	599
Subject Index.		625

Contributing Authors

Donald M. Bers, Ph.D.
Professor and Chair of Physiology, Loyola University Chicago, Stritch School of Medicine, Maywood, Illinois

James M. Downey, Ph.D.
Professor of Physiology, College of Medicine, University of South Alabama, Mobile, Alabama

Gerd Heusch, M.D., Ph.D., M.D.(Hon)
Professor and Director, Institute for Pathophysiology, University Clinic Essen, Essen, Germany

Gary D. Lopaschuk, Ph.D.
Professor and Director, Cardiovascular Research Group, Heritage Medical Research Centre, University of Alberta, Edmonton, Alberta, Canada

David J. Paterson, D.Phil.
Joint Director, Burdon Sanderson Cardiac Science Centre, Professor of Cardiovascular Physiology and Fellow of Merton College, University of Oxford, Oxford, England

Mark G. Perlroth, M.D.
Professor of Physiology and Medicine, Division of Cardiovascular Diseases, Department of Medicine, Stanford University School of Medicine, Stanford, California

Michael M. Sack, M.D., Ph.D.
Mitochondrial Genomics Laboratory, Cardiovascular Branch, National Institutes of Health, Bethesda, Maryland

R. John Solaro, Ph.D.
University Professor and Head, Department of Physiology and Biophysics, University of Illinois at Chicago, College of Medicine, Chicago, Illinois

Foreword

Despite the extraordinary advances in cardiology during the past century, cardiovascular disease remains the most common cause of death and serious morbidity in the industrialized world and is increasing rapidly in developing nations. However, there is substantial cause for optimism; research on cardiovascular diagnosis and therapy has never been more active and productive, and it has brought great advances in clinical cardiology. Cardiovascular research is based increasingly on advances in basic science. For the past fifty years, physiology, the "queen of the biomedical sciences," provided the principal underpinnings to clinical developments in cardiovascular medicine. More recently, the applications of cellular and molecular biology to cardiovascular medicine have become increasingly evident. This anxiously awaited fourth edition of Professor Opie's masterful text, *Heart Physiology,* presents an appropriately expanded scientific base for cardiovascular disease.

This marvelous book is a concise, yet comprehensive, presentation of basic cardiovascular science. It presents, in a very readable and eminently understandable fashion, an extraordinary amount of important information critical to our understanding of how the cardiovascular system and its components function and malfunction. Professor Opie has the unique ability to explain in a straightforward manner the key principles of modern cardiovascular science without oversimplifying this complex subject.

While the fourth edition of this now well-established book builds on the strengths of its predecessors, it has been completely revised and largely rewritten. It is as current as last month's journals. The excellent explanatory diagrams (an Opie trademark) are even better than in previous editions and serve to make even the most complex concepts understandable. In preparing this edition, Professor Opie has enlisted the collaboration of eight distinguished coauthors. Yet, Opie's strong guiding hand remains clearly apparent throughout the book. This provides the unusual combination of the authority of a multiauthored text and the clarity of a single accurate voice. In an era of multiauthored texts, which are often disjointed and present information that is repetitive and sometimes even contradictory, it is refreshing to have a body of information that speaks with a single, authoritative, respected, and accurate voice. *Heart Physiology* is such a book.

This magnificent edition of *Heart Physiology*, clearly the finest yet, will be of immense value and interest to students and teachers of cardiovascular science, and to the many scholarly practitioners of cardiovascular medicine and surgery who wish to move beyond practice guidelines and understand the underlying cellular and physiologic bases of cardiovascular disease and its treatment.

Eugene Braunwald, M.D.
Harvard Medical School
Boston, Massachusetts

Foreword

The explosive growth of science has made the single-authored cardiology text a rarity. On the one hand, details of molecular biology and signal transduction are becoming critical to the understanding of heart disease pathology; on the other, definitive tests of the clinical relevance of these fundamental concepts are coming from a growing list of clinical trials. However, the interplay between basic science and clinical experience often generates counterintuitive findings. Concepts of disease once viewed as obvious have turned out to be either wrong or, at best, oversimplifications, while the clinical presentation in patients with heart disease commonly obscures the underlying pathophysiologic mechanisms. The patient with heart failure, for example, suffers from more than a weakened myocardium, as evidenced by the dismal results of virtually every clinical trial of inotropic therapy and by growing evidence that drugs that weaken the failing heart prolong survival and improve symptoms. Myocardial infarction, we now know, is not primarily a disorder of the heart, but instead is a consequence of blood vessel disease—the heart being the victim of coronary artery occlusion. And clinical trials of drugs intended to prevent sudden cardiac death have demonstrated that modification of abnormal ion channel function can be more proarrhythmic than antiarrhythmic.

There are many reasons why so many of our attempts to apply basic science to clinical cardiology have yielded counterintuitive results. The failure of inotropic drugs to improve outcome in heart failure reflects the fact that the failing heart is deteriorating progressively, and that energy starvation probably plays a role in causing cell death. Limiting myocardial infarct size is generally impossible after coronary artery occlusion, unless flow to the ischemic myocardium can be restored. Efforts to prevent lethal arrhythmias by administering drugs that eliminate nonlethal ectopy generally worsen outcome because these drugs depress conduction elsewhere in the heart, thereby initiating lethal arrhythmias.

These and other errors do not reflect flaws in either clinical observations or basic "facts;" instead, they occur because causal links between basic mechanisms and disease are generally more complex than can be recognized intuitively. This, in turn, reflects the many gaps that remain in our understanding of pathophysiology. Yet it is an oversimplification to assume that the more we know the better able we will be to manage the cardiac patient. In spite of the dazzling technology now available for diagnosis and treatment of heart disease, real understanding of the mechanisms responsible for heart disease often requires information that is not easily retrieved from the literature. Moreover, to meet the challenges posed by the cardiac patient, we must identify, interpret, integrate, and then apply the appropriate basic science knowledge for each clinical situation. This is best done at the bedside by an informed clinical scientist, rather than in a conference room by a committee.

The ability to integrate basic science and clinical cardiology is facilitated by an authoritative single-authored text that shifts effortlessly and naturally between these two aspects of cardiology. Lionel Opie, who for more than 30 years has made original contributions to our understanding of the mechanisms responsible for clinical heart disease, meets this need. His fourth edition of *Heart Physiology: From Cell to Circulation* demonstrates Professor Opie's broad and expert view of cardiology, his ability to integrate basic science and clinical medicine and, above all, the lucidity of his writing.

Arnold M. Katz, M.D., D.Med.(Hon.)
Professor of Medicine Emeritus
University of Connecticut
Farmington, Connecticut

From the Introduction to the First Edition

Richard J. Bing, M.D., doyen of cardiac metabolism and physiology, founder of the School of Modern Cardiac Metabolism, and Professor Emeritus, University of Southern California, turned 94 in October 2003. He remains active and continues contributing to the International Society of Heart Research. The following is an extract from his Introduction to the first edition of this book:

"Evolution of science, like biological evolution, develops by a zigzag course of trial and error; the errors are soon forgotten though they serve as stepping-stones to new progress. The factors which determine both scientific progress and scientific error are dependent on the ability of the brain to be analytical, curious, critical, observant, and imaginative. These are constant factors—qualities of the human brain which have evolved together with other properties of mind and body. There are, on the other hand, variables which determine progress in the natural sciences. Techniques and the spirit of the period, together with the personality of the scientist, make up these variables. Endowed with these constants, and blessed or cursed by these variables, the human mind attempts to discover single stones in the mosaic of the biological system, or if graced with a flash of genius, it can visualize whole parts of nature's mosaic.

A glance into the early beginnings of cardiac physiology and metabolism is not amiss, because we find that the pioneers wrestled with the same ideas that occupy us today, and that an astonishing amount of scientific truth is contained in early publications. Much of this important work, dating from the 1870s to 1920, was summarized in a remarkable fashion by Tigerstedt in 1923, in a volume on the physiology of the circulation. Tigerstedt himself was an outstanding investigator, to whom we owe the discovery of renin. One section of this remarkable book deals with the "chemical conditions for cardiac action."

His book contains a wealth of information, for example: the Langendorff perfusion method was first introduced in 1890 by Martin and Applegarth of Johns Hopkins in Baltimore; Langendorff had no knowledge of this work when he described his perfusion method in 1895. Particularly fascinating is the story of the discovery of the role of calcium ions. It is interesting that Ringer was first misled by the use of sodium chloride-enriched tapwater which contained, without his knowledge, not only calcium chloride but also potassium chloride which antagonized the calcium effect. A year later, Ringer discovered that the arrested heart could be made to beat again by the addition of calcium chloride. He concluded in 1883 that calcium is absolutely essential for maintenance of cardiac contraction. Thus Ringer established that calcium increased the force of contraction and prolonged systole. Yet excess calcium could result in contracture of the heart and could diminish the duration of diastole.

What distinguishes the present volume from the early publication by Tigerstedt, are the continuous advances in physical and biological chemistry, molecular biology, electron microscopy, electrophysiology, and myocardial mechanics. In bringing together these basic disciplines into a volume that can be assimilated by clinical cardiologists and medical students, the present work achieves a milestone.

Richard J. Bing, M.D.

Preface

Encouraged by the public reception of the former editions, the author has spared neither labour nor expense to render this as perfect as his opportunities and abilities would permit. The progress of knowledge is so rapid, and the discoveries so numerous, both at home and abroad, that this may rather be regarded as a new work than as a re-publication of an old one. On this account, a short enumeration of the more important changes may possibly be expected by the reader.
William Withering (discoverer of digitalis),
In *Botany, Third Edition,*
London: Calldel and Davies, 1801

Like Withering, over 200 years ago, I once again am excited by the impossible task of keeping up with the rapid progress of knowledge and discoveries in physiology and pathophysiology of the heart. To bring these changes to students and fellows, six crucial changes have been made in this fourth edition:

1. Co-authors. Frankly admitting that no one person can deal with the astounding amount of new research since 1997, the following experts have graciously agreed to be co-authors of specific chapters: Dr. James Downey, President of the International Society of Heart Research (Chapter 5); Dr. Donald Bers, author of *"Excitation–Contraction, Coupling and Cardiac Contractile Force"* (Chapter 6); John Solaro, co-editor of the *"American Society of Physiology Handbook of Physiology, Cardiovascular System Section, 2002"* (Chapter 8); Michael Sack, former director of the Hatter Institute for Cardiology Research and now at the National Institutes of Health, Bethesda, Maryland (Chapter 9); Professor Gerd Heusch, Director of the Institute of Pathophysiology, University Clinic Essen, Germany (Chapters 10, 17 and 19); Dr. Gary Lopaschuk, Professor and Director, Cardiovascular Research Group, University of Alberta, Canada (Chapter 11); Mark Perlroth, Professor of Medicine, Stanford University Medical Center, Stanford, California (Chapter 12); and David Paterson, Professor of Cardiovascular Physiology, University of Oxford (Chapters 14 and 15).

2. There is a new chapter on cell signaling, one of the most active areas of research in molecular physiology and, it must be confessed, one of the most confusing. There are downward signals, upward signals, "cross-talk" is common and, in my view, "backchat" is unavoidable.

3. The material on electricity has been reorganized with the help of Dr. James Downey. There are many more ECG illustrations, both in the section on the physiology of ECG (Chapter 4) and in the section of arrhythmias (Chapter 20). The ECG remains a fundamental entry point to cardiac physiology for both students and cardiologists in training.

4. New illustrations abound. Once again I must stress the creative capacity of my artist and colleague, Jeanne Walker, in helping me to produce what is arguably the most unique aspect of this book, namely the simple didactic illustration. About 60% of the illustrations are new or very substantially altered.

5. Color illustrations. The section of color plates has been doubled, also emphasizing that the major teaching method of this book is by visual impact.

6. References. It has been impossible to list all the references that I should have included. There is so much new work since 1997 that each chapter warrants, at a minimum, 100 references. My apologies to those eminent authors who have inevitably been left out. I realize this is a sure way of making enemies, but the book has to be kept to proportion.

What remains unchanged is the original intent of the book: to explain cardiac function to a wide range of potential readers, including fellows in cardiology, research students, and advanced medical students.

Because the drawings and color plates constitute a diagrammatic text that can stand alone, and because of the greater emphasis on the circulation, this book should be seen as a companion and not as competitor to Arnold Katz's classic book, *Physiology of the Heart*. The topic of the present *Heart Physiology* makes it a natural companion to Eugene Braunwald's classic, *Heart Disease*, now in its 7th edition, Hurst's long-running *The Heart,* in its 10th edition, and an innovative newcomer, Eric Topol's *Textbook of Cardiovascular Medicine,* now in its 2nd edition.

Lionel H. Opie, M.D., D.Phil.
2003

Acknowledgments

Further crucial acknowledgments are due to Ms. Jeanne Walker, a wonderful medical illustrator without peer, and to Mr. Victor Claasen, better than a computer in remembering and retrieving references. Without the expert secretarial assistance of Sylvia Dennis, this book could not have been completed expeditiously. I am most grateful to my colleagues in the Hatter Institute for all they have taught me.

I was privileged to complete the last edition of this book in Merton College, Oxford, a most historic, scholarly, and beautiful institution, of which William Harvey was Warden many years ago. Then, jumping ahead to the memory of a modern cardiological pioneer, this fourth edition was written in the Chris Barnard Building of the University of Cape Town, with Table Mountain towering overhead.

> *The heart, with the veins and arteries and the blood they contain, is to be regarded as the beginning and the author, the fountain and original of all things in the body, the primary cause of life.*
>
> *William Harvey, 1628*
> *Warden, Merton College, Oxford University*

PART I
Basic Cardiovascular Physiology

1

Introductory Cardiovascular Concepts

No understanding of the circulatory reactions of the body is possible unless we start first with the fundamental properties of the heart muscle itself, and then find out how these are modified, protected and controlled under the influence of the mechanisms—nervous, chemical and mechanical—which under normal conditions play on the heart and blood vessels.

E. H. Starling (1)

FROM PREHISTORY TO HARVEY

The existence of the heart was well known to the ancient Greeks, who gave it the name *kardia*, as in cardiac, tachycardia, and bradycardia. Aristotle thought that the heart was the seat of the soul and the center of man. The Romans modified *kardia* to *cor*, the latter word still surviving in cordial greetings and in cor pulmonale. The old Teutonic word *herton* also is derived from cor and gives us *heart* via the medieval English *heorte*.

Galen (ca. 200 A.D.), the father of experimental physiology, knew that the heart set the blood in motion. He discovered that arteries contained blood and not air. Yet he thought that there were pores between the left and right side of the heart and that a "vital spirit" was formed in the lungs by a mixture of blood and air. Such was Galen's authority that his views on the circulation became dogma, dispelled only by the careful anatomic dissections of Vesalius (1514–1564), who worked at Padua in Italy and clearly showed that there were no pores in that part of the heart (the septum) separating the left and right sides.

The critical point that the circulations of the left and right heart are separate was grasped by Servetus (1511–1553): "The connection between the cavities of the heart is not established through the median partition of the heart; a wonderful track conducts the blood, which flows in a long detour from the right of the heart to the lung and becomes red; at the moment of relaxation it reaches the left cavity of the heart."

Servetus hid this brilliant passage in a book of theology in which he criticized the Trinity, thereby falling foul of the Calvinist rulers of Geneva, who burnt him

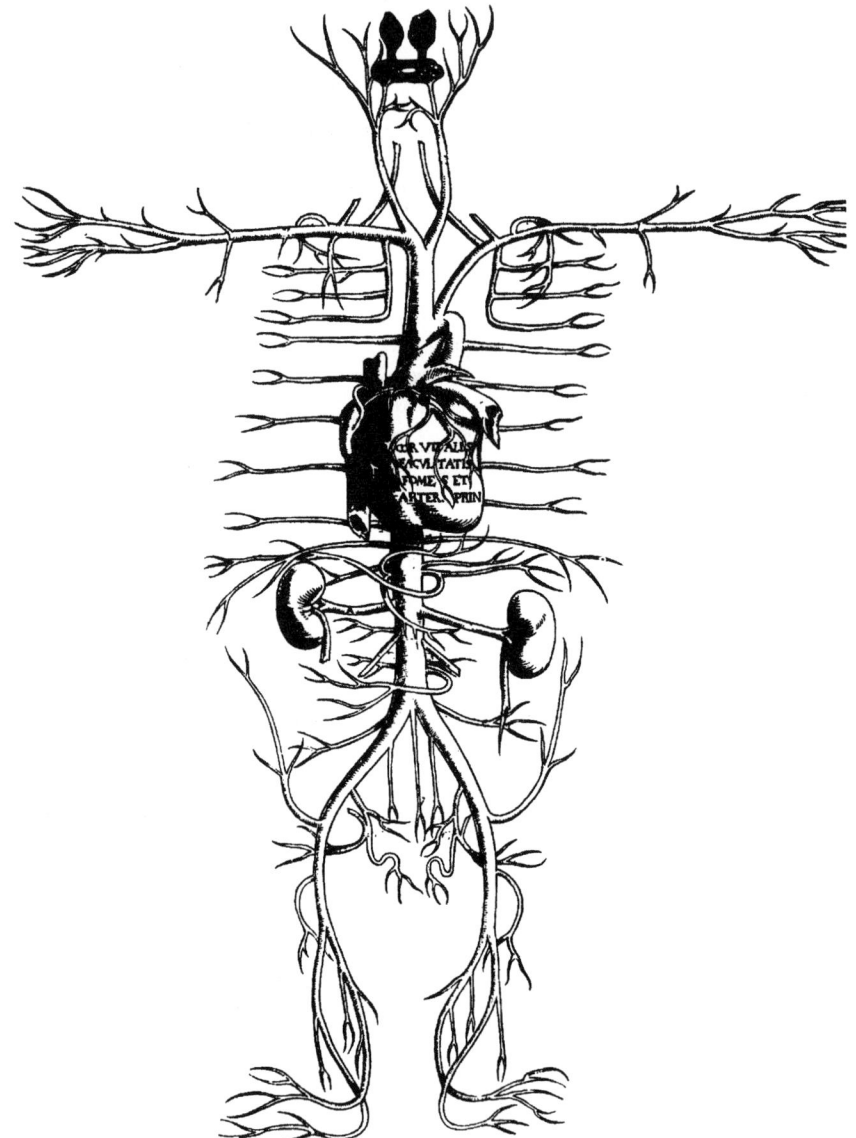

FIG. 1-1. The heart at the center of the circulation, as drawn by Vesalius (1514–1564) in his *Tabulae Anatomicae*.

at the stake. In 1571, an Italian, Cesalpino, described the function of valves: "Special membranes at the openings of the vessels prevent blood flowing back so that there is perpetual movement of the blood from the vena cava through the heart and lungs into the aorta."

The basis of modern concepts of the circulation was laid by Harvey (1578–1657), who reasoned that the circulation of the blood was caused by pumping of the heart. His *Anatomical Treatise on the Motion of the Heart and Blood in Animals* appeared in 1628 and is probably the most important single volume in the history of cardiology. Born in England and trained in Padua before returning to London, he must have been influenced by Vesalius' masterly drawing of the circulation (Fig. 1-1). Thus, it is to Harvey and his predecessors that we owe our knowledge of the heart as a mechanical pump. His concepts provide the foundation for our modern understanding of the fundamental facts of the circulation (Fig. 1-2).

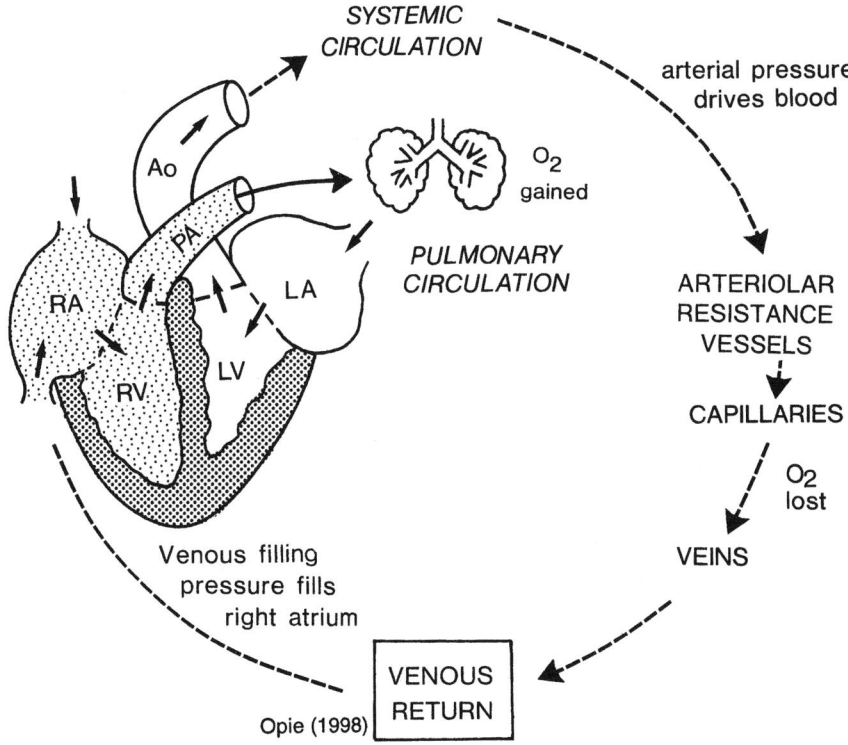

FIG. 1-2. Normal circulation. Harvey wrote in 1628: "These are then the very elements...of the passage and circulation of blood, from the right auricle into the right ventricle; from the right ventricle by way of the lungs into the left auricle; thence to the left ventricle and aorta; whence by the arteries at large through the tissues into the veins, and by the veins back again...to the base of the heart." Harvey used the term auricle, which is now replaced by the modern word atrium. *RA*, right atrium; *RV*, right ventricle; *PA*, pulmonary artery; *LA*, left atrium; *LV*, left ventricle; *Ao*, aorta; O_2, oxygen. The dotted contents of the right atrium, right ventricle, and pulmonary artery represent deoxygenated blood.

An original of his book is closely guarded in the library of Merton College, Oxford University, England, where he became Warden.

BASIC ANATOMY OF THE HEART

Left Side of the Heart

In the lungs, venous blood received from the right side of the heart, is oxygenated and then flows into the *left atrium* of the heart, which is a thin-walled muscular chamber continuously receiving blood from the lungs. From the left atrium, blood enters the much thicker *left ventricle*. For the left ventricle to fill in this way requires that the valve lying between the left atrium and the left ventricle, namely the *mitral* or *bicuspid valve*, should be open (Fig. 1-3). That only happens when the pressure in the left ventricle is very low, as during its relaxation phase called *diastole* (from the Greek for apart + send). The large anterior and small posterior cusps of this valve are sometimes thought to resemble a bishop's miter, hence the term *mitral*. Each cusp is a thin, flexible sheath of connective tissue, secured at its base to the mitral valve annulus. The latter is a ring of connective tissue surrounding the opening between the atrium and the ventricle. The *chordae tendineae* are the thin, tendinous structures linking the free

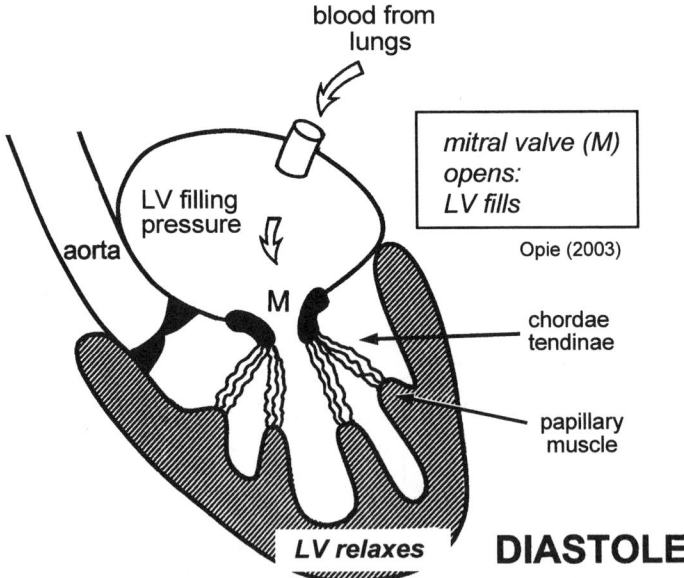

FIG. 1-3. Diastole, the ventricular relaxation phase. Note the role of the mitral valve in diastole, opening to allow blood flow between left atrium and left ventricle. According to a simplification of the Starling law, the more blood that enters the left ventricle, the more strongly the ventricle contracts to eject more blood into the aorta.

1. INTRODUCTORY CARDIOVASCULAR CONCEPTS

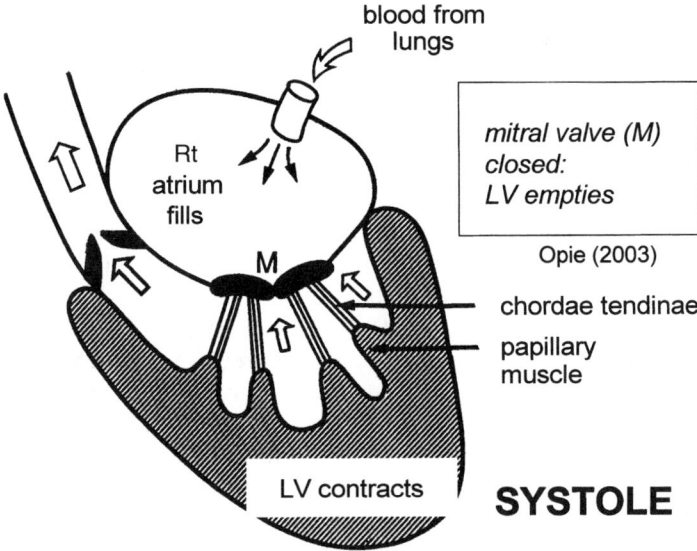

FIG.1-4. Systole, the ventricular contraction phase. The role of the mitral valve in systole. The left ventricular contraction increases the left ventricular pressure above that in the left atrium and the mitral valve shuts. The chordae tendineae become tense, which prevents the mitral valve from being pushed into the left atrium. The closed mitral valve and the increased pressure in the left ventricular force the blood into the aorta to be distributed to the circulation (see Fig. 1-2). *LV*, left ventricle.

ends of the cusp to the *papillary muscles*, which are long muscular projections of the inner wall of the ventricle. During left ventricular contraction or *systole* (Greek for contraction), the increased pressure in the left ventricle forces the two cusps of the mitral valve together, which then closes (Fig. 1-4). Thus, blood in the left ventricle is prevented from reentering the atrium. During systole, the papillary muscles also contract to tense the chordae tendineae, so that the mitral valve closes properly and is not forced into the atrial cavity.

Left ventricular contraction not only abruptly shuts the mitral valve but very shortly thereafter forces open the *aortic valve*, located at the base of the aorta, so that blood is expelled into the aorta (Fig. 1-4) from where it travels throughout the circulation to reach all parts of the body.

Transmural Distribution of Fibers in the Left Ventricle

The left ventricular wall, approximately three times thicker than that of the right ventricle, has its fibers distributed in various layers. The inner and outer layers run longitudinally in the direction from the apex of the heart to the base; the center fibers run circumferentially, and intervening layers have intervening patterns. The result of this change in muscle fiber pattern is that when the left ventricle contracts, it not only squeezes out the blood from the ventricle, but it twists and turns toward the chest wall so that the apex of the heart can be felt from the outside as the *apical impulse* (or apex beat). The overall effect of left ventricular contraction can be summarized as a reduction in both length and diameter of this chamber.

Right Side of the Heart

The systolic ejection of blood from the left ventricle provides enough force to drive the blood through the branches of the aorta, eventually to reach the minute vessels called the *capillaries* from where deoxygenated blood is returned by the venous system to the right atrium of the heart (Fig. 1-5). The right atrium, like the left, is a thin-walled muscular chamber that receives the venous return from the large veins of the circulation. The two main veins entering the right atrium are the *superior vena cava* and the *inferior vena cava*, which drain the upper and lower limbs, respectively. In addition, the right atrium receives blood from the coronary sinus, which is the main vein draining the heart muscle itself.

Blood flowing into the right atrium must thereafter enter the right ventricle through the *tricuspid valve* (three cusps), which is open during right ventricular diastole, when the right ventricle fills with blood. The tricuspid valve is closed when the right ventricle contracts. (Note the analogy to mitral opening and closing and to left ventricular relaxation and contraction.) The principles of right ventricular contraction are similar to those described for the left ventricle, except that the right ventricle is much thinner because it only has to drive blood into the lungs and not around the whole body, as in the case of the left ventricle. Therefore, the right ventricle must generate less pressure than the left. The contracting right ventricle forces venous blood to enter the pulmonary vascular tree. This blood is then oxygenated in the capillaries of the lungs to return to the left atrium and thereby to complete the circulation.

Pericardium

The *pericardium* is a thin, fibrous, bag-like structure within which the heart lies. The pericardium almost entirely surrounds the heart except for the sites of entry and exit of the great vessels. The pericardium is composed of two layers, one of which lies on the outer surface of the heart and the other is in contact with the surrounding lungs and other tissues. The two layers are separated by a small amount of lubricating fluid to allow movement of the heart during contraction and relaxation to occur without disturbance of the surrounding lungs. Normally, the pericardium does not interfere with the mechanical function of the heart, but when it is diseased, then cardiac filling can be compromised.

Endocardium

The *endocardium*, which covers the inner surface of the heart, has a large surface area because of the many papillary muscles and the irregular pattern of the

1. INTRODUCTORY CARDIOVASCULAR CONCEPTS

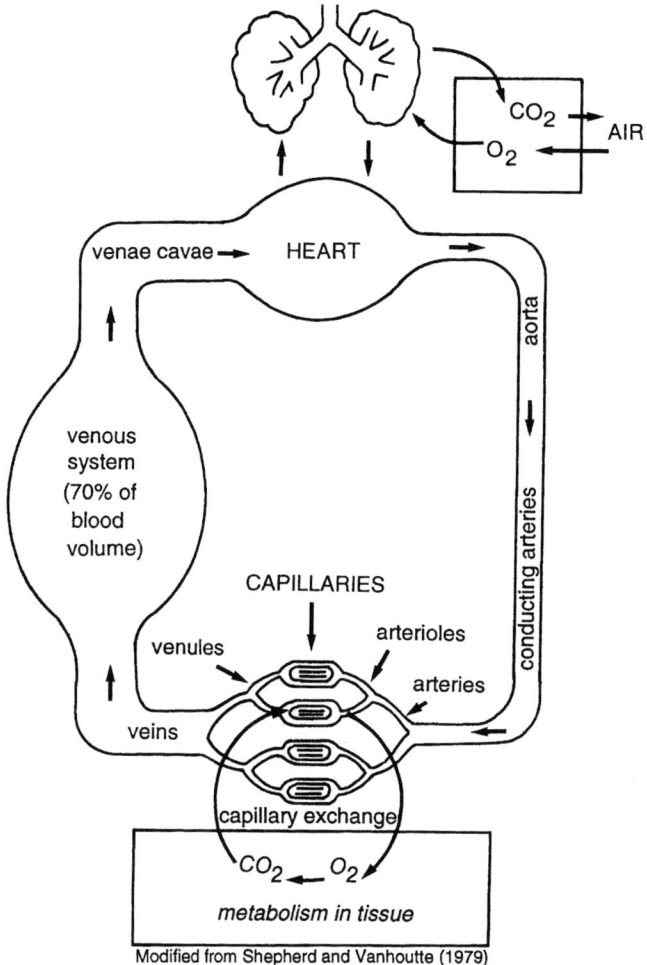

FIG. 1-5. Role of heart in transport of oxygen. Schematic diagram shows how the pumping heart conveys oxygenated blood to the peripheral circulation. Note the role of the capillaries in allowing rapid gas exchange, with diffusion of oxygen to the various tissues and collection of the carbon dioxide produced during metabolism in the tissues. The veins function as both collecting and storage systems. For the latter reason, they are called venous capacitance veins. (Modified from Shepherd JT, Vanhoutte PM. *The human cardiovascular system. Facts and concepts.* New York: Raven Press, 1979.)

inner wall of the left ventricle (Fig. 1-3). Previously thought to be inert, the endocardium is now suspected of being metabolically active and thereby contributing to the regulation of left ventricular contraction. For example, experimental removal of the endocardium alters the pattern of the relaxation phase of the left ventricle.

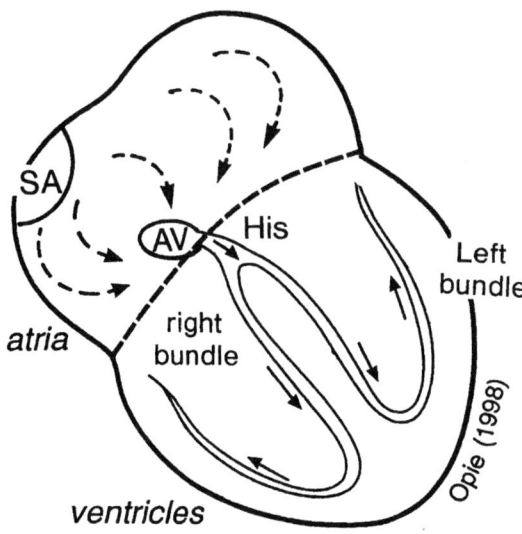

FIG. 1-6. Schematic of conduction system. The spontaneous origin of the electrical impulse is in the sinoatrial node in the right atrium, from where the impulse travels over the atrial walls to be collected in the atrioventricular node, thence to pass down the His bundle and into the left or right bundle before eventually reaching the ventricular myocardium. This path is followed during every heartbeat. *SA*, sinoatrial; *AV*, atrioventricular.

Conducting System

Each time the heart beats, ventricular contraction is triggered by a wave of electricity, which arises spontaneously in a collection of specialized cells in the right atrium (Fig. 1-6). These cells are collectively called the *sinoatrial node* or sinus node because they are situated near the coronary sinus (into which veins from the heart muscle drain). From the sinoatrial node the electrical impulse spreads rapidly through the left and right atria, to be collected in a second node, the *atrioventricular node*. The impulse slows down in this node and then again speeds up along a specialized bundle of conducting fibers, the *His bundle*, before dividing into two major branches, the left and right bundles, by which the electrical impulses spread throughout the ventricles to trigger ventricular contraction. This series of electrical events is repeated with every heartbeat.

ANATOMY OF THE CIRCULATION

There are two anatomically separate vascular beds or circuits through which blood is driven (Fig. 1-2). The left ventricle drives blood through the *systemic circulation*, and the right ventricle drives it through the *pulmonary circulation*. In each case, the vessels connecting the ventricle to capillaries of that circulation have to withstand more pressure and are thicker than the vessels leading from the capillaries to the atrium. The former vessels are called *arteries* and the latter *veins*. In the systemic circulation, arteries convey oxygenated blood from the left ventricle to the capillaries, whereas the veins carry the deoxygenated blood from the capillaries to the heart. In the pulmonary circulation, the arteries are again by definition those vessels conveying blood from the right ventricle to the pulmonary capillaries. Because this blood has reached the right ventricle from the systemic veins and is deoxygenated, the blood in the pulmonary arteries is deoxygenated in contrast to the blood in all the other arteries, which is oxygenated. Similarly, blood leaving the pulmonary capillaries by the pulmonary veins to the heart is oxygenated, in contrast to blood in all the other veins, which is deoxygenated.

Microcirculation

When blood is ejected from the left ventricle, it enters the aorta, which divides into many arteries that eventually become the smaller *arterioles* before reaching the capillaries (Fig. 1-5). In the *capillaries*, which are the exchange vessels, oxygenated blood becomes deoxygenated as the oxygen leaves the red cells and enters the tissue by diffusion. It is also here that nutrients such as glucose and fatty acids (Chapter 11) leave the blood to provide for the energy needs of the tissues of the body, whereas products of metabolism such as carbon dioxide and some waste products leave the tissues. The capillaries are therefore crucially concerned with the metabolism of all organs and tissues of the body. Metabolism includes all those processes whereby the carbon atoms from glucose and fatty acids interact with the oxygen to form carbon dioxide and energy. The importance of the capillaries is underscored as follows: "The heart and vasculature exist for one fundamental purpose: the delivery of metabolic substrates to the cells of the organism. This delivery takes place across the thin walls of the capillaries, which thus subserve the ultimate function of the cardiovascular system" (2).

The deoxygenated venous blood leaving the capillaries enters the veins, which constitute a low-pressure, large-volume system, containing most of the blood volume. Taken together, the veins constitute the *venous capacitance system*. From that reservoir, blood reaches the right atrium by the large veins or vena cava. At the start of exercise, blood is forced out of the venous capacitance system by muscular contraction and by nervous influences, so that more blood is returned to the right atrium. This increased *venous return* stimulates the heart to contract more forcefully.

Arteriolar Resistance

Because of the crucial role of the capillaries, it would intuitively be expected that there would be a way in which the rate of blood flowing through these vessels could be carefully controlled. For example, during exercise, more blood must flow through the capillaries to meet the much higher demand of the exercising muscles for oxygen.

Arterioles are small arteries approximately 30 µm in lumen diameter with relatively thick muscular walls. They constitute the major resistance against which the ventricles pump, and collectively they constitute the *peripheral or systemic vascular resistance* (Fig. 2-15). If the arterioles dilate, the vascular resistance falls and more blood enters the capillaries.

Regulation of the degree of arteriolar dilation or constriction is extremely complex, involving nervous, hormonal, and metabolic control (Chapter 2). When there is excess arteriolar constriction (high systemic vascular resistance), then the pressure inside the arterial tree rises, as in a disease called hypertension. Conversely, a number of vasodilator drugs and exercise can reduce the systemic vascular resistance.

Arterial Blood Pressure

The pressure pattern in the circulation varies from high arterial to low venous values and can be measured invasively at any point by insertion of a needle connected to a pressure transducer. The pressure changes quite abruptly at the level of the arterioles, the site of the major resistance component of the systemic vascular resistance (Fig. 1-7). The aorta has the crucial function of transforming the abrupt increase and decrease of pressure in the left ventricle to a smoother pressure pattern with a much higher diastolic value (Fig. 1-8). This "pressure-

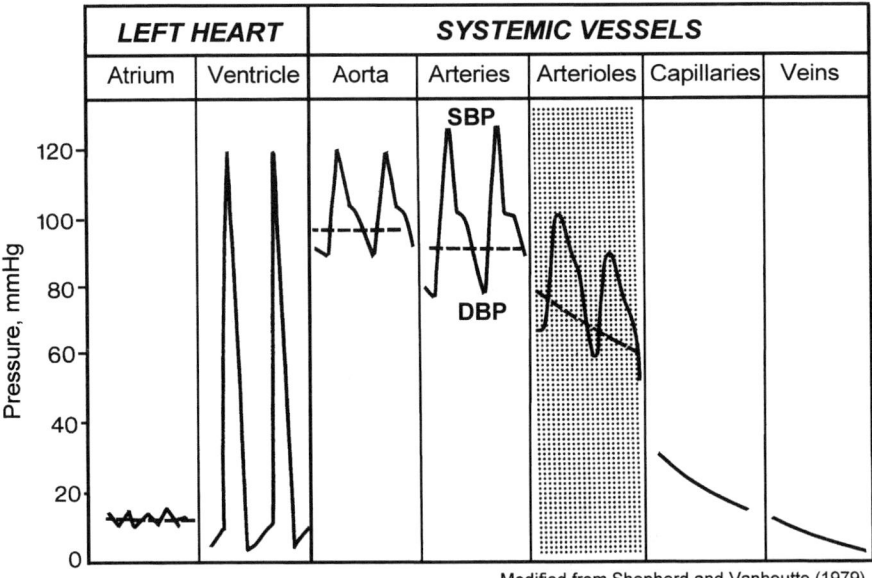

FIG. 1-7. The arterial pressure pattern changes quite abruptly at the level of the arterioles, where the systemic vascular resistance is generated. The pressure then becomes very low in the capillary and veins. (Modified from Shepherd JT, Vanhoutte PM. *The human cardiovascular system. Facts and concepts.* New York: Raven Press, 1979.)

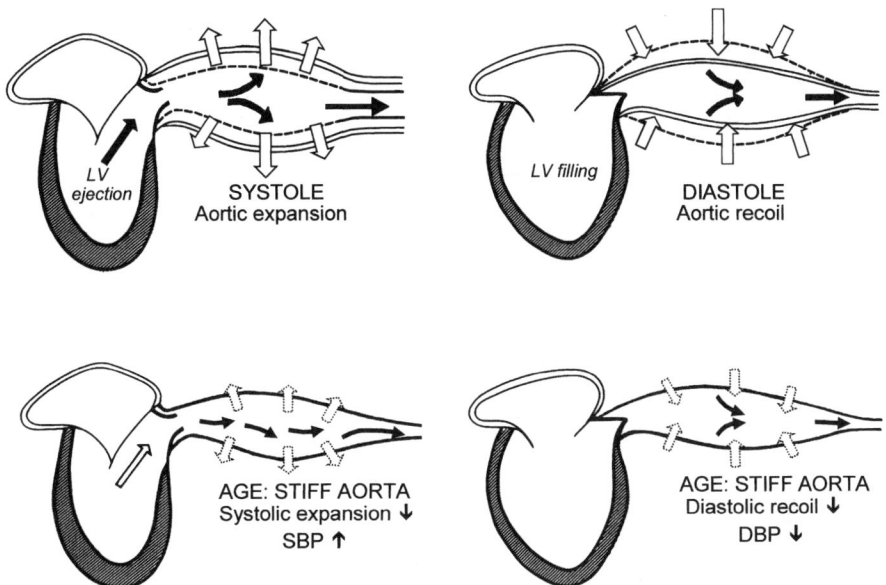

FIG. 1-8. The aorta. The pressure-equalizing or buffering function of the aorta. During ventricular systole, the stroke volume ejected by the ventricle results in some forward capillary flow, but most of the ejected volume is stored in the elastic arteries. During ventricular diastole, the elastic recoil of the arterial wall maintains blood flow throughout the remainder of the cardiac cycle. (Modified from Berne RM, Levy MN, eds. *Physiology*. St. Louis: Mosby, 1983.)

smoothing" function is crucial because a relatively high diastolic pressure is required to help transfer the blood to various organs, particularly the heart.

The peak pressure in the major arteries is actually higher than that in the aorta, probably partly due to the increasing resistance offered by the decreasing and tapering arterial lumen and partly due to variations in the transmission velocity of the blood. Clearly, therefore, the arterial blood pressure will vary according to the site of its measurement. In humans, the standard noninvasive technique involves measurement of the arterial blood pressure in the brachial artery. By using a cuff that automatically inflates at preset intervals (e.g., every 10 to 20 minutes) and records the sound electronically, a 24-hour ambulatory blood pressure can be obtained. This pressure is usually simply called the blood pressure. The pattern shows marked diurnal variations and is influenced by the subject's emotional status and exercise (Fig. 1-9). During the daytime, when stimulatory nervous activity dominates, the blood pressure values are much higher than at night, when inhibitory nervous activity dominates. Changes in the pulse rate accompany those in the blood pressure, so that emotional excitement or the stimulus of waking in the morning leads to an increase in both, whereas at night, the heart rate and blood pressure both decrease.

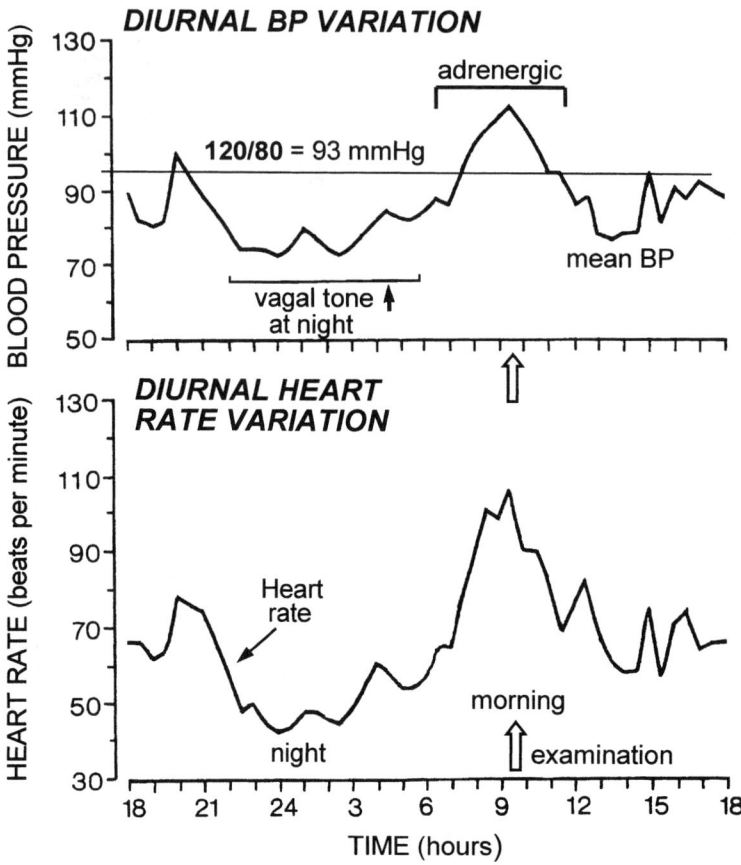

FIG. 1-9. Diurnal pattern of blood pressure and heart rate. Variation throughout 24 hours (diurnal) taken by an ambulatory machine. The mean blood pressure values are shown, not the systolic and diastolic. A commonly accepted normal blood pressure value of 120/80 mmHg corresponds with a mean value of 93 mmHg. The typical trace shows low blood pressure and heart rate during sleep, which increase before and during waking, with further increases before and during emotional stress (e.g., student examination).

SUMMARY

The basic function of the heart is to act as a pump that ejects blood from the thick-walled left ventricle, to be propelled throughout the body, ultimately to reach the peripheral circulation. There, in the capillaries, oxygen is removed to nourish the various organs and tissues of the body. The deoxygenated venous blood flows back to the right side of the heart to be ejected from the right ventricle to the lungs, once more to be oxygenated and to enter the left atrium and left ventricle.

STUDENT QUESTIONS

1. Describe the function of the valves separating left atrium and left ventricle.
2. Define systole and diastole.
3. Describe in outline the pulmonary circulation.
4. What is the role of the arterioles?
5. Why are capillaries important?

CARDIOLOGIST-IN-TRAINING QUESTIONS

1. When the heart contracts, the left ventricular cavity becomes smaller, yet systolic contraction can be felt on the precordium as the apical impulse. Why?
2. Describe the typical diurnal (24-hour) blood pressure and heart rate variation. Can you explain the physiologic changes that occur?
3. How does diastolic recoil of the aorta contribute to the blood pressure changes with aging?
4. Describe the changes in blood pressure that occur with aging. What is the origin of these changes?

REFERENCES

1. Starling EH. On the circulatory changes associated with exercise. *J R Army Med Corps* 1920;34: 258–272.
2. Levick JR. Vascular smooth muscle. In: *An introduction to cardiovascular physiology*. London: Butterworths, 1991:171–175.
3. Shepherd JT, Vanhoutte PM. *The human cardiovascular system. Facts and concepts.* New York: Raven Press, 1979.
4. Berne RM, Levy MN, eds. *Physiology*. St. Louis: Mosby, 1983.

2

Control of the Circulation

Physiology is the logic of life.
Persson (1)

Control mechanisms are the key to the regulation of this logic. Such controls may be exerted either at the central nervous system level or at the periphery. In addition to control by the autonomic nervous system, locally produced metabolites convey integrative signals during specific physiologic changes and challenges. Messages that play a major role in regulating the circulation reach the heart from the central nervous system along the autonomic pathways, which function independently of the conscious nervous system (hence the name autonomic). The two divisions of the autonomic nervous system have opposite functions. First, the adrenergic or sympathetic nervous system is able to release its excitatory messengers, *epinephrine* and *norepinephrine*, in "sympathy with" states of excitation, such as waking up, the start of exercise, and during emotional stress (Fig. 2-1). Second, the parasympathetic system acts alongside (Greek, *para*, beside) the adrenergic nervous system to release its own transmitter, acetylcholine. Alternate names are the cholinergic nervous system and the vagal nervous system (Fig. 2-2).

ADRENERGIC AND CHOLINERGIC EFFECTS

Each system has a particular intensity of stimuli flowing down (*neural traffic*) to the terminal nerve fibers or neurons (or *varicosities*), which lie close to the cells of the organ to be controlled. These terminal neurons liberate their primary messengers, or *neurotransmitters*, mainly norepinephrine and acetylcholine, which travel across the short distance called the *synaptic gap* or *synaptic junction* (*synapse*, join) to the external cell membrane of the heart or the vascular smooth muscle. These neurotransmitters act on receptors that are specific sites on the cell membrane. The tight molecular fit between the stimulant molecule (*agonist*) and the receptor gives rise to the *"key and lock"* model.

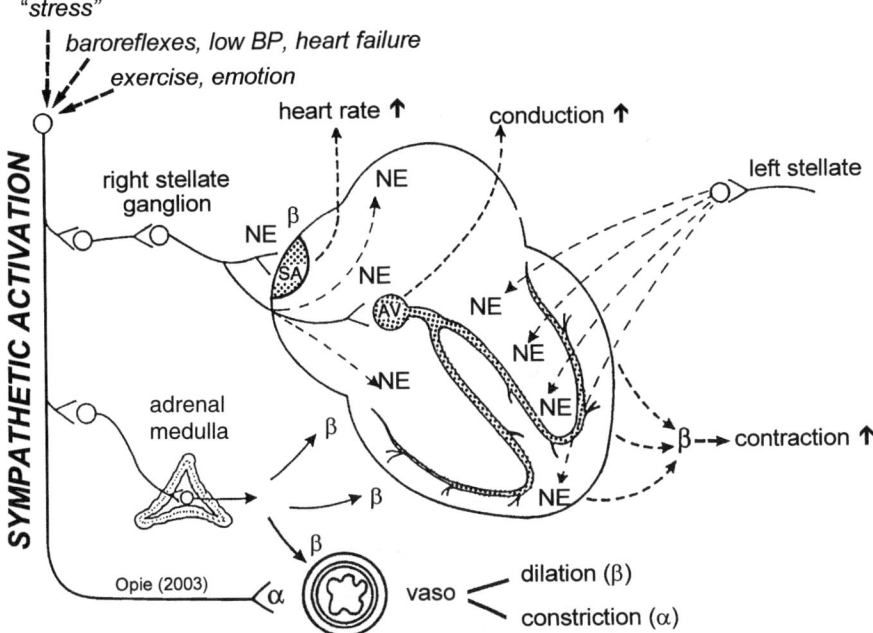

FIG. 2-1. Mechanisms of sympathetic stimulation by stress, emotions, or exercise, acting via (a) a collection of nerve cells (right stellate ganglion) to increase release of norepinephrine to areas of sinus and atrioventricular nodes, (b) another collection of nerve cells, the left stellate ganglion, to increase release of norepinephrine to the left ventricle, and (c) the adrenal medulla to release epinephrine to all parts of the heart and to the arterioles (shown in cross-section). The cardiac receptors stimulated by norepinephrine and epinephrine are the β-adrenergic receptors. The vascular receptors stimulated are the norepinephrine-mediated α-adrenergic vasoconstrictive receptors and the epinephrine-mediated vasodilatory receptors. As a consequence of these changes, the heart rate increases, as does the rate of conduction of the electrical impulse through the atrioventricular node and the conduction system. At the same time, the force of contraction increases. The changes in the blood vessel are complex and contradictory. Vasoconstriction or vasodilation may dominate, or there may be no overall change. For baroreflexes, see Figure 14-2. NE, norepinephrine; SA, sinoatrial; AV, atrioventricular, E, epinephrine.

Receptors

Two major types of such receptors have been defined by the specific nature of the cardiovascular reactions evoked by infused catecholamines (2). Those receptors concerned with enhanced contractility and heart rate are called *β-adrenergic receptors* and those concerned with increasing the tone of arterioles are called *α-adrenergic receptors*. *Cholinergic receptors* respond to their messenger *acetylcholine* and in general have the opposite effect of adrenergic stimulation (Table 2-1). For example, β-adrenergic stimulation increases the heart rate, whereas cholinergic stimulation decreases it (Figs. 2-1 and 2-2). Cholinergic

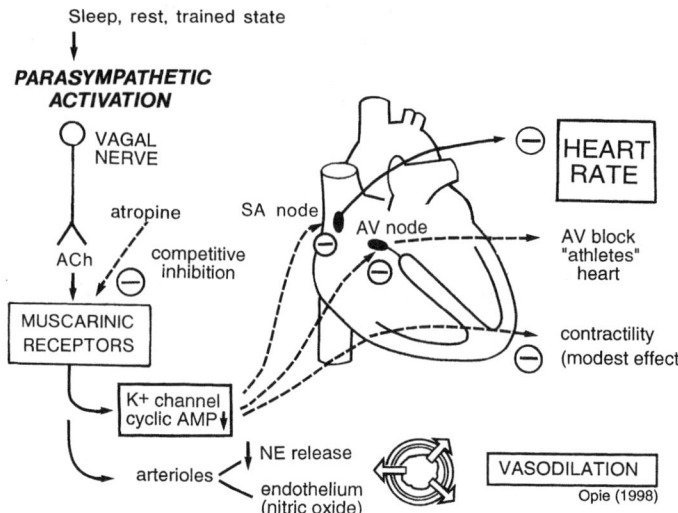

FIG. 2-2. The parasympathetic or cholinergic system, acting via the muscarinic receptors, has inhibitory effects on the heart. The major site of action of parasympathetic control of the heart appears to be the sinoatrial node, where it decreases the heart rate in contrast to sympathetic stimulation (Fig. 2-1). It also decreases the force of ventricular contraction. Another parasympathetic effect is inhibition of the atrioventricular node. In trained athletes, parasympathetic activity increases to slow the heart rate. In overtraining, the atrioventricular node can be inhibited to block the conduction of the impulse from the sinoatrial node to the ventricles, an example of atrioventricular block (Fig. 5-21).

TABLE 2-1. Proposed patterns of receptor stimulation to explain opposite effects of sympathetic adrenergic and parasympathetic cholinergic stimulation on the heart and circulation

	β-Adrenergic	α-Adrenergic	Cholinergic
Heart			
SA node pacemaker	+	0	−
AV node conduction	+	0	−
His Purkinje system conduction	+	0	−
Myocardial contraction[a]	+	0, +	−
Peripheral circulation[b]			
Coronary arterioles	Dilate	Constrict[e]	Dilate
Skeletal muscle	Dilate ($β_2$)	Constrict[e]	Dilate
Splanchnic flow	Dilate[d]	Constrict[f]	0
Renal flow[c]	Constrict	Constrict	0
Colon and genitals	Dilate	Constrict	Dilate

The above patterns are inferred from the known properties of adrenergic and cholinergic receptors in isolated systems and from the effects of infusions into a human of epinephrine (chiefly β stimulation), norepinephrine (combined cardiac β stimulation and vascular α stimulation), and acetylcholine (inhibition of release of norepinephrine from nerve terminals).
[a]Cholinergic effects are controversial. For recent evidence, see reference 2a.
[b]See pages 116–124 in reference 14. For modifications, see below.
[c]Reference 2b.
[d]Reference 15.
[e]During exercise, direct α-mediated vasoconstriction is overridden by β-mediated increased force of myocardial contraction and production of vasodilator metabolites.
[f]Splanchnic flow decreases as plasma norepinephrine increases (8).
SA, sinoatrial; +, stimulation; −, inhibition; 0, no effect; AV, atrioventricular.

receptors are also called *muscarinic receptors* because they respond to the complex chemical compound muscarine derived from some mushrooms.

Effects of Infusion of Catecholamines

The similar chemical structures of norepinephrine and epinephrine give rise to the family name of *catecholamines*. Barcroft and Swan (3) found that an infusion of epinephrine (also called *adrenaline*) increased the heart rate and systolic blood pressure (BP) but decreased the diastolic value while augmenting blood flow in the arms and legs (Fig. 2-3). The β-adrenergic receptors can be further separated into those with a cardiac stimulatory effect (β_1-adrenergic receptors) and those found mainly but not exclusively at extracardiac sites such as the arterioles (β_2-adrenergic receptors), where they cause vasodilation. During physiologic exercise, such as vigorous cycling, most but not all the hemodynamic changes can be explained by an increase in plasma epinephrine levels (4). The increased amount of blood ejected from the heart in systole overrides the arteriolar dilator effect to increase the systolic BP, whereas in diastole, the arteriolar dilation tends to decrease the diastolic BP (Fig. 2-3). Thus, the mean BP may not increase much. Two of the major effects of epinephrine are an increase in cardiac output and an increase in limb blood flow, the latter as a result of arteriolar vasodilation (Fig. 2-4).

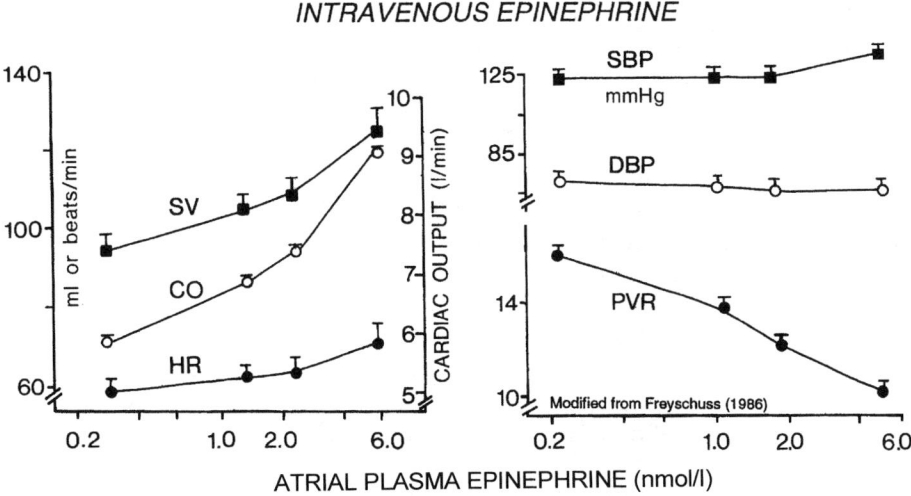

FIG. 2-3. Infusion of epinephrine (adrenaline) with effects on the heart rate, stroke volume, cardiac output, systolic blood pressure, diastolic blood pressure, and peripheral vascular resistance in healthy adults. HR, heart rate; SV, stroke volume; CO, cardiac output; SBP, systolic blood pressure; DBP, diastolic blood pressure; PVR, peripheral vascular resistance. (Modified from Freyschuss U, Hjemdahl P, Juhlin-Dannfelt A. Cardiovascular and metabolic responses to low dose adrenaline infusion: an invasive study in humans. *Clin Sci* 1986;70:199–206.)

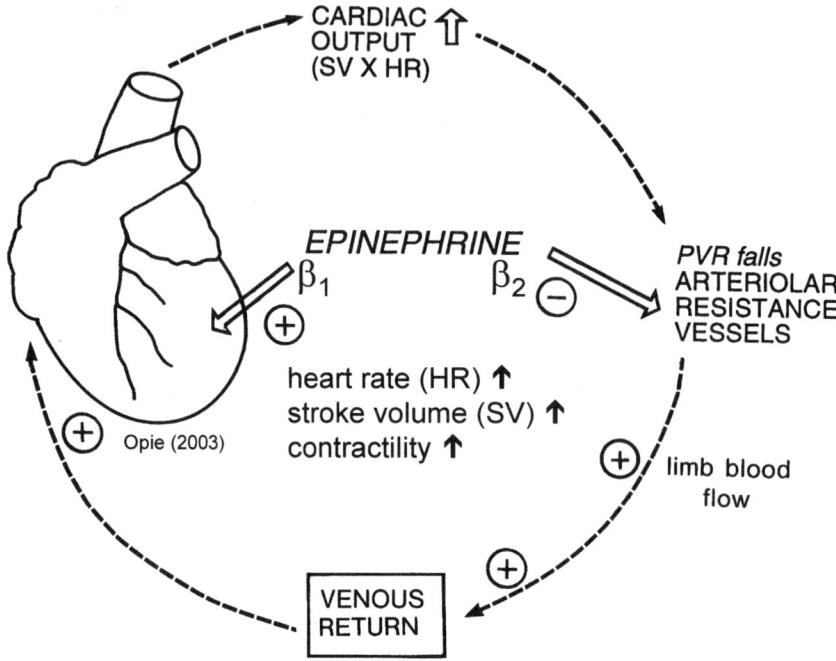

FIG. 2-4. Schema of effects of epinephrine on the circulation. Epinephrine, released from the adrenal gland in response to emotion or exercise, has a stimulatory effect on myocardial β-receptors. Epinephrine decreases systemic vascular resistance by its effects on $β_2$-adrenergic receptors. The net result is that the diastolic blood pressure decreases. The systolic pressure may, however, increase because of the increased cardiac output.

Infusion of Norepinephrine

Norepinephrine (also called noradrenaline), like epinephrine, increases the heart rate but, in contrast to epinephrine, reduces limb blood flow and increases both systolic and diastolic BP (Fig. 2-5). The major reason for these differences lies in the dual effect of norepinephrine, stimulating both myocardial β-adrenergic receptors and arteriolar α-adrenergic receptors. The latter effect, being vasoconstrictive, causes the arterioles to contract, thereby increasing the resistance against which the heart works (Fig. 2-6). Despite the direct β-adrenergic–mediated increase in heart rate as a result of stimulation of the sinoatrial node, the heart rate decreases after an initial transient increase. The explanation for this phenomenon is the existence of a pressure-sensitive control mechanism located in the *baroreceptors* (Greek, *baro*, pressure), as shown in Fig. 14-2.

Sympathetic Stimulation

When the sympathetic nerves to the heart but not to the peripheral circulation are stimulated, then β-adrenergic effects predominate (Fig. 2-7). There is a

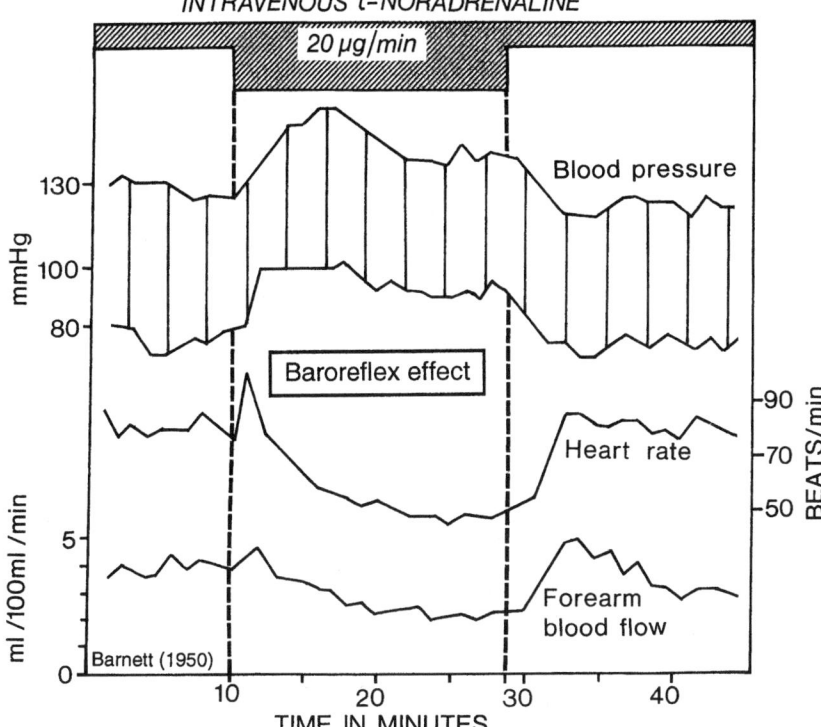

FIG. 2-5. Effect of norepinephrine (noradrenaline) on circulation. Intravenous infusion in humans. (Modified from Barnett AJ, Blacket RB, Depoorter AE, et al. The action of noradrenaline in man and its relation to phaeochromocytoma and hypertension. *Clin Sci* 1950;9:151–179.)

marked increase in the heart rate, left ventricular pressure, and the index of left ventricular contractile activity. The BP increases abruptly because much greater cardiac output has been ejected into the same vascular bed. During exercise, when such β-adrenergic stimulation of the heart is accompanied by a mixture of peripheral effects, α-adrenergic vasoconstriction tends to be offset by β-adrenergic vasodilation.

Signal Systems

The opposite effects of sympathetic and parasympathetic stimulation on myocardial contraction and arteriolar tone can be explained in terms of intracellular signal systems (Fig. 2-8). These signals link receptor occupation to the change in biologic function, such as muscular contraction, vasoconstriction, and vasodilation. When β-adrenergic receptors are occupied, the mem-

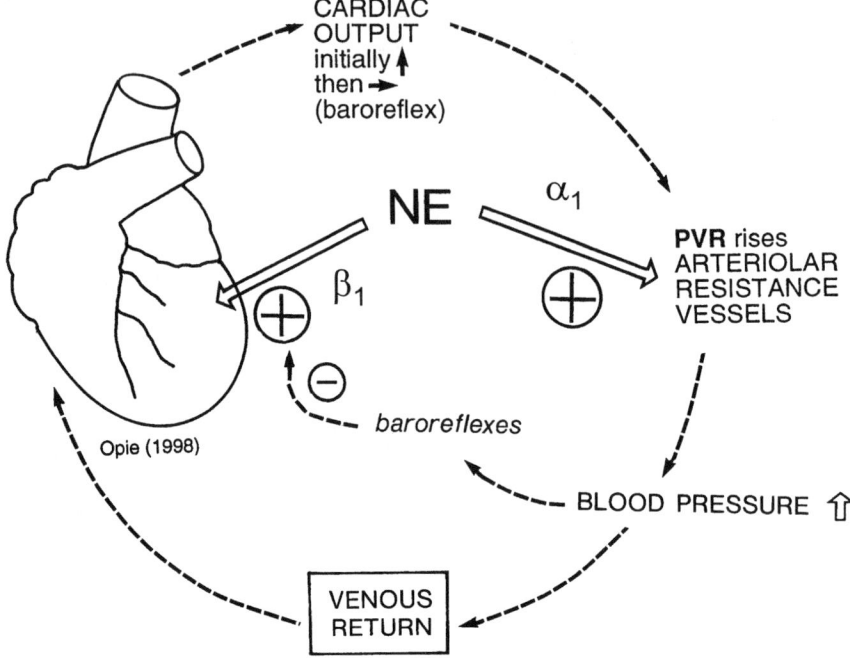

Fig. 2-6. Schema of norepinephrine effects on the circulation. Note β-adrenergic effects on the myocardium to increase heart rate and contractility, which initially increase cardiac output. In addition, the afterload increases as a result of α-adrenergic–mediated stimulation of arteriolar resistance vessels with an increase in peripheral vascular resistance. The net effect is that the blood pressure increases so that the baroreflexes are stimulated to slow the heart rate. In the end, the cardiac output is unchanged or might even decrease. *NE*, norepinephrine; *PVR*, peripheral vascular resistance.

brane-bound enzyme adenylate cyclase is stimulated into activity by one of a superfamily of proteins, the stimulatory G protein G_s (Fig. 7-2). The result is conversion of adenosine 5′-triphosphate (ATP) into cyclic adenosine 3′,5′-monophosphate (cAMP), the second messenger that in turn promotes calcium entry into the myocardial cell by increasing the opening of the calcium channel. Enhanced release of stored calcium from the sarcoplasmic reticulum follows next, so that cytosolic calcium increases more as the force of contraction increases.

Parasympathetic stimulation leads to an opposite series of events. Occupation of the muscarinic receptor by the neurotransmitter acetylcholine interacts with the inhibitory G protein G_i to decrease activity of adenylate cyclase. The result is less formation of cAMP, leading to decreased contractile force, most marked when there is increased sympathetic tone (5).

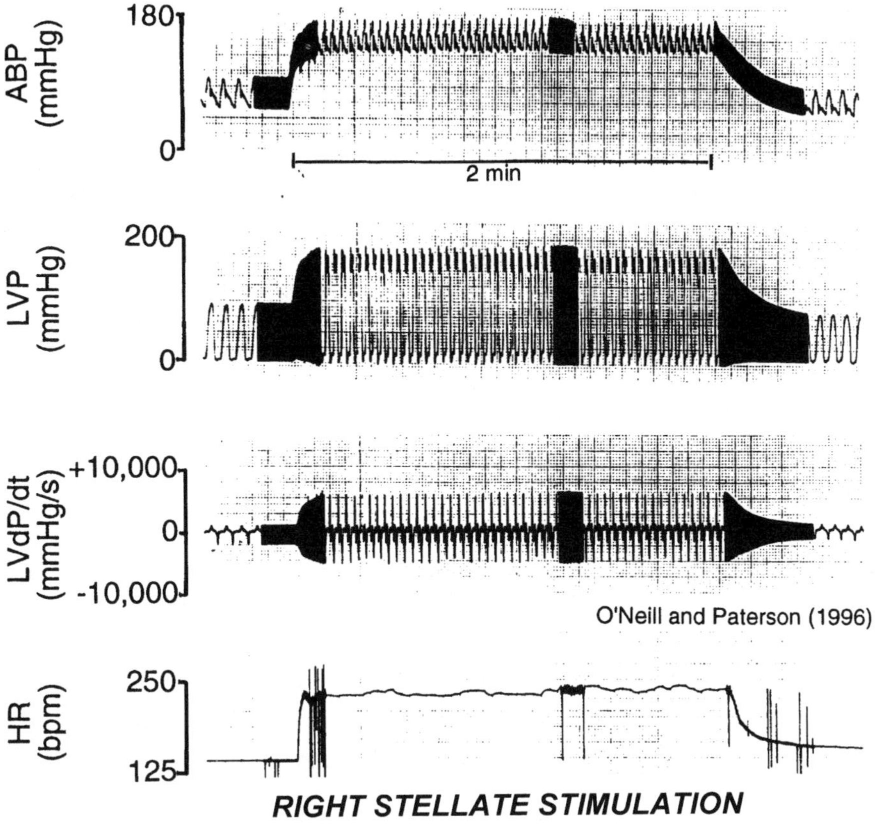

RIGHT STELLATE STIMULATION

FIG. 2-7. Effect of rapid sympathetic stimulation of the right stellate (sympathetic) ganglion on the heart in the absence of any changes in peripheral vascular resistance. *HR*, heart rate; *LVP*, left ventricular pressure; an index of contractility, i.e., LVdP/dt, left ventricular rate of pressure increase as a function of time; *ABP*, arterial blood pressure. (Courtesy of Prof. David Paterson, University Laboratory of Physiology, Oxford, England.)

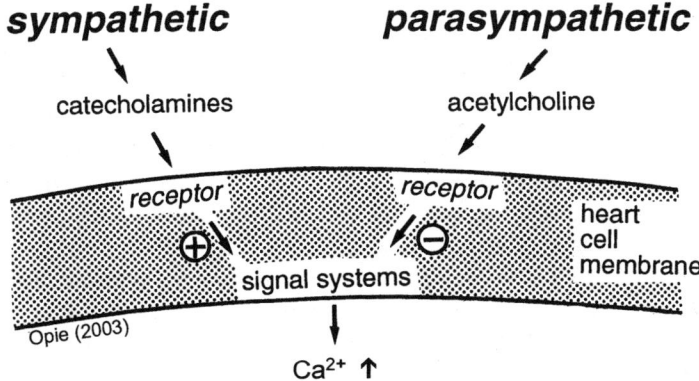

FIG. 2-8. Opposing autonomic effects of sympathetic and parasympathetic systems.

Sinus Node Pacemaker Activity

Similar systems work in the case of the sinus (sinoatrial) node (Figs. 2-1 and 2-2) with β-adrenergic stimulation increasing the heart rate because cAMP, the second messenger, enhances the rate of spontaneous pacemaking. The latter is a complex event, dependent on at least three currents (Chapter 5), thereby providing fail-safe mechanisms to prevent sinus arrest, which is one cause of sudden cardiac death. Cholinergic stimulation via acetylcholine slows the pacemaker rate by decreasing formation of cAMP. This sequence lessens the degree of increase in the heart rate achieved by β-adrenergic stimulation. In addition, acetylcholine directly inhibits the sinus node (Fig. 5-4).

Vascular Control

Of particular importance is the diameter of the small arteries (arterioles) that control the resistance against which the heart works (the peripheral vascular resistance). Control of this site cannot be simplified into opposing effects of the sympathetic and parasympathetic systems. Rather, vasoconstrictors and dilators act in opposing ways (Fig. 2-9). Although norepinephrine acting by α_1-adrenergic receptors causes vasoconstriction, almost paradoxically, circulating norepinephrine and epinephrine cause vasodilation acting through the β_2-receptors, which increase cAMP in vascular smooth muscle. The latter change, for complex reasons, causes vasodilation rather than the expected vasoconstriction. Parasympathetic stimulation causes vasodilation via nitric oxide released from the inner lining of the blood vessels (endothelium), if the endothelium is not damaged. Signals emanating from the endothelium play a major role in regulation of vascular tone. Such signals include nitric oxide, released not only in response to acetylcholine but also during exercise. Adenosine is a further vasodilatory local mediator. Control of vascular smooth muscle tone is extremely complex but of great importance because of the role of the peripheral vascular resistance in determining the load against which the heart works and in setting the BP.

Release of Norepinephrine from Terminal Adrenergic Nerves

During the sympathetic adrenergic response, norepinephrine is released from small swellings, the *terminal varicosities*, lying on minute end branches of the neurons of the adrenergic nervous system (Fig. 2-9). Norepinephrine is synthesized in the varicosities via two compounds called dopa and dopamine and ultimately from the amino acid tyrosine, which is taken up from the circulation. Such synthesis takes place only in the sympathetic nerve terminals, not in the ordinary myocardial cells. The norepinephrine thus synthesized is stored within the terminals in *storage granules* (or *vesicles*) to be released on stimulation by an adrenergic nervous impulse. Thus, when central stimulation increases during excitement or exercise, an increased number of adrenergic impulses liberate an

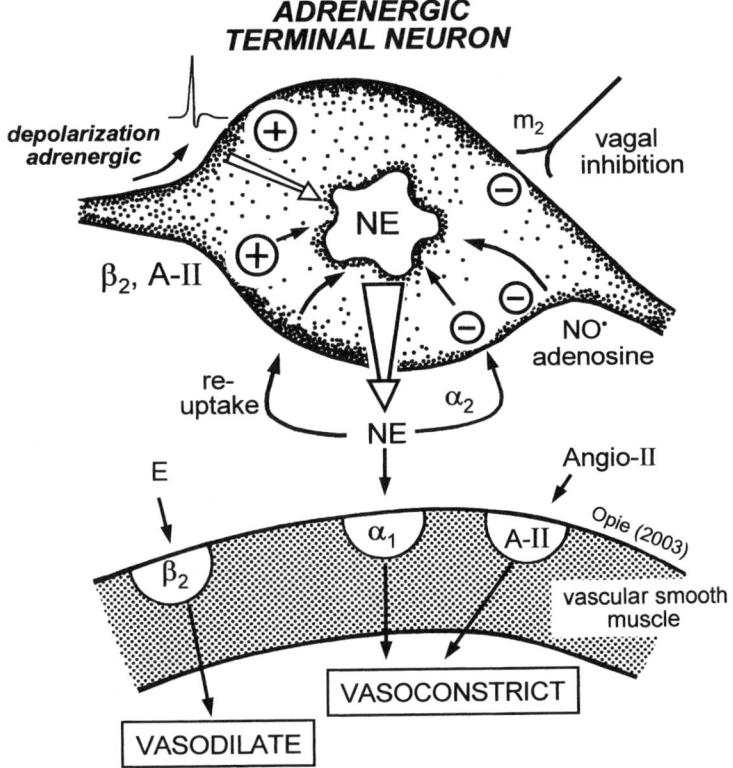

FIG. 2-9. **Role of neuromodulation in arteriolar constriction and dilation.** Norepinephrine is released from the storage granules of the terminal sympathetic neurons into the synaptic cleft that separates the terminals from the arterial wall. Norepinephrine has predominantly vasoconstrictive effects acting via postsynaptic α_1-receptors. In addition, norepinephrine stimulates presynaptic α_2-receptors to invoke feedback inhibition of its own release, to modulate excess release of norepinephrine. Parasympathetic cholinergic stimulation inhibits the release of norepinephrine and thereby indirectly causes vasodilation. Circulating epinephrine stimulates vascular vasodilatory β_2-receptors but also presynaptic receptors on the nerve terminal that promote release of norepinephrine. Angiotensin II, formed ultimately in response to renin released from the kidneys, is also powerfully vasoconstrictive, acting both by inhibition of norepinephrine release (presynaptic receptors, schematically shown to the left of the terminal neuron) and also directly on arteriolar receptors. E, epinephrine; NE, norepinephrine; A-II or *angio-II*, angiotensin II; M_2, muscarinic receptor, subtype 2.

increased amount of norepinephrine from the terminals. Most of the released norepinephrine is taken up again by the nerve terminal varicosities to reenter the storage vesicles or to be metabolized. At least some of the released norepinephrine interacts with the specific vascular α-receptors, and another fraction enters the circulation to account for the increased blood norepinephrine levels found during states of excitement or stress or exercise.

TABLE 2-2. *Presynaptic receptors and their effects on release of norepinephrine from terminal neurons*

Presynaptic receptor	Agonist	Source of agonist	Effect on NE release
M_2	Acetylcholine	Cholinergic	−
α_2	NE	Adrenergic terminal	−
A-II	Angiotensin II	Renin–angiotensin system	+

NE, norepinephrine; −, inhibits; +, enhance; agonist, messenger or hormone stimulating receptors; M_2, cholinergic cardiac muscarinic; α_2, α_2-adrenergic.

Feedback Inhibition of Presynaptic Receptors

There are two types of α-adrenergic receptors. Those situated on the sarcolemma are called *postsynaptic* or *postjunctional receptors*, whereas those situated on the terminal varicosities are called the *presynaptic* or *prejunctional receptors* (Fig. 2-9). Norepinephrine can inhibit its own release, acting on the α_2-adrenergic receptors. Anatomically these are presynaptic α-receptors (Table 2-2). *α_1-Adrenergic receptors* are situated on the arteriolar sarcolemma and therefore called *postsynaptic receptors* (Table 2-3). Norepinephrine stimulates these receptors to cause vasoconstriction.

Neuromodulation is the process whereby the release of norepinephrine from the terminal neurons is either increased or decreased. The most powerful neuromodulator stimulating the release of norepinephrine is *angiotensin II*, the circulating vasoconstrictor that helps to control the BP. Negative neuromodulators, decreasing the release of norepinephrine, include the local messengers adenosine and nitric oxide formed during exercise. Norepinephrine release is also lessened when there is increased cholinergic activity, as at night, when the muscarinic presynaptic receptors on the terminal neurons are stimulated (Fig. 2-9).

Overall Adrenergic Effects on Vascular Beds

Adrenergic stimulation has very complex overall effects on various vascular beds and on the cardiovascular system (Tables 2-1 and 2-4). In vascular smooth

TABLE 2-3. *Postsynaptic receptors and their proposed effects on cardiac or vascular cytosolic calcium levels (Ca^{2+}) and on cardiovascular function*

Postsynaptic receptor	Cardiac Ca^{2+}	Vascular Ca^{2+}	Overall CV effect
α_1	(+)	++	PVR ++
β_1	++	(−)	CO ++
β_2	+	−	CO +, PVR −
A-II	(+)	++	PVR ++

For receptor agonists, see Figure 2-8.
CV, cardiovascular; (+) or (−), controversial and/or modest effect; +, increased; −, decreased; PVR, peripheral (systemic) vascular resistance; CO, cardiac output.

TABLE 2-4. *Effects of adrenergic stimulation by norepinephrine and epinephrine on vascular tone[a]*

Norepinephrine
  Released from terminal neurons
    Vasoconstriction throughout vascular bed
  Circulating
    Vasoconstriction of cutaneous, splanchnic, and renal beds
    Venoconstriction
Circulating epinephrine
  Predominant β_2 vasodilatory effect
    Muscular arterioles (heart and skeletal muscle)
  Predominant α vasoconstrictor effect
    Other resistance vessels and veins
Overall effect: vasodilatory[b]

---

[a]Tone, from Greek *tonos* (something stretched).
[b]Stratton et al. (1985), Freyschuss et al. (1986).

muscle, the α_1-mediated vasoconstrictive effects of norepinephrine are opposed by circulating epinephrine, which is simultaneously released (e.g., during exercise) and stimulates vasodilatory β_2-receptors. In arterioles of the splanchnic bed, epinephrine also stimulates α_1-adrenergic receptors to cause vasoconstriction, thereby helping to divert blood from nonmuscular to muscular tissues (6). Although norepinephrine can stimulate the vasodilatory β_2-receptors, the reasons for its overall vasoconstrictor effect are thought to be (a) that the α_1-receptors are anatomically closer than the β_2-receptors to the sites of norepinephrine release from the terminal neurons, (b) β_2 stimulation at the presynaptic receptor on the terminal neuron gives positive neuromodulation, leading to the release of norepinephrine (Fig. 2-9), and (c) the α_1-adrenergic vascular receptors may be greater in number or activity than the vasodilatory β-receptors. Note that the vasoconstrictor role of the β_2-receptor on the terminal neuron is controversial, although supported by recent data on humans (7). Furthermore, the overall effects of sympathetic stimulation on the arterioles differ from individual to individual. In those who are hypertensive or who may be prone to develop hypertension, vasoconstrictive effects appear to predominate.

Why does blood flow during exercise increase only in those muscles that are actually used, whereas the flow decreases in those that are not being used (6,8)? Even when the vasodilatory β_2-receptors are experimentally blocked, there is still an increase in muscle blood flow during exercise (9). Thus, the explanation may lie in the production of vasodilatory local metabolites by the exercising muscles.

BAROREFLEXES AND CENTRAL CONTROL

When the BP increases excessively, pressure-sensitive cells in the aortic arch and the carotid artery (in a small dilation called the carotid sinus) respond by conveying impulses to a central coordinating nucleus in the brainstem, called the nucleus solitarius. From here, the vagal nucleus is stimulated to send out vagal stimuli to decrease the heart rate and to decrease the force of contraction of the left ventricle (Fig. 2-10). Furthermore, the sympathetic nucleus is inhibited to lessen the degree of sympathetic stimulation of the heart. All these changes will in turn lower the cardiac output so that the BP then decreases toward the normal range: increased BP → carotid baroceptors → nucleus solitarius in the brainstem → vagal nucleus → vagal stimulation and sympathetic inhibition → slower heart rate and less force of cardiac contraction → lower cardiac output → BP decreases to appropriate levels.

This sequence explains the *reflex bradycardia* that can be expected during an acute elevation of arterial BP as a result of stimulation of the baroreceptors in response to peripheral α_1-adrenergic vasoconstriction during an infusion of norepinephrine (Fig. 2-5). Conversely, the low BP after hemorrhage or in heart failure causes a *reflex tachycardia*. Regarding BP, the major role of the carotid sinus reflex is to smooth out acute changes in the BP (10).

An interesting application of the principles of baroreflex control is the use of *carotid sinus massage* in the therapy of some types of tachycardia that originate

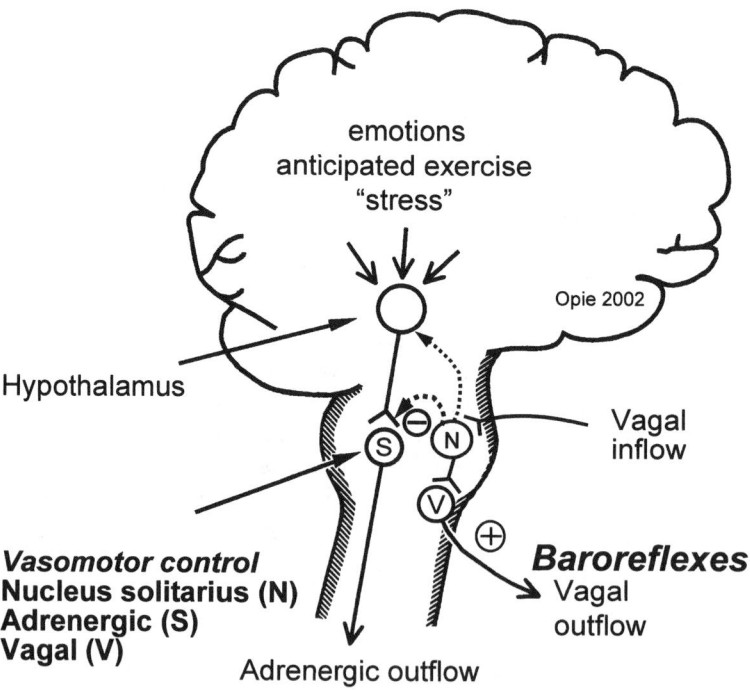

Fig. 2-10. Medullary autonomic control centers. Example of reflex changes if blood pressure is too high and increased vagal and decreased sympathetic activity is required to decrease the blood pressure. *S*, sympathetic adrenergic vasomotor center; *N*, nucleus solitarius (solitary nucleus); *V*, vagal nucleus (nucleus ambiguus).

above the ventricle, i.e., supraventricular tachycardias. External manual stimulation of the mechanoreceptors in the carotid sinus provokes the afferent stimuli, which travel to the vagal nucleus to stimulate the efferent limb so that there is increased vagal inhibition of both sinus and atrioventricular nodes, which in turn helps to terminate the tachycardia (Fig. 20-5)

Vasodilatory Local Messengers

During exercise, adrenergic outflow is increased. Stimulation of the heart by β-receptors leads to an increase in frequency and force of contraction (Fig. 2-7), yet simultaneously α-adrenergic stimulation will tend to constrict the resistance arterioles (Fig. 2-6). Therefore, exercise should be associated with an inevitable increase in BP. The reason that this does not happen is because vasodilatory messengers are locally formed during muscle metabolism and act on the arterioles to vasodilate. Together with epinephrine-induced $β_2$-receptor stimulation, they account for the decrease in peripheral vascular resistance during exercise. Similar messengers are thought to account for the increase in coronary blood flow, also occurring during exercise (Chapter 10). Of particular current interest is the proposed role of a relatively newly defined messenger, nitric oxide, manufactured at several sites including the vascular endothelium (Fig. 2-11). The stimulus to such release of nitric oxide during exercise is not fully known. Hypothetically, a low tissue oxygen tension, occurring as oxygen is used during exercise, could stimulate the synthesis of nitric oxide (11). Alternatively, the increased rate of blood flow during exercise causes a mechanical effect on the endothelium (shear stress) that liberates nitric oxide. Another vasodilatory messenger is adenosine, a metabolite formed as the rate of breakdown of the high-energy phosphate compound ATP exceeds the rate of its resynthesis during exercise.

Neuroregulation by Local Messengers

Both adenosine and nitric oxide are local messengers, being small molecules that very significantly influence local autonomic control of the arterioles. For example, adenosine is a direct vasodilator by its actions on the adenosine receptor on vascular smooth muscle cells and acts as a negative neuromodulator, thereby inhibiting release of norepinephrine (Fig. 2-9).

Nitric oxide not only acts as a local messenger to convey signals from the endothelium to vascular smooth muscle, but it also is a modulator at "every known level of neurogenic control" (1). It is a unique messenger for three reasons. First, it is a gas. Second, it is a free radical and therefore highly interactive. Third, it only acts in the local vicinity where it is formed. After it escapes into the blood, its half-life is extremely limited as it is promptly neutralized in the circulating blood by hemoglobin (12). Physiologically, nitric oxide can be synthesized not only in the vascular endothelium but also in the nerve terminals of the nitric oxide–releasing nerves (*nitroxidergic nerves*) as well as in other sites in the

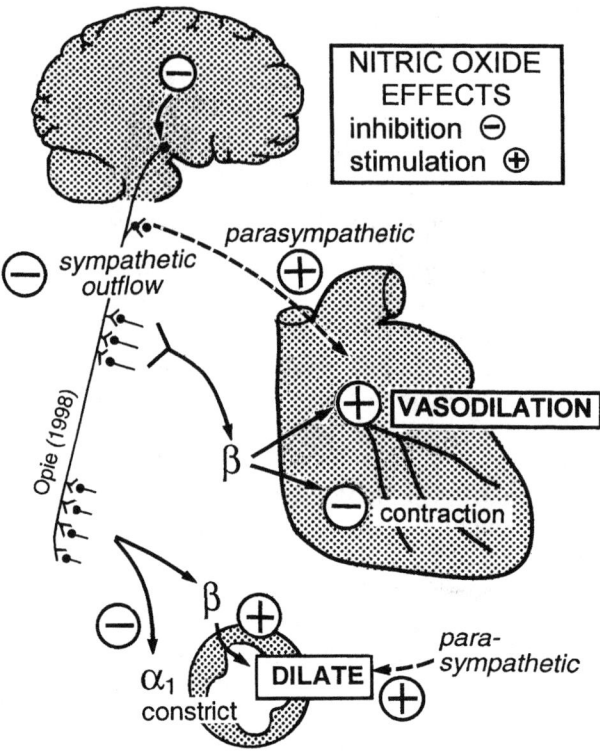

FIG. 2-11. Nitric oxide effects on circulation. Proposed sites at which the local messenger nitric oxide can alter autonomic effects on the cardiovascular system. [For details, see Persson (1).]

nervous system. Pathologically, nitric oxide can be synthesized in myocardial cells to inhibit contraction in some disease states. In general, nitric oxide acts on the autonomic nervous system at several levels to inhibit sympathetic outflow and to lessen the release of norepinephrine from terminal neurons (Fig. 2-1). These are all vasodilatory effects. Nitric oxide also mediates parasympathetic-induced vasodilation because it enhances the relapse of acetylcholine.

BLOOD VOLUME CONTROL: ROLE OF RENIN–ANGIOTENSIN SYSTEM

Besides the fight-or-flight adrenergic reaction, primitive humans needed defense against lack of water and salt. If the blood volume decreases excessively, the circulation must fail. To help regulate the blood volume, there is an important physiologic control mechanism, the *renin–angiotensin system*. Renin is an enzyme liberated from the kidneys in response to a low renal perfusion, low blood volume, low BP, or sodium depletion. These changes release renin, which stimulates the conversion of a polypeptide called angiotensinogen to angiotensin I in the liver. Angiotensin I circulates and is converted to angiotensin II by the activity of the angiotensin-converting enzyme found in the capillary bed of the lung and elsewhere. Angiotensin II is a powerful vasoconstrictor (Fig. 2-12). Hypothetically, the regulatory role of this system might have evolved as follows. When early hunters lacked water, their blood volume would tend to decrease, with a consequent decrease in BP and stimulation of renin release from the kidneys. In today's world, trauma and blood loss unfortunately still occur.

The low blood volume caused by blood loss invokes a compensatory angiotensin II–mediated vasoconstriction to increase the BP (Fig. 14-5). In addition, angiotensin II helps to keep up the blood volume by releasing from the adrenal cortex the hormone aldosterone, which acts on the kidneys to retain sodium, and antidiuretic hormone, which retains water. The renin–angiotensin system is also stimulated in severe exercise, presumably to help conserve sodium and water lost by sweating (Fig. 15-5). However, activity of the renin–angiotensin system may have adverse effects in chronic disease states, aggravating conditions such as hypertension (Fig. 14-6) and heart failure (Fig. 16-14).

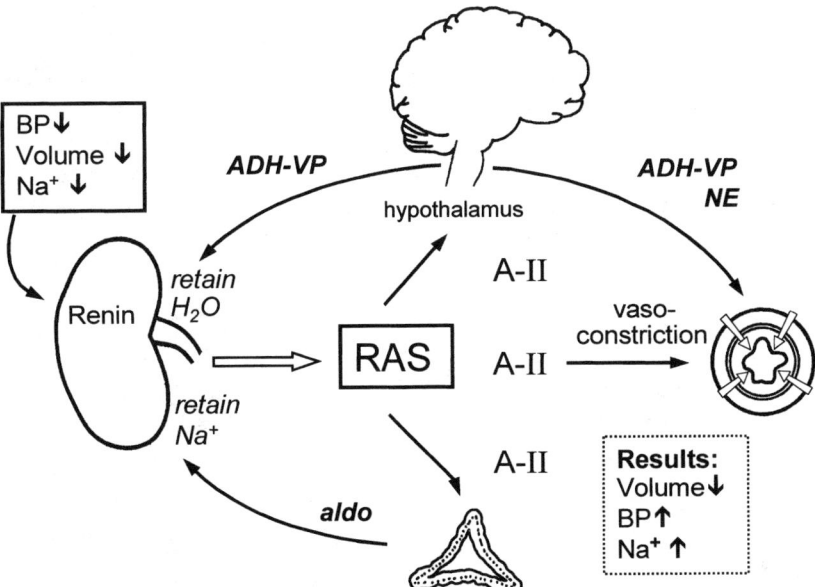

FIG. 2-12. Blood volume control systems. In response to low blood volume or blood pressure or with sodium depletion, the kidney releases renin (Fig. 16-21) that stimulates the renin–angiotensin system with increased formation of vasoconstrictive angiotensin II. Angiotensin II also releases aldosterone from the adrenal cortex to retain sodium and water. A third action of angiotensin II is the release of antidiuretic hormone, also called vasopressin, from the hypothalamus. By the antidiuretic effect, water is retained and by the effect of vasopressin, vasoconstriction is increased. *NE*, norepinephrine; *aldo*, aldosterone; *RAS*, renin–angiotensin system; *A-II*, angiotensin II; *ADH*, antidiuretic hormone; *VP*, vasopressin.

REDISTRIBUTION OF BLOOD DURING EXERCISE

Apart from the heart and lungs, the internal organs of the body do not require increased blood flow during exercise. Such organs are the liver, kidneys, stomach, and intestines. In these organs, blood flow actually decreases during exercise, which helps to direct the blood volume to the muscular organs undergoing increased metabolic activity, such as the heart and skeletal muscle. The mechanisms of such redistribution of blood are several: (a) the absence of vasodilatory metabolites in nonmuscular, nonexercising intraabdominal organs (6); (b) the continued vasoconstrictive effects of norepinephrine in these nonexercising organs; and (c) the capacity of epinephrine to stimulate vasoconstrictive α-receptors rather than vasodilatory β_2-receptors in the arterioles of these organs (Table 2-4).

PERIPHERAL VASCULAR RESISTANCE

Total peripheral vascular resistance (PVR), also called systemic vascular resistance, is crucial to the control of the circulation (Fig. 2-13). It is calculated from the formula: BP = CO × PVR. Therefore, CO = PVR/BP and PVR = BP/CO, where CO is cardiac output per minute (stroke volume × heart rate). The BP is the difference between the mean pressures in the aorta and in the right ventricle, and the cardiac output is the product of the stroke volume and the heart rate. The standard approach to the measurement of these entities and of PVR has been the use of invasive catheterization techniques. At present, noninvasive echocardiographic methods (using ultrasound principles) are increasingly used even though they are less accurate. Physiologically, PVR is low during and just after exercise or when the ambient temperature is high (peripheral vasodilation helps cutaneous heat loss). PVR is high in the cold or when the body is deprived

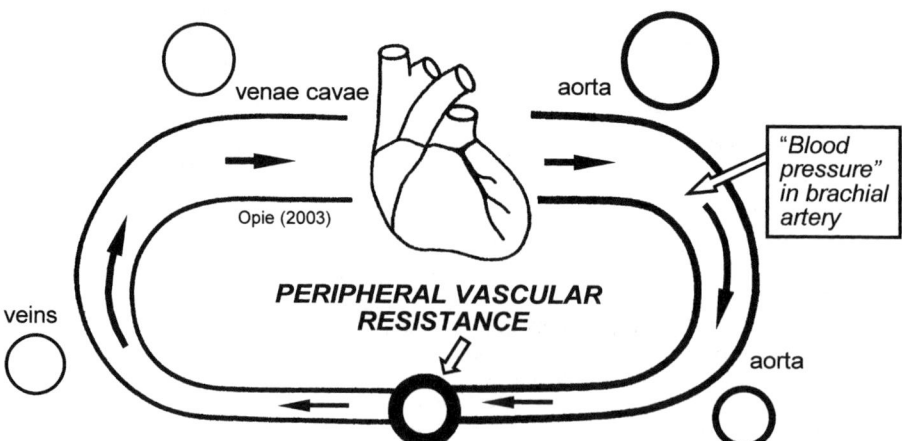

FIG. 2-13. Schematic role of peripheral vascular resistance (also called systemic vascular resistance or total peripheral resistance) in the circulation.

of fluid and the blood volume is low because there is stimulation of the system that ultimately forms angiotensin II (Fig. 2-12). Three disease states that increase PVR to an abnormal degree are arterial hypertension, severe heart failure when the heart contracts too feebly to keep up the BP so that the baroreflexes are stimulated and adrenergic activity increases, and when the heart develops a shock-like state (cardiogenic shock), as in a massive heart attack with myocardial infarction (Chapter 18), and intense reflex adrenergic stimulation is evoked.

Blood flow through the arterioles occurs because the pressure gradient at the arterial end is higher than at the capillary end (Fig. 1-5). Apart from the pressure differences, a crucial factor is the radius of the blood vessel, which is regulated by the balance of vasodilatory and vasoconstrictive effects and, therefore, at least in part by the autonomic nervous system. In idealized conditions with blood flowing smoothly (*laminar flow*) in a rigid tube, resistance to flow through that vessel is inversely proportional to the fourth power of the tube's radius (Fig. 2-14). Hence,

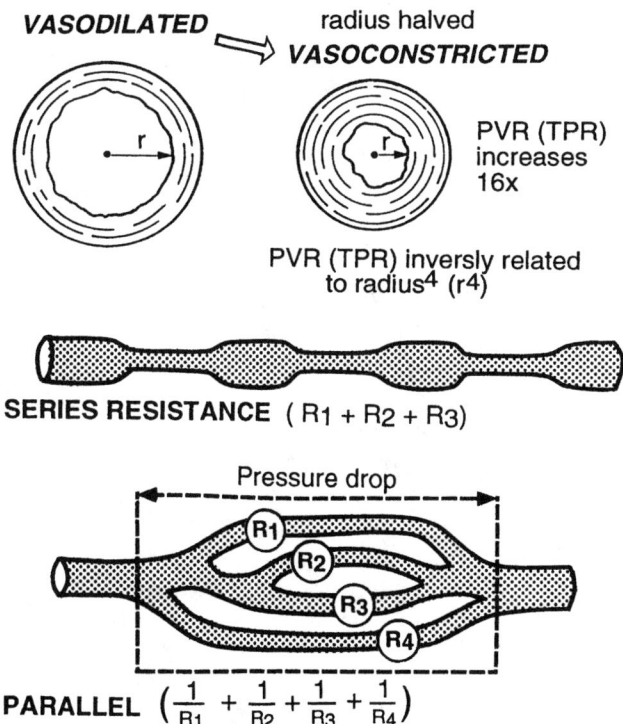

FIG. 2-14. Poiseuille law. Top: The major factor governing the resistance of the arterioles is the radius is shown. Peripheral vascular resistance is inversely related to the fourth power of the radius (r^4). **Bottom:** Most of the resistance arterioles in the circulation are in parallel and constitute the peripheral vascular resistance (peripheral vascular resistance = total peripheral resistance). At the level of the arterioles, the resistance is largely governed by the radius in such a way that resistance increases in proportion to the fourth power of the radius. *PVR*, peripheral vascular resistance; *TPR*, total peripheral resistance; *r*, radius; *R*, resistance.

reduction of the diameter of the arterial lumen is the most powerful determinant of resistance to flow.

Technically, the resistance of a rigid tube can be given by the Poiseuille law, whereby $R = P/Q = (8 \times \text{viscosity} \times \text{length})/r^4$, where R is resistance, Q is flow, r is radius, and P is the pressure decrease over the length of the tube (Fig. 2-14).

Normally, the blood viscosity is not an important variable and the length factor does not change, so that it is the radius that is dominant among the factors regulating vascular resistance. In the presence of vascular disease, such as coronary stenosis, turbulent blood flow will increase the resistance further.

Altered arteriolar diameter not only regulates PVR but changes the pattern of blood flow distal to the arteriole. Because the flow through the arteriole is highly dependent on the radius (according to the Poiseuille equation), more blood reaches the capillaries during vasodilation. Thus, during exercise, increased capillary flow delivers more oxygen to exercising tissues.

THE MICROCIRCULATION

Because arterioles and capillaries act so closely in concert, they constitute what is called the *microcirculation* (Fig. 2-15). To carry out its specialized functions, the capillaries have walls that are only one cell thick (Fig. 2-16). There are three possible modes of exchange across the capillary walls. The first is through pores between cells, the second through small pores within the cells, and the

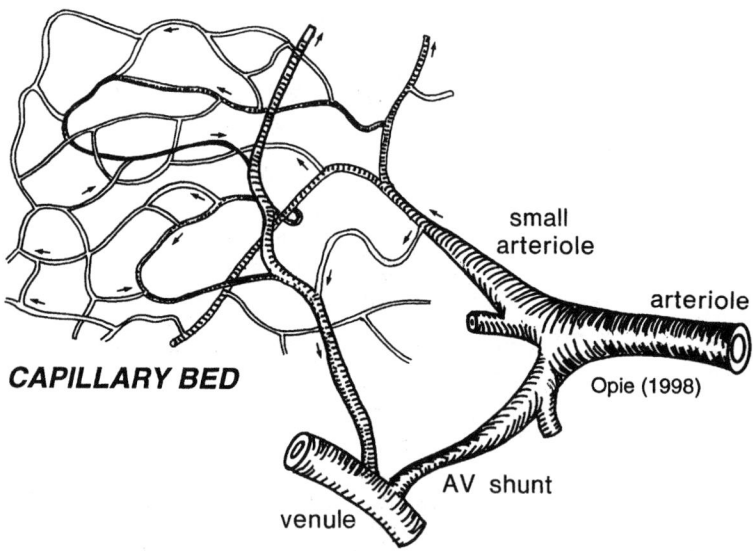

FIG. 2-15. The microcirculation, which includes the arterioles and the capillary bed. Note the existence of arteriolar-venule (*AV*) shunts, which can open or close to increase the amount of blood actually in the capillary bed.

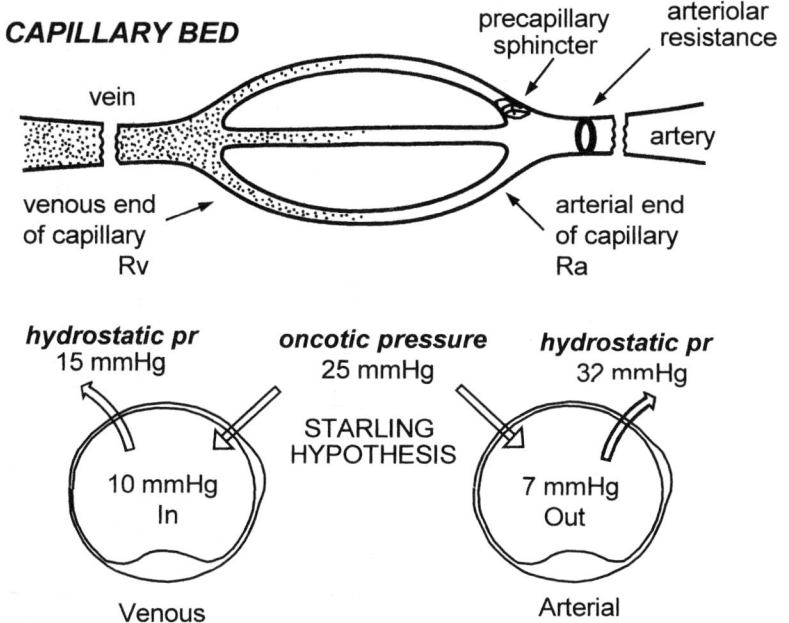

FIG. 2-16. Capillary bed and the Starling hypothesis. The blood flow to the capillary bed is regulated by the arteriolar resistance (*Ra*), the activity of the precapillary sphincters, by atrioventricular shunts, and the resistance at the venous end (*Rv*). The Starling hypothesis (also called Starling principle) for the regulation of fluid transfer states that the major pressure forcing fluid out is the hydrostatic pressure (related to the blood pressure and greater at the arterial end) versus the plasma protein oncotic pressure that is the force bringing fluid back into the capillaries.

third by means of vesicles. Gases, such as oxygen and carbon dioxide, readily flow by diffusion through the pores, as do small molecules such as glucose and lactate. Transport of complex molecules, such as fatty acids, may require transport by *vesicles*. The latter are small, pinched-off fragments of the cell membrane that can entrap a large molecule, close up, and hypothetically transport the molecule across to the opposite side of the cell where the vesicle can reopen to release the transferred molecule. This proposed role of vesicles is, however, controversial.

Oxygen, diffusing from the capillaries, is used in the mitochondria, which are intracellular organelles (Fig. 3-4) in which the oxygen is converted by a series of metabolic steps to CO_2 and water, and energy in the form of ATP is produced. This CO_2 diffuses from the mitochondria back to the capillary blood, and the water joins the total body water. For such energy production to occur also requires that the potential fuels for the heart, such as glucose and fatty acids, must be broken down into much simpler components of only two carbons, which can then enter the mitochondria and participate in energy production.

Starling Hypothesis for Fluid Exchange

Although the great English physiologist Starling is much better known for his "law of the heart" (next section), he made an even earlier contribution to cardiovascular physiology in the Starling hypothesis or principle that describes the forces that regulate the passage of fluid across the capillary endothelium. The most important force that moves fluid out is hydrostatic pressure, related to BP (Fig. 2-16). A typical value for the hydrostatic pressure at the arterial end of the capillary would be 32 mmHg. Conversely, the oncotic pressure, i.e., the osmotic pressure of the plasma proteins, is the force drawing in the fluid from the extravascular space. This is 25 mmHg, so that at the arterial end, there is a net force of 7 mmHg forcing fluid out. At the venous end of the capillary, the hydrostatic pressure has decreased to 15 mmHg, whereas the oncotic pressure remains at 25 mmHg. Therefore, there is a net inward gradient of 10 mmHg. Thus, overall, although there is considerable exchange between the fluid within the capillary and that in the pericapillary spaces, there is no net outward movement of this fluid. The situation is changed in severe heart failure when less blood is pumped out of the left ventricle so that more accumulates in the left atrium. Gradually, the back pressure builds up to increase the hydrostatic pressure in the pulmonary capillaries, thereby exceeding the oncotic pressure. This series of events forces fluid into the extravascular pulmonary spaces and the pulmonary alveoli (the small terminal branches of the bronchial tree). The result is a fluid-filled lung with severe shortness of breath, a condition called acute pulmonary edema.

The Starling "Law of the Heart"

During exercise, more venous blood is returned to the right atrium. The reason is that more blood is squeezed out of the venous capacitance vessels by the contracting skeletal muscle and that there is also an increase in the *venous tone* (an increase in tension in the muscle walls) induced by autonomic activation (Table 2-2). In addition, the cardiac output increases substantially, so that the venous return must also increase by the same amount. To maintain balance in the circulation, the greater venous return must in some way stimulate the heart to contract (Fig. 2-13). This mechanism is known as the Starling law: "Within physiological limits, the larger the volume of the heart, the greater the energy of its contraction and the amount of chemical change at each contraction."

The latter conclusion was reached in Starling's fundamental lecture on the law of the heart, given at Cambridge, England, in 1915 and published in 1918 (13). He was aware of the longitudinal fibrils constituting muscle and proposed that "lengthening the muscle increases the extent of the active surface," very similar to the modern concept of cross-bridge interaction. He also gave an early view on molecular mechanisms in heart failure, proposing that the "concentration of active molecules becomes less," which leads to the modern view that there are abnormalities of the calcium cycle in heart failure.

The most important proposal made by Starling was that the heart volume and hence the length of the heart muscle fiber could be increased by an increased venous filling pressure, now often termed the preload (Chapter 12).

Left Ventricular Failure

When the left ventricle fails, as after a prolonged pressure overload (Chapter 16), it sets in chain a similar sequence of events. The failing left ventricle is unable to pump sufficiently strongly to maintain the arterial BP. This tendency to an excessively low BP (arterial hypotension) elicits powerful protective reactions that maintain the BP, including stimulation of the baroreflexes and release of the adrenergic hormones that stimulate the β-adrenergic receptors in the kidneys to release renin and at the same time stimulate the α-adrenergic receptors in the arterioles to constrict. Although these mechanisms help to maintain the BP, they decrease the caliber of the arterioles against which the heart must work, thereby actually exaggerating the degree of heart failure.

These concepts show how the function of the heart cannot be separated from the control of the circulation. Starling emphasized that the circulation could control the heart by variations in the load. The heart, in turn, can send biochemical signals to the circulation by means of the baroreflexes, the adrenergic hormones, and the renin–angiotensin system.

CORONARY CIRCULATION

From the metabolic point of view, the circulation could be regarded as a system for the transfer of energy from the heart to the organs of the periphery (Fig. 2-17). In the heart, the oxygen taken up is used for the oxidation of the major fuels, glucose, and fatty acids, with the production of CO_2, H_2O, and energy-rich ATP. Myocardial contraction uses ATP and provides the mechanical energy to drive blood through the circulation and to deliver oxygen to the various tissues. Just as the general systemic circulation conveys oxygenated blood to the tissues of the body, so the coronary circulation takes oxygen to the heart muscle (Fig. 2-17). Anatomically, oxygenated blood leaves the aorta just above the aortic valve through two small openings called ostia, from which flow the left and right coronary arteries convey blood to the heart muscle. The left coronary artery subserves mainly the large left ventricle, whereas the right serves chiefly the smaller right ventricle, although this pattern is variable. Each artery splits into smaller branches and then into arterioles and capillaries, following the pattern already described for the systemic circulation. From the capillaries run small veins called venules that empty into veins, which ultimately collect in the coronary sinus to enter the right atrium. The major coronary arteries run on the surface of the heart sending branches down so that the arterioles actually lie within the myocardium. During exercise, when the oxygen requirement of the heart

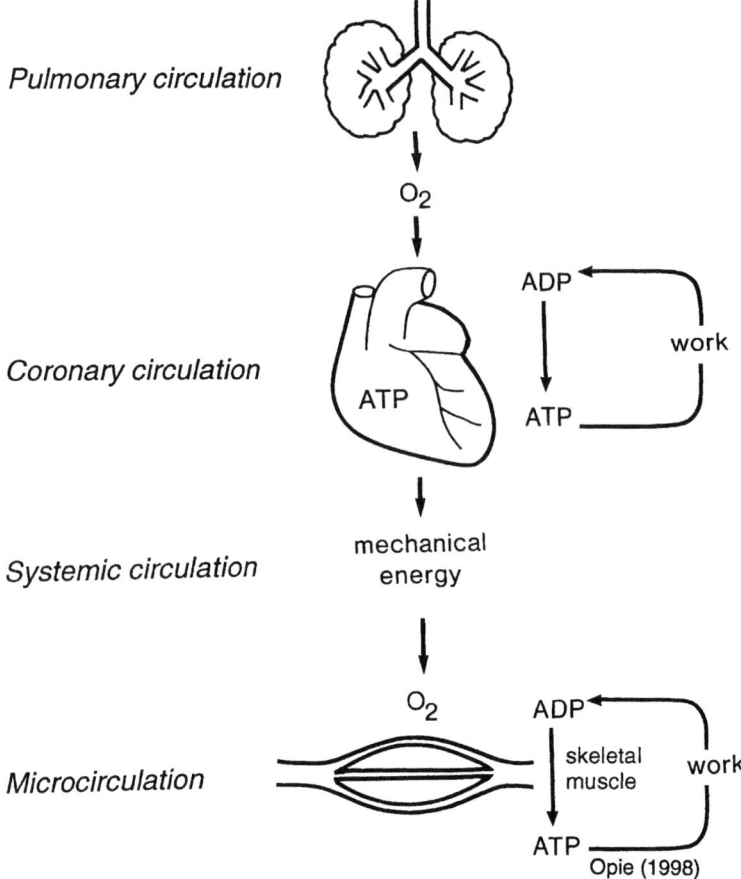

FIG. 2-17. The circulation and adenosine 3′,5′-triphosphate (ATP) transfer. Links between the pulmonary circulation, coronary circulation, systemic circulation, and microcirculation. In essence, ATP produced in the myocardium as a result of the oxygen delivered by the coronary circulation is broken down and the power is transferred to mechanical energy that propels blood through the systemic circulation to deliver oxygen to the capillaries and thence to the tissues where ATP is formed from adenosine 5′-diphosphate (*ADP*). In that way, the whole circulation acts as an ATP transferral system.

increases considerably, the coronary flow rate also increases to deliver the increased oxygen needed. Although the coronary arteries do not have extensive major branches joining up with each other, i.e., there are no large *collaterals* (width, laterally), yet at the level of the small arterioles, such connections do exist to open up during exercise, thereby increasing the blood flow through the capillary bed.

SUMMARY

1. *The heart and circulation work in concert.* The activity of the autonomic nervous system links the heart rate and contractile response of the heart to the requirements of the peripheral tissues via the peripheral circulation.
2. *The autonomic nervous system has two major branches:* the adrenergic or stimulatory system and the cholinergic or inhibitory system. The adrenergic system liberates two neurotransmitters, epinephrine and norepinephrine, whereas the cholinergic neurotransmitter is acetylcholine.
3. *These neurotransmitters may have opposing effects on the heart and circulation.* Epinephrine stimulates β-adrenergic receptors in the heart to increase heart rate and force of contraction. Epinephrine also dilates the arterioles by their β-adrenergic receptors. Although circulating norepinephrine stimulates β-receptors, locally released norepinephrine has a powerful arteriolar vasoconstrictive effect, the result of α_1-adrenergic stimulation.
4. *Acetylcholine is the neurotransmitter of the parasympathetic (cholinergic) nervous system.* It decreases the heart rate and the force of ventricular contraction. It also is an indirect arteriolar vasodilator by inhibiting the release of vasoconstrictive norepinephrine from the nerve terminals.
5. *The baroreflexes link the heart and circulation.* When the arterial pressure is low, then baroreflexes are stimulated to activate adrenergic vasoconstriction and to increase the heart rate. Converse changes occur when the BP is too high, e.g., after an experimental infusion of norepinephrine.
6. *During exercise, the activity of the adrenergic autonomic nervous system increases.* The heart rate increases, contractility increases, and more blood is pumped from the heart (cardiac output increases). This blood is redistributed in the tissues according to the needs during exercise. More blood is required in the myocardium and skeletal muscle, so that the arterioles to these tissues vasodilate during exercise. Conversely, arterioles serving those organs such as the kidney, which do not need more blood during exercise, are vasoconstricted.
7. *The heart pumps against the PVR, created by the highly muscular small-bore arterioles.* Their constriction or dilation explains an increase or decrease in PVR because that resistance is inversely related to the fourth power of the radius (Poiseuille law). Hence, only small changes in the arteriolar radius have major consequences.
8. *The PVR is influenced by the both autonomic nervous system and local messengers.* For example, norepinephrine released from the terminal neurons of the sympathetic nervous system is vasoconstrictive, whereas the local messengers adenosine and nitric oxide are vasodilatory. Formation of these local messengers may account for arteriolar vasodilation during exercise, which allows more blood to be brought to the functioning skeletal muscles and also helps to decrease the BP, thereby avoiding an excessive hypertensive response during exercise.

STUDENT QUESTIONS

1. What are the divisions of the autonomic nervous system, and what are the associated receptors?
2. What are the major cardiovascular effects of stimulation of each branch of the autonomic nervous system?
3. How do epinephrine and norepinephrine differ in their effects on the circulation?
4. Outline how messenger systems act to decrease or increase heart rate.
5. What is neuromodulation?

CARDIOLOGIST-IN-TRAINING QUESTIONS

1. Describe the effects of stimulation of the right sympathetic nerves on the cardiovascular system.
2. Distinguish between the Starling principle (or hypothesis) and the Starling law of the heart.
3. Describe the various receptors found on the adrenergic terminal neuron and how they affect the release of norepinephrine. What are the anticipated changes in BP in response to stimulation of each of these receptors?
4. Describe in detail the neurohormonal response to sodium depletion.
5. What is the Poiseuille law, and what is its relevance to the control of BP?

REFERENCES

1. Persson PB. Modulation of cardiovascular control and their interaction. *Physiol Rev* 1996;76: 193–244.
2. Ahlquist RP. A study of the adrenotropic receptors. *Am J Physiol* 1948;153:586–600.
2a. Lewis, ME, et al. Vagus nerve stimulation decreases left ventricular contractility *in vivo* in the human and pig heart. *J Physiol* 2001;534:547–552.
2b. Werko L, Bucht H, Josephson B, et al. The effect of noradrenalin and adrenalin on renal hemodynamics and renal function in man. *Scand J Clin Lab Invest* 1951;3:255–261.
3. Barcroft H, Swan HJC. *Sympathetic control of human blood vessels*. London: Edward Arnold, 1953.
4. Stratton JR, Pfeifer MA, Ritchie JL, et al. Hemodynamic effects of epinephrine: concentration-effect study in humans. *J Appl Physiol* 1985;58:1199–1206.
5. Nakayama Y, Miyano H, Shishido T, et al. Heart rate-dependent vagal effect of end-systolic elastance of the canine left ventricle under various levels of sympathetic tone. *Circulation* 2001;104: 2277–2279.
6. Taylor J, Hand GA, Johnson DG, et al. Augmented forearm vasoconstriction during dynamic exercise in healthy older men. *Circulation* 1992;86:1789–1799.
7. Azevedo ER, Kubo T, Mak S, et al. Nonselective versus selective β-adrenergic receptor blockade in congestive heart failure. *Circulation* 2001;104:2194–2199.
8. Rowell LB. *Human circulation, regulation during physical stress*. New York: Oxford University Press, 1986.
9. Lund-Johansen P. Central haemodynamic effects of β-blockers in hypertension. A comparison between atenolol, metoprolol, timolol, penbutolol, alprenolol, pindolol and bunitrolol. *Eur Heart J* 1983;4[Suppl D]:1–2.
10. Smit AA, Timmers HJ, Wieling W, et al. Long-term effects of carotid sinus denervation on arterial blood pressure in humans. *Circulation* 2002;105:1329–1335.
11. Park KH, Rubin LE, Gross SS, et al. Nitric oxide is a mediator of hypoxic coronary vasodilation. Relation to adenosine and cyclooxygenase-derived metabolites. *Circ Res* 1992;71:992–1001.

12. Schechter AN, et al. Hemoglobin and the paracrine and endocrine functions of nitric oxide. *N Engl J Med* 2003;348:1483–1485.
13. Starling EH. *The Linacre lecture on the law of the heart*. London: Longmans, Green, 1918.
14. Shepherd JT, Vanhoutte PM. *The human cardiovascular system. Facts and concepts*. New York: Raven Press, 1979.
15. Freyschuss U, Hjemdahl P, Juhlin-Dannfelt A. Cardiovascular and metabolic responses to low dose adrenaline infusion: an invasive study in humans. *Clin Sci* 1986;70:199–206.
16. Barnett AJ, Blacket RB, Depoorter AE, et al. The action of noradrenaline in man and its relation to phaeochromocytoma and hypertension. *Clin Sci* 1950;9:151–179.

3
Heart Cells and Organelles

Striated muscle cytoarchitecture: an intricate web of form and function.
Clark et al. (1)

Thus far, the theme has been developed that myocardial contraction plays a crucial role in the regulation of the circulation by ejection of blood from the left ventricle and that the tone of the peripheral arterioles provides much of the resistance against which the heart works. The emphasis of this chapter is on the general organization of myocardial contractile cells and the properties of their supporting cells. Comparisons and contrasts are also made between myocardial and vascular smooth muscle cells because the peripheral and coronary circulations crucially govern myocardial function.

Most of the heart is made up of contractile muscle cells, also known as *myocytes* or, more specifically, *cardiomyocytes*. The rest consists of pacemaker and conducting tissues (which are concerned with the generation and propagation of the heart's electrical activity), blood vessels, and the extracellular space (Table *3-1*). Myocytes constitute approximately 75% of the total volume of the

TABLE 3-1. *Cells of the heart*

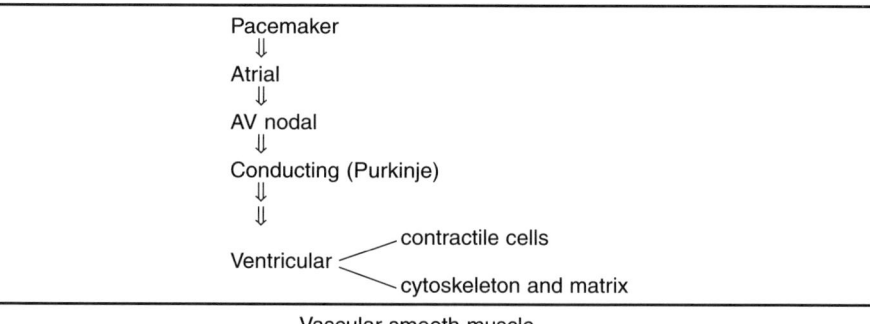

Top panel shows the cells concerned with initiation and conduction of the cardiac impulse to the ventricular contractile cells. Cytoskeletal and matrix cells give support. Vascular smooth muscle and other vascular cells regulate the load against which the heart contracts.
AV, atrioventricular.

myocardium (2). A *myofiber* is composed of a group of myocytes held together by surrounding connective tissue (frontispiece). Additional strands of collagen connect myofibers to each other. The myocytes are filled with bundles of contractile proteins, each bundle called a *myofibril*.

WORKING VENTRICULAR MYOCYTES

Although there are many different cell types in the heart, the ventricular myocytes, by their contraction, propel the blood throughout the body. These working myocytes are described, followed by atrial cells and then vascular smooth muscle cells. The individual ventricular myocytes that account for more than half of the heart's weight are roughly cylindrical in shape. Those in the atrium are quite small, less than 10 μm in diameter and approximately 20 μm in length. Relative to the atrial cells, the ventricular myocytes are large, measuring approximately 10 to 25 μm in diameter and 50 to 100 μm in length (Table 3-2). Early in life, there are vast numbers of myocytes in the heart, possibly as much as 6×10^9 cells. Millions of cells are lost for every year of life, so that the centenarian has only approximately one-third of the original number of heart cells left (3).

When examined under the light microscope, these cells have cross striations and are branched. Each myocyte is bounded by an external membrane called the *sarcolemma* (Latin, *sarco*, flesh; *lemma*, thin husk) and is filled with rod-like bundles of *myofibrils* (Color Plate 8-1). The latter are the contractile elements. The sarcolemma of the myocyte invaginates to form an extensive tubular network (*T tubules*) that extends the extracellular space into the interior of the cell (Color Plate 8-1). The nucleus, which contains almost all the cell's genetic infor-

TABLE 3-2. *Microanatomy of contractile and conducting (Purkinje) cells*

	Ventricular myocyte[a,b]	Atrial myocyte[a,c]	Purkinje cells[a,d]
Shape	Long and narrow	Elliptical (oval)	Long and broad
Length (μm)	50–100	~20	150–200
Diameter (μm)	10–25	5–6	35–40
T tubules	Plentiful	Rare or none	Absent
Intercalated disk and gap junction	Prominent end-to-end transmission	Side-to-side as well as end-to-end transmission	Very prominent; abundant gap junctions; fast end-to-end transmission
General appearance	Mitochondria and sarcomeres, very abundant; rectangular branching bundles with little interstitial collagen	Bundles of atrial tissue separated by wide areas of collagen	Fewer sarcomeres, paler

Note that the length of isolated myocytes from rat and human ventricles is similar, as is sarcomere length (see ref. 1e). Note differences from vascular smooth muscle cells (see ref. 1f).

[a–d]See references 1a–1d.

mation, is often centrally located. Some myocytes have several nuclei. Interspersed between the myofibrils and immediately beneath the sarcolemma are many *mitochondria*, the main function of which is to generate the energy, in the form of adenosine 5′-triphosphate (ATP), needed to maintain the heart's function and viability.

Cytosol

The sarcolemma separates the intracellular and extracellular spaces. Within the sarcolemma, the contractile apparatus and various organelles do not lie loose but are contained in a fluid microenvironment with a specific content of ions, especially potassium, calcium, and sodium. The intracellular fluid, together with the proteins in it, is the *cytoplasm*, also called the *sarcoplasm*. Its fluid component, excluding the proteins, is called the *cytosol*. As is common usage in physiology and medicine, the term fluid is used even though liquid is strictly correct. It is the much higher intracellular, rather than extracellular, concentration of potassium ions that gives cardiac (and other) cells their specific electrical properties; whereby the inner side of the sarcolemma is negatively charged, and the outer side has positive charges, thereby conferring a state of *polarization*. It is also in the cytosol that the concentrations of calcium ions increase and decrease to cause cardiac contraction and relaxation. The proteins of the sarcoplasm contain many specialized molecules, including enzymes that act to accelerate the conversion of one chemical form to another, thereby eventually producing energy. For example, glucose taken up from the circulation by cardiomyocytes is broken down by a series of enzymes to become much smaller molecules that can enter the mitochondria, where they are broken down further with the eventual production of ATP.

Within the cell, mitochondria, the contractile mechanism, and the nucleus are not simply suspended or distributed in cytosolic space. Increasingly, the cytoplasm is seen as having a highly organized *cytoskeleton* (skeleton within the cell) that "guides" message-carrying molecules toward those "significant other" molecules with whom they really want to link. Scaffolding proteins provide preferred docking sites for intracellular messengers such as cyclic adenosine 3′,5′-monophosphate (Fig. 2-11). Energy can be directed from the site of production to where it is needed. In brief, the cytoplasm is no longer a "well-mixed bag" (4).

Myofibrils and Contractile Proteins

The major function of myocardial myocytes lies in the contraction–relaxation cycle. The two chief contractile proteins, located within the myofibrils, are the thick *myosin filaments* and the thin *actin filaments* (Latin, *filament*, delicate thread). During contraction, the filaments slide over each other without the individual molecules of actin or myosin actually shortening (Fig. 3-1). As they slide, they pull together the two ends of the fundamental contractile unit called the *sar-*

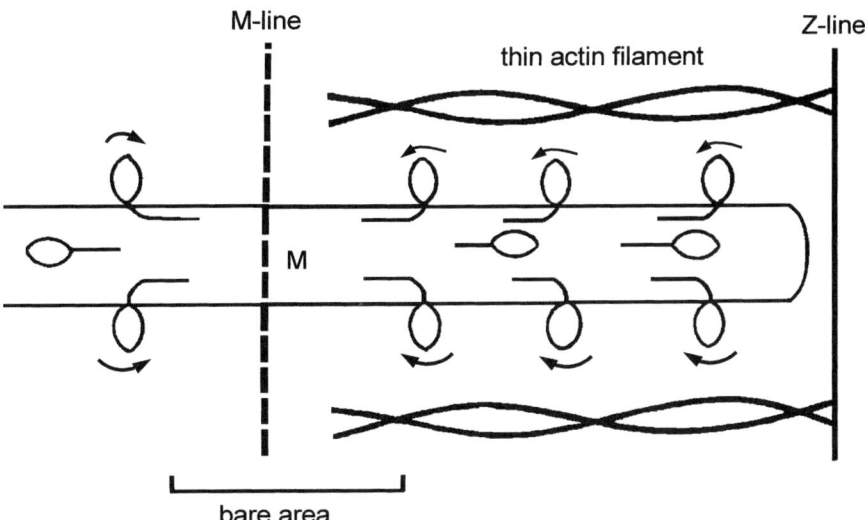

FIG. 3-1. Schematic concept of contractile proteins. A thick myosin filament (*M*) stretches to either side from the central M line and lies in between two much thinner actin filaments. The latter consist of two twisting chains and extend inward from the Z lines on either side of the myofibril. During cardiac contraction, myosin heads "flex" to interact with actin filaments to move the Z lines closer together.

comere (Latin, *mere*, part). On electron microscopy (Fig. 3-2), the sarcomere is limited on either side by the *Z line* (Z, abbreviation for German *Zückung*, contraction) to which the actin filaments are attached. These are also called *Z bands* or *Z disks*. Conversely, the myosin filaments extend from the center of the sarcomere in either direction toward but not actually reaching the Z lines. A third major protein, *titin*, attaches the myosin filaments to the Z lines. Titin is a macromolecule of high molecular weight that has expansile properties and contributes to the mechanical stretch capacity of the myocardium.

The site where the myosin and actin filaments overlap is called the *anisostropic* or *A band*, which shows up darkly on electron microscopy in contrast to the lighter zones of *isotropic* or *I bands* on either side, which contain only actin filaments. These bands have different light-scattering properties, the A bands being more powerful in this regard than the I bands. In the center of each A band, there is a relatively clear zone known as the *H zone* (German, *helle*, clear). Here, only myosin is present because the overlapping of the thin and thick filaments falls short of this region. Each H zone contains a central dark region, the *M line*, which contains M-line proteins that appear to extend across the filaments as if to hold them in their correct anatomic position.

Cross-bridge cycling is the entire process whereby the myosin heads interact with the actin filaments (Fig. 3-3). The cycle is initiated by an increase in cytoso-

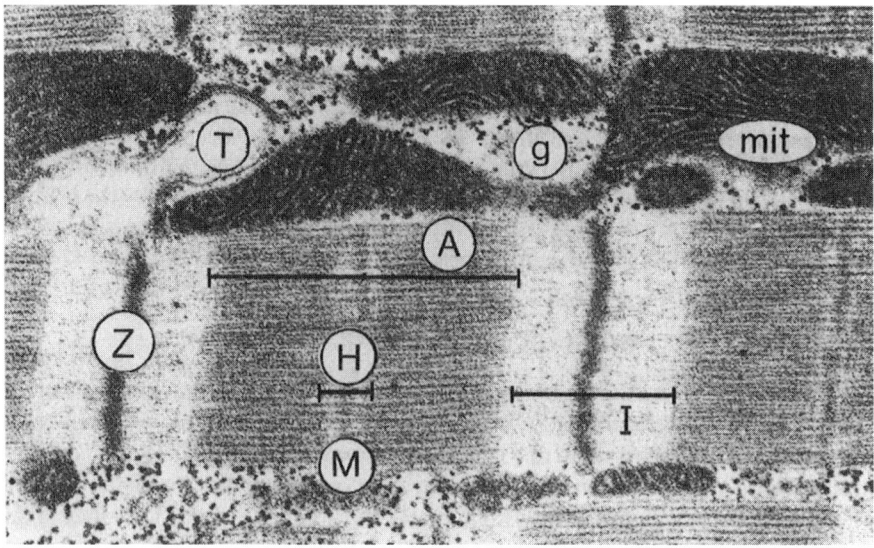

FIG. 3-2. Myofibrils and sarcomeres. Longitudinal section of rat papillary muscle shows regular arrays of myofibrils divided into sarcomeres (Color Plate 1). The sarcomere is the contractile unit between the Z lines (Z). Note the presence of numerous mitochondria (*mit*) sandwiched between the myofibrils, and the presence of T-tubules (*T*), which penetrate into the muscle at the level of the Z bands. This two-dimensional picture should not disguise the fact that the Z line is really a Z disk. For description of A, I, and H zones (*H*), see text. M, M band; g, glycogen granules. Original magnification ×32,000. (Courtesy of Dr. J. Moravec, Dijon, France.)

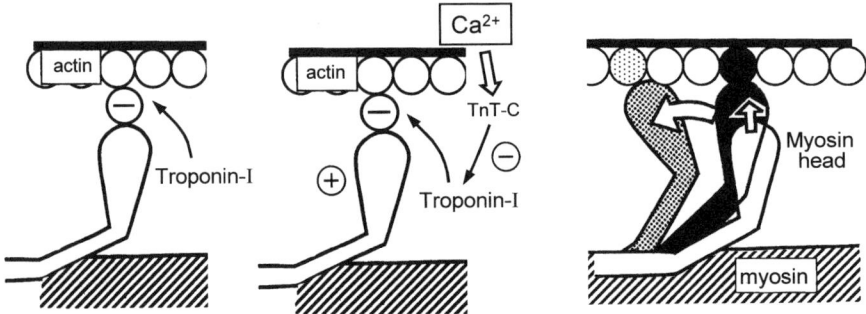

FIG. 3-3. Cross-bridge contraction phase. Schematic of interaction between myosin head and actin filament during contraction. **Left:** The inhibitory effect of troponin I on the interaction between the myosin head and the actin filament. **Middle:** The arrival of calcium ions at the start of systole that combine with troponin C (*Tn-C*), thereby relieving the inhibition exerted by troponin I. **Right:** Illustration of how the myosin head flexes to interact with one of the actin units (*black*). During flexion, this unit is moved along (new position indicated by *dotted circle*). Then the myosin head relaxes, thereby able to restart the cycle. There are many different myosin heads interacting, some in flexion and some in extension. The whole process occurs throughout the period of contraction during the availability of calcium ions.

lic calcium in response to the wave of electricity that reaches the ventricular myocytes from the conduction system. The process is called *cross-bridge cycling*. As the actin filaments move inward toward the center of the sarcomere, drawing the Z lines closer together, the sarcomere shortens. Relaxation takes place when ATP attaches to the myosin head.

Mitochondria

Mitochondria occupy a large proportion (Table 3-3) of each myocyte. They are wedged in between the myofibrils, presumably so that the chief source of energy supply is close to the chief site of energy use. Mitochondria are often described as the powerhouses of the cell, producing the energy (as ATP) that the cells need to survive and function (Fig. 3-4). Much of the molecular machinery that is responsible for producing this energy is located on the inner multifolded membrane containing the *cristae* (Latin, *crista*, crest), which occupy a vast membrane area compared with other cell membranes (Table 3-4). The enzymes located here

TABLE 3-3. Cardiac organelles and their function[a]

Organelle	Percentage of cell volume	Function
Myofibril	~50[b]	Interaction of thick and thin filaments during contraction cycle
Mitochondria	~60 in humans[c] 16 in neonates[b] 33 in adults[b] 23 in adult men[c]	Provide ATP chiefly for contraction
T system	1[d]	Transmission of electrical signal from sarcolemma to cell interior
Sarcoplasmic reticulum	33 in neonates[b] 2 in adults[b]	Takes up and releases Ca^{2+} during contraction cycle
Terminal cisternae	0.33 in adults[d]	Site of calcium storage and release[e]
Rest of network	Rest of volume	Site of calcium uptake en route to cisternae
Sarcolemma	Very low	Control of ionic gradients; channels for ions and action potential; maintenance of cell integrity; receptors for drugs and hormones
Nucleus	5	Protein synthesis
Lysosomes	Very low	Intracellular digestion and proteolysis
Sarcoplasm (cytoplasm)	12[d]	Provides cytosol in which rise and fall of ionized calcium occurs; contains other ions and small molecules
Sarcoplasm with nuclei	18 in humans[c]	Gene regulation

Note that the extracellular space occupies approximately 75% of the total heart volume.
[a]Composition and function of rat ventricular heart cell with some data for humans modified from reference 2a.
[b]Reference 2b, [c]Reference 2c, [d]Reference 2a, [e]Reference 2d.
ATP, adenosine 5'-triphosphate.

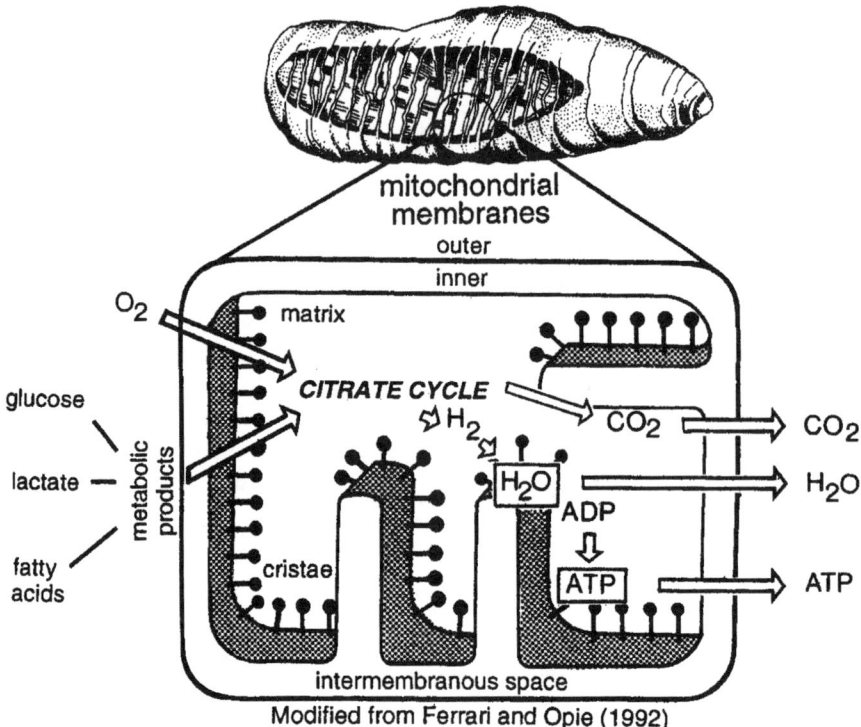

FIG. 3-4. Mitochondrial structure and function. The traditional cocoon mitochondrion is shown. In the production of adenosine 5'-monophosphate (*ATP*), simplified metabolic products derived from the major fuels and oxygen taken up by the myocardium are able to enter the citrate cycle, which produces ATP, CO_2, and H_2O. The cristae on the inner surface of the inner mitochondrial membrane are the site of ATP synthesis. Each crista resembles a button projecting from the inner membrane and contains the enzymes involved in ATP synthesis. ADP, adenosine 5'-diphosphate.

TABLE 3-4. *Membrane areas of ventricular cells*[a]

	Area/volume (μm^2 membrane area/μm^3 cell volume)
External sarcolemma	0.3
External sarcolemma plus T tubules	0.4 (or more)[b]
Sarcoplasmic reticulum	1.2
Mitochondrial cristae	11.0

[a]From reference 2a.
[b]Other workers estimate that the T-tubules increase the area/volume ratio by several times.

promote the activity of the citrate cycle, originally described by the Nobel prize winner Sir Hans Krebs in a famous paper that was rejected by *Nature*. The energy that is released during the transfer of these hydrogen atoms to oxygen is harnessed for the synthesis of ATP; hence, the term *oxidative phosphorylation*.

In addition to the generation of ATP, cardiac mitochondria have another important role. They can potentially accumulate calcium. This process helps to prevent the level of calcium in the cytosol from becoming too high in conditions of calcium overload, as during severe lack of oxygen.

Sarcolemma and Glycocalyx

Because actin and myosin only contract in the presence of calcium ions, one of the major functions of the sarcolemma is to regulate with precision the intracellular calcium ion concentration. The extracellular concentration of calcium is approximately 1,000 times higher than the intracellular value, so that the sarcolemma must be impermeable to calcium ions, only allowing the passage of minute amounts required to trigger some intracellular events concerned with contraction. The sarcolemma, via its pumps and exchangers (Chapter 4), maintains major differences in the ionic composition of intracellular and extracellular fluids. Lying between the sarcolemma and the extracellular space is a "twilight zone," the glycocalyx, which appears to help in the regulation of calcium ion entry into the myocytes.

The *glycocalyx* is the outermost layer of the cell, consisting chiefly of complex carbohydrates called polysaccharides, often associated with proteins (glycoproteins). The latter have negative electrical charges that act to trap positively charged ions such as the calcium ions. Experimentally, the glycocalyx can be peeled away from the underlying sarcolemma by completely removing and then reintroducing extracellular calcium (the calcium paradox). Loss of the protective glycocalyx allows a normal concentration of extracellular calcium, otherwise harmless, to flood into the cardiac myocytes, causing massive damage.

The *lipid bilayer* is immediately within the glycocalyx and is usually regarded as the only true component of the sarcolemma. The lipid bilayer is similar in composition to most external cell membranes, so that the general term *plasmalemma* is also used. Chemically, the *phospholipids* are the major constituent of this membrane. These lipids have a phosphate group that joins their *hydrophilic* (water-loving) heads with the *hydrophobic* (water-repelling) fatty acid tails, the latter pointing inward toward each other. Molecules with such opposite charges are called *amphiphiles* (Latin, *amphi*, on both sides). When the sarcolemma breaks down in severe ischemia, liberation of amphiphiles can alter the balance of intracellular charges to have potentially toxic effects.

Integral proteins have highly specialized and varied functions. They are tightly held (hence the term integral) in the sarcolemma by the side chains of their amino acids, which bind to the lipid tails in the center of the bilayer. Integral proteins control the flow of ions across the sarcolemma, some acting as ion channels, others as ion exchangers, and yet others as ion pumps (Chapter 4).

Calcium ions bind to external binding sites on the sarcolemma and glycocalyx, both to the complex lipids containing phosphate groups (phospholipids) of the outer layer of the sarcolemmal bilayer and, in a more diffuse fashion, to the negatively charged proteins of the glycocalyx. In some way, not fully understood, the wave of excitation can allow such "bound" calcium ions to enter through those integral proteins that function as calcium channels.

Channels and Ion Transport

Ion-selective channels are examples of membrane proteins. They "open" as the wave of electrical excitation travels across the myocardium to allow a controlled and sequential passage of minute amounts of sodium, calcium, and potassium ions across the sarcolemma, which is otherwise relatively impermeable to these ions. Thus, during electrical excitation, the opening of ion-selective channels alters the charges across the sarcolemma. This highly regulated series of changes in electrical charge (or potential) is called the *action potential*.

Sodium channels open first to bring in positively charged sodium ions at an extremely rapid rate, thereby causing the equally rapid upstroke phase of the action potential. The entry of these positive charges causes the sarcolemma to lose its resting negative charge or polarity (Fig. 4-1), thereby becoming *depolarized*. *Calcium channels* are relatively selective for the entry of calcium ions that occurs somewhat more slowly and when most of the rapid entry of the sodium ions has ceased. Calcium ion entry accounts for at least part of the flat phase (*plateau*) of the action potential. *Potassium channels* are highly complex in their number and function, but some of them open toward the end of the action plateau phase of the action potential to carry positive charges outward across the sarcolemma, thereby terminating the action potential. Although the function of each of these channels is complex, a reasonable simplification would be as follows. Opening of the sodium channel is crucial for the swift conduction of the electrical impulse throughout the heart. By rapidly changing the electrical charge across the sarcolemma, sodium entry creates conditions suitable for onward transmission of the impulse (Fig. 5-7). Entry of calcium ions is concerned with the triggering of the contractile cycle (Color Plate 8-1). Outward flow of potassium ions, by restoring the normal electrical charge of the cell membrane, prepares the myocardial cells for the next wave of depolarization.

Transverse Tubular System and Caveolae

The sarcolemma does not just line the outer surface of the cardiac myocyte but penetrates into the intracellular space to form a series of tube-like invaginations (Fig. 3-5). The *T-tubules* bring intra- and extracellular domains together in the closest possible contact, short of fusing them together. The salient features of the T-tubules are as follows:

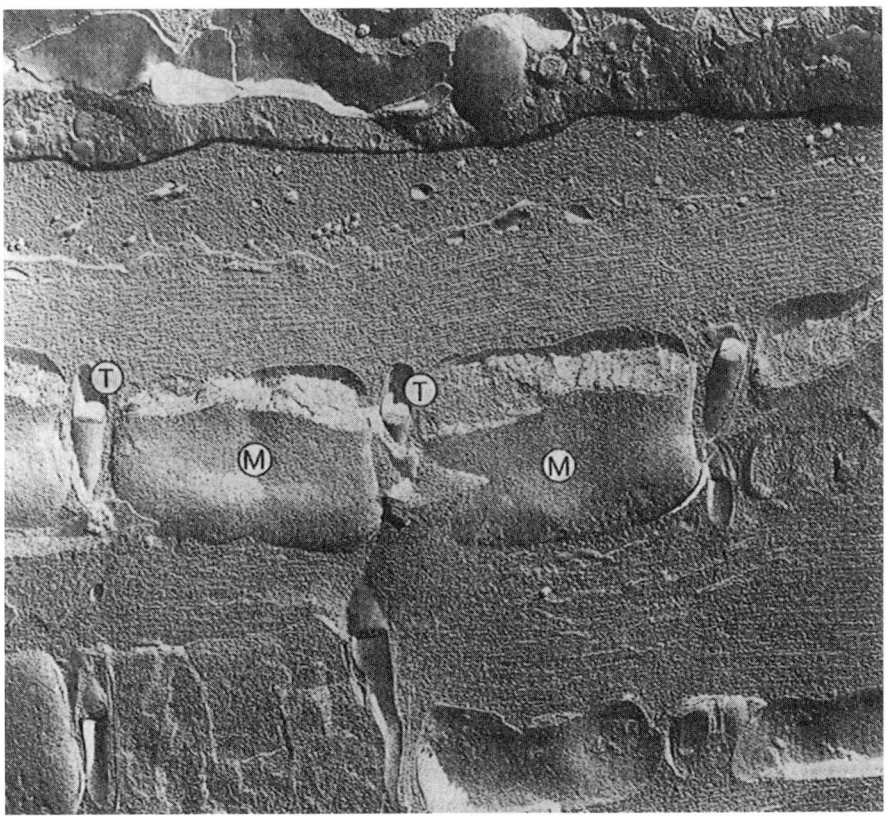

FIG. 3-5. T-tubule system. The extensive network lies between mitochondria (*M*) and penetrating the rows of sarcomeres at the Z lines, delineated by a freeze-fracture micrograph. The lumen of the T-tubules (*T*) is continuous with the extracellular space and brings the extracellular fluid into the ventricular myocyte. For the relationship between T-tubules and sarcoplasmic reticulum, see frontispiece. Original magnification ×31,580. (From Scales DJ. Aspects of the mammalian cardiac sarcotubular system revealed by freeze-fracture electron microscopy. *J Mol Cell Cardiol* 1981;13:373–380, with permission.)

1. Because the T-tubules are an extension of and have the same ultrastructure as the cell surface, they increase the surface area of the cell, at least by 30% (Table 3-4) and possibly much more, thereby facilitating the spread of the excitatory stimulus to within the cell.
2. The lumen of the T-tubules at the surface of the cell is relatively wide, which ensures that an adequate supply of oxygen and nutrients contained in extracellular space becomes available for transfer to intracellular space. Nonetheless, fluid in the T-tubules is not exactly the same in composition as that in the extracellular space because communication is not entirely free.
3. T-tubules contain a particular type of calcium channel (the L type) that responds to the wave of electrical excitation and depolarization by allowing

the entry of calcium ions. These activate the sarcoplasmic reticulum (SR) to release much more calcium (for details, see next section). Not surprisingly, T-tubules are absent in noncontractile cells such as Purkinje fibers (5).
4. T-tubules are subject to extreme mechanical forces during systole and diastole, yet the lumen always remains open. Such stability is explained by their subcellular scaffolding closely resembling that of the sarcolemma (see section describing costameres) (5).

Caveolae (Latin, small caves) are small folds that project inward from the sarcolemma to increase the membrane surface area. They contain the protein caveolin. Their function remains hotly debated and may include many functions such as signal transduction, production of nitric oxide, and membrane stabilization by linkage to dystrophin and other anchoring proteins. One proposal is that the calcium ion influx that releases calcium from the SR originates from the mouth of the caveolae in cells that lack T-tubules such as vascular smooth muscle cells and neonatal cardiomyocytes (6).

Sarcoplasmic Reticulum

The SR is crucial for the regulation of calcium ion movements within the cell. Cardiac SR can be sedimented from suitably treated cells by ultracentrifugation. When isolated, the SR takes on the appearance of small vesicles or granules. These still have the capacity for active transport and release of calcium, which is crucial for the regulation of cardiac contraction and relaxation. Calcium ions stored within the SR are released by the entry of a relatively small number of calcium ions from the T-tubules. As cytosolic calcium increases, the cross-bridge cycle is triggered. Reuptake of calcium ions by the SR lowers the cytosolic calcium ion concentration to cause relaxation. Anatomically, the SR is a fine network (Latin, *reticulum*, small network) spreading throughout the myocytes, demarcated by its lipid bilayer, which is rather similar to that of the sarcolemma. Parts of the SR lie in very close apposition to the T-tubules (Fig. 3-6). Here the tubules of the SR expand into bulbous swellings, still hollow, that lie along the inner surface of the sarcolemma or are wrapped around the T-tubules. These expanded areas of the SR have several names: *subsarcolemmal cisternae* (Latin, baskets) or *junctional components*. The combination of one cisterna and the T-tubule is a *diad*. In skeletal muscle, the cisternae occur in pairs lying astride the T-tubule, the three components having the appearance of *triads*. The function of diads and triads is to release calcium to initiate the contractile cycle. The close physical contact between the cisternae and the sarcolemma is made even more intimate by the development of small electron-dense feet found at coupling sites. The *foot structure*, also called the *junctional channel complex*, facilitates communication between the T-tubules and the SR. Thus, the wave of depolarization when it reaches the T-tubules has only to send its messenger (calcium) on a short journey across the foot space to the calcium release channel of the SR, from where the calcium that triggers contraction originates.

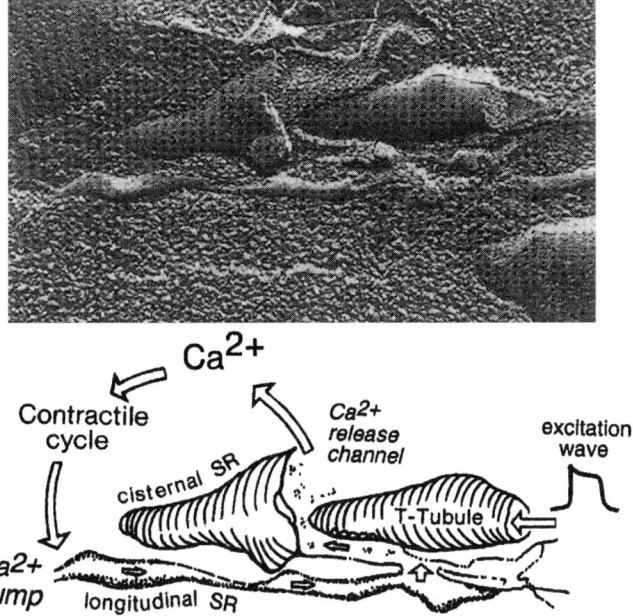

FIG. 3-6. Calcium kinetics and sarcoplasmic reticulum (*SR*). Release of calcium from the cisternal or junctional component of the SR is rapid. In the heart, it is potentiated by entry of calcium from the T tubule, around which the cisternal SR is wrapped. The uptake of calcium, which causes relaxation of the contractile proteins, probably occurs through the tubular network of the SR. Original magnification ×86,400. (Freeze-fracture electron micrograph from Scales DJ. Aspects of the mammalian cardiac sarcotubular system revealed by freeze-fracture electron microscopy. *J Mol Cell Cardiol* 1981;13:373–380, with permission.)

The second part of the SR, the *longitudinal* or *network SR*, consists of ramifying tubules (Color Plate 8-1) and is concerned with the uptake of calcium ions from the cytosol to initiate relaxation. At the start of diastole, the calcium pump located on this part of the SR, rapidly transfers enough calcium from the cytosol to the interior. Such calcium then flows along the longitudinal tubules of the SR to reach the cisternae, then again to be released by the next wave of depolarization. (Note that these longitudinal tubules of the SR have a completely different function from those of the T-tubules).

The Nucleus

Cardiac myocytes usually contain only one nucleus, although binucleate and multinucleate cells are also found. Nuclei usually are located near the center of the cell and account for approximately 5% of the cell's volume. Almost all the genetic information that is needed for each myocyte to maintain and repair its structure is contained in its nucleus or nuclei. The nucleus is surrounded by an envelope formed by two membranes that are each approximately 10 nm thick. This envelope is perforated at frequent intervals, and the pores are believed to be responsible for the selective passage of chemical materials into and out of the nucleus.

The major role of the nucleus is to control the systems responsible for tissue maintenance and repair. The genetic information that is required for this process is stored as sequences of bases in DNA. The actual process of protein synthesis takes place in the cytosol on very small particles called *ribosomes*. There must be a system that allows the coding information stored in the genes to be transferred to the amino acid assembly sites on the ribosomes. This function of information transfer is performed by a special form of ribonucleic acid called *messenger RNA* (mRNA), which leaves the nuclei throughout the nucleus pores, carrying within it the required coding sequence. mRNA is bound to ribosomes free in the cytosol or attached to a net-like system known as the *rough endoplasmic reticulum*. These bound ribosomes are lined up on the outside of the endoplasmic reticulum, giving the rough appearance. (Note the important distinction between the endoplasmic reticulum and the SR). Hence, mRNA molecules originating in the nucleus alert the ribosomes to the particular amino acid sequences that are required. Another form of RNA, *transfer RNA*, supplies the required amino acids in activated form to the ribosomes, where the amino acids are joined together in the sequence dictated by mRNA. Once assembled, the proteins fold, associate with others, and are distributed throughout the cell. The *Golgi apparatus* is functionally associated with the endoplasmic reticulum. It is concerned with the processing and completion of those proteins due for secretion from cells or for incorporation into lysosomes or membranes of the cell.

Communication between Cardiomyocytes

Where the ends of neighboring cardiac myocytes make contact with one another, the sarcolemma becomes highly specialized and altered in nature to form the *intercalated disk* (Fig. 3-7). In addition, the disks run longitudinally between myocytes to provide lateral contact. The disks consist of three main specialized components: the gap junctions chiefly found in the longitudinal part of the disk, the fascia adherens junctions, and the desmosomes found chiefly in the transverse part. Gap junctions ensure rapid electrical communication between cells so that the whole heart behaves as a unified *syncytium*, (Greek, *syn*, together; *cyte*, cell). Adherens junctions and desmosomes ensure that the mechanical forces generated by the individual cells are transmitted throughout the myocardium. The summation of these forces results in cardiac contraction (Fig. 1-4).

Gap junctions are microchannels passing through the longitudinal part of the intercalated disk to allow physical communication of the cytosol of one cell with that of the next. These structures are also called *nexus junctions* (Latin, *nexus*, bond). They constitute a small but critical part of the disk, perhaps 5%, where

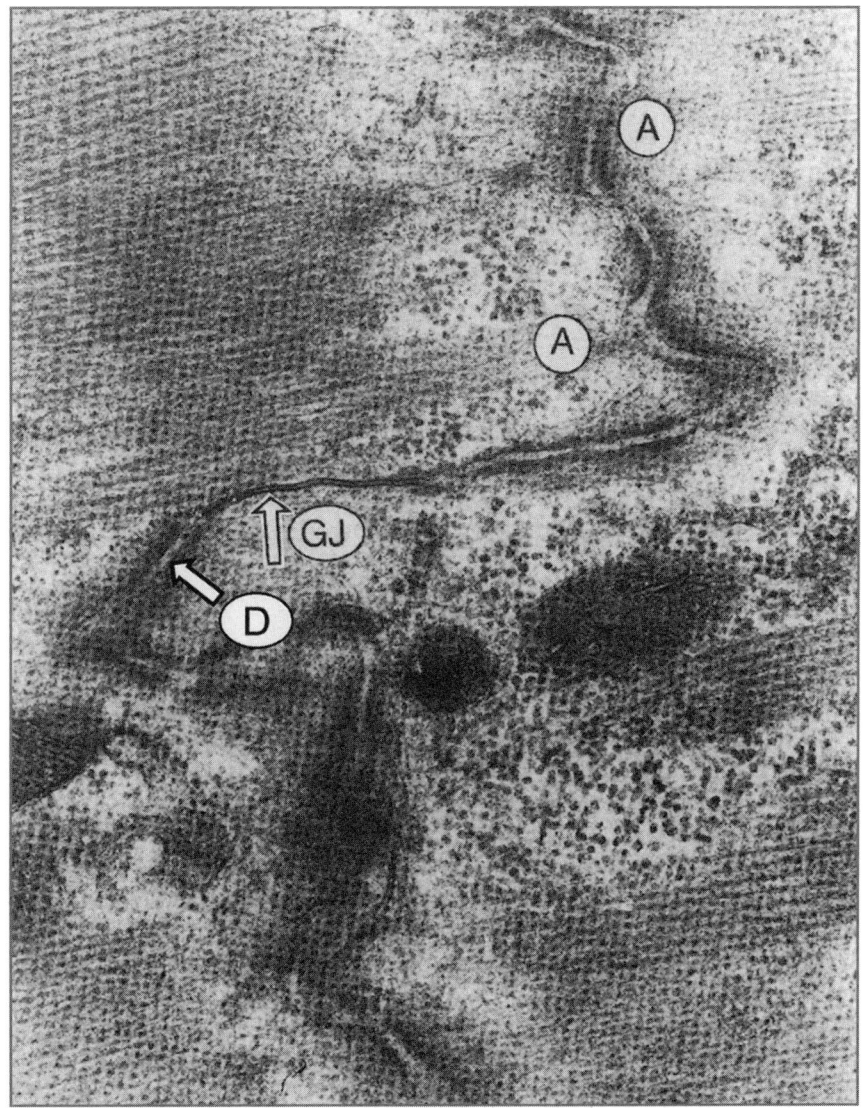

FIG. 3-7. Intercalated disk that connects adjacent ventricular myocytes. The disk serves to anchor actin filaments, to bind cells to each other, and to communicate between cells. *A*, actin filaments inserting into fascia adherens; *GJ*, gap junction; *D*, desmosome, classically located at 45 degrees to the actin filaments. Original magnification ×43,000. (Courtesy of Dr. J. Moravec, Dijon, France.)

the space between the opposing surfaces of the adjacent cells (Fig. 3-7) is reduced to only 1 or 2 nm. The microchannels connect the facing membranes of the opposing cells to transport small molecules and ions from cell to cell and also act as low-resistance electrical pathways (Fig. 3-8). The molecular structures of the gap junction proteins (*connexins*) have now been identified (7). Six connexin proteins constitute one hemichannel or *connexon*, and two connexons, one from each cell, constitute the gap junction channel. The channels cluster in gap junction plaques. Small molecules pass through.

Connexin 43 is the major protein isoform found in the ventricles and allows the easier passage of larger molecules of other isoforms found in the atrium (7). Connexins are not static molecules but have very short half-lives (1 to 5 hours), thereby indicating active participation in cellular responses. The depolarizing sodium current can spread rapidly and directly from cell to cell through the gap junction channels, aided by the close association of sodium channels and connexin 43 (8). Connexons are very sensitive to an abnormal increase in cytosolic calcium concentrations, as may occur in ischemia. Then the connexons close and seal off the damaged cells. Gap junctions also occur laterally between adjacent

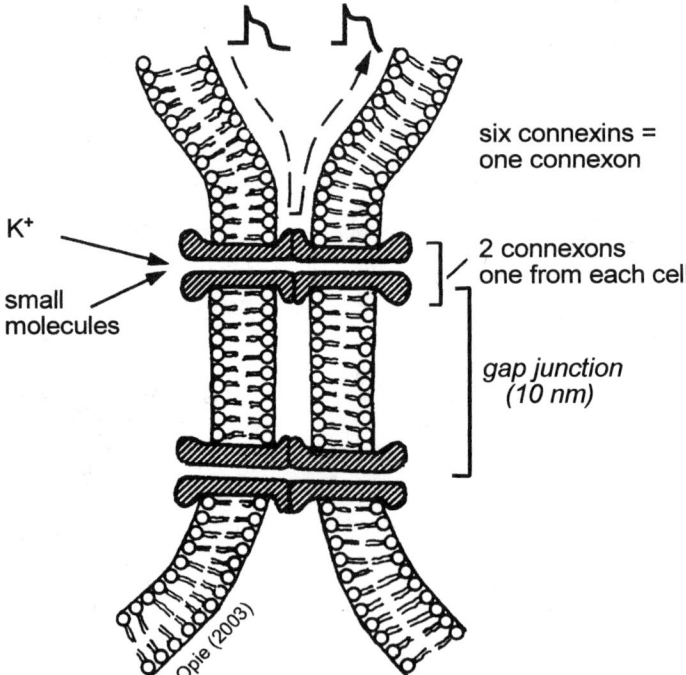

FIG. 3-8. Gap or nexus junction where the distance between the adjacent cells is reduced to only 1 or 2 nm. Note that two connexons, one from each cell, form the microchannels that allow end-to-end and side-to-side electrical and ionic communication between cells. Gap junctions are particularly prominent in Purkinje fibers.

cardiomyocytes, allowing lateral connection, especially in atrial cells where side-to-side connections are frequent, and aid in rapid conduction of depolarization through the atria.

The *fascia adherens junctions* of the transverse portion of the disk are where the actin filaments are inserted (Latin, *fascia*, band, i.e. the adherent band). Hence, the intercalated disks are the terminal anchors (1). The associated proteins include N-cadherin, catenin, vinculin, and α-actinin (Fig. 3-9). The cell adhesion molecule A-CAM (also called N-cadherin) links two adjacent myocytes across the extracellular space, thus being an important structural protein of the adherens junction. Vinculin forms another part of the attachment complex linking via α-catenin to N-cadherin in the adherens junction.

Desmosomes are another type of adherens junction (Fig. 3-7). In cardiomyocytes, they are localized to specialized areas on the intercalated disks to function as "integrators of mechanical integrity" (1). They do this by providing insertion sites for desmin-containing intermediate filaments, thereby facilitating the formation of a transcellular cytoskeletal network that promotes longitudinal force transmission (Fig. 3-10). Also attached to the desmosomal plaque are the cytoplasmic tails of other desmosome-associated proteins such as desmoplakin (the most abundant) and the desmosomal cadherins.

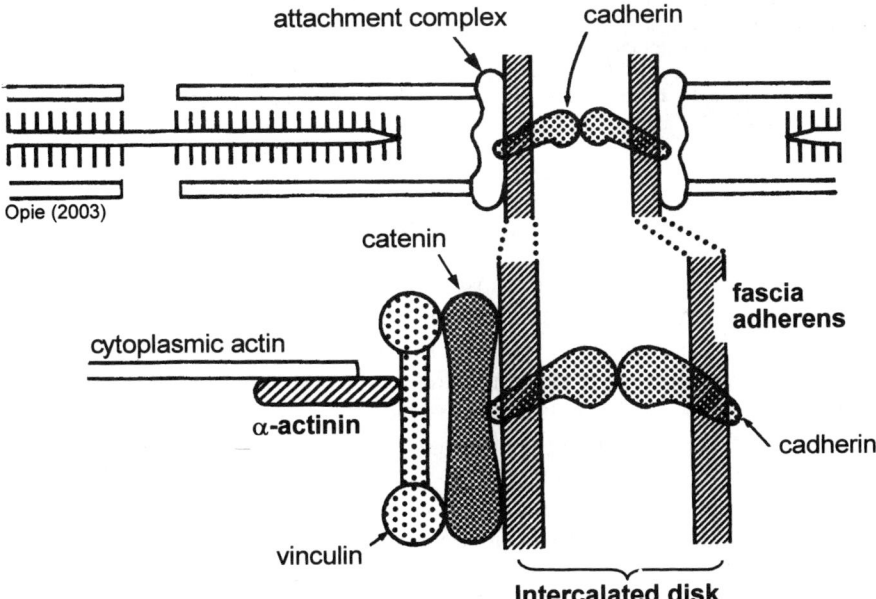

FIG. 3-9. Proteins of the fascia adherens of the intercalated disks, joining the ends of cardiac myocytes. N-cadherin (A-CAM, the adherens junction cell adhesion molecule) is calcium dependent and links the two adjacent intercalated disks. Vinculin binds other vinculin molecules (and a closely related protein, α-catenin), α-actinin, and talin, thereby anchoring the actin filaments to the fascia adherens.

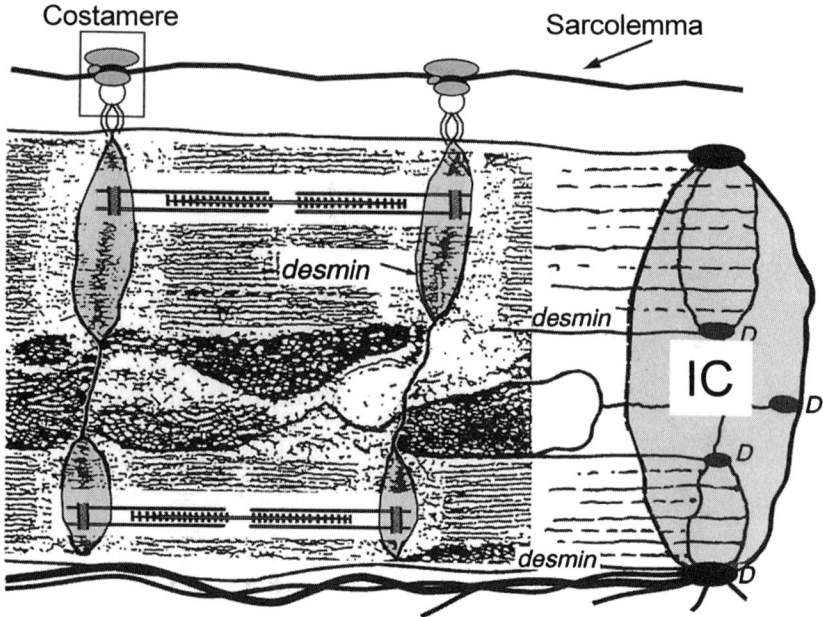

FIG. 3-10. Desmin in cardiomyocyte cytoskeleton. Note desmosomes (*D*), joined by desmin, that longitudinally link cell membranes through intercalated disks (*IC*) (see also Figure 3-7). Desmin joins all longitudinally, running between the myofiber and transversely to encircle myofibers at the Z bands (*Z*). *M*, mitochondria. For further details, see color figures in Fatkin D, Graham RM. Molecular mechanisms of inherited cardiomyopathies. *Physiol Rev*, 2002;82:945 and Color Plate 8-11.

CARDIOMYOCYTE CYTOSKELETON

The term cytoskeleton includes those proteins that connect the contractile system to the sarcolemma, connect sarcomeres to each other, and connect cells to the extracellular structures (Table 3-5). As the sarcomere contracts, the cytoskeleton provides spatial stability and transmits lateral forces from the Z line to the sarcolemma and beyond to the extracellular matrix (ECM) (Fig. 3-11). Among these force-conducting proteins are desmin filaments attached to the Z bands and actin filaments attached to α-actinin molecules that lie within the Z bands (9). Without the cytoskeleton, contraction of the sarcomere would be a solitary event that could not result in ventricular contraction. *Costameres* (Latin, *costa*, a rib) are the key rib-like subsarcolemmal structures that link the sarcomeres to the ECM. The cytoskeletal thin (actin) and intermediate filaments stretch from the sarcomere to attach to the costameres. *Intermediate filaments* are strong rope-like polymers approximately 10 nm in diameter that are easily deformed but resist rupture. An example is *desmin*, which is organized in a three-dimensional network of interconnecting transverse and longitudinal fibers to form

TABLE 3-5. Major proteins of the cytoskeleton and intercalated disks

Name	Where found	Molecular properties	Proposed function
Desmin[a] (Fig. 3-12, Color Plate 8-11)	Major part of intermediate filaments; joins Z lines to sarcolemma	MW, 55 kd; relatively flexible; hollow core; 7–11 nm thick	Connects Z lines to each other and to the sarcolemma via the costameres[b]; stabilizes sarcomeres during contraction
Vinculin[a,c] (Figs. 3-11, 3-13)	Attaches Z lines to talin and integrin complex of costamere; in VSM-dense bands	MW, 122 kd; like a balloon on a string, 8-nm globular head; 19-nm tail	Stabilizes sarcomere by binding sites: vinculin-vinculin, α-actinin, and talin; part of integrin signaling system
N-cahedrin[c] (Fig. 3-11)	Fascia adherens of the intercalated disk	MW, 135 kd; glycoprotein, calcium dependent	Links two adjacent cells across the EC space at the intercalated disks
Integrin[c] (Fig. 3-13)	Transmembrane protein with cell surface adhesion receptors	MW, 130–160 kd; external globular head with ligand-binding site; small IC domain with talin-binding site	Internal talin binding; external binding to collagen, laminin, and fibronectin (all three in the extracellular space)
Talin[c] (Fig. 3-13)	With integrin in cell-to-matrix junctions	MW, 213 kd; elongated	Links integrin and vinculin in cell-to-matrix junctions
α-Actinin[c] (Figs. 3-11, 3-13)	With vinculin in cell-to-matrix junctions; Z bands; dense bodies in VSM cells	MW, 95 kd; rod-like ~4 nm in diameter and 40 nm in length	Links tails of actin fibers at Z bands and cross-links actin filaments; links actin to dense bodies in VSM
Spectrin[d]	Sarcolemma (costamere)	α and β subunits; rod-shaped tetrameres; each ~240 kd	Links Z line to sarcolemma via ankyrin
Catenin[e] (Fig. 3-11)	Fascia adherens, desmosomes	MW, ~100 kd	Modulates attachment sites of actin and desmin
Dystrophin[e] (Color Plate 8-11)	Binds to cytosolic actin and to dystroglycans in sarcolemma	MW, 427 kd; flexible elongated; similar to spectrin	Actin–dystrophin–dystroglycans complex anchors the entire myofibril to sarcolemma
Connexin 43[e] (Fig. 3-10)	Major component of gap junction	MW, 43 kd; part of gap junction channel	Six connexins = one connexon; two connexons = one gap junction channel

[a]Reference 8a, [b]Reference 1, [c]Reference 8b, [d]Reference 8c, [e]Reference 8d.
MW, molecular weight; EC, extracellular; VSM, vascular smooth muscle; IC, intracellular.

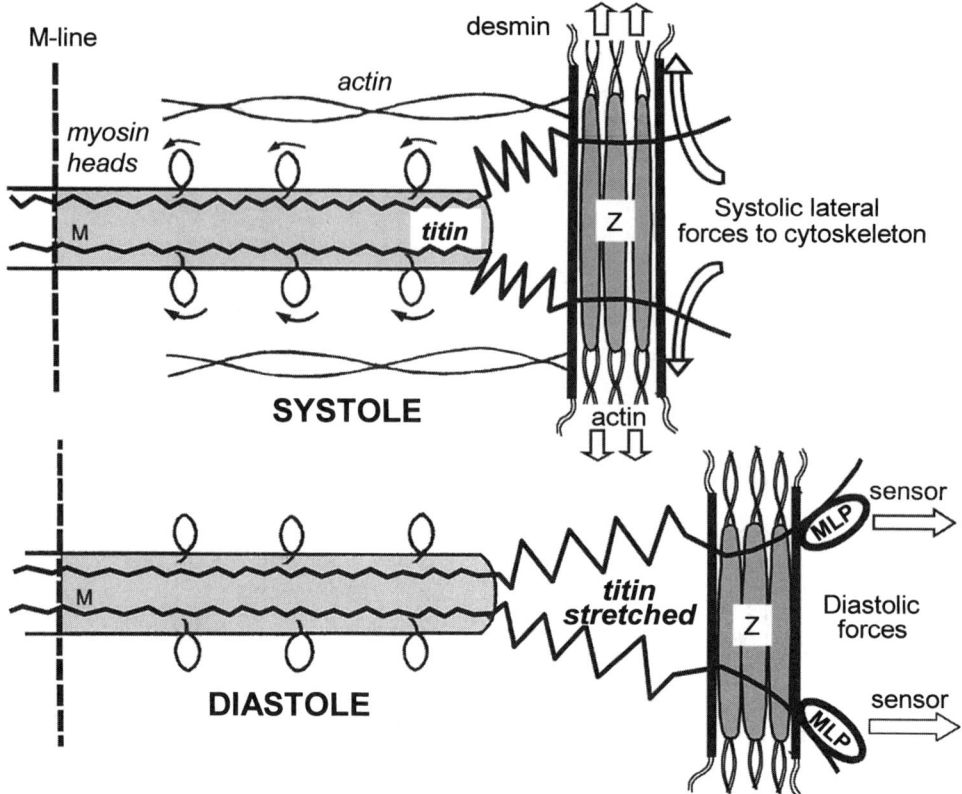

FIG. 3-11. Transmission of mechanical forces from sarcomere. During systole, the sarcomere has shortened as result of myosin head flexion and movement of actin filaments toward the M line (Fig. 3-2). Horizontal force is exerted on the Z line, which in turn transmits lateral force to the sarcolemma by the thin and intermediate filaments, cytoplasmic actin, and desmin. In diastole, as the sarcomere stretches, the elastic segment of titin expands and transmits force via muscle LIM protein (MLP), which acts as a mechanical sensor. When continued, as in as sustained volume overload, muscle LIM protein stimuli may induce myocyte lengthening as in the dilated failing heart. For further details, see Knoll R, Hoshijima M, Hoffman HM, et al. The cardiac mechanical stretch sensor machinery involves a Z disc complex that is defective in a subset of human dilated cardiomyopathy. *Cell* 2002;111:943.

ring-like bands around the myofibrils at the Z-line level that connect to the costameres (Color Plate 8-11).

Integrin Linkage Complex of Costameres

Costameres consist of at least three cytoskeletal protein networks that link the Z and M lines of the sarcomeres to the ECM and to each other (Color Plate 8-11). Chief among these are the integrin-based complex, also called the focal adhesion complex, and the dystroglycan complex (1). Less clear is the role of the spectrin complex. In addition to their physical stabilizing function, costameres allow external communication beyond the sarcolemma by the *integrin* molecules that extend from the *focal adhesion complexes* of the costamere through the sarcolemma to link to the external laminin and collagen matrix. Internal forces, such as those generated during systole, can thereby be conducted outward (Fig. 3-11), while external mechanical forces, such as pressure overload, can be communicated inward to stimulate the signaling systems initiated by *focal adhesion kinases* that ultimately lead to hypertrophy. Thus, the integrins mediate a two-way signaling system, both outside in and inside out (10). *Vinculin* is an elongated molecule, like a balloon on a string, which has binding sites for other vinculin molecules for α-actinin and for talin (Fig. 3-12). It links the sarcomere via cytoplasmic actin and α-actinin to talin and hence to integrin and extracellular laminin. In ischemia sustained beyond 120 minutes, vinculin is destroyed, allowing the sarcolemma to rupture more easily, thereby liberating intracellular enzymes and hastening cell death.

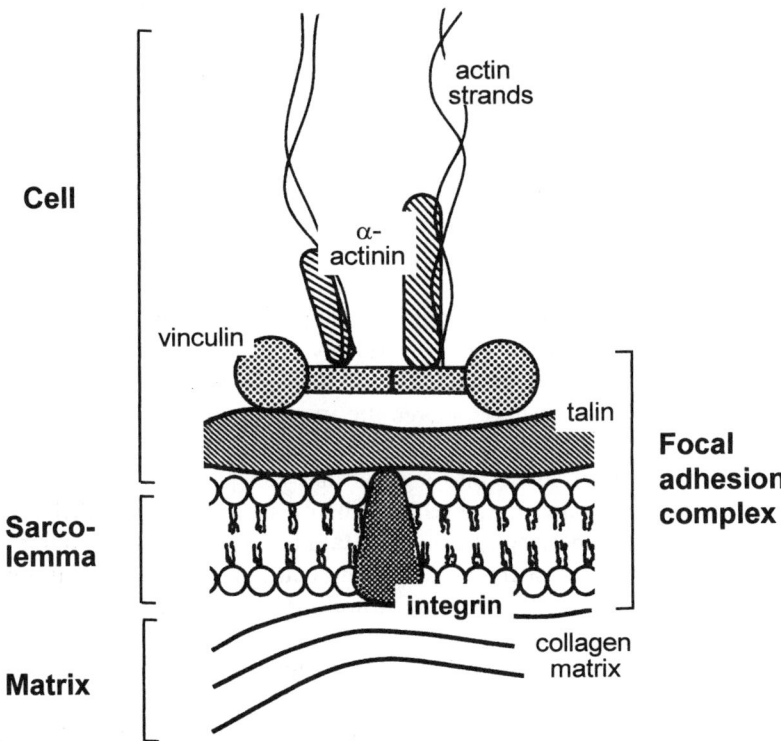

FIG. 3-12. Proteins of the cell-to-matrix junctions. Integrin, the transmembrane protein, links vinculin and talin to the collagen matrix. For costamere, see Color Plate 8-11. (Modified from Ganote C, Armstrong S. Ischaemia and the myocyte cytoskeleton: review and speculation. *Cardiovasc Res* 1993;27:1387–1403.)

Dystroglycan Complex

This transmembrane complex also transmits lateral force from the sarcomere to extracellular laminin. The core component is dystrophin, a large protein that links cytoplasmic actin to the sarcolemmal transmembrane dystroglycan (with α and β components) and the adjacent sarcoglycans (Color Plate 8-11). The latter are small glycosylated transmembrane proteins that, if mutated, can give rise to hamster cardiomyopathy. In ways not fully understood, dystrophin links to other components of the costamere such as vinculin and spectrin (1). Cleavage of dystrophin by a virus infection weakens the cytoskeleton and explains some cases of dilated heart failure (cardiomyopathy) (Chapter 16).

Spectrin Complex

Spectrin is a prominent component of the costameres (Color Plate 8-11). Speculatively, spectrin may link the sarcolemma to the muscle LIM protein (MLP) at the Z line where it is part of the titin complex (Fig. 3-11). It is proposed that cytoplasmic actin links MLP to spectrin and from there via ankyrin to the sarcolemma, perhaps to a sodium-potassium pump (1). MLP acts as a sensor during diastolic stretch, as occurs during volume overload of the heart (Fig. 3-8). In knockout models, the heart fails and dilates.

EXTRACELLULAR MATRIX

The cardiac connective tissue, a major component of the ECM, has an important supportive mechanical role by surrounding the various types of cells found in the heart and binding them to each other so that force transmission is uniform throughout the myocardium. The connective tissue is produced largely by fibroblastic cells and contains collagen as well as other important matrix proteins such as laminin (Table 3-6). Fibroblasts are the most numerous cell type found in the myocardium, which underscores the importance of the ECM (11). This network also has additional and important functions in translating signals induced by mechanical stress into signals that can promote cell growth (11). Thus, the ECM participates in the remodeling of the myocardium that accompanies left ventricular hypertrophy and heart failure. Collagen is a major determinant of myocardial tissue stiffness, and as it accumulates, myocardial mechanical function deteriorates (Fig. 16-8). On boiling, collagen becomes gelatinous, which explains the name (Greek, glue + production).

Fibrosis (fibrous tissue formation) is regulated at least in part by increased activity of the renin–angiotensin–aldosterone system, which includes local production of angiotensin II (12). Collagen forms *collagen fibers*, which are present in the extracellular space and lie close to the surface of the myocytes, forming an important part of the ECM within which the myocytes lie (Fig. 3-13). Collagen fibers extend from the surface of the cells to the tissue skeleton as well as

TABLE 3-6. *Major proteins of the extracellular matrix*

Name	Where found	Molecular properties	Proposed function
Collagen[a]	Collagen matrix (Fig. 3-11)	MW, 95–180 kd; helical structure of 3 polypeptide chains, each of ~1,000 amino acids. Type I: thick fibers, major part of collagen; Type III: thinner fibers, 10% of total	Links myocytes, prevents excess stretch, transmits force from myofilaments to ventricular or vascular wall; provides elasticity to aorta; in excess, causes myocardial fibrosis and contractile dysfunction; determines stiffness of myocardium
Fibronectin[b]	EC matrix	Two large chains linked by disulfide bonds; MW of each, 220 kd	Essential meshwork for organization of other matrix proteins including collagen[c]
Elastin[d]	Vessel walls; subendocardial myocardium	MW, ~140 kd with elastic links between subunits	Major source of elasticity of arterial matrix; in atheroma, lipid content increases

[a–d]See references 10a–10d.
MW, molecular weight; EC, extracellular.

from cell to cell. These fine fibers and filaments act as "struts" to hold the myofibrils in position so that the pattern of contraction is orderly. The collagen matrix probably limits the amount that the heart can be dilated in diseased states (Fig. 16-8). The major types of cardiac collagen fibers are collagen types I and III. Collagen I is organized into thick bundles and is strong enough to resist tensile stretch, even in the volume-overloaded heart. Collagen III cross-links with collagen I. Another type of collagen, type IV, is a major component of *basement membranes*, where it attaches to the extracellular glycoproteins fibronectin and laminin. Hypothetically, the increased collagen and greater severity of fibrosis in diseased states are linked to a marked increase in myocardial stiffness and depressed systolic and diastolic function.

Elastic fibers containing *elastin* (Table 3-6) are found in close approximation to collagen, for example, around the collagen skeleton, on the surface of capillaries, and around the myocytes. These elastic fibers have properties similar to those of polymeric rubber, accounting for a part of the elasticity of the myocardium. Another component of the elasticity resides in the cross-bridges, so that the myocardium becomes less elastic as the cross-bridges interact during systole. A third elastic component lies in the titan molecules that link myosin filaments to the Z lines.

Glycoproteins, also called *proteoglycans*, are proteins of one or more attached short sugar chains, such as chondroitin and heparan sulfate as well as fibronectin and laminin. *Fibronectin* is a glycoprotein that influences cellular properties, including growth and hormonal repair, through an interaction with fibronectin

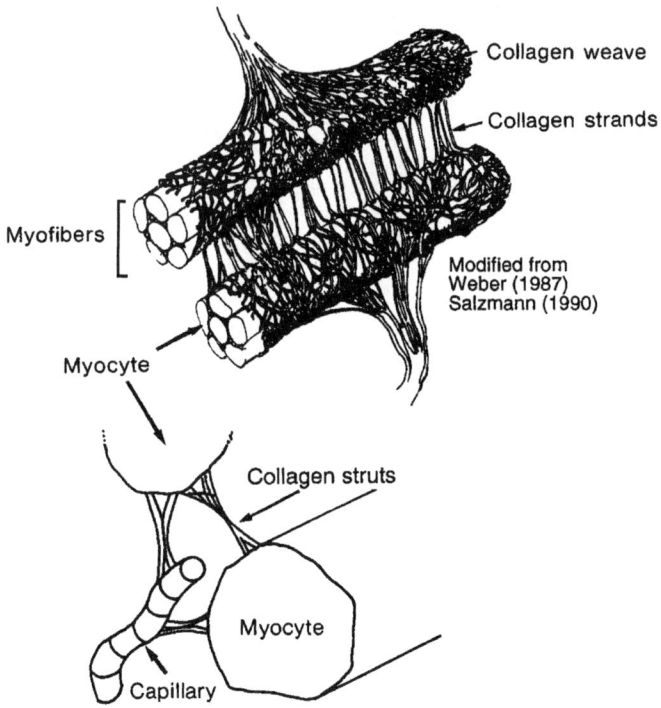

FIG. 3-13. Collagen matrix of the normal left ventricle. Groups of myocytes held together by the collagen weave are termed myofibers. Myofibers are connected to one another by strands of collagen, whereas connections between myocytes and those between myocytes and their adjacent capillaries are by struts of collagen. Collagen is a basic protein of white fibrous material. On boiling, collagen becomes gelatinous, which explains the name (collagen = glue + production, from the Greek). (Modified from Weber KT, Clark WA, Janicki JS, et al. Physiologic versus pathologic hypertrophy and the pressure-overloaded myocardium. *J Cardiovasc Pharmacol* 1987;10[Suppl 6]:S37–S49 and Salzmann JL, Labopin M, Belichard P, et al. Collagen remodelling in cardiac hypertrophy. In: Swynghedauw B, ed. *Research in cardiac hypertrophy and failure*. London: INSERM/John Libbey Eurotext, 1990:293–306.)

cell surface receptors. Hence, fibronectin increases after experimental myocardial infarction, possibly the result of synthesis by cardiac fibroblasts. *Laminin* is a glycoprotein of the basement membrane that has a molecular weight almost double that of fibronectin and is composed of three subunits linked by disulfide bonds. *Cardiac fibroblasts* are mesenchymal cells that potentially produce components of the ECM, including collagen and fibronectin, in response to simulation by growth factors and/or angiotensin II.

The *matrix metalloproteinases* include the various enzymes that break down all types of collagen (*collagenases*) and other components of the ECM including laminin, fibronectin, and other glycoproteins. The balance between the synthesis of ECM collagen and other components as stimulated by growth factors, angiotensin II, and aldosterone versus degradation by the metalloproteinases has important implications for the mechanical properties and hence the function of the myocardium (Fig. 16-8).

ATRIAL CELLS

Atrial cell contraction helps to fill the left ventricle during the relaxation phase (Fig. 1-3) so that the force of contraction that must be developed is low because the left ventricular diastolic pressure is only just more than zero. Thus, in contrast to ventricular myocytes, atrial cells do not have prominent myofibrils, and other specialized structures concerned with contraction such as T tubules are rare. Atrial cells are smaller than ventricular cells, and elliptical rather than rodlike in shape (Table 3-1). There is also a prominent collagen matrix, which may help to avoid overdistention of the atria. To help spread the electrical impulse rapidly throughout the atria, there are side-to-side and end-to-end gap junctions between the cells. Whether there are, in addition, specialized conduction pathways in the atria is still controversial.

VASCULAR SMOOTH MUSCLE CELLS

The main function of these cells is to maintain vascular tone and hence to regulate peripheral vascular resistance. There are two types of contraction, phasic and tonic, the latter being sustained. Vascular smooth muscle cells differ from myocardial cells in several important ways (Fig. 3-14). First, they are approximately fusiform in shape, which allows them to form the muscular tube of the arteries. These cells are 100 to 500 μm in length and approximately 5 to 6 μm in diameter. There is a very large surface-to-volume ratio, made even larger (approximately 70%) by the appearance of numerous prominent surface vesicles, the cave-like caveolae. These probably have a function similar to that of T tubules in myocardial cells conveying surface electrical charges to the SR (13). A second difference is that vascular smooth muscle cells do not need to respond rapidly to a wave of depolarization because contraction and relaxation are so much slower. Thus, the SR is relatively poorly developed. Nonetheless, it remains the chief organelle concerned with the regulation of cytosolic calcium concentrations. Organelles such as the Golgi apparatus, mitochondria, and lysosomes are situated mainly in the *sarcoplasmic core* where they surround the nucleus (13).

The *myofilaments* lie in the more peripheral part of the cell, away from the central organelles. Force transmission from the contractile myofilaments to the cell surface takes place by insertion of actin filaments into the subsarcolemmal dense bands. Dense bands and bodies contain α-actinin, which helps to crosslink the actin filaments as in the Z lines of striated muscle.

The *action potential* is different in shape from that of myocardial cells. Starting from a less negative voltage, the upstroke is much slower because the sodium channel that is associated with rapid conduction in cardiac cells is so low in its

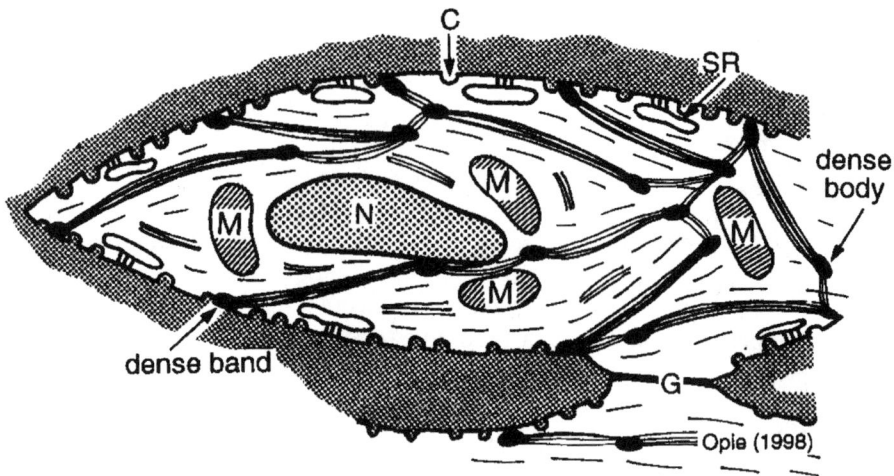

FIG. 3-14. Structure of vascular smooth muscle cell. Note the absence of well-defined muscular striations, with prominent caveolae (*C*), the relative absence of mitochondria (*M*), the dense bands or bodies, and the gap junctions (*G*) between adjacent cells. *SR*, sarcoplasmic reticulum; *N*, nucleus.

activity in vascular smooth muscle cells. The plateau of the action potential is not sustained, in part because the opening of the calcium channel is brief. Outward depolarizing potassium currents play a major role in terminating the action potential and maintaining the resting potential, as in cardiac cells. The depolarizing calcium current can be "opened" not only by voltage but by occupation of several receptors that respond to vasoconstrictive agonists such as α_1-adrenergic stimulation, endothelin, or angiotensin II.

In *vascular disease,* vascular smooth muscle cells can have an important synthesis role. In normal adult vascular smooth muscle cells, this system is quiescent, yet it can be activated to play an important role in the pathologic growth of vascular cells that occurs in atheroma formation and restenosis (Figs. 10-11 and 17-12). These muscle cells contain prominent nuclei and retain the capacity to reproduce themselves by hyperplasia. They can also grow larger by hypertrophy in response to the sustained intraarterial pressure found in systemic hypertension. They can manufacture all the principal components of the vascular matrix and its connective tissue, including collagen and the elastic fibers, thereby contributing to vascular damage in atherosclerosis.

SUMMARY

1. *The basic unit of the contracting myocardial cell is the myocyte,* consisting mainly of the contractile proteins. Z lines terminate the myocyte on either side. Thin actin filaments extend inward from the Z lines and interdigitate with the thicker and much larger myosin filaments. The latter extend from

the center of the myofibril toward the Z lines without touching them. Myosin fibers are indirectly linked to the Z lines by large titin elastic molecules. When contraction is initiated by the arrival of calcium ions, the myosin heads flex to move the actin fibers in such a way that the Z lines come closer together.

2. *To regulate the intracellular concentration of calcium ions requires a series of interacting events.* The external cell membrane or sarcolemma has specialized proteins embedded in its lipid bilayer that act as channels. The calcium channels allow entry of relatively small amounts of calcium ions during each wave of electrical excitation. The electrical impulses are conveyed to the interior of the myocytes by invaginations of the sarcolemma called T tubules. These lie close to that part of the SR (the cisternae or junctional component) that stores calcium ions. The SR and the adjoining T tubules are physically linked by specialized structures called feet, which are thought to "guide" calcium ions entering the myocyte through the T tubule to the specific receptor that releases calcium from the SR. This increase in internal cytosolic calcium concentration triggers contraction.

3. *Relaxation of the contractile proteins* is achieved by the uptake of calcium ions into the longitudinal component of the SR, in which the calcium ions travel back to the storage sites on the cisternae to await the arrival of the next excitation wave.

4. *Communication between myocytes occurs at the gap junctions* at the ends and sides of the cells where minute conducting channels lie in specialized proteins called connexons. These regulate the passage of ions and small molecules from one cell to the next. In addition, the electrical impulses pass preferentially along the gap junctions.

5. *The cytoskeleton* within each cardiac myocyte supports the contractile proteins and links them to the Z lines. Other parts of the cytoskeleton link the myocytes to the ECM via integrin molecules that span the sarcolemma.

6. *The ECM binds groups of myofibers together* and provides a framework for the contracting cells. Furthermore, this ECM is alive and reactive. When fibrous tissue is abnormally increased in amount, myocardial contraction and relaxation are impaired.

7. *Atrial cells differ ultrastructurally from ventricular cells* in that they are smaller with smaller T tubules and less prominent sarcomeres. Atrial cells also have prominent side-to-side gap junctions. These differences may explain the lesser force of atrial contraction and the far more rapid conduction of the electrical impulse through atrial than through ventricular contractile cells.

8. *Vascular smooth muscle cells are different* in shape, ultrastructure, and function from striated myocardial cells. These cells are adapted to much slower rates of contraction and relaxation and to the maintenance of sustained tonic contractions, thereby helping to regulate the resistance against which the heart pumps out blood.

9. *The cardiac conduction system* is composed of cells that have poorly developed contractile structures and are adapted to rapid conduction (Table 3-2).

ACKNOWLEDGMENT

Prof. Jutta Schaper and Dr. Sawa Kostin, Max Planck Institute, Bad Nauheim, Germany, generously provided valuable advice and criticism.

STUDENT QUESTIONS

1. Describe the major features of the ultrastructure of the myofiber.
2. Describe in outline form the interaction between the thick and thin filaments during contraction.
3. What are T tubules? Do they have any role in the contractile cycle?
4. Describe in outline form the major functions of the SR.
5. How do conducting cells differ in their ultrastructure from ordinary contracting myocardial cells? What are these conducting cells called?
6. How do atrial cells differ in their ultrastructure from ventricular cells? Are there any functional consequences of these differences?

CARDIOLOGIST-IN-TRAINING QUESTIONS

1. Describe in outline form the actin–myosin interaction during the cardiac contraction cycle.
2. What are T tubules and what role do they play in initiating cardiac contraction?
3. What are the anatomy and function of the SR?
4. How do atrial and ventricular cells differ?
5. How do cells communicate with each other?
6. How is contraction of the sarcomere linked to the ECM? Why are these links important?

REFERENCES

1. Clark KA, et al. Striated muscle cytoarchitecture: an intricate web of form and function. *Annu Rev Cell Dev Biol* 2002;18:637–706.
1a. Legato. *The myocardial cell for the clinical cardiologist.* Mount Kisco, NY: Futura, 1973.
1b. Laks MM. et al. Myocardial cell and sarcomere lengths in the normal dog heart. *Circ Res* 1967;21: 671–678.
1c. McNutt NS, Fawcett DW. The ultrastructure of the cat myocardium. II. Atrial muscle. *J Cell Biol* 1969;42:46–67.
1d. Sommer JR. Ultrastructural considerations concerning cardiac muscle. *J Mol Cell Cardiol* 1982;14 [Suppl 3]:77–83.
1e. Moody CJ, et al. Functional and autoradiographic evidence for endothelin 1 receptors on human and rat cardiac myocytes. Comparison with single smooth muscle cells. *Circ Res* 1990;67:764–769.
1f. Somlyo AP, Somlyo AY. In: Fozzard HA, et al., eds. *The heart and cardiovascular system*, 2nd ed. New York: Raven Press, 1991:1295–1324.

2. Brilla C, Janicki JS, Weber KT. Impaired diastolic function and coronary reserve in genetic hypertension. Role of interstitial fibrosis and medial thickening of intramyocardial coronary arteries. *Circ Res* 1991;69:107–115.
2a. Page E, McCallister LP. Quantitative electron microscopic description of heart muscle cells. Application to normal, hypertrophied and thyroxin-stimulated hearts. *Am J Cardiol* 1973;31:172–181.
2b. David H, et al. Morphometric characterization of left ventricular myocardial cells of male rats during postnatal development. *J Mol Cell Cardiol* 1979;11:631–638.
2c. Schaper J. et al. Ultrastructural morphometric analysis of myocardium from dogs, rats, hamsters, mice, and from human hearts. *Circ Res* 1985;56:377.
2d. Page E. Distribution, surface density and membrane area of diadic junctional contacts between plasma membrane and terminal cisterns in mammalian ventricle. *Circ Res* 1979;45:260–267.
3. Olivetti G, Melissari M, Capasso, JM, et al. Cardiomyopathy of the aging human heart. Myocyte loss and cellular hypertrophy. *Circ Res* 1991;68:1560–1568.
4. Weiss JN, et al. The cytoplasm. No longer a well-mixed bag. *Circ Res* 2001;89:108–110.
5. Kostin S, et al. The internal and external protein scaffold of the T-tubular system in cardiomyocytes. *Cell Tissue Res* 1998;294:440–460.
6. Löhn M, et al. Ignition of calcium sparks in arterial and cardiac muscle through caveolae. *Circ Res* 2000;87:1034–1039.
7. Delmar M. Connexin diversity. Discriminating the message [Editorial]. *Circ Res* 2002;91:85–86.
8. Kucera JP, et al. Localization of sodium channels in intercalated disks modulates cardiac conduction. *Circ Res* 2002;91:1176–1182.
8a. Schaper J. et al. Impairment of the myocardial ultrastructure and changes of the cytoskeleton in dilated cardiomyopathy. *Circulation* 1991;83:504–514.
8b. Yoshida K, et al. Reperfusion of rat heart after brief ischemia induces protolysis of calspectin (nonerythroid spectrin or fodrin) by calpain. *Circ Res* 1995;77:603–610.
8c. Kostin S, et al. The protein composition of the normal and diseased cardiac myocyte. *Heart Failure Reviews* 1998;2:245–260.
9. Ganote C, Armstrong S. Ischaemia and the myocyte cytoskeleton: review and speculation. *Cardiovasc Res* 1993;27:1387–1403.
10. Ross RS, et al. Integrins and the myocardium. *Circ Res* 2001;88:1112–1119.
10a. Weber KT, et al. Collagen network of the myocardium: function, structural remodeling and regulatory mechanisms. *J Mol Cell Cardiol* 1994;26:279–292.
10b. Coller BS. In: *The heart and cardiovascular system, 2nd edition*. Fozzard HA, et al., eds. New York: Raven Press, 1991:219–273.
10c. Knowlton AA. Rapid expression of fibronectin in the rabbit heart after myocardial infarction with and without reperfusion. *J Clin Invest* 1992;89:1060–1068.
10d. Robert L, Birenbaut P. In: Camilleri JP, ed. *Diseases of the arterial wall*. London: Springer-Verlag, 1989:44–54.
11. Spinale FG. Bioactive peptide signalling within the myocardial interstitium and the matrix metalloproteinases [Editorial]. *Circ Res* 2002;91:1082–1084.
12. Weber KT, Sun Y, Katwa LC, et al. Connective tissue: a metabolic entity? *J Mol Cell Cardiol* 1995; 27:107–120.
13. Forbes MS. Ultrastructure of cardiac muscle and blood vessels. In: Sperelakis N, et al., eds. *Heart physiology and pathophysiology*, 4th ed. San Diego: Academic Press, 2001:71–98.
14. Scales DJ. Aspects of the mammalian cardiac sarcotubular system revealed by freeze-fracture electron microscopy. *J Moll Cell Cardiol* 1981;13:373–380.
15. Jorgensen AO, Broderick R, Somlyo AP, et al. Two structurally distinct calcium storage sites in rat cardiac sarcoplasmic reticulum: an electron microprobe analysis study. *Circ Res* 1988;63:1060–1069.
16. Weber KT, Clark WA, Janicki JS, et al. Physiologic versus pathologic hypertrophy and the pressure-overloaded myocardium. *J Cardiovasc Pharmacol* 1987;10[Suppl 6]:S37–S49.
17. Salzmann JL, Labopin M, Belichard P, et al. Collagen remodelling in cardiac hypertrophy. In: Swynghedauw B, ed. *Research in cardiac hypertrophy and failure*. London: INSERM/John Libbey Eurotext, 1990:293–306.

PART II

Electrophysiology and Electrocardiogram

4

Channels, Pumps, and Exchangers

Sodium channels are dynamic molecules that drastically change their structural confirmation on a sub-millisecond time scale.

Balser (1)

The two crucial qualities of the sarcolemma are the capacity to maintain vast gradients of ions and enzymes between the intracellular and extracellular environments (Fig. 4-1) and the capacity to respond to the wave of depolarization by the brief opening and closing of highly specific ion channels. Several major consequences follow, including the triggering of the contractile mechanism in the case of cardiomyocytes.

When the electrical charge is not flowing, during diastole, the inside of the cell is negatively charged and the outside is positively charged so that the sarcolemma is *polarized*. This polarity is lost and reversed during the ionic movements that accompany the wave of electrical excitation, a process called *depolarization*. The juxtaposition of the depolarized and polarized cells allows current to flow between these cells with differing polarities so that the current spreads further and other adjacent cells become depolarized (Chapter 5). The initial phase of depolarization, by changing the membrane potential from its resting negative value, allows the opening of *voltage-gated channels* for sodium and calcium ions that carry positive charges within the cell, which explains the temporary reversal of polarity. Thereafter, the outward flow of potassium ions is the major factor causing *repolarization*. This sequence of electrical changes during the cardiac action potential can be divided into five arbitrary phases: 0, 1, 2, 3, and 4 (Fig. 4-2). There are substantial differences between Purkinje cells, adapted for fast conduction of the cardiac impulse, and ventricular cells, adapted to generate pressure (Fig. 4-3). During the rapid phase of initial depolarization (phase 0), the Purkinje cells reach a greater positive value and then repolarize much more rapidly (phase 1) before the plateau phase (phase 2) is reached. The greater phase 0 is understandable because the main task of Purkinje fibers is to rapidly conduct the wave of excitation. The duration of the action potential is longer in Purkinje fibers (Fig. 5-6), so that repolarization (phase 3) is relatively slower in these fibers. At the junction of the Purkinje network and the ventricu-

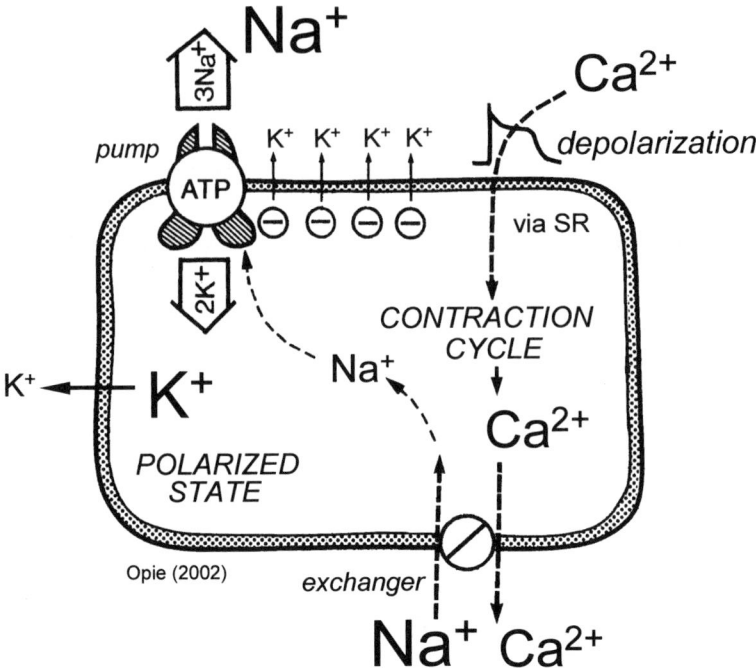

FIG. 4-1. Ionic balance in a cardiomyocyte. The potassium concentration is much higher inside than outside the cell, whereas sodium is much higher outside than inside the cell. These differential concentrations are maintained by the activity of the sodium–potassium pump using energy in the form of adenosine 5'-triphosphate (*ATP*). A high internal potassium concentration in turn promotes outward transsarcolemmal diffusion of a relatively minute number of potassium ions, thereby creating a negative charge within the sarcolemma and hence the polarized state. Note calcium ion entry during the action potential leading to contraction and outward transport of the calcium ions that have entered the cell by the sodium–calcium exchanger.

lar muscle, the longer Purkinje action potential duration means that the Purkinje cells have a longer refractory period (Fig. 20-4) that hypothetically helps to guard against reentry of the electrical impulse as it travels toward the ventricles (for reentry and arrhythmias, see Figure 20-2).

It should be stressed that the ionic movements accompanying the waves of excitation involve only minute numbers of ions across the sarcolemma, whereas the overall cell content of these ions remains virtually unchanged. Thus, the opening of sodium and calcium channels during depolarization leads to a small net gain of these ions. To restore ionic balance, calcium ions leave the cardiomyocyte as sodium ions enter through the sodium–calcium exchanger. Sodium ions are therefore gained by both the sodium channel and this exchange system. Activity of the sodium–potassium pump is then required to pump sodium out of the cell against a concentration gradient (Fig. 4-4).

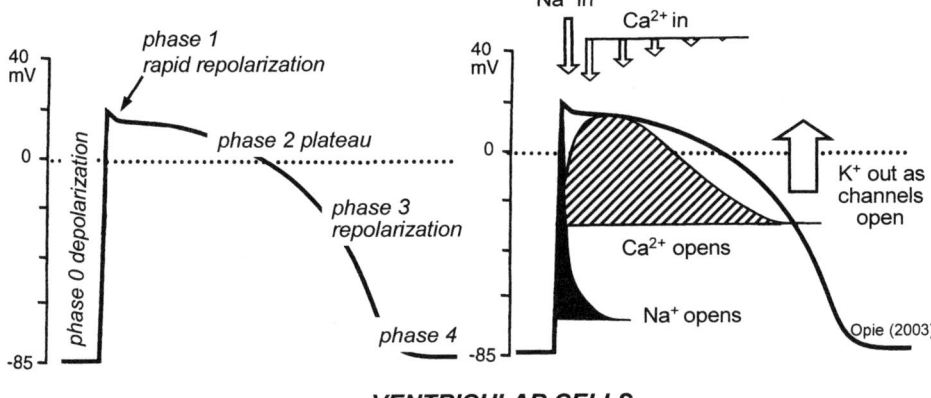

FIG. 4-2. Action potential phases and currents. The four phases of the cardiac action potential **(left)** and the underlying currents **(right)**. The rapid entry of sodium ions accounts for the initial phase of rapid depolarization of the action potential. Calcium ions enter chiefly by the slow calcium channel. After entry of positively charged sodium and calcium ions, the cell is fully depolarized. Then potassium channels open. The outward flow of positively charged potassium ions largely explains repolarization. Finally, the cell reenters the state of polarization.

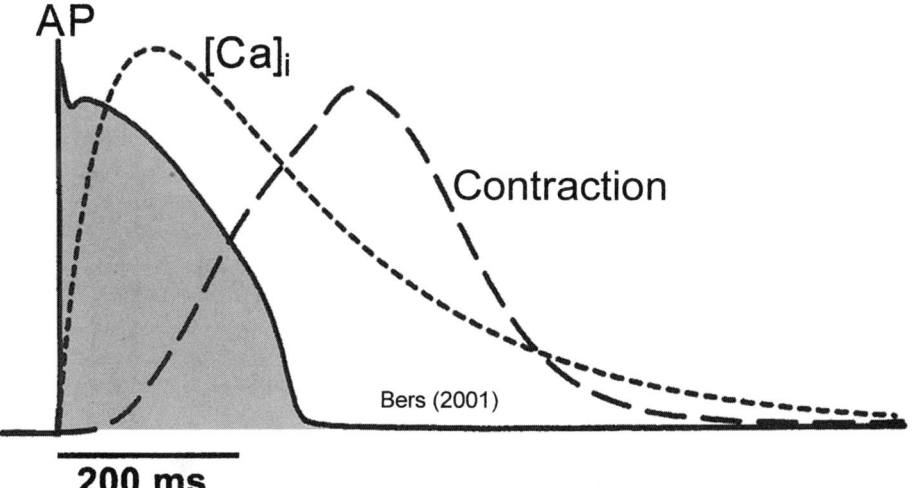

FIG. 4-3. Ventricular action potential, cytosolic calcium (Ca_i), and contraction. Note that in this rabbit ventricular myocyte muscle preparation, there is no perceptible delay between rapid depolarization of the action potential (phase 0, Fig. 4-2) and the start of the calcium transient, although the sodium channel opens before the calcium channel. The delay between the peak of the calcium transient and the peak of muscle contraction is because the calcium ion concentration has to increase to a particular critical value to trigger the actin–myosin interaction. (From Bers DM, *Excitation contraction coupling and cardiac contractile force*, 2nd ed. Dordrecht: Kluwer, 2001:229, with permission.)

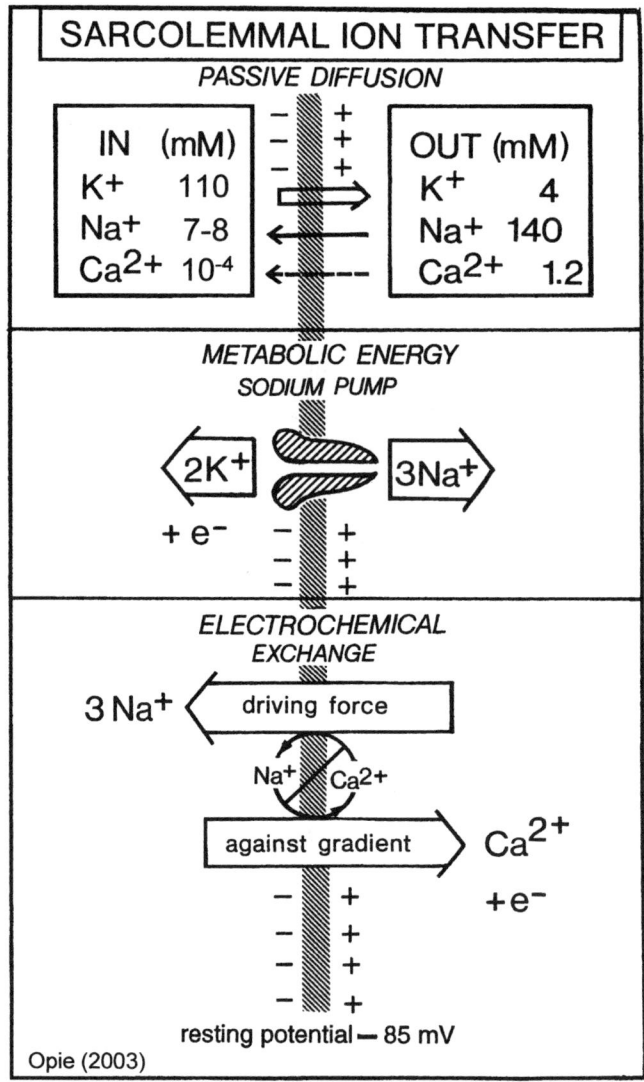

FIG. 4-4. Nonchannel ion transfer across the sarcolemma. Note the roles of passive diffusion, sodium–calcium exchange, and sodium–potassium pump (sodium pump). The intracellular concentrations are an approximation for those free to act, i.e., the activities. The sodium–calcium exchange can reverse according to the transmembrane potential and the relative concentrations of each ion on each side of the membrane (see text). For transfer of ions by channel opening and closing during action potential, see Figure 4-2.

RESTING MEMBRANE POTENTIAL

Starting with a hypothetical resting cell with equal concentrations of the principal charge-bearing ions (Na^+, K^+, Cl^-) on either side of the sarcolemma, it is interesting to see how the resting membrane potential could be generated. The calcium ion can be left out of consideration because its permeability is so low. The sodium–potassium pump localized to the sarcolemmal membrane (Table 4-1) will actively transfer potassium ions inward to give a high intracellular potassium concentration. As potassium accumulates in high concentrations on the inner surface, some of the ions will start to move back again to the outer surface because the sarcolemma is normally relatively highly permeable to potassium ions, i.e., the *conductance* to K^+ is high. As these K^+ ions cross the sarcolemma, they leave behind unbalanced negative charges so that the cell becomes polarized with a resting membrane potential of approximately −85 mV in the case of the ventricular myocyte. Only a small fraction of the total cell K^+ ions are involved in the generation of the resting membrane potential. To depolarize fully requires less than 1μmol/kg of electrically unbalanced K^+ movement (2) compared with the ventricular content of 70 mmol/kg (Table 4-2). The apparent paradox is that the high internal concentration of potassium, a positively charged ion within the cell, is associated with a negative internal charge at the inner layer of the sarcolemma, as just described.

By contrast, sodium ions pumped out of the cell accumulate on the outer surface of the sarcolemma and tend to diffuse inward (Fig. 4-4). The latter process is much slower than the outward diffusion of potassium ions because the sarcolemma is so much less permeable to sodium than to potassium. Therefore, sodium ions contribute little to the resting membrane potential. A theoretical

TABLE 4-1. *Approximate density of channels, pumps, and receptors in ventricular sarcolemmal membrane*

	Per square micron of sarcolemma
Sodium-potassium pump	~400
Sodium channel	16
Calcium channel (DHP binding sites)[a]	25
Calcium channel (L-type)[b]	1.2
Calcium channel (T-type)[b]	0.1
Potassium channels	
ATP sensitive[c]	10
I_{K1} or I_{Kir} (inward rectifier)[d]	1
I_K or I_{Kv} (delayed rectifier)[d]	1
β-Adrenergic receptor	2
Muscarinic receptor	6

[a]References 1a, 1b.
[b-d]See reference 1c–1e.
DHP, dihydropyridine.

TABLE 4-2. *Intracellular and extracellular concentrations of ions in normal heart ventricles*

Ion	Extracellular concentration		Ventricular values		
	Total (mmol/L)	Ionized (mmol/L)	Ventricular content (mmol/kg wet wt)	Ionized concentration (mmol/L)	Activity (mmol/L)
Na^+	140	140	40[a]	~20[b]	~7–8
K^+	4	4	70[a]	~140[b]	~100–110
Mg^{2+}	1.20	0.60	8	~17[c,d]	~0.6–0.9[c,d]
Ca^{2+}	2.50	1.25	0.6[e]	0.0002–0.001[e]	no data
Cl^-	140	140	25	~25[f]	~20[b]

[a–d]See reference 2a–2d.
[e]Reference 2e, Figure 6-3.
[f]Reference 2f.

example may be given. Let 400,000 Na^+ and K^+ ions be pumped by the sodium pump per millisecond per unit area (3). Suppose that of the 400,000 K^+ ions pumped inward, 200 K^+ ions will diffuse outward. By contrast, supposing that only four Na^+ ions diffuse inward owing to a much lower conductance than that of potassium (Fig. 4-4), there would now be a charge difference of 196 negative ions on the inside of the sarcolemma. This difference in charges causes the electrical potential. The actual contribution of potassium to this potential can be calculated by the Nernst equation $E_m = -61.5 \log K_i/K_o$, where K_o is the external potassium ion concentration, K_i is the internal potassium ion concentration (Table 4-2), and E_m is the electrical potential. If the external potassium were 4 mmol/L and the internal value 140 mmol/L, the calculated *equilibrium potential* for potassium would be −93 mV. A better value for the active intracellular K^+ concentration is 110 mmol/L. For this value of the *internal potassium activity* and the same external potassium concentration, the calculated potential difference caused by potassium is −88.4 mV, close to the measured diastolic potential in human ventricular cells of approximately −80 mV (4). Over a range of internal potassium values, the potassium equilibrium potential remains approximately 10 mV lower than the equilibrium potential (5). The difference is in part explained by contribution of the permeabilities of sodium and chloride ion, as given by the far more evolved Goldman field equation (6). An additional and variable complexity is that the sodium pump generates a small hyperpolarizing current.

CURRENT FLOW THROUGH CHANNELS

Ions will only permeate the membrane by some type of carrier, such as a channel, exchanger, or pump. If through a channel, this occurs only when the channel is in the open state. Ion movement through open channels is governed by two factors: (a) the potential (electrical driving force) across the membrane and (b) the concentration gradient across the membrane for that particular ion. These two factors provide the net *driving force*. The current-carrying capacity of the sarcolemma is influenced by three factors: I = N × i × p, where I is the total current (over the whole of the sarcolemma), N is the number of open channels, i is the current through each of the channels, and p is the probability of channel opening.

The word *potential* is derived from potent, meaning power. The resting membrane potential is the electrical driving force across the membrane resulting from the charge differences.

Current literally means running in Latin. An electrical current is a flow of electricity due to the difference in potential between two points or poles. This difference is measured in volts. The actual amount of current flow depends not only on the voltage but also on the resistance to flow and is measured in *amperes*. One ampere is when 1 V acts through a *resistance* of 1 Ω. The *voltage* is the electrical force resulting from the differences in potential across the sarcolemma. The voltage actually causes the current to flow as, for example, when sodium ions enter the cell (Fig. 4-2). During the passage of the electrical wave, as the inner layer of the sarcolemma becomes depolarized, the sodium channel is opened by the process of *voltage activation*.

STRUCTURE OF CHANNELS

Ion channels are pore-forming membrane proteins that span the lipid bilayer to allow a highly selective pathway into the cell when the channel changes from a *closed* to an *open state*. A simplified model of how channels open and close during the voltage changes associated with the action potential was initially evolved from electrophysiologic considerations and is the basis of the current molecular proposal. Hypothetically, each channel is guarded by two or more *gates* that control its opening and closing (Fig. 4-5). Ions can pass through the channel only when both gates are open, a process that responds to changes in the voltage, both being *voltage-operated gates*. When both activation and inactivation gates are open, the inward flow of sodium or calcium ions through their respective channels to produce the sodium and calcium inward currents.

Molecular Structure of Ion Channels

Modern techniques of molecular biology and immunology have allowed cloning and sequencing of channel proteins (7). From the evolutionary point of view, perhaps a very simple potassium channel served as the basis from which more complex channels evolved (Fig. 4-6). There is a striking molecular similarity between the sodium and calcium channels. This conservation of structure is probably common to all voltage-gated ion channels and suggests that there is

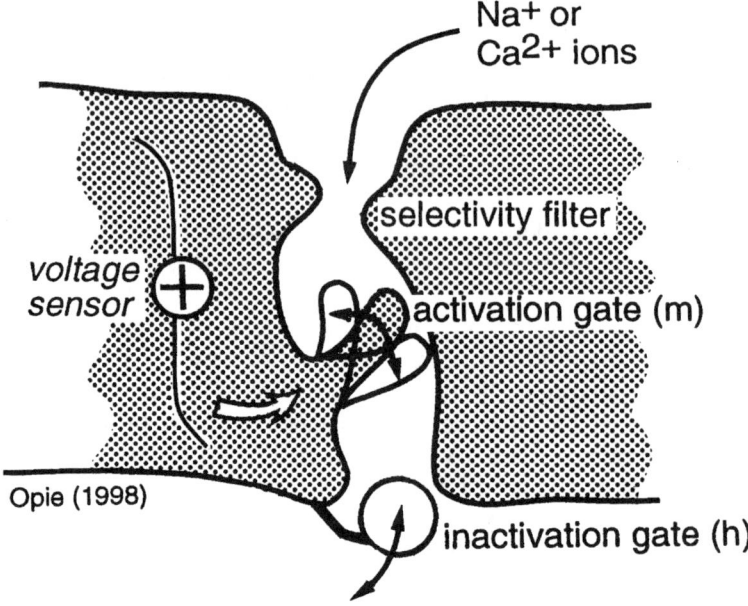

FIG. 4-5. Channel pore model shows activation and inactivation gates. The selectivity filter allows a specific ion to enter. The voltage sensor is a highly charged segment (helix) of the membrane-spanning domain (Fig. 4-6) responding to the voltage changes during depolarization and repolarization. The sensor tells the activation and inactivation gates to open and close.

a gene superfamily. Both sodium and calcium channels have four repeating transmembrane domains in their major α_1 subunit, very similar to each other in structure. When antibodies are directed against these domains, the channel is inactivated (8), suggesting that crucial properties such as voltage sensitivity are located within these structures. In addition to the major α_1 subunit, both sodium and calcium channels contain a number of other subunits of ill-defined function, such as the β subunit.

Each of the four transmembrane domains is made up of six helices. In each domain, one specific helical segment called S4 is rich in amino acids, highly positively charged, and acts as the *voltage sensor* (Fig. 4-6). As the wave of depolarization reaches the ion channel, the charges on the voltage sensor respond and include conformational changes in the channel *pore* that admits the ions and is thought to be formed by the four domains that make one α_1 subunit; these domains are folded in on each other, somewhat like four cans placed next to each other to form the channel pore between them (Fig. 4-7). Technically, one functioning sodium or calcium pore is formed by the "union" of four H5 or P loops, each lying between helices S5 and S6 of each of the four domains that make one α_1 subunit (7). In the case of the voltage-operated potassium channel

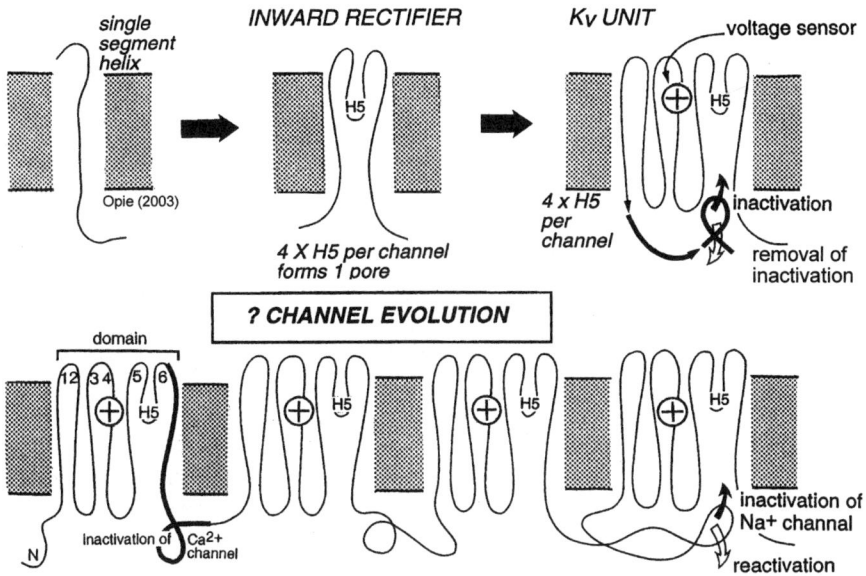

FIG. 4-6. **Possible channel evolution.** Hypothetically, primitive cells required potassium entry to act as a molecular signal. The simplest structure is with a single transmembrane helix (span) previously thought to be a channel and called K_{MIN}. It cannot function on its own. Next came the inward rectifier, with two spans and one H5 loop; four of these are required to function. Potassium channel structure became progressively more complex until evolving into the voltage-dependent potassium channel K_V. Even this cannot function on its own but requires four pore-forming subunits with four pore (P or H5) loops to make one functioning channel (i.e., four × six spans = 24 spans). Sodium and calcium channels are more highly evolved, serving functions such as conduction (sodium) and contraction (calcium). Both consist of a long polypeptide chain, with four transmembrane domains. Each domain consists of six helices or spans with a total of 24 spans. Helix S4, the fourth span, is highly charged (+ sign in figure) and thought to be the voltage sensor that activates the pore that transmits the ions (Fig. 4-5).

K_V, there are four separate subunits, each with six segments, that make up one pore (Fig. 4-6).

Gating Kinetics

Functionally, the Hodgkin–Huxley hypothesis proposes that opening and closing of channels can be explained by three sequences, resting, activated, and inactivated, involving two gates (9). Most but not all channels are activated by depolarization and at negative membrane potentials are in the *resting state*, with the activation (m) gate shut and the inactivation (h) gate open. Early during depolarization, both gates are open (Fig. 4-5) and the current flows (the *active state*). With increasing depolarization, the inactivation gate shuts, the current ceases to flow, and the channel becomes inactivated. With repolarization, the m gate

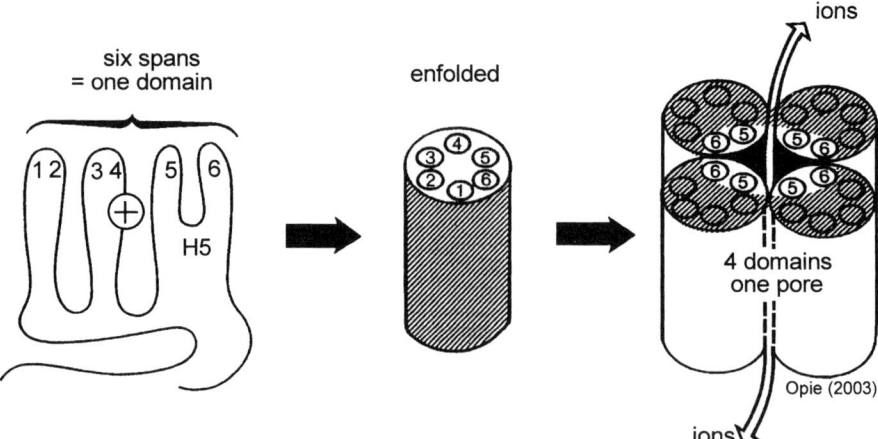

FIG. 4-7. Ion channel structure and function. The basic structure is six transmembrane spans and one pore-forming loop (H5). Four of these domains, when enfolded, make one channel pore, each contributing their S5 and S6 spans with linking H5 loops. The resultant functional pore allows the transmission of ions. For sodium and calcium channels, four domains are joined by linker loops to make one α_1 subunit (Fig. 4-6), whereas for potassium, each six-span domain is a separate subunit (Fig. 4-15).

rapidly closes (deactivation), while the h gate recovers from inactivation and opens. Thus, the channel has resumed the resting state. Each of these states is thought to be interchangeable in response to voltage (resting to active state and vice versa) or continued depolarization (conversion to inactivated state) or repolarization (reconversion to resting state). More complex models may be more accurate (10).

The movement of an ion across these gates at any given instant depends on the voltage and the time after the onset of depolarization. In technical terms, this process is both *voltage-gated* and *time-dependent*. The time factor is of considerable importance because the calcium channels only start to open fully by the time most of the sodium channels have already closed. It is thought that only a small percentage of the potentially active channels operate at any one time.

In a single myocyte, there are many thousands of each type of ion channel, constituting a *multichannel preparation* that behaves in a complex way, being a summation of the behavior of the many thousands of individual channels in that cell. Each individual channel is, at any given time and at any given voltage, either open or closed (Figs. 4-8 and 4-9). Opening takes place in bursts (Fig. 4-9). When depolarization is initiated, the individual sodium channels are more likely to be in the open state, so that there is an increased *probability of channel opening*. Then, as depolarization proceeds and the membrane potential approaches zero and becomes positive, the individual sodium channels are more likely to be closed (Figs. 4-8 and 4-9).

4. CHANNELS, PUMPS, AND EXCHANGERS

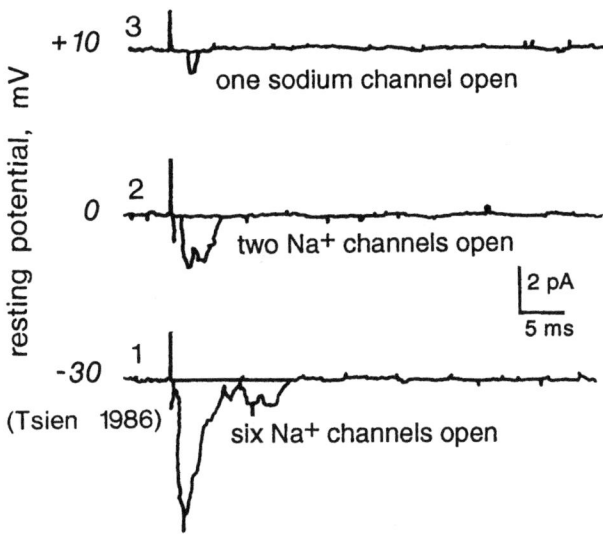

FIG. 4-8. Sodium current in single channels. The patch recordings are the summated values of single channels. The membrane potential just before depolarization (holding potential, V_m) was made progressively more positive (1 = –30 mV; 2 = 0 mV; 3 = +10 mV) in relation to the resting potential. The I_{Na} generated in single channels was recorded when the cell depolarized to a value 40 mV greater than the resting membrane potential. Straight and noisy lines indicate average baseline and single channel current levels, respectively. As the holding potential was made less negative, the number of sodium channels that opened in response to the test depolarization decreased (from six to two to one). (From Tsien R. Excitable tissues: the heart. In: Andreoli T, et al., eds. *Physiology of membrane disorders.* New York: Plenum Press, 1986:475, with permission.)

Incorporated into models of the channel are *selectivity filters*, which govern the specificity for ions. The calcium channel is far more selective for calcium ions than is the sodium channel for sodium ions. In reality, selectivity depends on the properties of specific amino acids, such as glutamate, that make up the lining of the channel pore (11).

Molecular Mechanisms for Gating

The voltage-gated sodium, calcium, and potassium currents, which pass through channels that respond to voltage changes, stand in contrast to the *ligand-operated channels*. Ligands (Latin, *ligare*, bind) bind to the cell membrane at receptor sites and then convey the signal to the channel gate usually by a specialized protein, crucial to the process of intracellular signaling, called the G protein. Examples are ligand-gated and G-dependent potassium channels (Table 4-3).

Voltage-gated channels (such as those for sodium, calcium, and some potassium currents) have two molecular "gates." The *voltage sensor*, located on the S4

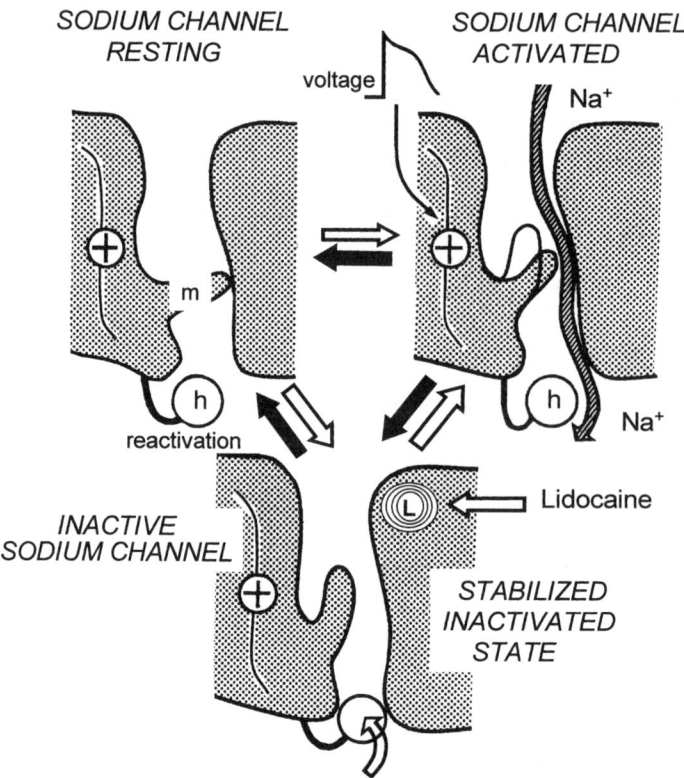

FIG. 4-9. Resting, activated, and inactivated sodium channels. Hypothetically, the sodium channel can exist in any of three states. In the polarized (resting) state, the m gate is closed and the h gate is open. On depolarization, the m gate opens while the h gate closes somewhat later. On repolarization, the m gate closes rapidly, a process called deactivation, while the h gate recovers from inactivation to enter the resting state. Each of the above arrows is reversible; the change from resting to activated state and inactivated state to resting occurs during the normal cardiac cycle. A sodium channel inhibitory drug such as lidocaine keeps the channel in the inactivated state so that channel activation is largely inhibited. These proposed concepts are based on the Hodgkin–Huxley model (41).

TABLE 4-3. *Control of cardiac ionic channels*

Voltage-gated channels
   Sodium channel
   Calcium channel
   Some potassium channels
Ligand-gated (G-dependent) channels
   Acetylcholine-sensitive K channel
   Adenosine-sensitive K channel
   ATP-sensitive K channel
Stretch-activated channels (mechanoreceptors): controversial
   Nonselective channels[a]
   Specific channels (e.g., swelling-operated Cl⁻ channel)

[a]Reference 11a. For G proteins, see Figure 7-2.

span, responds to changes in voltage to "open the pore" and explains the *activation gate*, previously called the m gate. Activation and inactivation are now seen as changes in the molecular configuration of the pore. In the case of the sodium channel, the *inactivation gate (h gate)* may open and close according to the "ball-and-socket" model. Inactivation can be linked to outward movement of the linker between domains III and IV, thereby acting as a "lid" to occlude the pore (1). In the case of the calcium channel, inactivation is associated with the sixth transmembrane-spanning segment (S6) of the first domain (Fig. 4-6). Thus, the mechanism of inactivation is not ball and chain (12) but might involve a molecular conformational reshuffle of the channel. In the case of the potassium channel, the amino terminal region of the channel protein may plug the channel from within (13).

SODIUM CHANNEL

Effects of Depolarization

One of the first events in response to the onset of depolarization of phase 0 of the action potential is opening the sodium channel (Figs. 4-2 and 4-7) when the voltage reaches −70 to −60 mV, which is its *threshold of activation* (Table 4-4). On depolarization, sodium channels drastically change their structural conformation within submilliseconds (1). The voltage sensors on the four charged S4 spans or segments (Fig. 4-6) respond ultrarapidly by a concerted outward movement that leads to further molecular changes and opening of the channel pore (Fig. 4-7). Thus, sodium current flows inward very rapidly during the first millisecond of depolarization (Fig. 4-9). At the same time, depolarization triggers "fast inactivation," proceeding more or less simultaneously with activation. Inactivation has two time constants. The first time is less than 1 milliseconds, switching off the sodium current very rapidly. The second component is much slower, at approximately 4 milliseconds and may account for the combined but constantly decreasing sodium inflow during the later stages of the action potential. This is the slow or late sodium current $I_{Na(s)}$ or $I_{Na(l)}$ (14).

Sodium Conductance Versus Current

The sodium channel can exist in any of three hypothetical states: resting, activated, and inactivated (Fig. 4-10). Depolarization changes the resting state to the activated state. The conductance increases and sodium ions flow inward. The conductance is a measure of the permeability of the membrane to an ion and helps to determine the rate of current flow. Thus, $I_{Na} = gNa(V_m - E_{Na})$, where I_{Na} is sodium current flow, gNa is sodium conductance, V_m is voltage across the membrane, and E_{Na} is the sodium equilibrium or reversal potential. The latter depends on the concentration of ions on either side of the sarcolemma. In the resting state, between depolarizations, the reversal potential is +40 mV for

TABLE 4-4. Contrasting properties of sodium and calcium channels

Property	Sodium channel	Calcium channel
Ion specificity	Sodium	Calcium
Inhibitors	Tetrodotoxin; lidocaine, quinidine, and other class I antiarrhythmics	Ca^{2+} antagonists (L channel); nickel, mibefradil (T channel)
Physiologic occurrence	Atrial, Purkinje, and ventricular tissue	Nodal and vascular tissue; as component of normal atrial, Purkinje or ventricular action potential
Effect of β-adrenergic receptor stimulation[a]	Increases (controversial)	Enhances Ca^{2+} entry by opening channels
Threshold of activation	−70 to −60 mV	−60 to −20 mV (−60 mV, T-type channel in SA node; −30 mV, L-type channel in ventricles)
Time constant of activation inactivation	<1 msec (fast)	10–20 msec
	4 msec (slow)[b]	50–500 msec
Overshoot	+20 to +35 mV	0 to +15 mV
Maximal rate of depolarization	100–1,000 V/sec (phase 0)	1–10 V/sec
Type of conduction	Fast (0.3–3.0 msec)	Slower (0.01–0.10 msec)
Role in arrhythmias	Ventricular tachyarrhythmias; ectopic activity; possibly in ischemia as inhibited fast responses	Slow conduction predisposes to reentry; role in early ischemic or reperfusion arrhythmias

For L and T calcium channels, see Table 4-5.
Electrophysiologic data modified from reference (39).
[a]By increasing internal sodium, Na/Ca exchange increases with a positive inotropic effect.
[b]This value refers to membrane potentials more positive than −20 mV, with even longer times reported.
SA, sinoatrial.

sodium. At the start of phase 0 depolarization, I_{Na} is large because the conductance is high and the voltage across the sodium channel is also high. I_{Na} decreases as depolarization proceeds (Fig. 4-8) because (a) the voltage across the sodium channel V_m decreases, and, therefore, the potential approaches E_{Na}, the reversal potential for sodium, and (b) the inactivation "gates" start to shut, thereby decreasing sodium conductance (Fig. 4-10). Hence, the driving force decreases, and the flow of sodium ions slows and then stops. In the meantime, the calcium conductance has increased.

Clinical Applications

Antiarrhythmic agents that inhibit the sodium channel are known as *class I antiarrhythmics* and include lidocaine, quinidine, and others (Fig. 4-9). Lidocaine probably indirectly prolongs the inactivation state of the channel, perhaps by interacting with the S4 sensor, to prolong the inactive state (1). *Tetrodotoxin* is a highly toxic experimental inhibitor of the sodium channel. More physiolog-

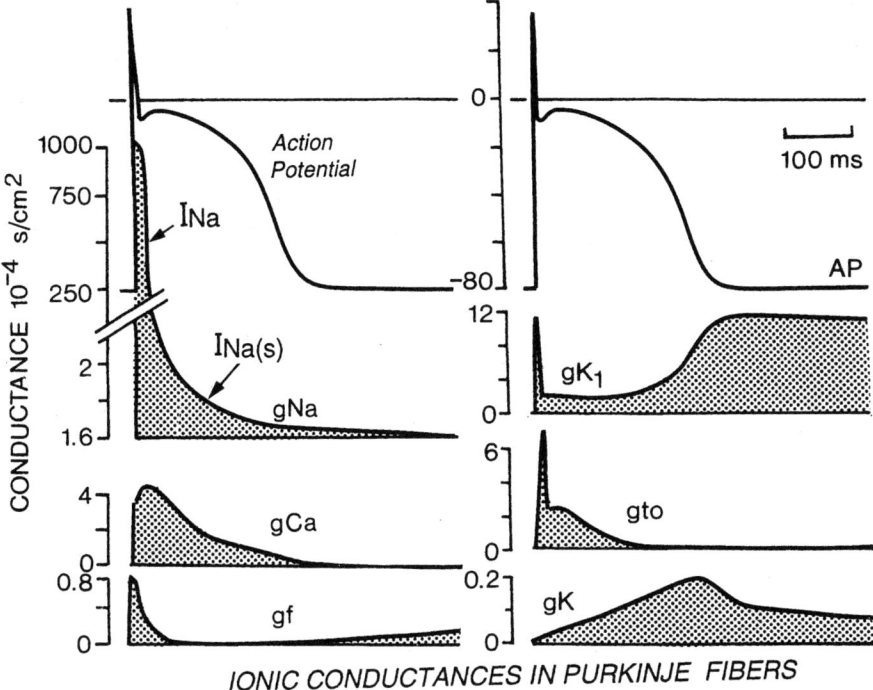

FIG. 4-10. Ionic conductances during action potential. How changing conductances contribute to shape of cardiac action potential of Purkinje fibers is illustrated. Computed action potential and ionic conductances (g) per unit of membrane surface. Note the extremely large initial peak of sodium conductance (gNa), approximately 250 times that of Ca conductance (gCa), and corresponding to the fast phase of the inward sodium current (I_{Na}). Thereafter, a slower phase follows ($I_{Na(s)}$). gf, conductance for current I_f found in Purkinje and pacemaker cells (Fig. 5-3). gK_1 is the conductance of the inward rectifier potassium current (K_{ir}) that decreases during depolarization. g_{to} is the conductance of the transient outward potassium current (I_{to}) in atria and Purkinje fibers (Fig. 4-2) and causes prominent phase 1. gK is the conductance of the voltage-gated delayed rectifier (I_K or I_{Kv}). (Modified from unpublished data of A. Coulombe and from data of Prof. E. Coraboeuf, Paris.) See also Fig. 20-9.

ically, the sodium channel can be totally inhibited by increasing the extracellular potassium to depolarizing *hyperkalemic* values, which remove the potential difference from within to outside the cell. The result is inhibition of cardiac contraction with cardiac arrest *(cardioplegia)*.

Ionophores

Ionophores are compounds that enhance the flow of ions along their electrochemical gradient. They enter membranes to act as pathways for ions. For example, *monensin* is a sodium ionophore and *nigericin* is a potassium ionophore. Although such compounds are not used in clinical practice, they have important physiologic and pharmacologic implications. For example, an unexpected effect of monensin is to promote release of atrial natriuretic peptide from the atria.

CALCIUM CHANNEL

Although the calcium ion concentration in the extracellular space outside the heart cell is higher than that inside, a large concentration gradient is maintained because the sarcolemma is virtually impermeable to calcium. To achieve the correct voltage required to open the calcium channel needs a greater degree of depolarization than to open the sodium channel. Some calcium also enters through reversal of the sodium–calcium exchange system, especially during the early phase of the plateau of the action potential (see Sodium–Calcium Exchange section).

Molecular Structure of the Calcium Channel

There are four subunits of the cardiac L-type calcium channel (α_1, α_2, β, and δ), the type that is found in ventricular cells. The combined molecular weight is 220 kd. In the α_1 subunit (molecular weight, 165 kd), there are four repeating domains, each of six helices, similar to that of the sodium channel, and suggests a common gene (Figs. 4-6 and 4-11). The major evident difference from the sodium channel lies in the established phosphorylation sites of the calcium channel protein, almost all located on the C terminal tail. In addition, there are critical differences between sodium and calcium channels in the amino acid structure of the channel pores, probably in the descending loop located between helices S5 and S6 of each domain. Thus, the presence or absence of glutamate residues in the structure of the channel pore can determine specificity for calcium ions (11). The β subunit of the calcium channel appears to interacts with the α_1 subunit to make more binding sites available for calcium antagonist drugs (15).

Calcium Permeation

The major functional property of the calcium channel is to regulate the entry of calcium ions. This process is inhibited when calcium antagonist drugs (calcium channel blockers) bind to their binding sites on the calcium channel protein. One model for the physiologic function of the calcium channel (Fig. 4-12) proposes that the channel is opened as depolarization reaches a critical threshold potential that converts the resting channel to the actived state, when both the activation (d) gate and the inactivation (f) gate are open. At this time, the hypothetical gates have a greater probability of being in the open rather than in the closed state. It should be remembered that they are opening and closing continuously in bursts of activity. The calcium ions flow during a particular time (time dependent) and until a particular voltage is reached (voltage dependent) during the depolarization

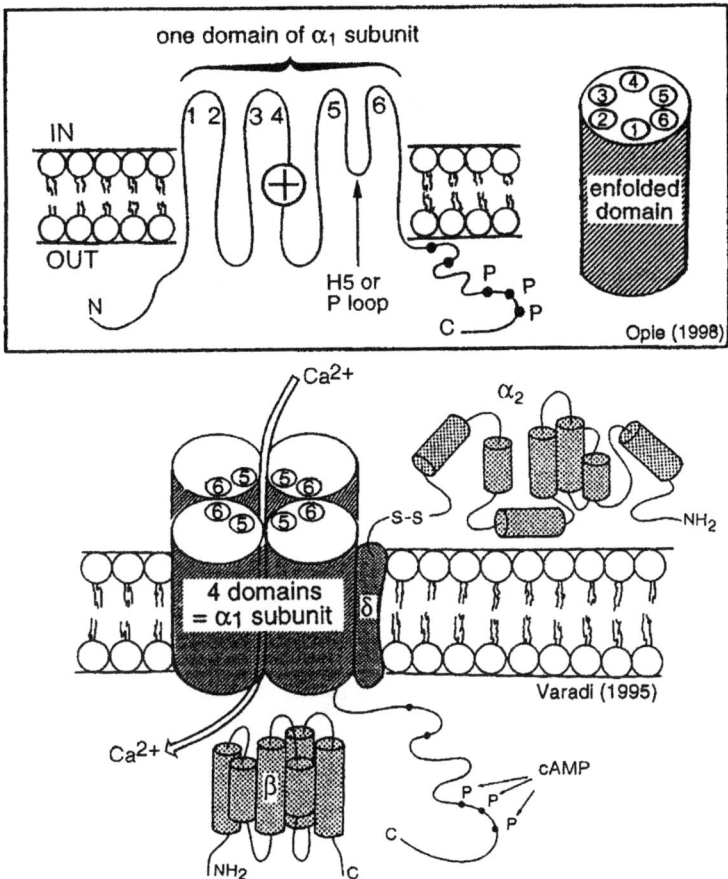

FIG. 4-11. Calcium channel structure. Top: The molecular structure of one domain of the α_1 subunit of the calcium channel is shown. Note the voltage sensor on segment S4 and the pore-forming loop (H5 or P) between S5 and S6, as for the sodium channel (Fig. 4-6). Four enfolded domains **(top, right)** arranged around the channel pore make up one α_1 subunit **(bottom)**. The major differences from the sodium channel lie in the nature of the C terminal chain, in the phosphorylation (P) sites on the C terminal chain, the mechanism of inactivation, and the existence of a large β subunit. The latter binds to the α_1 subunit to change its properties and to increase sensitivity to calcium antagonist drugs. The functions of the α_2 subunit and the δ subunit are not known. The γ subunit, present in skeletal muscle, is absent in heart and vascular smooth muscle. During β-adrenergic stimulation, cyclic adenosine 3′,5′-monophosphate (*cAMP*) phosphorylates several sites on the C terminal chain of the α_1 subunit to increase the probability of calcium channel opening (Fig. 4-13). (**Bottom** modified from Varadi et al. *Trends Pharmacol Sci* 1995;16:43.)

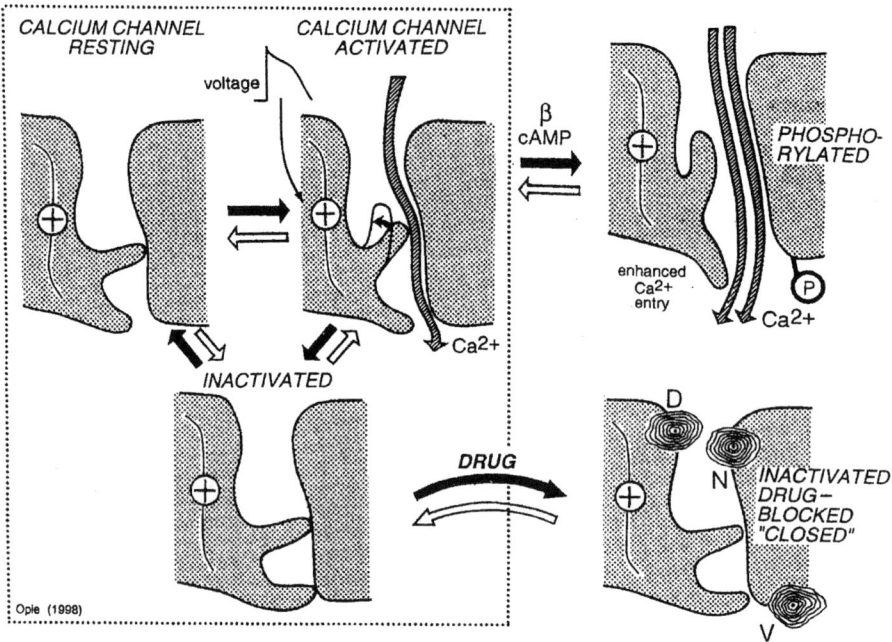

FIG. 4-12. States of the calcium channel. The channel can go through the same cycle and state changes as in Fig. 4-19, changing from the resting to the activated and inactivated states in response to voltage. Calcium antagonist drugs (N, nifedipine and other dihydropyridines; D, diltiazem; V, verapamil) can bind to various schematic sites to induce the drug-blocked inactivated state. β-adrenergic (β) activation by formation of cyclic adenosine 3′,5′-monophosphate (cAMP) promotes calcium channel phosphorylation (P) and probability of the open state.

process. Then, most of the gates come to be in the closed state, and the channel is inactivated. Calcium channels are also inactivated by the internal subsarcolemmal concentration as it increases in response to calcium release from the sarcoplasmic reticulum. The mechanism of this inhibition may be via binding of calcium ions to calmodulin. The calcium-calmodulin then inactivates the channel (16). Therefore, calcium entry by the L channels may be self-regulatory.

Calcium Channel Phosphorylation

The α_1 subunit (organ specific subunit) of the calcium channel can be phosphorylated especially in the C terminal tail (Fig. 4-11). This process occurs in response to catecholamine stimulation, which increases internal cyclic adenosine 3′,5′-monophosphate to activate a kinase enzyme that transfers a phosphate group from adenosine 5′-triphosphate (ATP) to the calcium channel. Thereby, the electrical charges near the inner mouth of the nearby pores are altered to induce changes in the molecular conformation of the pores. Ultimately, there is an increased probability of opening of the calcium channel, of importance in helping to cause an enhanced inotropic response during β-adrenergic stimulation. One of two mechanisms may explain what is happening. Either the time that the channel remains in the open state is increased so that more calcium ions flow with the same degree of voltage activation or phosphorylation may bring into play calcium channels that were otherwise inactive.

T- and L-Type Calcium Channels

There are two major subpopulations of calcium channels relevant to the cardiovascular system: *T channels* and *L channels* (17). A third population of N channels is found in nervous tissue. The T (transient) channels open at a more negative voltage (Fig. 4-13), have shorter bursts of opening, and do not interact with calcium antagonist drugs. Because they open at a more negative voltage than the L channels, the T channels account for the earlier phase of the opening of the calcium channel during early depolarization of the sinoatrial node and, hence, of initiation of the heart beat (Fig. 5-2). They also occur in the atrioven-

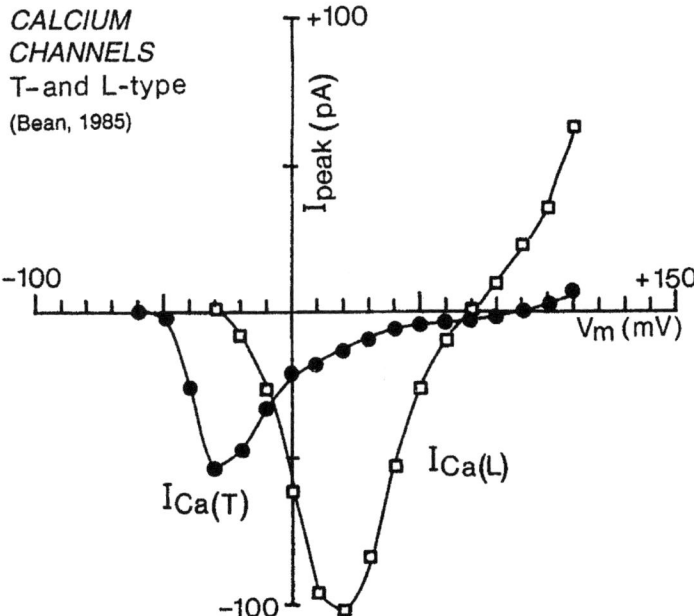

FIG. 4-13. Calcium channel subtypes. Contrasts between the transient calcium channel [$ICa(T)$] and the long-lasting calcium channel [$ICa(L)$]. Voltage-current relationship is shown for the dog atrial cells exposed to an external calcium concentration of 5 mmol/L. Note that the transient channel opens at a more negative voltage than the long-lasting channel and therefore opens first during the depolarization process. The transient channel also starts to close earlier and reaches a lower peak current flow. (Modified from Bean BP. Two kinds of calcium channels in canine atrial cells. Differences in kinetics, selectivity and pharmacology. *J Gen Physiol* 1985;86:1–30.) Also see computer calculations of Lipscombe (19).

TABLE 4-5. Contrasting properties of T and L calcium channels

	T-type	L-type
Voltage of activation	"Low"	"High"
Activation threshold: SA node[a]	−60 to −50 mV	−40 mV (much lower, $Ca_v1.3\alpha$)[b]
Activation threshold: atria[c]	−50 mV (not human)	−30 mV
Activation threshold: ventricles[d]	Absent except in LVH (−40 mV)[e]	−30 to −35 mV
Channel conductance (pS)[f]	8	25
Mean open time	Short, 1–2 msec	Very short, <1 msec
Inactivation kinetics[g]	Rapid	Slow
Channel blockers	Nickel, amiloride, mibefradil[h]	Classic calcium antagonists, such as verapamil, nifedipine, and diltiazem
β-Receptor stimulation[c]	No effect	Major effect
Calcium agonist (Bay K 8644)	No effect	Channel opens

[a]Guinea pig sinoatrial node cells (18a).
[b]Reference 19.
[c]Dog atrial myocytes (17).
[d]Guinea pig ventricular myocytes (18b).
[e]Reference 18c.
[f]pS = pico siemens; 1 siemen = 1 mho (18d).
[g]Activation and inactivation voltages and kinetics depend on surface potential and hence on concentration and type of external divalent ions. For other circumstances and values, see reference 18e.
[h]Reference 18f.
LVH, left ventricular hypertrophy.

tricular node and in Purkinje cells. T channels are not found in human atrial or ventricular cells (18). In left ventricular hypertrophy, T channels develop as part of the fetal growth program. T channels are also of considerable importance in the initiation of contraction in vascular smooth muscle.

The L (long-lasting) channels open at a less negative "higher" voltage (Table 4-5), thus accounting for the later phases of calcium channel opening. Controversially, a subdivision of L channels may open at low voltages close to those opening the T channels (19). The L channels have two patterns in which their gates work (modes of gating). Mode 1 has short bursts of opening, and mode 2 has longer periods of opening. Calcium channel blocking drugs change the mode of opening to a preponderance of mode 1, so that the amount of calcium entering through the channel is reduced.

Calcium Channel Blocking Drugs

The transmembrane-spanning helices are probably the sites to which these calcium antagonist drugs bind. The chief drug categories are the dihydropyridines, such as nifedipine and amlodipine, and the nondihydropyridines verapamil and diltiazem, giving rise respectively to the N, V, and D binding sites. Some properties of these drugs are similar, and others differ. The shared properties are peripheral vasodilation, with use in hypertension, and coronary dilation, with use in angina pectoris. There are additional binding sites to which other new calcium antagonist drugs such as amlodipine may also bind. It is likely that the drug binding sites differ somewhat from organ to organ. For example, some calcium channel blockers act more specifically on the vascular tissue than on the myocardium, which is important in hypertension when peripheral arteriolar dilation is a crucial property.

POTASSIUM CHANNELS

Understanding the vast number of potassium channels can be simplified by their division into two distinct molecular families: voltage-gated (or voltage-operated) channels and inward rectifier channels (20). These are designated K_v and K_{ir}, respectively, the latter often called the K_1 channels (Table 4-6). Both families of potassium channels help to control the outward flow of potassium ions (Fig. 4-14), especially during repolarization (K_v) and in the maintenance of the resting membrane potential (K_{ir}).

Why Are There So Many Potassium Channels?

Seen from an evolutionary perspective, a very simple K^+ channel, probably with only two transmembrane helices (spans), might first have come into existence to generate the resting membrane potential of primitive cells (Fig. 4-6). This simple structure is now called the inward rectifier, K_{ir}. Another member of this family, the ATP-sensitive K^+ channel, (K_{ATP}), evolved to stop the potassium leak induced by hypoxic damage. When the beating heart emerged, the K_v superfamily (Fig. 4-15) came into existence with its voltage sensor on an adjacent transmembrane span (S4). Hypothetically, transmembrane segments (or spans) S2 and S3 evolved to protect the voltage sensor S4 from the irrelevant charges of the lipid bilayer. Members of the K_{ir} family evolved into another superfamily (Fig. 4-16), including K_{ACh} and K_{ADO} that help to decrease the heart rate by responding, respectively, to acetylcholine and adenosine. To achieve a functioning potassium channel pore requires the combination of multiple subunits, i.e., either four subunits each of six spans or the combination of four units each of only two spans (Figs. 4-15 and 4-16). Such variable combinations mean that a great molecular diversity of potassium channels is possible.

Voltage-Operated or Delayed Rectifier K^+ Channels

These channels conduct two potassium currents that make major contributions to repolarization (Table 4-6), hence playing an important role in regulating the duration of the action potential. These currents only activate slowly in response to the voltage changes initiated by depolarization, which explains the alternate name *delayed rectifier currents*. Separate genes encode the slow and fast repo-

TABLE 4-6. Currents associated with normal cardiac action potential

Current	Abbreviation	Qualities
Fast inward sodium current	I_{Na}	Responsible for upstroke of action potential; abolished by tetrodotoxin; inhibited by class I antiarrhythmic agents; 4 units each of 6 transmembrane spans
Inward calcium current	I_{Ca}	Important for plateau phase of cardiac action potential; involved in excitation–contraction coupling; increased by β-stimulation; 4 units each of 6 transmembrane spans
Subtype T channel	$I_{Ca(T)}$	Transient calcium current, opening at low voltages; may be important in sinus node depolarization
Subtype L channel	$I_{Ca(L)}$	Long-duration calcium current, admitting major calcium ion flow, inhibited by standard calcium antagonists; Note pacemaking subtype, $Ca_v 1.3\alpha$
Potassium currents		
Background K current (inward or anomalous rectifier)	I_{K1} or I_{Kir}	Helps to regulate RMP and contributes to late phase 3 repolarization; previously thought to be time independent; above RMP, outward potassium current; below RMP, strong inward current with rectification that augments flow; depolarization shuts channel, current flows again during repolarization to help end action potential; not a pacemaker current
Voltage-gated K currents (delayed rectifier)	I_K or I_{Kv} includes rapid (K_r) and slow (K_s) currents	Outward potassium current chiefly responsible for repolarization; voltage gated; enhanced by increased internal calcium[a]; activated by depolarization (fully active at −10 mV) and deactivated by full repolarization; time dependent; promotes spontaneous depolarization as it decays; 6 transmembrane spans; 2 divisions, K_r (rapid, HERG) and K_s (slow); molecular basis of each identified[b]
Early transient outward K current	I_{to}	Prominent in Purkinje cells, atrial cells, and epicardial ventricular cells; causes obvious phase 1; shortens action potential duration; inhibited in heart failure and LV hypertrophy
Other currents		
Diastolic pacemaker current in SA node or Purkinje fibers	I_f	Inward "funny" sodium (and potassium) current; increased by β-stimulation; causes automaticity in SA node or injured Purkinje fibers
Sodium–calcium exchange	$I_{Na/Ca}$	Contributes to late phase of cardiac action potential plateau (Na^+ inward)
Chloride current	I_{Cl}	Inward flow of negative charges; shortens action potential duration during adrenergic activation
Pump current	$I_{Na/K}$	Greater outflow of charges as $3Na^+$ versus inflow of $2K^+$; electrogenic

For review, see reference 18.
[a]Reference 20a.
[b]Reference 27.
RMP, resting membrane potential; HERG, human ether-à-go-go-related gene; LV, left ventricular; SA, sinoatrial.

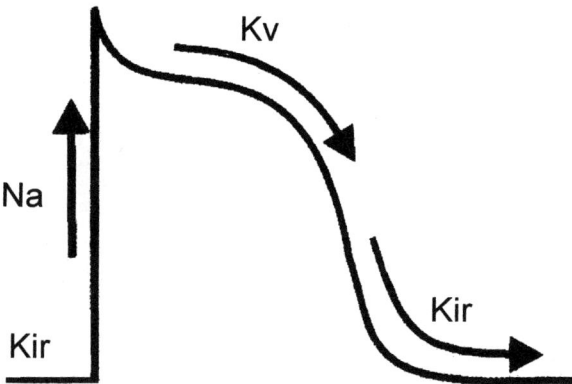

FIG. 4-14. **Contributions of major divisions of potassium channels** to the shape of ventricular action potential. Note further division of K_v into rapid and slow components.

larizing complements K_s and K_r (Fig. 20-9). Either gene may be defective, giving rise to two different types of long QT syndrome (Fig. 20-10).

The Slowly Repolarizing K⁺ Channel, K_s

The K_s channel responds to β-adrenergic stimulation, being enhanced four- to sixfold (21). This acceleration has both physiologic and pathologic significance. During a physiologic tachycardia, the time between beats is shortened, thereby threatening coronary flow that occurs chiefly in diastole. Hence, the β-mediated shortening of the action potential is essential to allow adequate coronary flow. In disease, such as long QT syndrome, sympathetic stimulation fails to abbreviate the action potential yet accelerates the advent of the next depolarizing, with risk of serious arrhythmias and cardiac death (Fig. 20-11). The class III antiarrhythmics inhibit K_r but not K_s channels (Fig. 20-9).

The HERG Channel K_r

The superfamily that includes this channel is sometimes called the *shaker family* because this current was first cloned in a mutant of the fruitfly *Drosophila*. When this channel is genetically absent from the fruitfly, exposure to ether provokes spasms of muscular shaking. In humans, the gene that expresses this channel is HERG (human ether-à-go-go–related gene), which, when mutated, gives abnormalities of the K_r current that explain one type of the congenital human long QT syndrome. The latter predisposes to potentially fatal arrhythmias (Fig. 20-10). More common is the acquired form of the long QT syndrome resulting in an apparently unpredictable manner from a variety of structurally unrelated and potentially fatal drugs. Such drugs interact with

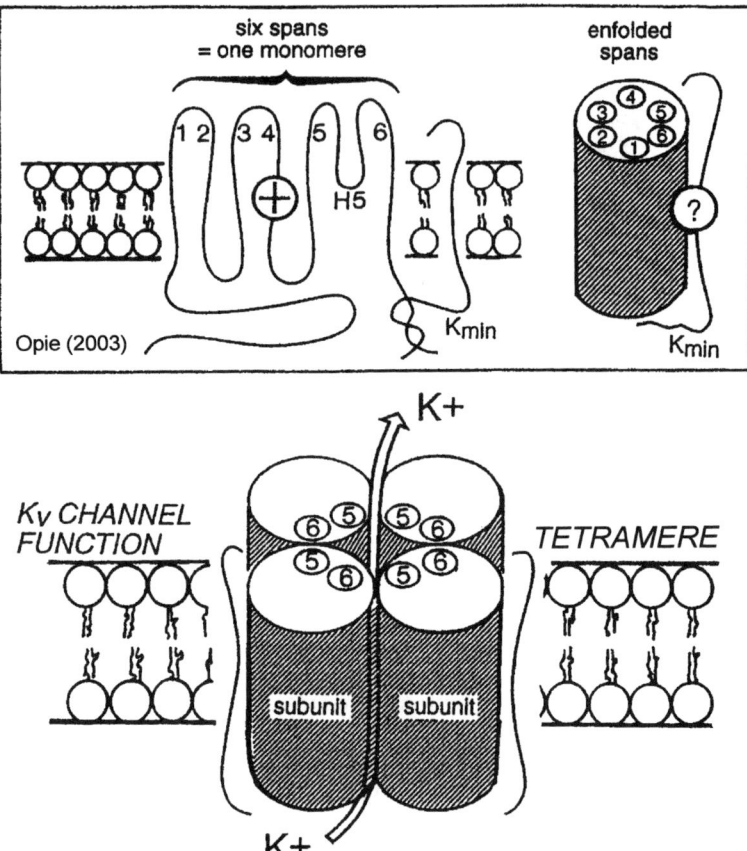

Fig. 4-15. Structure of voltage-operated potassium channel. This channel (K_v) consists of four unlinked subunits. Each of these potassium channel subunits is composed of a transmembrane domain with a positively charged S4 helix, similar to the voltage sensor of sodium and calcium channels (Fig. 4-6). Four subunits, each a monomomere, make a functional, voltage-sensitive potassium channel (heterotetramere is a combination of four different subunits) with one functional pore. The single transmembrane span (K_{min}) interacts with the last of the other six spans to produce one subunit, to produce the slow component of K_v.

specific aromatic amino acids not found in other potassium channels but present in the pore structure and the neighboring transmembrane domain of the HERG channel (22).

The Inward Rectifier Superfamily, K_{ir}

Potassium channels of this family set the resting membrane potential of cardiac myocytes. Structurally, this is an extremely simple channel with only two transmembrane helices and one pore (Fig. 4-16). The gene expressing this chan-

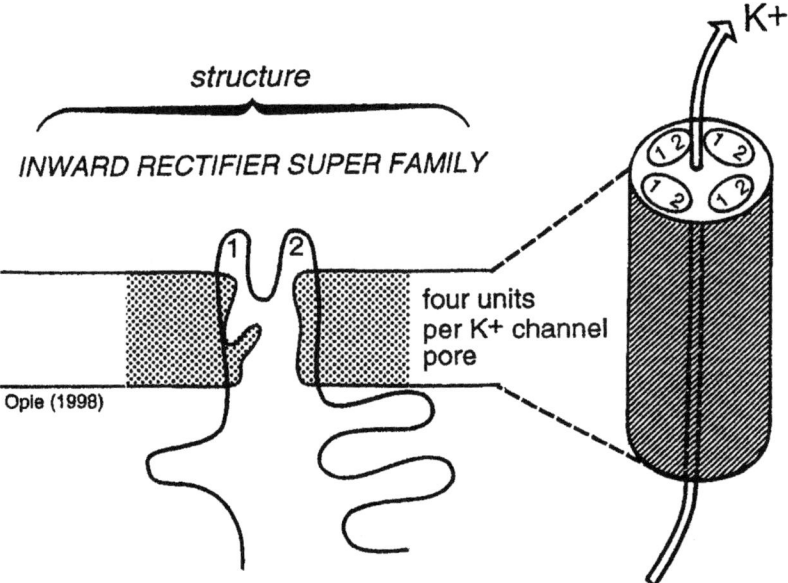

FIG. 4-16. Inward rectifier superfamily, having only two transmembrane spans (*1* and *2*) and the loop (*H5*), that participates in the pore. The illustration on the right shows that four of these simple structures are required to make one functioning channel pore that passes potassium ions.

nel is probably Kir2.1 (23). The channel passes an *outward current* when the membrane potential is above the potassium equilibrium potential (E_k) to contribute to the repolarization phase of the action potential and to help end the action potential, thereby regaining the resting membrane potential (Fig. 4-17). Conversely, this same channel potentially passes a large *inward* K^+ current when the cell membrane is hyperpolarized (i.e., when the resting membrane potential is below −85 mV), and this inward current helps to maintain the high internal K^+ activity and hence the membrane polarity. The unusual nature of the current flow, which is much larger in one direction, has given rise to the name *anomalous rectifier*. Hypothetically, naturally occurring *polyamines*, such as spermine and spermidine, can plug the inner side of the pore when the K^+ flux is directed outward to reverse the direction of current flow. Mg^{2+} ions have a similar but much less powerful effect (23).

The Transient Outward Potassium Current, I_{to}

This voltage-gated potassium current largely accounts for the very early repolarization after the peak of the upstroke of the action potential. This current is especially prominent in atrial, Purkinje, and subepicardial ventricular cells (Fig. 4-2), giving the typical "spike-and-dome" appearance (24). The notch created by

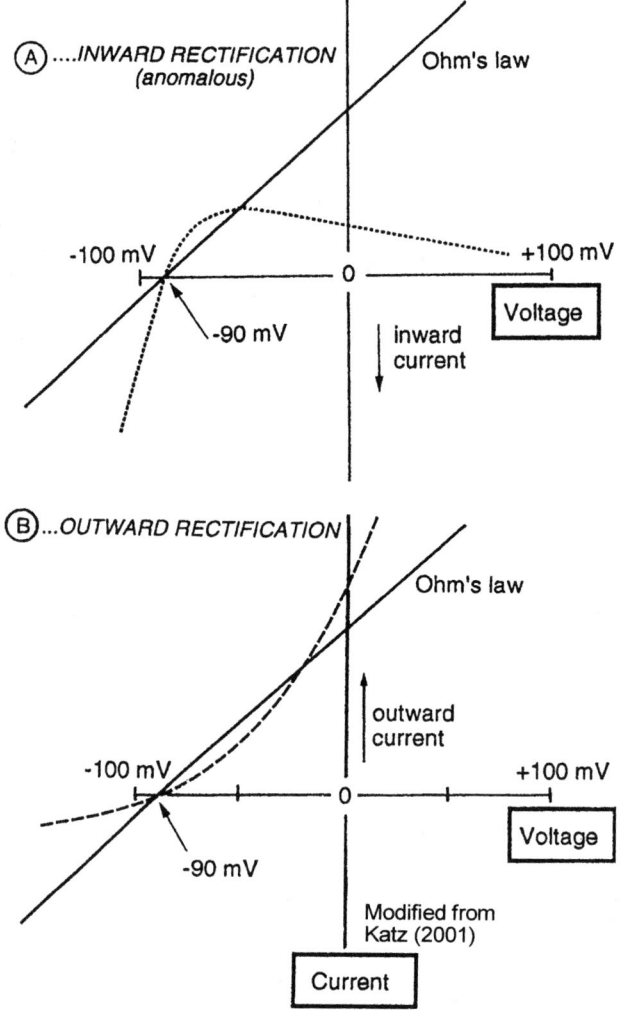

FIG. 4-17. Inward versus outward rectification. Current-voltage relationships show the effects of changing membrane potential (*abscissa*) on the ionic currents (*ordinate*) generated by three different types of potassium channels. Inward currents are downward, and outward currents are upward. All potassium currents are zero at approximately −90 mV, the equilibrium potential for potassium. An ohmic current **(A)** is a linear function of membrane voltage because resistance is constant. Inward (anomalous) rectification **(A)** occurs when depolarization causes potassium channels to close, thereby decreasing outward current. Outward rectification **(B)** occurs when depolarization opens potassium channels and so increases outward current. Thus, outward rectification favors outward current, whereas inward rectification favors inward current. (Modified from Katz AM, *Physiology of the heart*, 3rd ed. Philadelphia: Lippincott Willilams & Wilkins, 2001:482, with permission.)

4. CHANNELS, PUMPS, AND EXCHANGERS

I_{to} resets the action potential to the early phase of the plateau. I_{to} also contributes to phase 2 repolarization (Fig. 20-9) because the action potential duration is prolonged when this current is inhibited, as in left ventricular hypertrophy (Fig. 13-11). The molecular correlate for this current in the human heart is the Kv4.3 potassium channel gene. Strong expression of I_{to} in rats and mice explains why the action potential duration in these species is so short. In a variety of diseases such as left ventricular hypertrophy, heart failure, and myocardial infarction, this current is suppressed so that the action potential is prolonged (Fig. 13-11). The proposed mechanism is local activation of the renin–angiotensin system with increased production of angiotensin II (25).

Ligand-Operated Members of K_{ir} Superfamily

Ligand-operated channels, also part of the K_{ir} superfamily (26), include the muscarinic- and adenosine-operated channels found in nodal tissue and the atrium (Table 4-7). The muscarinic-operated channel, operated by the M_2-receptor, is

TABLE 4-7. Ligand-operated and additional potassium currents

Current	Abbreviation	Qualities
Ligand-operated G protein–gated K channels (inward rectifier family)		
Acetylcholine sensitive	I_{kACh}	Activated by acetylcholine muscarinic receptors (m_2) in nodal, Purkinje and atrial cells; not in ventricles; time independent; when current switched on in nodal cells, spontaneous depolarization is delayed; heteromultimer of 2 distinct inwardly rectifying subunits[a]
Adenosine sensitive	I_{kADO}	Probably same as I_{kACh}; adenosine stimulates time-independent potassium current
ATP regulated	I_{kATP}	ATP inhibits in physiologic concentrations; decrease in ATP/ADP ratio and adenosine activate; inhibited by sulphonylureas, activated by K channel activators; structure part of inward rectifier family[b]
Additional K currents		
Calcium activated	Ik_{Ca} or BK_{Ca}	Important in vascular smooth muscle, to hyperpolarize and thereby to inhibit calcium channel; vasorelaxation; large conductance ("big" channel)
Sodium activated[c]	I_{kNa}	Activated when internal sodium rises as in ischemia or during sodium pump inhibition
Fatty acid activated[c]	I_{kFFA}	Activated by increased internal free fatty acids (FFA) during sustained ischemia

[a]Reference 26.
[b]Reference 25a.
[c]For further details, see reference 18. For encoding gene and coactivation by Cl^-; see reference 25b.
ATP, adenosine 5'-triphosphate; ADP, adenosine 5'-diphosphate.

LIGAND OPERATED K⁺ CHANNEL

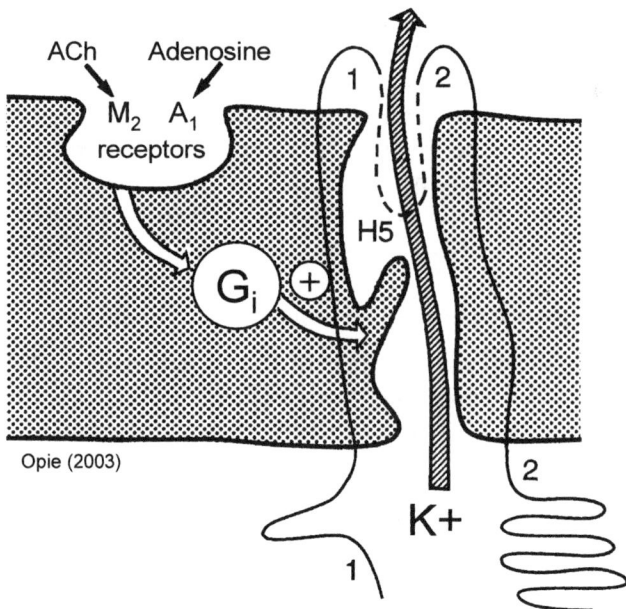

FIG. 4-18. Ligand-gated potassium channels. These channels are part of the inward rectifier superfamily. This drawing shows the proposed control mechanisms in response to acetylcholine (*ACh*) and adenosine, both of which slow the heart rate. m_2, muscarinic receptor subtype 2; A_1, adenosine receptor subtype 1; G_k, G protein controlling activity of this potassium channel.

linked to the channel by the inhibitory G protein G_i (Fig. 4-18). Hence, this K⁺ channel is also called GIRK₁ (G protein–activated inward rectifying K₁ channel). The current conducted is sensitive to acetylcholine, I_{kACh}. The adenosine-sensitive K⁺ current, I_{kADO}, probably identical to I_{kACh}, responds to the adenosine receptor A_1 rather than to the muscarinic receptor and is also linked to the channel by means of G_i. Both of these currents function to increase outward potassium flow in nodal tissue and therefore to hyperpolarize. Thus, the membrane potential is moved away from the threshold for spontaneous firing so that the discharge rate of nodal tissue slows and the heart rate decreases.

The Smallest Potassium Channel Structure, K_{min}

Previously thought to be an extremely primitive channel K_{min}, this single strand of only one helix with 130 amino acids is now known to be a regulator of the slow component of the delayed rectifier current K_s (Fig. 4-15). From the molecular point of view, K_{min} is coexpressed with one functioning six-membrane spanning "standard" potassium K_s channel (27).

The Largest Conductance Potassium Channel, BK_{Ca}

This calcium-activated potassium channel, part of the delayed rectifier superfamily, is probably of major importance in vascular smooth muscle. The concept is that cytosolic calcium building up during opening of the vascular calcium channels in turn opens this channel. The result is a large efflux of potassium ions so that the vascular cell hyperpolarizes and the calcium channel closes. This channel has by far the largest conductance for potassium, meaning that when the channel is open, much more potassium can flow through it than in the case of the other potassium channels.

ATP–Sensitive Potassium Channel

This channel represents a hybrid between the K_{ir} superfamily and the totally different ABC (ATP binding cassette) family (Fig. 4-19). The latter provides two binding sites, one for SUR (sulfonylureas, epitomized by the oral antidiabetic agent glibenclamide) and the other for ATP. The K_{ir} component of the channel forms the channel pore as a heteromultimer of four subunits, each of only two helices. Also participating in this functioning channel pore are four peripore structures each constituted by the two transmembrane-spanning domains (SUR component and the ATP-binding site component). Because the K_{ir} component of the channel is controlled by the binding of internal ATP, it is called the K_{ATP} channel. Technically, the inward rectifier concerned is Kir6.2 (28).

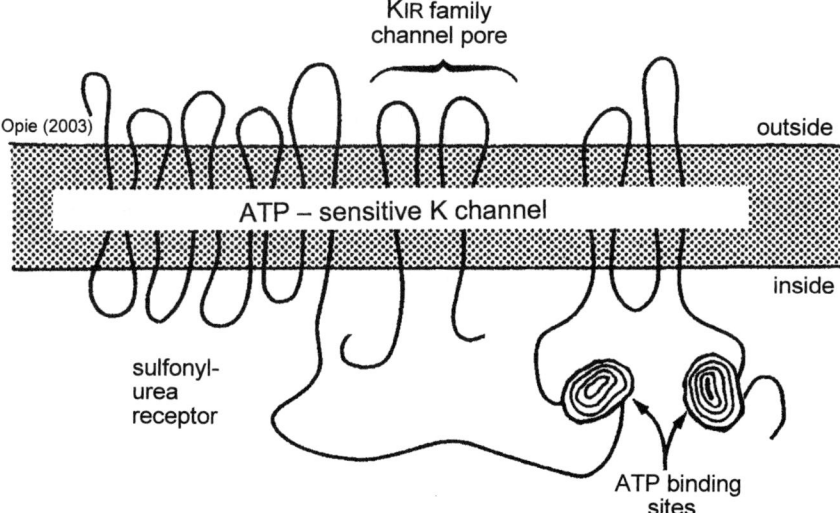

FIG. 4-19. Hybrid composition of adenosine 5'-triphosphate (*ATP*)–sensitive potassium channel, which represents a union between a member of the inward rectifier K_{IR} family and the ABC superfamily (ATP binding cassette). On the left is the sulfonylurea receptor and on the right, the ATP binding sites. The actual channel pore is composed of four K_{IR} subunits.

There is no obvious physiologic role for K_{ATP} in cardiac myocytes. Rather, they may be "metabolic sensors" that link cytosolic energy metabolism to membrane electrical activity (29). Pathophysiologically, one hypothesis is that they act as "alarm systems." As ATP breaks down in response to severe ischemia and the subsarcolemmal ATP decreases, the channel opens with outward passage of K^+ ions and their accumulation on the outside of the cell. This process causes loss of normal membrane polarization with a decreased contractile response and an induced state of inactivity or rest. The channel is very sensitive to ATP inhibition (30) so that there must be powerful deinhibitors that come into play. During anoxia or ischemia, this channel opens relatively rapidly, much before the ATP has decreased to the very low levels required for channel opening. The current hypothesis is that subsarcolemmal ATP decreases and ADP increases markedly while the overall bulk of ATP is still relatively well preserved (29). Probably the ATP inhibition is relieved by local accumulation of adenosine 5'-diphosphate (ADP), adenosine, and lactate (18). Another powerful reliever of the ATP inhibition is phosphoinositol diphosphate, formed during α-adrenergic or angiotensin II signaling (18).

The function of K_{ATP} in vascular smooth muscle is much clearer. There, in response to the formation of adenosine, this channel opens and participates in coronary vasodilation. Adenosine formed during myocardial hypoxia or during vigorous work is thought to diffuse from the cardiac myocyte to the K_{ATP} channel on vascular smooth muscle cells to relieve the inhibition by ATP and to allow channel opening. The egress of potassium ions opening causes hyperpolarization that in turn leads to vasodilation by inactivation of the calcium channels. (This vasodilatory mechanism is distinct from the interaction of adenosine with I_{kADO}, described in the next section, although both mechanisms lead to hyperpolarization.)

The *clinical implications* of the inhibition K_{ATP} by sulfonylureas relate to their use as oral agents in the therapy of maturity-onset diabetes mellitus. These drugs, such as glibenclamide, inhibit K_{ATP} and promote coronary vasoconstriction. They also lessen ischemic loss of potassium and early ischemic arrhythmias (31). They inhibit the protective phenomenon of preconditioning (Fig. 19-19). Other drugs known as the *potassium channel openers*, such as pinacidil, cromakalim, minoxidil, diazoxide, and the mixed nitrate-potassium opener nicorandil, all induce coronary dilation by promoting K_{ATP} opening. By mechanisms not fully understood, these drugs protect ischemic myocardial cells.

Ischemia-Induced Potassium Current Flow

In ischemia, not only does the ATP-sensitive potassium channel open, but several other new channels may come into operation (Fig. 4-20). A *sodium-activated potassium current*, responding to an increase in internal sodium, may become important in ischemia, when internal sodium is known to increase. Its existence remains controversial. Likewise, the fatty acid–activated potassium

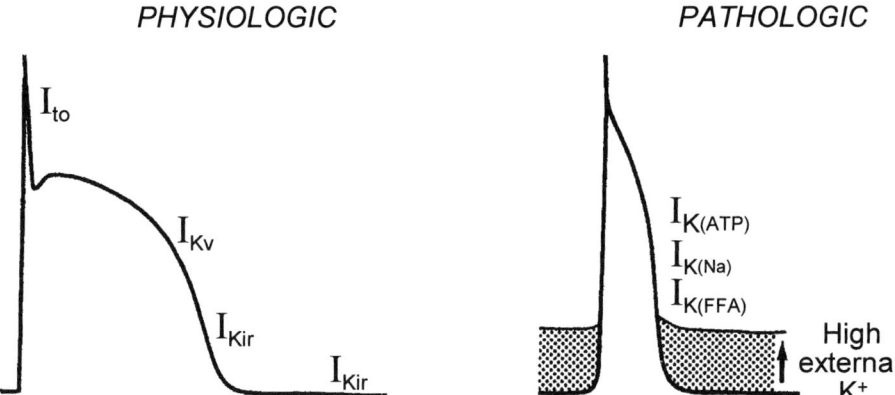

FIG. 4-20. Physiologic versus pathologic potassium channels. Note contribution of potassium channels to repolarization process. **Left:** In physiologic conditions (Purkinje cell), I_{to} causes the early phase of repolarization, I_K (I_{Kv}) and I_{K1} (I_{Kir}) contribute to repolarization, and I_{K1} maintains the negative resting potential. **Right:** In pathologic/anoxic conditions, the action potential duration is markedly shortened by $I_{K(ATP)}$ with contributions from $I_{K(Na)}$ and I_{KFFA}. For details, see Carmeliet (18).

channel also appears to respond to changes in ischemia when there is a buildup of fatty acid metabolites (18).

Rectification of Potassium Currents

Normally, the relationship between the voltage and current is a straight line (Ohm law). When a current can pass through the channel in both directions, but the flow in one direction is greater, then this selective process is called rectification (Fig. 4-17). The channel rectifies in an inward direction when the voltage decreases to less than the equilibrium potential for potassium (at approximately −90 mV). At a molecular level, the concept is that the inward current "unplugs" an internal divalent ion such as magnesium that would normally block the channel pore. Because of the marked deviation of the voltage-current relationship for the K_{ir} channel, this potassium current is also called the *anomalous rectifier*. Outward rectification occurs when the major current flow is in the outward direction but the voltage is more positive than zero.

CHLORIDE CHANNELS

The role of chloride currents in the heart remains unclear, especially because one of the proposed chloride currents has more correctly been identified as the potassium current I_{to}. In general, the existence of chloride currents in the human has not been confirmed. One chloride current is activated by calcium, another is swelling operated, and yet another is activated by β-adrenergic stimulation (Fig.

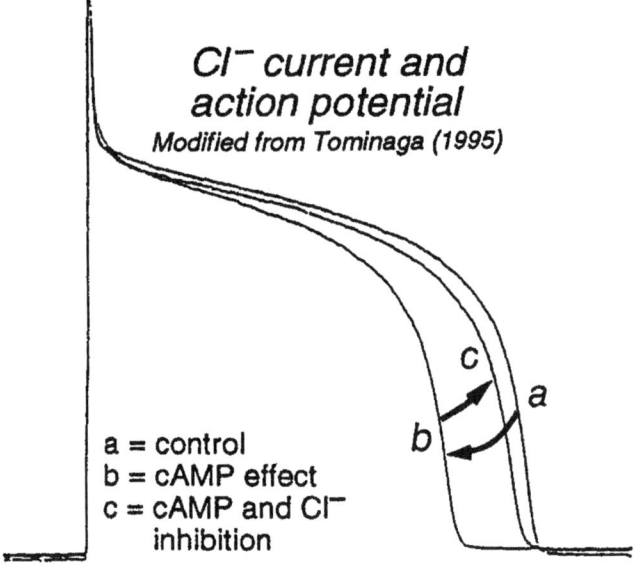

FIG. 4-21. Inward chloride (Cl^-) flux. There are several of such inward fluxes. This figure shows the role of one of them in shortening the action potential duration during catecholamine β-adrenergic stimulation. In response to cyclic adenosine 3′,5′-monophosphate, the action potential duration shortens from a to b. When the chloride current is blocked, the action potential duration widens from b to c. This abbreviation of the action potential is especially important during β-adrenergic stimulation when the heart rate increases and the duration of the cardiac cycle decreases. For further details, see Tominaga et al. *Circ Res* 1995;77:417.

4-21). By promoting influx of chloride ions with negative charges, there is in effect an outward repolarizing current. β-Adrenergic stimulation also stimulates repolarizing potassium currents. Without these compensatory mechanisms that shorten the action potential duration, β-adrenergic stimulation, as in exercise, would widen the action potential by enhanced opening of the calcium channel, thereby shortening diastole and limiting coronary blood flow.

VENTRICULAR ACTION POTENTIAL

The characteristic appearance of the ventricular action potential can now be interpreted in greater detail in terms of opening and closing of the sodium, calcium, and potassium channels just discussed. The rapid phase of depolarization of the action potential (phase 0) is the result of the flash opening of the sodium channels (Fig. 4-10). Sodium conductance first increases very rapidly, as does the flow of the inward current (I_{Na}), to peak within less than 1 millisecond and then to fall off equally rapidly. This flash of inward sodium movement, carrying positive charges, fully depolarizes the cell, causing the rapid upstroke or *phase 0* (for the four phases, see Fig. 4-2).

In the meantime, the much slower L calcium channels have already started to open, with the L type opening at approximately −30 to −35 mV (Table 4-5). By contrast, T-type channels are normally absent from ventricular cells. As the sodium current fades away, it is replaced by flow of the L-type calcium current (I_{Ca} or I_{si}, slow inward current), which forms most of the plateau. From the peak of depolarization, the overshoot is lost (phase 1), and in the case of atrial and Purkinje tissue and subepicardial ventricular cells, the transient outward potassium current I_{to} flows at this stage. In the remaining ventricular myocardium, I_{to} is not as strong. Therefore, phase 1 is much better defined in atrial and Purkinje fibers than in the ventricular myocardium (exception: epicardial cells, Fig. 4-22). As soon as phase 1 has passed, a relatively flat plateau forms (phase 2), which merges into the phase of rapid repolarization (phase 3).

Phase 3 is complex in origin. It determines the action potential duration (Table 4-8). One of the major proposals is that as a result of the initial depolarization (phase 0), potassium currents are activated after a delay (I_{kr}, I_{ks}, and I_{k1}), thereby terminating the action potential. A second proposal is that the calcium channel closes in response to increased internal calcium (32), so that there is no more influx of calcium. Third, the inward current generated by sodium–calcium exchange ceases and becomes an outward current (see next section). Fourth, an inward flow of negatively charged chloride ions might contribute, especially dur-

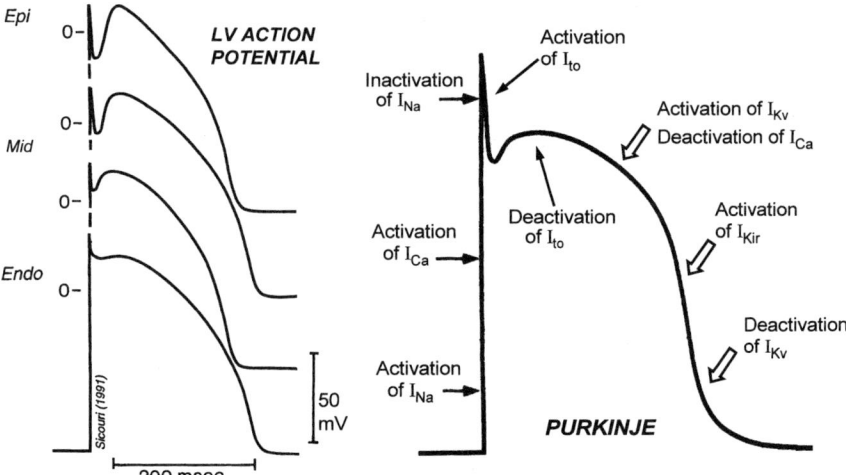

FIG. 4-22. **Contrasting ventricular and Purkinje action potential patterns. Left:** Left ventricular action potential, comparing epicardial, mid-myocardial, and endocardial patterns. Note prominent spike-and-dome pattern in epicardial (*Epi*) cells, the result of activity of the early repolarizing potassium current (I_{to}). *Mid*, mid-myocardial; *Endo*, endocardial. For technical details, see Sicouri and Antzelevitch, Circ Res 1991;68:1729. **Right:** The currents associated with the Purkinje fiber action potential are shown: I_{Na}, sodium current; I_{Ca}, calcium current; I_{to}, transient outward current; I_K or I_{Kv}, voltage-gated or delayed rectifier potassium current; I_{K1} or I_{Kir}, background potassium current or inward rectifier. For further details, see Hauswirth et al. (41).

TABLE 4-8. Currents terminating action potential plateau

Increased outward positive currents
 Potassium current I_k (to lesser extent I_{k1})
Decrease of inward positive currents
 L-calcium current
 Na/Ca exchange current (sodium entry)
 Slow decay phase of sodium current
Increase of inward negative current
 Chloride current $I_{Ca(cAMP)}$

---

ing catecholamine stimulation (Fig. 4-21). Once the action potential is over, the resting membrane potential is restored and maintained (phase 4). During this diastolic phase of electrical rest, the activity of the sodium–potassium pump and the various exchange systems restore any remaining ionic balance across the sarcolemma. In atrial and ventricular cells, when the resting membrane potential has been regained, it remains stable throughout diastole so that these cells cannot fire spontaneously. In the sinoatrial and atrioventricular nodes, spontaneous diastolic depolarization can occur (phase 4) by complex mechanisms (to be described in Chapter 5). Such depolarization is known as phase 4 depolarization and is relatively slow when compared with the rapid depolarization of phase 0.

SODIUM–CALCIUM EXCHANGE

Sodium–calcium exchange has an important role in the normal cardiac action potential, excitation-contraction coupling, and the arrhythmias of heart failure (33). Three sodium ions are exchanged with one calcium ion through a process not requiring energy but responsive to the membrane potential and the concentration of sodium and calcium ions on each side of the membrane. Because three Na^+ ions exchange with one Ca^{2+}, the exchange is *electrogenic* in the direction of sodium transport.

Any lingering doubt about the existence of the exchanger has been set to rest by Nicoll et al. (34) who cloned its structure. There are 970 amino acids, with a molecular weight of 108 kd, and part of the structure has homology to the sodium pump. There is a large cytoplasmic domain of 520 amino acids to which calmodulin binds. The meaning of this potential control mechanism is still unclear. There are now several relatively specific peptide inhibitors of sodium–calcium exchange (16).

Because sodium and calcium ions can move either inwardly or outwardly, in part in response to the membrane potential (Fig. 4-23), there must be a specific membrane potential at which the ions are so distributed that they can move one way as easily as the other. This *reversal potential* ($E_{Na/Ca}$) could theoretically be calculated from the concentrations of sodium and calcium ions on each side of the membrane. Yet the subsarcolemmal sodium and calcium ion concentrations (more correctly, their activities) are not known. The reversal potential may be halfway between the resting membrane potential and the depolarized state (16).

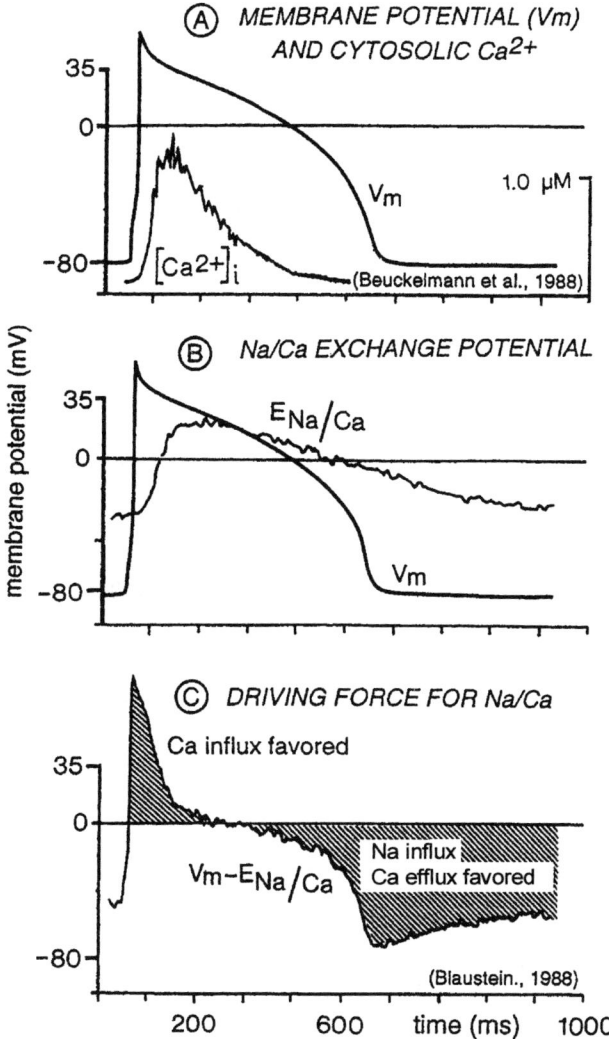

FIG. 4-23. Sodium–calcium exchanger and action potential. Proposed role during various phases of the cardiac ventricular action potential. **A:** Relationship between action potential and internal calcium. **B:** The potential for the sodium–calcium exchanger ($E_{Na/Ca}$). Note that early, soon after the onset of rapid depolarization, conditions are such that Ca^{2+} influx is favored **(C)**, whereas later during phase 3 of the action potential (Fig. 4-2), conditions favor Ca^{2+} efflux and therefore Na^+ influx. Because three sodium ions are exchanged for one calcium ion, there is a net inward current flow that contributes to the late phase of the action potential. Recent data suggest an abrupt increase in submembrane internal calcium within one millisecond of L-channel opening, thereby abbreviating the influx of calcium via this exchanger (44). V_m (Modified from Blaustein MP. Sodium/calcium exchange and the control of contractility in cardiac muscle and vascular smooth muscle. *J Cardiovasc Pharmacol* 1988;12[Suppl 5]:S56–S58.)

Changing the membrane potential from the resting value of, for example, −85 mV to +20 mV in the phase of rapid depolarization affects the sodium–calcium exchange in such a way that sodium ions tend to exit and calcium ions to enter, sometimes called reverse mode sodium–calcium exchange. Predisposing to this early outward movement of sodium ions is their internal accumulation in a small subsarcolemmal space (see fuzzy space, later in this section). During this early phase of the action potential plateau, calcium ions enter both by the exchange mechanism and through the calcium channel (Fig. 4-23).

Consequently, the rapid accumulation of calcium ions within the subsarcolemmal space changes the balance of charges in such a way that the tendency is for calcium ions to leave and for sodium ions to enter. Therefore, during the late phase of the action potential plateau, it is postulated that the exchanger operates in the forward mode (or inward mode) to promote an inward sodium current, thereby contributing to the late phase of the action potential duration (16).

The above-simplified scheme of sodium and calcium ion movements during the action potential is derived from first principles. The scheme does not reflect hard experimental data apart from the changes in the membrane potential during the action potential pattern development and the internal overall cytosolic calcium ion concentration. Other factors must be extrapolated or calculated from computer models.

The driving force of the exchanger is $E_m - E_{Na/Ca}$, where E_m is the membrane potential and $E_{Na/Ca}$ is the reversal potential for the current carried by the sodium–calcium exchanger. This reversal potential is $3E_{Na} - 2E_{Ca}$, which in turn depends on the voltage differentials and transmembrane activities of sodium and calcium ions, all of which are constantly changing. When E_m is more positive than $E_{Na/Ca}$, sodium ions tend to be driven out, and when E_m is more negative than $E_{Na/Ca}$, calcium ions tend to leave (Fig. 4-23).

Postulated Role of Exchanger in Arrhythmias

Repetitive rhythmic activity of the sodium–calcium exchanger may explain some triggered arrhythmias (Fig. 20-8). Calcium entry will be associated with egress of calcium ions and electrogenic entry of sodium ions. The further postulate is that there should be recycling of the excess of cytosolic calcium ions in and out of the sarcoplasmic reticulum, which would cause a rhythmic inward current, the *transient inward current*. There is good evidence of the activity of this current in digitalis-induced ventricular arrhythmias and increasing evidence of its role in ischemic and reperfusion arrhythmias.

RESTITUTION OF IONIC BALANCE
Sodium and Calcium

As a direct result of the rapid opening of the sodium channel followed by the slower opening of the calcium channel, each action potential will lead to an early gain of sodium ions and a later gain of calcium ions. The sodium–calcium exchanger can theoretically correct both of these ionic imbalances. Early activity of the exchanger, soon after the onset of sodium influx through the sodium channel, will theoretically help to extrude the sodium ions just gained. Later operation of the sodium–calcium exchange in the forward mode will help extrude the calcium ions already gained. There is at present no proof that these neat hypothetical balancing acts actually occur; yet the concept is attractive. Computer calculations suggest that sodium–calcium exchange continues, even when the cell is fully repolarized, to help the cytosolic calcium revert to the resting (diastolic) levels (16). Of the calcium ions entering the cytosol to initiate systole, approximately 75% are liberated from the sarcoplasmic reticulum and approximately the same percentage returns to the sarcoplasmic reticulum (Fig. 6-2). The other 25% enters from the T tubule by either the L channels or the sodium–calcium exchanger. Approximately the same amount leaves the myocyte by the sodium–calcium exchanger functioning in the opposite direction. Thus, the sodium–calcium exchanger helps to restitute the ionic imbalances created by the sequential opening of the sodium and calcium channels and the calcium transient that underlies excitation–contraction coupling.

Potassium

During the repolarization phase of the action potential, there is a net, albeit small, loss of potassium ions through the open potassium channels. To pump these ions back into the cell against a large concentration gradient requires the activity of the sodium pump.

SODIUM–PROTON EXCHANGE AND ACID-BASE HOMEOSTASIS

The internal pH (pH_i) is more alkaline than can be expected if protons (H^+) were passively distributed across the cardiac cell membrane (35). Therefore, protons must be transported out of the myocyte. Such transport is achieved by the electroneutral one-for-one exchange of Na^+ and H^+ (Fig. 4-24). The activity of this exchanger (also called an antiporter) is driven by the gradient of sodium ions, much higher outside than inside the myocyte (Fig. 4-4). The function of the exchanger can be defined by a number of inhibitors, including the diuretic amiloride and the specific inhibitor HOE 694.

This exchanger corrects an acid load during ischemia and acidosis by transporting protons (H^+) out of the cell while transporting Na^+ into the cell. The resultant increase of internal sodium can be dealt with either by the operation of the sodium–calcium exchanger or by the sodium–potassium pump. The former promotes calcium entry with a risk of arrhythmias and contracture (Fig. 20-13). Pathologically, the exchanger may mediate some of the adverse effects of chronic β-adrenergic stimulation, presumably by indirectly promoting calcium entry via the sodium–calcium exchanger (36).

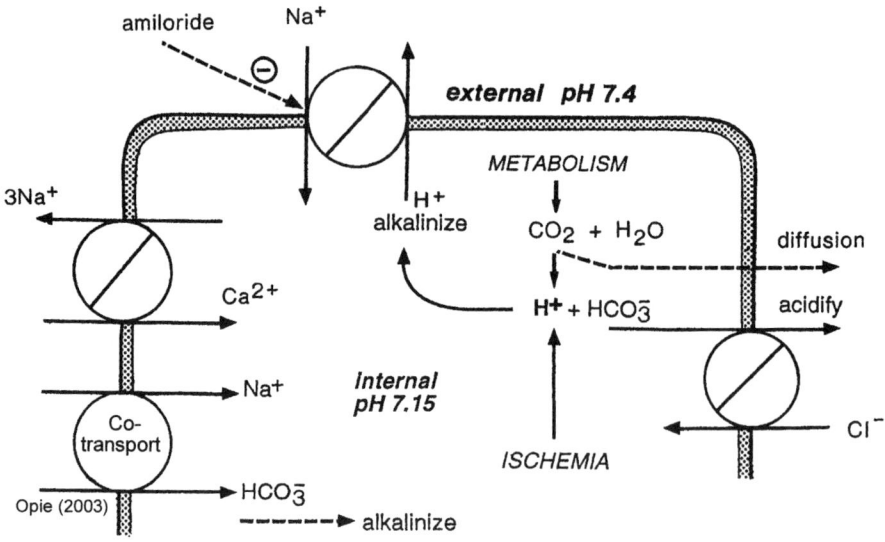

FIG. 4-24. Intracellular acid-base homeostasis. Proposed role of sodium–hydrogen exchanger and interaction with sodium–calcium exchanger. The sodium–HCO$_3$ cotransporter and chloride–HCO$_3$ exchanger act to alkalinize and acidify, respectively.

SODIUM–POTASSIUM PUMP

To reiterate, the resting heart cell sarcolemma is relatively impermeable to sodium ions but becomes highly permeable with the opening of the sodium gate initiated by depolarization. Even more sodium ions enter during the later phase of the action potential plateau by sodium–calcium exchange. All such sodium ions must eventually be returned to the extracellular space or the cell will be overloaded with sodium, with the further threat of absorption of water by osmosis, which could burst the overloaded cells. Most of this influx of sodium across the sarcolemma is corrected by the activity of the sodium–potassium pump. A lesser component is linked to the sodium–calcium exchange system when it transiently functions to extrude sodium from the cell during the early phase of the action potential (Fig. 4-23).

The sodium–potassium pump uses energy to extrude sodium out of the cell and potassium into the cell against the electrochemical gradients (Fig. 4-25). Although commonly called the sodium pump, more accurate names are the sodium–potassium pump or the Na$^+$/K$^+$-ATPase. The pump is activated by internal sodium or external potassium and uses energy in the form of ATP complexed to magnesium. Binding sites for ATP, Na$^+$, K$^+$, and digitalis have been identified.

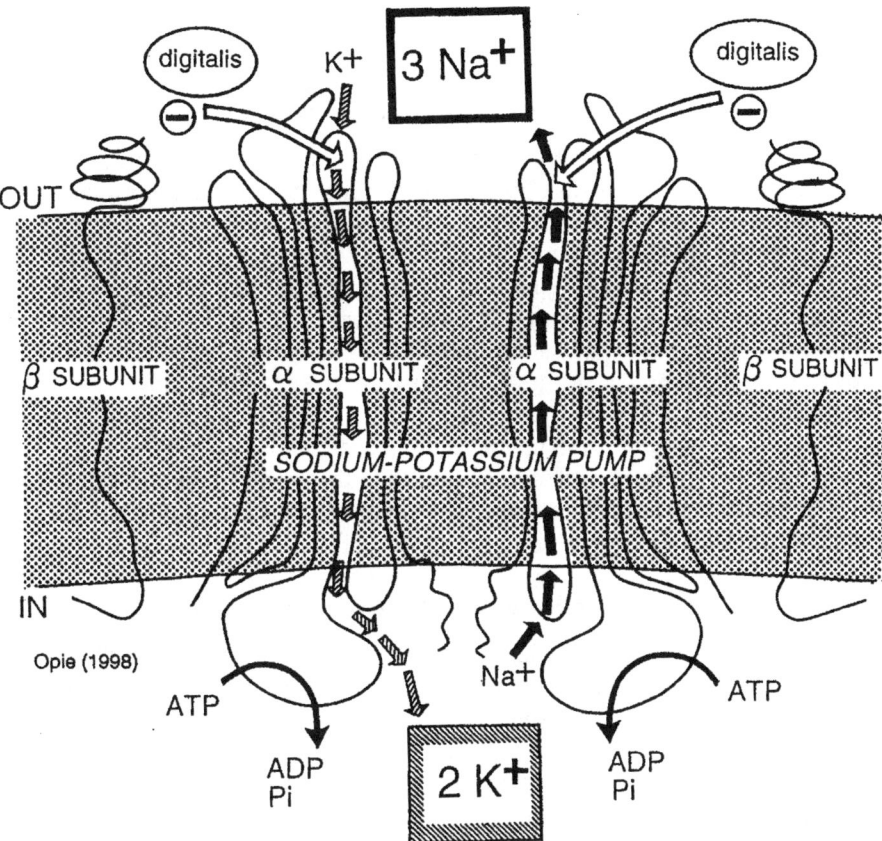

FIG. 4-25. Sodium pump function and structure. The sodium pump (also called the Na+/K+ ATPase) transports three sodium ions outward and two potassium ions inward. In structure, the pump is thought to consist of two α subunits, each of molecular weight approximately 112,000, and of two surrounding β subunits of molecular weight approximately 35,000. The ionic channel is located in the α domain, which also has (1) the external digitalis binding site, (2) the external potassium binding site, (3) the internal sodium binding site, and (4) the adenosine 5′-triphosphate (*ATP*) hydrolysis site. Note that external potassium inhibits the binding of digitalis. *ADP*, adenosine 5′-diphosphate; P_i, inorganic phosphate.

$$3 \ (Na^+) \ in \rightarrow 3 \ (Na^+) \ out$$

$$2 \ (K+) \ out \rightarrow 2 \ (K^+) \ in$$

$$MgATP^{2-} \rightarrow MgADP^{1-} + P_i^{2-} + H^+$$

One ATP molecule is used per transport cycle. The ions are first secluded within the pump protein, then extruded to either side. One positive charge must leave the cell for each three sodium ions exported because only two potassium ions are imported, so that the pump is *electrogenic*. The outward current thus generated is called I_P. It makes a relatively small but definite contribution to the normal resting negative membrane potential (Fig. 4-4) and to repolarization (37).

Sodium Pump Activation by Ions

The sodium–potassium pump is asymmetrically situated in the sarcolemma so that sodium-activation sites are located on the internal surface and most of the potassium activation sites are on the external surface (Fig. 4-25). The pump is activated as the internal sodium increases, e.g., after repetitive openings of the sodium channel. According to the fluid mosaic model of the cell membrane, the lipid bilayer is interspersed with globular proteins, some of which penetrate the membrane. The sodium–potassium pump is probably such a protein. When K^+ binds to the outside or Na^+ to the inside surface, the enzyme changes its molecular configuration, which is transmitted to other subunits of the sodium pump, which also change their configuration to the active form. ATP binds to the enzyme to form a phosphorylated intermediate that breaks down to provide the energy required for transport of sodium and potassium ions against a concentration gradient. Thus, the pump is activated, and 3 Na^+ exchanged for 2 K^+.

Molecular Structure of the Sodium Pump

The α subunit consists of a long polypeptide chain, with N and C terminal units, and a molecular weight of approximately 112 kd. There are at least six and possibly eight transmembrane spanning units (Fig. 4-25). External digitalis and potassium binding sites are located on the external hinges between the transmembrane units, whereas sodium binds to an inner hinge. The hydrolytic site for ATP is also defined. The significance of the phosphorylation sites remains unknown. Phosphorylation does not explain the stimulating effects of β-adrenergic activity on the pump (37).

Significance of the Digitalis Effect

Digitalis-type compounds have been used for the failing heart since 1785. They include digitalis leaf, previously used, and now digoxin and ouabain. They all inhibit the sodium–potassium pump to increase internal sodium. The "reverse mode" sodium–calcium exchange is thereby promoted with an increase in internal calcium and a positive inotropic effect. The significance is twofold. First, digoxin improves the contractile state of the myocardium. Second, digitalis compounds are frequently used in pharmacologic experiments to eliminate the effects of this pump, thereby uncovering the role of the exchange systems.

CALCIUM PUMPS

Energy in the form of ATP is required to transport calcium ions against the large concentration gradients that exist between the relatively low calcium ion levels in the cytosol and the much higher values in the sarcoplasmic reticulum or extracellular space. The sarcoplasmic reticulum contains a battery of these calcium pumps. These pumps are switched on by a membrane protein called *phospholamban* (Greek, *phospho*, phosphate; *lamban*, receptor), which requires a phosphate group for its maximal activity (Fig. 6-9). Such phosphorylation is achieved by either catecholamine β-adrenergic stimulation or an increased cytosolic calcium ion concentration. Therefore, the increase of calcium ions associated with systole will stimulate the uptake of calcium into the sarcoplasmic reticulum to help to initiate diastole. Catecholamine stimulation will further accelerate the uptake of calcium ions into the sarcoplasmic reticulum to shorten diastole and accelerate relaxation so that the left ventricle can fill better. Another type of calcium pump, also ATP dependent, plays a small role in calcium extrusion from the cytosol (Fig. 6-2).

MAGNESIUM

Magnesium is an important constituent of the cytosol and is essential for numerous enzymatic reactions (including the sodium pump, myosin ATPase, oxidative phosphorylation, and various enzymes of glycolysis). The vital functions of ATP and other adenine nucleotides are carried out in their ionized forms chelated with magnesium. The total magnesium in the cell is approximately 8 mmol/L/kg wet weight with a calculated overall intracellular concentration of approximately 17 mmol/L (Table 4-2). Of this, approximately 10 mmol/L should be bound to adenine nucleotides and a small proportion to mitochondria (12% of total) and myofibrils (2% of total). To measure the true intracellular magnesium concentration is very difficult. The activity might be approximately 0.6 mmol/L, although the values are controversial. This value may increase to 10 times during very severe ischemia, probably because of the breakdown of magnesium bound to ATP as total ATP decreases. The mechanisms regulating magnesium transport in and out of the heart cell are still obscure; an exchanger may be involved. Currently available data suggest that magnesium is not involved in the beat-to-beat regulation of contraction, although it is an important controller of the activity of some key enzymes.

NONSPECIFIC STRETCH CHANNELS

The potential links between stretch of the myocardium, as during sustained heavy heart work, and protein synthesis are unsolved, which is required to produce compensatory hypertrophy (Chapter 13). Several types of nonmyocardial cells, varying from simple protozoa to hair cells of the ear, have the capacity to translate mechanical cell deformation into activation of an ion channel and to allow the gated entry of ions. In the myocardium, such *stretch-activated channels* may act as mechanoreceptors and admit calcium ions (38) that in turn stimulate the growth factor calcineurin. During acute cardiac stretch, stretch-activated channels may help to increase the force of cardiac contraction (see Anrep effect, Chapter 13). Yet despite intense research, there is still no clear proof that stretch-activated channels exist in the heart.

ENERGY FOR ION FLUXES

Whenever an ion is transported against a concentration gradient, energy is required. To estimate how much ATP is expended on maintenance of ionic gradients is not easy and requires a number of assumptions. It is simplest to take the case of potassium ion flux via the sodium–potassium pump. The transport of 0.7 μmol of K^+/g per minute requires 0.35 μmol of ATP/g per minute or approximately 4 μL of O_2/g per minute. This contrasts with the oxygen uptake of the human heart in basal conditions of approximately 100 μL/g per minute. Thus, very roughly, as much as 4% of the energy needs of the heart might be expended on potassium movements by the pump. The same pump is ultimately responsible for balancing sodium ion movements. When based on the requirements to pump out the sodium that has entered, much higher estimates for energy needs, as high as 15%, are obtained (Table 4-9).

Estimates suggest that the entry and exit of calcium ions across the sarcolemma requires relatively little energy, not more than 3% of the myocardial ATP usage (Table 4-9). Intracellular calcium ion movements also need energy. Calcium uptake by the sarcoplasmic reticulum in diastole requires 1 mole/L ATP for 2 mole/L calcium. Such use of energy can concentrate calcium by 1,000 to 5,000 times within the sarcoplasmic reticulum. A significant percentage of the

TABLE 4-9. *Estimated adenosine 5'-triphosphate requirements for ion fluxes and phases of cardiac action potential*

		Effect of increasing beating rate[b]		
Ion	K^+-arrested heart[a] (μmol/g wet wt/min)	75 beats/min[b] μmol/min	150 beats/min[a] μmol/min	330 beats/min[a] μmol/min
Total sodium flux	Up to 0.1	3.1	6.2	13.6
Fast channel (I_{Na})	—	0.4	0.8	1.7
Potassium flux	Included in above	Included in above	Included in above	Included in above
Calcium flux				
Slow channel (I_{si})	—	0.1–0.5	0.2–1.0	0.4–2.2
Contractile Ca^{2+} flux	—			
For 50% tension	—	~2.4	—	—
For peak tension	—	—	—	~30
Total ATP needed	10	23	41	152
Percentage breakdown				
Na^+ flux by pump	Up to 1%	15%	15%	9%
I_{Na}	—	2%	2%	1%
I_{ca}	—	0.4%–2.2%	0.5%–2.4%	0.3%–1.5%
Average internal Ca^{2+} flux	—	5%	6%	—
Peak internal Ca^{2+} flux	—	—	—	20%

[a]Isolated rat heart.
[b]Dog heart.
Data based on Table 4-5 of reference 38a. Energy for sodium influx via sodium channel is that required for subsequent outward pumping.
ATP, adenosine 5'-triphosphate.

total oxygen uptake (as much as 20%) of the heart is required for the calcium uptake associated with the process of relaxation.

SUMMARY

1. *The myocardial sarcolemma takes up potassium and ejects sodium ions* to produce the resting negative membrane potential. This process is achieved by activity of the sodium pump (sodium–potassium ATPase), which stretches across the cell membranes.
2. *As the wave of electrical excitation arrives, it initiates depolarization,* which causes a current flow that opens the voltage-activated gates of the sodium channel to allow the ultrarapid entry of positively charged sodium ions (phase 0 of the action potential). As depolarization proceeds, the calcium channel opens, being activated by a less negative voltage than the sodium channel. After depolarization ceases, there is a brief period of rapid repolarization (phase 1) before the pattern of the action potential levels off to form the plateau phase (phase 2). The continued inflow of calcium ions causes the action potential plateau.
3. *There are two major types of potassium channels,* besides the inward rectifier: voltage gated and ligand gated. The voltage-operated channels respond to depolarization in an orderly, time-dependent way. The inward rectifier (I_{Kir}) is a background current that is not activated by a voltage-dependent gate or by any regular ligand. On depolarization, this channel shuts off because of its special rectification characteristics. In the later stages of repolarization, it opens again to help the cell regain the resting membrane potential.
4. *During diastole, potassium ions leave the cardiac myocytes* as a background current that maintains the resting membrane potential. During repolarization, the potassium current starts to flow again as the rectifying current that helps to terminate the action potential plateau (phase 3), so that the resting potential is regained (phase 4).

These descriptions apply to contractile myocardial cells and conducting Purkinje fibers, not to spontaneously firing nodal tissue, which is considered in the next chapter.

ACKNOWLEDGMENT

Prof. E. Carmeliet, Leuven, Belgium, kindly provided expert advice on this chapter.

STUDENT QUESTIONS

1. What is a voltage-dependent ion channel?
2. Describe the two types of calcium channels.
3. What are the two major mechanisms for regulation of potassium channel activity? Give the name and function of four specific potassium channels and the principles of their regulation.

4. What are the phases of the action potential and how is the action potential plateau regulated?
5. Briefly describe sodium–calcium exchange and its physiologic function.

CARDIOLOGIST-IN-TRAINING QUESTIONS

1. The resting membrane potential of ventricular cells is approximately −85 mV. Which are the crucial ions involved and what governs their transmembrane distribution?
2. What is a current and what is a channel? Describe the currents that explain the phases of the cardiac ventricular action potential.
3. How is a sodium channel pore formed? Which commonly used antiarrhythmic drug alters the probability of sodium channel opening? Give one hypothesis for its mode of action.
4. Calcium channel opening is enhanced by β-adrenergic stimulation and decreased by calcium antagonist drugs. Explain each of these changes.
5. Outline the major differences between each of the following potassium currents: delayed rectifier and its rapid and slow components, inward rectifier, transient outward current, and the ATP-regulated current.
6. What is the physiologic role of the sodium–potassium pump? Explain the clinical effects of one commonly used cardiac drug by referring to this pump.

REFERENCES

1. Balser JR. The cardiac sodium channel: gating function and molecular pharmacology. *J Mol Cell Cardiol* 2001;33:599–613.
1a. Aibo S, Creazzo TL. Comparison of the number of dihydropyridine receptors with the number of functional L-type calcium channels in embryonic heart. *Circ Res* 1993;72:396–402.
1b. Wibo M, et al. Postnatal maturation of excitation-contraction coupling in rat ventricle in relation to the subcellular localization and surface density of 1,4-dihydropyridine and ryanodine receptors. *Circ Res* 1991;68:662–673.
1c. Rose WC. Macroscopic and unitary properties of physiological ion flux through L-type Ca2+ channels in guinea pig heart cells. *J Physiol* 1992;456:267–284.
1d. Coetzee WA. ATP-sensitive potassium channels and myocardial ischemia. *Cardiovasc Drugs Ther* 1992;6:201–208.
2. Aksnes G. Why do ischemic and hypoxic myocardium lose potassium. *J Mol Cell Cardiol* 1992;24:323–331.
2a. Dalby AJ, et al. Effect of glucose-insulin-potassium infusions on epicardial ECG changes and on myocardial metabolic changes after coronary artery ligation in dogs. *Cardiovasc Res* 1981;15:588.
2b. Baumgarten, Fozzard. In: Fozzard et al., eds. *The heart and cardiovascular system*, 2nd ed. New York: Raven Press, 1991:963.
2c. Page E, Polimeni PI. Magnesium exchange in rat ventricle. *J Physiol* 1972;224:121.
2d. Steenbergen C, et al. Increase in the cytosolic free magnesium during ischemia. *Circulation* 1998;80[Suppl II]:11-19.
2e. Jennings RB, Shen AC. Calcium in experimental myocardial ischemia. *Myocardiology* 1972;1:639–655.
2f. Desilets M, et al. Chloride dependence of pH modulation by beta-adrenegic agonist in rat cardiomyocytes. *Circ Res* 1994;75:862–869.

3. Woodbury JW. Interrelationships between ion transport mechanisms and excitatory events. *Fed Proc* 1963;22:31–35.
4. McCullough JR, et al. Two stable levels of diastolic potential at physiological K^+ concentrations in human ventricular myocardial cells. *Circ Res* 1990;66:191–201.
5. Sheu S-S, et al. Intra- and extracellular K^+ and Na^+ activities and resting membrane potential in sheep cardiac Purkinje strands. *Circ Res* 1980;47:692–700.
6. Goldman DE. Potential, impedance and rectification in membranes. *J Gen Physiol* 1943;27:37–60.
7. Tomaselli GF, et al. Molecular basis of permeation in voltage-gated ion channels. *Circ Res* 1993;72:491–496.
8. Grant AO. Evolving concepts of cardiac sodium channel function. *J Cardiovasc Electrophysiol* 1990;1:53–67.
9. Katz AM. Cardiac ion channels. *N Engl J Med* 1993;328:1244–1251.
10. Bennett PB, et al. On the molecular nature of the lidocaine receptor of cardiac Na^+ channels. Modification of block by alterations in the a-subunit III-IV interdomain. *Circ Res* 1995;77:584–592.
11. Yatani A, et al. Single amino acid substitutions within the ion permeation pathway alter single-channel conductance of the human L-type cardiac Ca^{2+} channel. *Circ Res* 1994;75:315–323.
11a. Suleymanian MA, Clemo HF, Cohen MN, et al. Stretch-activated channel blockers modulate cell volume in cardiac ventricular myocytes. *J Mol Cell Cardiol* 1995;27:721–728.
12. Zhang J, et al. Molecular determinants of voltage-dependent inactivation in calcium channels. *Nature* 1994;372:97–100.
13. Jan LY, et al. Potassium channels and their evolving gates. *Nature* 1994;371:119–122.
14. Undrovinas AI, et al. Gating of the late Na^+ channel in normal and failing human myocardium. *J Mol Cell Cardiol* 2002;34:1477–1489.
15. Pragnell M, et al. Calcium channel beta-subunit binds to a conserved motif in the I-II cytoplasmic linker of the alpha$_1$-subunit. *Nature* 1994;368:67–70.
16. Bers DM. Na/Ca exchange and the sarcolemmal Ca-pump. In: Bers DM, ed. *Excitation-contraction coupling and cardiac contractile force*. Dordrecht: Kluwer Academic Publishers, 2001:133–160.
17. Bean BP. Two kinds of calcium channels in canine atrial cells. Differences in kinetics, selectivity and pharmacology. *J Gen Physiol* 1985;86:1–30.
18. Carmeliet E. Cardiac ionic currents and acute ischemia: from channels to arrhythmias. *Physiol Rev* 1999;79:917–1017.
18a. Hagiwara N, et al. Contribution of two types of calcium currents to the pacemaker potentials of rabbit sino-atrial node cells. *J Physiol* 1988;395:233–253.
18b. Doerr T, et al. Ionic currents contributing to the action potential in single ventricular myocytes of the guinea pig studied with action potential clamp. *Pflugers Arch* 1990;416:230–237.
18c. Nuss HB, Hauser SR. T-type Ca^{2+} current is expressed in hypertrophied adult feline left ventricular myocytes. *Circ Res* 1993;73:777–782.
18d. Lacinova L, Hofmann F. In: Sperelakis et al., eds. *Heart physiology and pathophysiology of the heart*, 4th ed. San Diego: Academic Press, 2001:247–257.
18e. Hess P. In: Zipes, Jaliffe, eds. *Cardiac electrophysiology. From cell to bedside*. Philadelphia: WB Saunders, 1990:10–17.
18f. Mishra SK, Hermsmeyer K. Selective inhibition of T-type Ca^{2+} channels by Ro 40-5967. *Circ Res* 1994;75:144.
19. Lipscombe D. L-type calcium channels. Highs and new lows [Editorial]. *Circ Res* 2002;90:933–935.
20. Deal KK, et al. Molecular physiology of cardiac potassium channels. *Physiol Rev* 1996;76:49–67.
20a. Nitta J, et al. Subcellular mechanism for Ca(2+)-dependent enhancement of delayed rectifier K^+ current in isolated membrane patches of guinea pig ventricular myocytes. *Circ Res* 1994;74:96–104.
21. Kurokawa J, et al. Molecular basis of the delayed rectifier current I_{KS} in heart. *J Mol Cell Cardiol* 2001;33:873–882.
22. Mitcheson JS, et al. A structural basis for drug-induced long QT syndrome. *Proc Natl Acad Sci U S A* 2000;97:12329–12333.
23. Lopatin AN, et al. Inward rectifiers in the heart: an update on I_{K1}. *J Mol Cell Cardiol* 2001;33:625–638.
24. Schram G, et al. Differential distribution of cardiac ion channel expression as a basis for regional specialization in electrical function. *Circ Res* 2002;90:939–950.
25. Oudit GY, et al. The molecular physiology of the cardiac transient outward potassium current (I_{to}) in normal and diseased myocardium. *J Mol Cell Cardiol* 2001;33:851–872.

25a. Ashford MJL, et al. Cloning and functional expression of rat heart K_{ATP} channel. *Nature* 1994;370: 456–459.
25b. Yuan A, et al. The sodium-activated potassium channel is encoded by a member of the Slo gene family. *Neuron* 2003;37:765–773.
26. Krapivinsky G, et al. The G-protein-gated atrial K^+ channel I_{kACh} is a heteromultimer of two inwardly rectifying K^+-channel proteins. *Nature* 1995;374:135–141.
27. Attali B. A new wave for heart rhythms. *Nature* 1996;384:24–25.
28. Philipson LH. ATP-sensitive K^+ channels: paradigm lost, paradigm regained. *Science* 1995;270: 1159.
29. Abraham MR, et al. Coupling of cell energetics with membrane metabolic sensing. *J Biol Chem* 2002;277:24427–24434.
30. Ferrero Jr JM, et al. Simulation of action potentials from metabolically impaired cardiac myocytes. Role of ATP-sensitive K^+ current. *Circ Res* 1996;79:208–221.
31. Kantor PF, et al. Reduction of ischemic K loss and arrhythmias in rat hearts. Effect of glibenclamide, a sulfonylurea. *Circ Res* 1990;66:478–485.
32. Anderson ME. Ca^{2+}-dependent regulation of cardiac L-type Ca^{2+} channels: is a unifying mechanism at hand? *J Mol Cell Cardiol* 2001;33:639–650.
33. Pogwizd SM, et al. Arrhythmogenesis and contractile dysfunction in heart failure. *Circ Res* 2001;88: 1159–1167.
34. Nicoll DA, et al. Molecular cloning and functional expression of the cardiac sarcolemmal Na^+-Ca^{2+} exchanger. *Science* 1990;250:562–565.
35. Fliegel L. Regulation of myocardial Na^+-H^+ exchanger activity. *Basic Res Cardiol* 2001;96:301–305.
36. Engelhardt S, et al. Inhibition of Na^+-H^+ exchange prevents hypertrophy, fibrosis and heart failure in β_1-adrenergic receptor transgenic mice. *Circ Res* 2002;90:814–819.
37. Glitsch HG. Electrophysiology of the sodium-potassium-ATPase in cardiac cells. *Physiol Rev* 2001; 81:1781–1826.
38. Suleymanian MA, et al. Stretch-activated channel blockers modulate cell volume in cardiac ventricular myocytes. *J Mol Cell Cardiol* 1995;27:721–728.
38a. Opie LH. *The Heart. Physiology, metabolism, pharmacology and therapy.* Grune & Stratton, 1984.
39. Rubart M, et al. Genesis of cardiac arrhythmias: electrophysiological considerations. In: Braunwald E, et al., eds. *Heart disease*, 6th ed. Philadelphia: WB Saunders, 2001:659–699.
40. Tsien R. Excitable tissues: the heart. In: Andreoli T, et al., eds. *Physiology of membrane disorders.* New York: Plenum Press, 1986:475.
41. Hauswirth O, Singh BN. Ionic mechanisms in heart muscle in relation to the genesis and the pharmacological control of cardiac arrhythmias. *Pharmacol Rev* 1979;30:5–63.
42. Lubbe WF. Potential arrhythmogenic role of cyclic adenosine monophosphate (AMP) and cytosolic calcium overload: implications for prophylactic effects of β-blockers in myocardial infarction and proarrhythmic effects of phosphodiesterase inhibitors. *J Am Coll Cardiol* 1992;19:1622–1633.
43. Blaustein MP. Sodium/calcium exchange and the control of contractility in cardiac muscle and vascular smooth muscle. *J Cardiovasc Pharmacol* 1988;12[Suppl 5]:S56–S58.
44. Weber CR, et al. Na^+-Ca^+ exchange current and submembrane [Ca^{2+}] during the cardiac action potential. *Circ Res* 2002;90:182–189.

5

Pacemakers, Conduction System, and Electrocardiogram

Lionel H. Opie and James M. Downey

No one ionic current alone is responsible for SA node pacemaking.
Irisawa et al. (1)

The cardiac electrical impulse is generated in the sinoatrial (SA) node, rapidly conducted through the atria to the atrioventricular (AV) node, where it undergoes filtration and delay. Then another phase of rapid conduction through the His bundle and bundle branches follows, finally leading to excitation–contraction coupling in the ventricular myocyte. The whole sequence can be monitored by the electrocardiogram (ECG). The initiator of these events lies in the automatic pacemaker activity of the SA node, in which there is spontaneous diastolic depolarization. The action potential, initiated in a small group of primary pacemaker cells in the center of the SA node, spreads through peripheral regions of this node to atrial tissue and then to the rest of the heart (2).

SINOATRIAL NODE AUTOMATICITY

How does the *internal time clock* of the sinoatrial node know to undergo regular diastolic depolarization at a regular interval and thereby satisfactorily to initiate the heartbeat? The explanation for the pacemaker current that underlies automaticity in the SA node has swung away from the idea that an outward potassium current is the dominant factor to emphasize the additional and more important role of inward currents. Nonetheless, the exact regulation of the repetitive spontaneous firing of the SA node, essential for the pumping action of the heart and hence for human and animal life, is still not fully understood.

Structure of the Sinoatrial Node

Anatomically, the human SA node is spindle shaped and measures approximately $20 \times 3 \times 1$ mm. It contains clusters of cells, poor in contractile filaments,

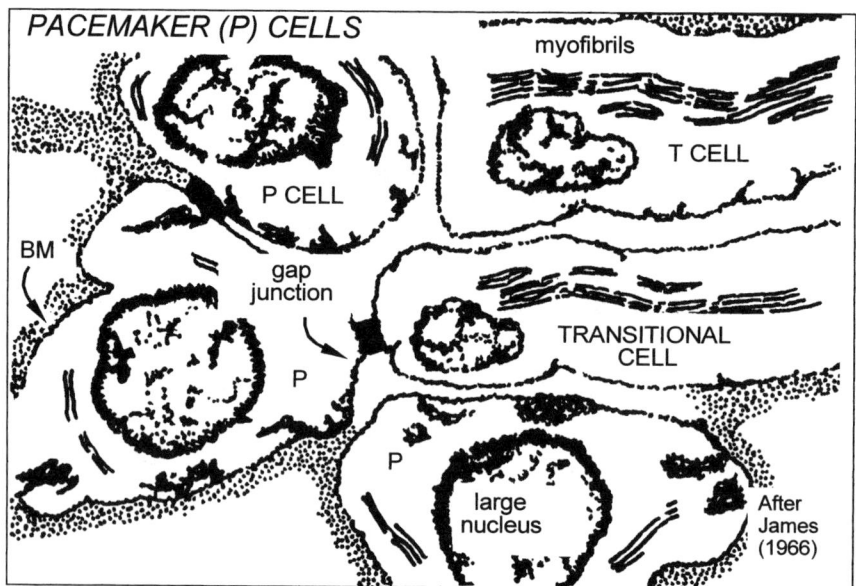

FIG. 5-1. P (pacemaker) cells of the sinoatrial node, where the heartbeat originates. These cells have few myofibrils, a large prominent nucleus, and occasional gap junctions joining the cells. Transitional T cells, closer to normal myocardial cells in histology, help to conduct the impulse away from the P cells. *BM*, basement membrane. (Modified from James et al., *Circulation* 1966;34:139).

where the automatic activity mostly resides in the *pacemaker* or *P cells* (Fig. 5-1). In contrast are *transitional cells*, which lie near the periphery of the node. Each cluster of P cells is enveloped by a basement membrane, and junctions between P cells are largely undifferentiated. P cells connect with each other by simple apposition of plasma membranes. The coordination is good enough for the transmembrane potential to change almost simultaneously in all P cells in one cluster. Synchronization between clusters of P cells occurs by conductance from a dominant pacemaker site, which shifts in response to physiologic stimuli, such as adrenergic or parasympathetic discharge (3). Because the autonomic nervous innervation is denser in the SA node than in the AV node, variations in autonomic tone have more influence on the activity of the pacemaker (SA node) rather than that of the filter (AV node).

DEPOLARIZING CURRENTS: INITIATORS OF THE HEARTBEAT

The crucial characteristic of SA tissue is the spontaneous diastolic depolarization in phase 4 of the action potential (Fig. 5-2). This depolarization starts at approximately −65 mV. When the *activation threshold* of the cell is reached at approximately −40 mV, the nodal cell fires and relatively rapid depolarization

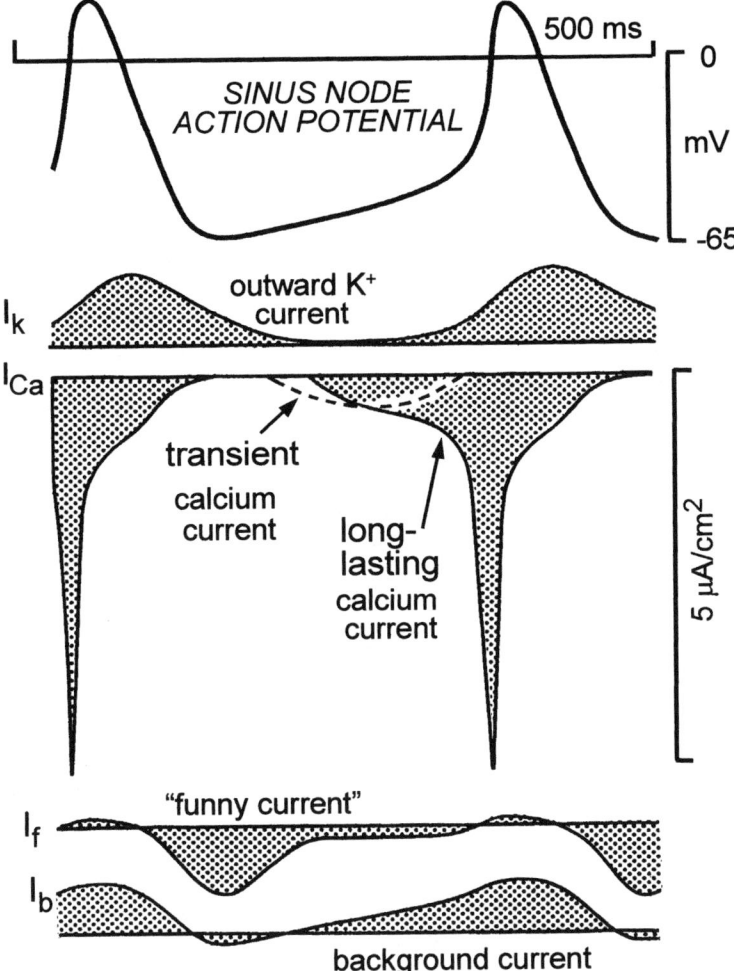

FIG. 5-2. Pacemaker currents in sinoatrial node. There are four proposed different pacemaker currents that explain "spontaneous depolarization." The repolarizing potassium current I_k is activated by full depolarization. Then, as the voltage decreases, it becomes inactivated and decays. At that time, I_f, the inward current evoked by hyperpolarization and increased by β-adrenergic stimulation, begins to flow (8) as does the postulated but controversial nonspecific inward current I_b. Approximately the same negative voltage range activates the transient inward calcium current I_{Ca-T}. Just when activation of the long-lasting calcium current I_{Ca-L} starts has not been determined, but it may be much sooner than previously thought (6). When depolarization reaches the threshold for activation of the nodal action potential at approximately −40 mV, there is major activation of I_{Ca-L} with greatly accelerated depolarization, typical of the upstroke of the action potential of the sinoatrial node. This model is based on, but substantially updated from, that of Yanagihara et al. (14).

initiates the nodal action potential. The pattern of this action potential differs markedly from that described in the previous chapter. The upstroke is markedly slower, and there is virtually no plateau. The former change is explained by the absence of the fast sodium current and the latter change by the rapid onset of potassium-dependent repolarization, the result of activation of the delayed rectifier potassium current (I_k) (Table 4-6). Regarding the crucial diastolic depolarization, the exact contribution of various currents is still controversial, as judged by various proposed models (4).

Delayed Rectifier Potassium Current (I_k)

The major potassium current in pacemaker cells is the delayed rectifier (I_k), whereas I_{k1} does not exist (1). Alterations in the rate of flow of this potassium current (I_k) are important in governing the pattern of the action potential of the SA node (Fig. 5-2). This current, also called I_{kv}, is activated by depolarization as reached at the apex of the action potential, so that it contributes to repolarization. With time (it is time dependent), it decays to allow inward currents to take over and to initiate the next wave of depolarization. Thus, the decaying potassium current is often emphasized in descriptions of SA automaticity (4,5).

Background Inward Current

This current remains when all others are blocked. Sometimes this current is called I_p (where p is pacemaker) or I_b (where b is background). The driving force is likely to be the spontaneous inward movement of sodium ions along their concentration gradient. The exact role of this background inward current is still controversial (4,6); a simplified proposal is shown in Fig. 5-2.

Slow Inward Nodal Calcium Currents

Calcium ions are essential for SA nodal pacemaker activity (2). The slow inward calcium current (I_{Ca}) explains the rising phase of the action potential. This current also contributes in part to the slowly rising depolarization phase (Fig. 5-2). Voltage clamp studies on SA cells show that the calcium current can be separated into (a) the transient component (I_{Ca-T}) with a threshold potential from approximately −60 to −50 mV or even lower (7) and (2) the long-lasting component (I_{Ca-L}) with a threshold of approximately −40 mV. A variant of I_{Ca-L}, encoded by a different gene, may be activated at lower voltages, down to approximately −60 mV to account for almost one-third of the diastolic inward current (6,7). Nonetheless, it is the transient T type that opens first because many studies show that it opens at a more negative voltage than I_{Ca-L}. Neither heart rate–lowering calcium antagonists (verapamil, diltiazem) nor β-adrenergic blockers inhibit the T current. In contrast, all these inhibit the L current that is obligatory for the relatively rapid upstroke of the SA nodal action potential. At the clinically used doses of these drugs, this inhibition is only partial, so that they slow but do not arrest the heartbeat. Beta-blockers slow the heart rate more because they also inhibit the inward current I_f.

Inward Current (I_f)

Voltage-clamp studies on the SA node T cells reveal an inward current that operates best in a voltage range more negative than that usually found in centrally located P-type SA cells. Because of its unexpected and *funny* properties, the new current was called I_f. The range of activation of this current (−90 to −50 mV) overlaps with, but does not coincide with, the normal diastolic voltage range of the spontaneously beating SA node. Thus, I_f may be fully operative only when the SA node is hyperpolarized, which explains the alternate name *hyperpolarization-activated cyclic nucleotide-gated current* (HCN). Probably both sodium and potassium ions can carry this current, although sodium ions may be dominant. The role of I_f as a potential pacemaker current remains controversial, although increasingly accepted. One important view is that I_f could be the major pacemaking current, its contribution often being overlooked (8). If the activation threshold for I_f in SA cells is only −35 to −45 mV, as sometimes claimed, I_f must be important in early depolarization (8). Strong evidence favoring its importance is that when the channel that mediates I_f is genetically ablated, then pacemaking is severely impaired, at least in neonatal heart cells (9). Alternatively, I_f may play a more major role only when β-adrenergic stimulation shifts the pacemaker focus from the dominant P cells of the SA node to the peripheral transitional cells, which have a lower negative resting membrane potential, more like that of the atrial cells. Similar pacemaker shifts may occur when the dominant pacemaker cells are injured by ischemia or inhibited by drugs.

Safety Factors in the Sinoatrial Node

In the SA node, the existence of at least four pacemaking currents (I_k, I_{Ca-T}, I_{Ca-L}, and I_f) as well as the background inward current as a fifth, plus some others not here considered (4) provides a safety factor so that inhibition of any one current still leaves several others to carry on the vital depolarizing function (Fig. 5-2). Which of these pacemaker currents is most important? Irisawa et al. (1) and others (6) propose that all four currents play a role. First, there is the decay of the outward K^+ current, I_k, already activated by the preceding nodal action potential. Then three currents depolarize to the threshold for spontaneous firing, namely, the background inward current, I_f, and both calcium currents.

Pacemaking Currents: Summary

Thus, there are many safety factors built into SA pacemaking. When "one pacemaking current fails, there is another waiting in the wings to take over" (1).

AUTONOMIC CONTROL OF SINOATRIAL NODE

The tachycardia of exercise or emotional excitement results from the combination of sympathetic stimulation and withdrawal of inhibitory parasympathetic (vagal) activity. Because vagal activity promotes bradycardia and adrenergic activity promotes tachycardia, it would be logical to suppose that these two contrasting effects on the heart rate could be explained by opposite effects on the SA node (Fig. 5-3). A simple hypothesis lies in the opposite effects on the formation of cyclic adenosine $3',5'$-monophosphate (cAMP) in sinus node cells (8). Thus

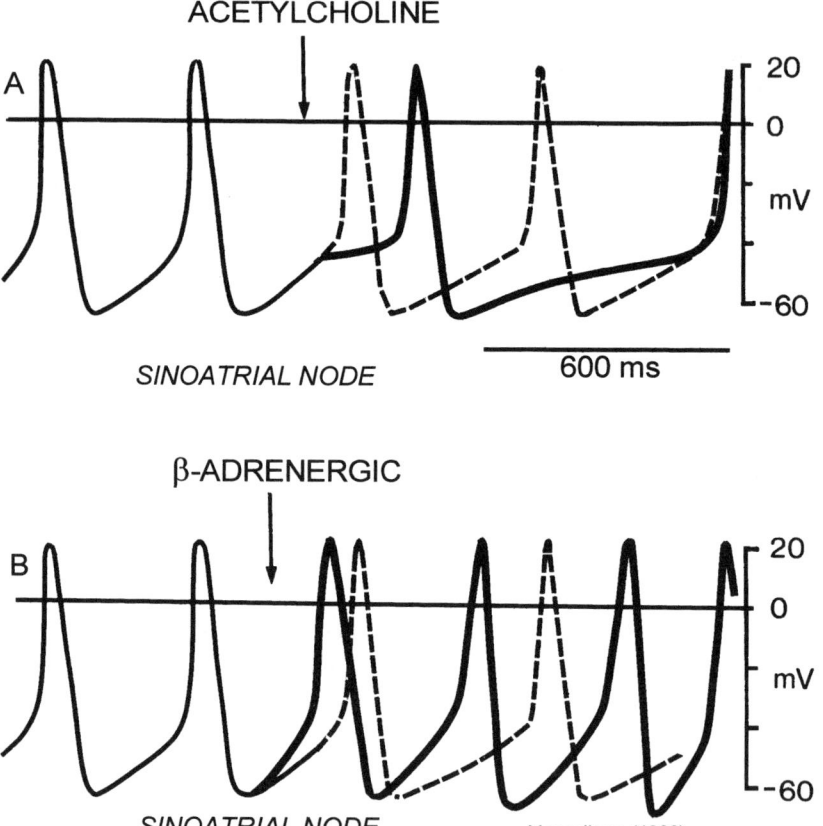

FIG. 5-3. Autonomic influences on sinus node. A: Increased vagal tone inhibits the sinoatrial node. The vagal neurotransmitter acetylcholine slows the heart rate (sinus bradycardia if fewer than 60 beats per minute) mainly by slowing the rate of diastolic depolarization. For basic traces, see Yanagihara et al. (14). **B:** Adrenergic stimulation of sinoatrial node. β-Adrenergic stimulation accelerates the cardiac pacemaker and increases its rate of firing (sinus tachycardia if more than 100 beats per minute) by multiple mechanisms including increased I_f and I_{Ca-L}. Intense β-receptor occupancy leads to hyperpolarization that further opens I_f. A pacemaker shift may be involved (see page 125).

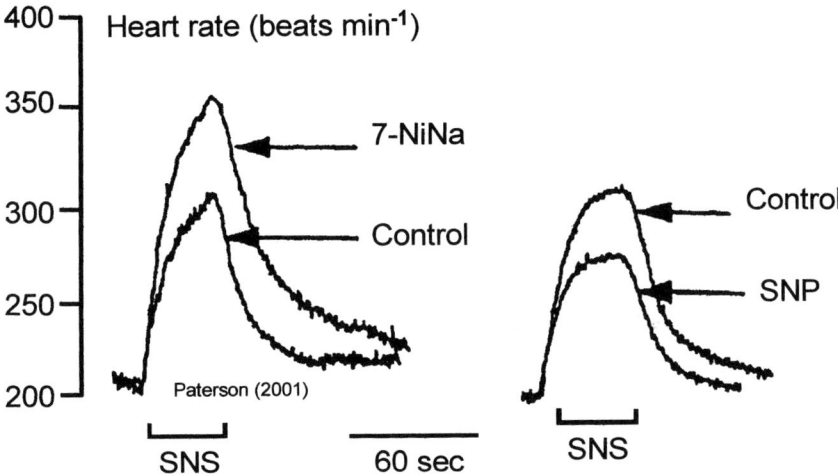

FIG. 5-4. Nitric oxide mediates cholinergic effects on sinoatrial node. Left: Sympathetic nerve stimulation increases the heart rate of isolated guinea pig atria. The inhibitory effect of nitric oxide limits the increase in rate because addition of 7-nitro indazole (7-NiNa), an inhibitor of nitric oxide synthase, further increases the rate. **Right:** Conversely, addition of the nitric oxide donor sodium nitroprusside decreases the heart rate. For schematic explanation of effects, see Figure 7-17. (From Paterson, *Exp Physiol* 2001;86:1, with permission.)

β-adrenergic stimulation acting via cAMP, increases the probability of opening of I_f and of the long-lasting inward calcium current (I_{Ca-L}). The transient component (I_{Ca-T}) is unaffected. The enhanced opening of I_f and of I_{Ca-L} causes the rate of diastolic depolarization to increase with more rapid SA node pacemaker firing. These same events are inhibited by vagal stimulation that releases nitric oxide at the nerve terminals to liberate acetylcholine and to slow the heart rate (Figs. 5-4 and 7-17).

Hyperpolarization Effects on the Sinoatrial Node

At higher concentrations of the autonomic messengers, hyperpolarization has added effects. Thus, intense vagal stimulation activates the *acetylcholine-regulated potassium channel* (Table 4-7), so that the outward potassium current I_{KACh} flows (Fig. 4-19). The potential of the membrane of the SA node is driven in a hyperpolarizing direction as the positively charged potassium ions leave the inner side of the sarcolemma. The more negative hyperpolarized voltage decreases the rate at which the activation threshold is reached. Of interest, adenosine, a breakdown product of adenosine 5′-triphosphate, activates the same channel. Marked adrenergic stimulation also hyperpolarizes the SA node by a *pacemaker shift* (3) from the normal dominant P cells to the more peripheral T cells (Fig. 5-1) that are more polarized in diastole. The consequent hyperpolarization changes the pacemaker potential in early diastole into the zone required

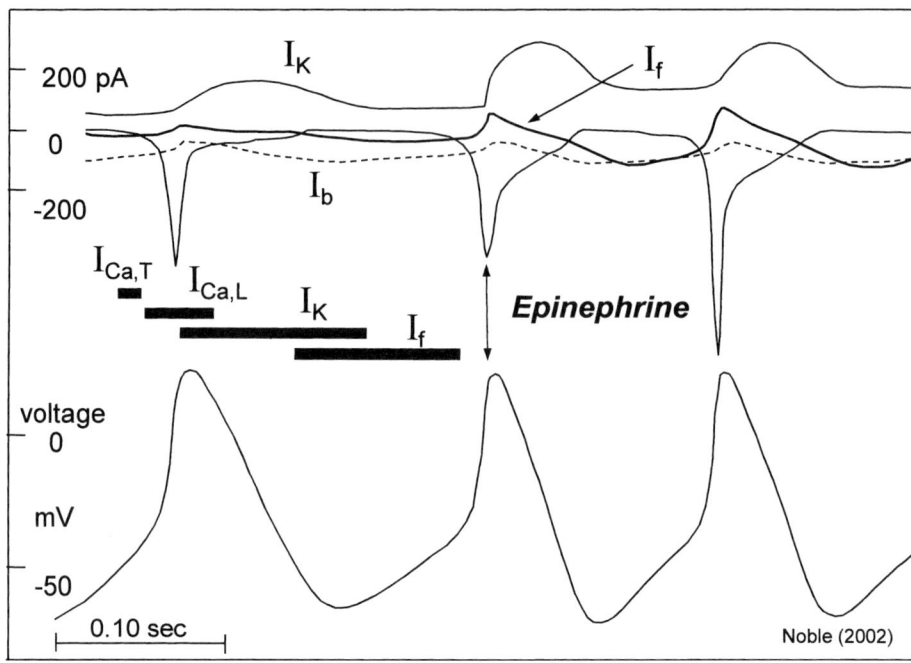

FIG. 5-5. Effect of epinephrine on pacemaker currents. Increased rate of sinoatrial discharge on addition of the β-adrenergic stimulant epinephrine is obtained by increased inward currents I_f and I_{ca-L} with increased outward current I_k. **Top:** Computer-calculated change in currents. Lower part shows the sinus node action potential (compare with Figure 5-3). For explanation of currents, see Figure 5-2. (Courtesy of Prof. D. Nobel, University Department of Physiology, Oxford, England.)

for increased activity of I_f (Fig 5-5), which therefore accelerates the rate of spontaneous depolarization. Thus, β-adrenergic receptor stimulation acts through multiple mechanisms to explain how exercise creates the tachycardia required to increase the cardiac output.

Intrinsic Heart Rate

This is uncovered when autonomic control is removed by the combined pharmacologic blockade of sympathetic β-adrenergic and parasympathetic vagal activity (10). In normal subjects, the intrinsic rate can be as much as 50% higher than the resting rate, showing that normally vagal inhibition is more powerful than adrenergic stimulation. In the presence of heart failure, the resting rate is increased because of the increased adrenergic tone required to maintain the blood pressure (Chapter 16). The ability of the heart rate to increase in heart failure is limited, which means that with exercise, the cardiac output cannot increase to the levels required for adequate muscle perfusion, and therefore fatigue sets in.

Overdrive Suppression

Overdrive suppression is the phenomenon whereby the pacing by the sinus node actually depresses the activity of other potential pacemaker cells, as found in the AV node and elsewhere. *Postpacing inhibition* is a closely related event whereby pacemaker activity is slow to resume when an induced tachycardia is terminated. When the sinus node is diseased, as in the *sick sinus syndrome* of the elderly, the SA node may suddenly slow and other pacemakers may not fire because of overdrive suppression resulting in cardiac arrest. The mechanism of overdrive suppression usually is studied in isolated Purkinje tissue, which is a potential subsidiary pacemaker with a prominent sodium channel. During overdrive suppression, induced by tachycardia, the slope of diastolic depolarization is decreased, and the voltage required to reach threshold is more positive. Hence, it is more difficult to initiate the action potential. Sinus arrest may be followed by periods of ectopic tachycardia in an apparent attempt to compensate. Adenosine accumulation, possibly also acting by hyperpolarization, is an alternate or additional cause of overdrive suppression, acting on the AV node.

PROPAGATION OF IMPULSE

After the impulse has formed in the SA node, it spreads very rapidly throughout the atrium to reach the AV node. In atrial tissue, the action potential has a different pattern, being dominated by a fast sodium channel that gives the rapid upstroke (Fig. 5-6). The action potential duration of atrial tissue is short (when measured at 50% of the peak amplitude) compared with that of the ventricles. The lesser force of contraction developed in the atria than in the ventricles can be related to the shorter action potential duration because the inward flow of calcium ions through the calcium channel is less. There are also fewer atrial T-tubules and L-type calcium channels, and there is less muscle.

The basic processes involved in depolarization and the spread of the wave of excitation should be recalled at this stage. When the electrical impulse arrives at the sarcolemma, it opens the sodium activation gate to cause depolarization to a less negative voltage, which in turn opens the calcium gate. Sodium and calcium ions enter, causing an internal microzone of positive changes within the cell. The crucial aspect of the spread of the wave of excitation is that positive ions will now be attracted to the negatively charged adjacent polarized cells (Fig. 5-7).

By these processes, the adjacent sarcolemma will tend to lose its polarity, which will then open more voltage-gated sodium channels with a further influx

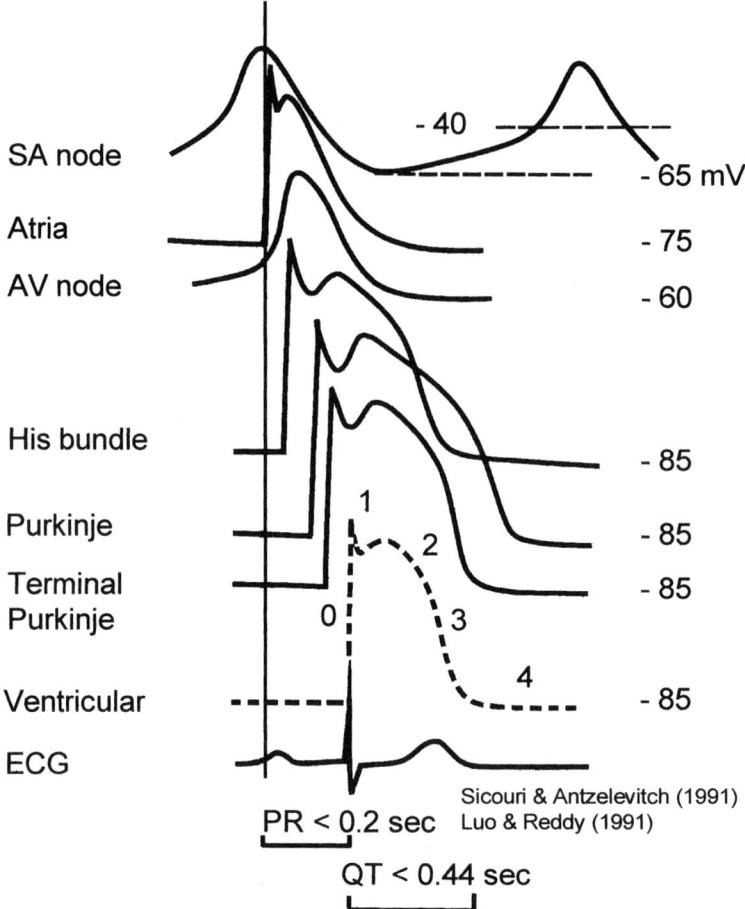

FIG. 5-6. Patterns of action potential as the impulse travels from the sinoatrial node to the ventricle. Note the relationship of each trace to the standard electrocardiographic pattern (bottom tracing). The values on the right indicate the resting membrane potential. For data on atria, atrioventricular node, and ventricles, see Wang et al. *Circ Res* 1996;78:697. For human atrial action potential, see Carmeliet. *Cardiovasc Drugs Ther* 1992;6:305. For ventricular action potential pattern, see Sicouri and Antzelevitch. *Circ Res* 1991;68:1729 and Luo and Reddy. *Circ Res* 1991;68:1501. AV, atrioventricular; PR, PR interval of the electrocardiogram; QT, QT interval of electrocardiogram.

of positive sodium ions. A self-perpetuating process occurs, and the impulse very readily spreads throughout the sarcolemma of a single heart cell and to adjacent cells via gap junctions (Fig. 3-9). The greater the rate of depolarization is, the more rapid the development of the charge differences between depolarized and polarized tissue and the more rapid the rate of conduction from cell to cell through the gap junctions of the intercalated disks (Fig. 3-9). Thus, conduc-

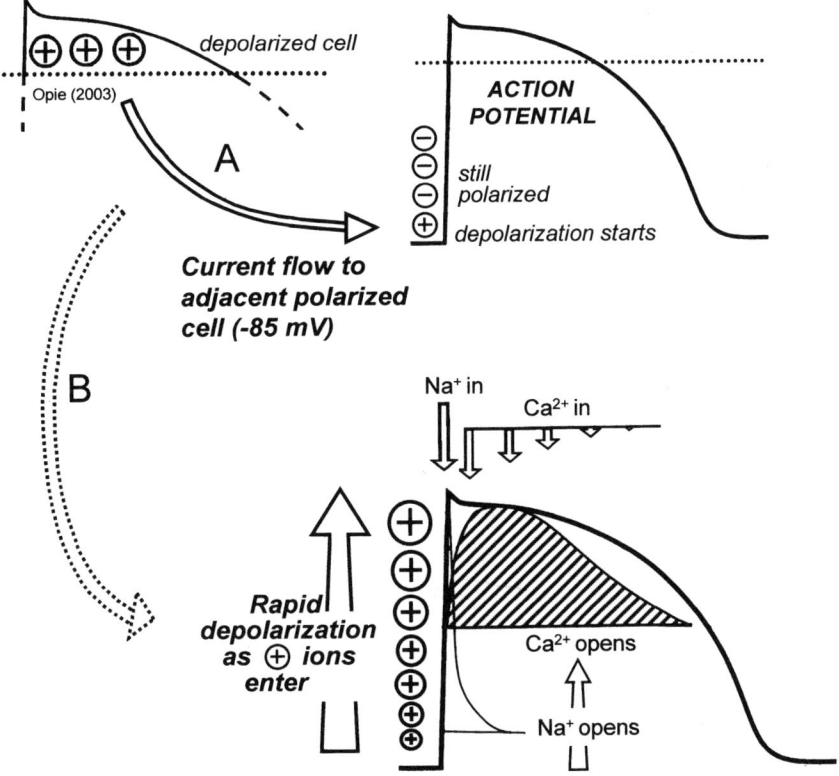

FIG. 5-7. Mechanism for spread of electrical impulse in relation to the ventricular action potential. After depolarization, a current will flow from positive to negative charges, thereby opening the sodium channel of the adjacent, previously polarized tissue and spreading the impulse rapidly.

tion of the wave of depolarization is rapid through tissues where the upstroke of the action potential is also rapid (considerable fast sodium channel activity), whereas conduction is slower through the AV node, where there is mainly calcium channel activity with a slower rate of depolarization (Fig. 5-8).

ATRIAL CONDUCTION

Are there specialized conducting fibers carrying the impulse through the atria from the sinus to the AV node? Three *internodal tracts* have been thought to serve as pathways that preferentially conduct the cardiac impulse through the atria. Histologically, they consist of cells somewhat similar to those of the Purkinje system. Physiologically, these cells are very insensitive to an increased extracellular potassium concentration, a property resembling that of the sinus

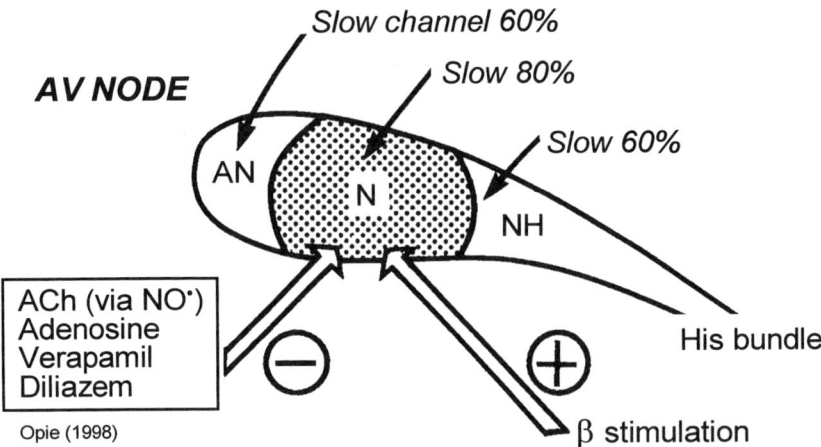

FIG. 5-8. Role of the slow calcium channel in the atrioventricular (AV) node. Note the possible contributions of slow calcium and fast sodium channels to the three parts of the AV node: the atrionodal zone (AN), middle zone of true nodal cells (N), and the nodal-His zone (NH). The figure does not distinguish between I_{Ca-T} and I_{Ca-L}. Note the effect of the inhibitory factors, such as acetylcholine (ACh), adenosine, and calcium channel blockers (verapamil, diltiazem), which slow conduction through the atrioventricular node. Conversely, β-agonists enhance conduction.

node. The pattern of atrial activation has been studied and displayed in the form of *isochrones* (11). Isochrones look like weather charts because of the wavy lines linking sites of simultaneous excitation as they radiate out from the SA node. The pattern of movement of isochrones shows how the impulse spreads. Such studies show that from the functional point of view, there are no narrow specialized atrial tracts. Rather, the entire atrial septum functions as a conduction system to take waves from the sinus to the AV node. According to this view, those atrial cells with specialized functional properties (resistance to high potassium, spontaneous diastolic depolarization) are not necessarily found in the three internodal tracts. By contrast, cardiac surgeons provide evidence of the importance of such pathways that, when damaged at operation, can promote atrial rhythm abnormalities.

ATRIOVENTRICULAR NODE

Atrial impulses cannot travel directly to the ventricles because of the connective tissue that separates the two chambers of the heart. Hence, the electrical impulse is collected in the AV node (Fig. 5-8), which is located in the right atrium just above the insertion of the tricuspid valve. From this node, the impulse continues along the bundle of His through the connective tissue separating the atria and ventricles. The AV node may be divided into three regions, atrionodal

(AN), nodal (N), and nodal-His (NH), based on the striking differences in the shape of the action potential rather than on anatomic grounds. Most of the cells of the AV node are slender transitional cells, similar to the T cells of the SA node. These are a few simple, rounded cells identical to the P cells of the sinus node, and at the margin of the node are ordinary working myocardial cells. As the AV node becomes transformed into the His bundle and conduction system, the cells become more linearly arranged, and their properties correspond more and more closely to fast conduction tissue.

Electrophysiologic Properties of the Atrioventricular Node

Many of the electrophysiologic properties of the AV node closely resemble those of the sinus node. In particular, there is a spontaneous slow diastolic depolarization with a slow upstroke, normally overridden by the sinus node. The AV node, however, can serve as a subsidiary but slower pacemaker when the main pacemaker in the sinus node fails to function. A second function of the AV node is to delay the rate at which the electrical impulse reaches the ventricles to ensure that the ventricles are relaxed at the time of atrial contraction (P wave), thereby helping to fill the ventricles. A third function of the AV node is to control the number and order of supraventricular impulses. The AV node responds in a highly complex way to the rate and type of electrical activation. Like other cardiac tissue, there is a built-in recovery time, i.e., the time lag before the next impulse can be processed, the *refractory period* (Fig. 20-4). In addition, short cycles, as when the heart rate is fast, advance the recovery time (facilitation), whereas, in contrast, sustained very fast impulses slow conduction (fatigue). All three properties are required to explain the great variation in the responses of the AV node, including the phenomenon of AV block (see later in this chapter).

Autonomic Control of Atrioventricular Node

The space just behind the AV node (*retronodal space*) is richly supplied with autonomic nerves. Here, adrenergic nerves deliver stimulatory sympathetic stimuli to the AV node to increase the rate of conduction (*positive dromotropic effect*), whereas vagal cholinergic nerves deliver inhibitory stimuli (*negative dromotropic effect*). These opposing effects are mediated by adrenergic stimulation and cholinergic inhibition of the L-type calcium current. When there is vagal stimulation, several mechanisms combine ultimately to inhibit the calcium current. As in the case of the SA node, interaction with G proteins inhibits the formation of cAMP and opens the K^+ channel, both of which tend to close the calcium channels. Also, as in the case of the SA node (Fig. 5-4), vagal stimulation of neuronal nitric oxide synthase forms nitric oxide, which in turn releases acetylcholine (Fig. 7-18) that tends to close the L-type calcium channels.

Inhibition of the Atrioventricular Node by Calcium Channel Blockers

The contribution of the long-lasting calcium current to the action potential is greatest in the central nodal zone (Fig. 5-8) where automaticity is absent and where the upstroke of the action potential increases most slowly. This is one of the few sites where conduction is by calcium channels rather than by sodium channels, hence the selectivity for the calcium channel blockers. Of these agents, verapamil and diltiazem are most inhibitory on the AV node. Most other drugs of the calcium channel blocker family do not inhibit the AV node sufficiently to have clinical effects on this node.

Inhibition of Atrioventricular Node by Adenosine

Adenosine, a breakdown product of adenosine 5'-triphosphate, both inhibits the L-type calcium current and hyperpolarizes the cell, the latter via the adenosine-sensitive potassium channel (Table 4-7). These effects, similar to those of acetylcholine, inhibit the AV node, which explains its pharmacologic effect in interrupting reentry pathways that travel through this node (Fig. 20-5). The adenosine effect occurs through the adenosine A_1 receptors, and then its inhibitory G protein targets the same K channel as does acetylcholine (Fig. 4-19).

HIS BUNDLE AND ITS BRANCHES: PURKINJE FIBERS

The His bundle, which divides into left and right bundles, runs from the AV node. It penetrates the connective tissue dividing atria and ventricles and is the only conducting connection between these chambers. The cells found in the common bundle and bundle branches are the characteristic Purkinje cells (Chapter 3). They are adapted to the rapid conduction of the electrical impulse as follows. First, these cells are approximately three times wider than the standard ventricular myocytes (Table 5-1), the principle being the resistance to electrical conduction decreases as the cellular diameter increases. Second, the sparseness of myofibrils and T tubules decreases the resistance to internal conduction. Third, Purkinje cells are packed tightly together so that the diameter effectively available for conduction is that of the entire bundle rather than of the individual components. Finally, there are numerous end-to-end gap junctions that facilitate faster conduction between cells. All these properties confer on Purkinje cells the ability to conduct electrical impulses extremely quickly (200 cm per second) to enable all the cells of the ventricles to be excited almost simultaneously.

Although Purkinje cells have the potential for spontaneous diastolic depolarization, two factors keep them from doing so. First, the rate of spontaneous firing is much slower than that of nodal tissue, being only approximately 30 per minute. Thus, the potential automaticity is overdriven by that of both the sinus and AV nodes. Second, although the Purkinje pacemaker current I_f operates at a negative voltage range, as found in normally polarized Purkinje fibers, such

TABLE 5-1. *The four pacemaker currents in sinoatrial node*

Current	Qualities	Proposed role
Outward decaying current I_k	Initial activation at −50 mV, fully activated at −10 mV[a]	Depolarization inactivates so that the inward currents take over
Inward background current I_p or I_b	Controversial role; may be substantial (6)	May contribute to spontaneous depolarization
Inward current I_f (Na⁺ and K⁺ ions)	Initially activated at hyperpolarizing voltages; range, −90 to −50 mV[b]; may be activated at less negative voltages (8)	May initiate spontaneous depolarization especially during β-adrenergic stimulation
Inward calcium currents I_{Ca-T} and I_{Ca-L}	I_{Ca-T} activated at −60 to −50 mV[c]	Contributes to diastolic depolarization
	I_{Ca-L} activated at −40 mV[c] or possibly as low as −60 mV (6); inhibited by Ca^{2+} and indirectly by beta-blockers	Accounts for steep upstroke of action potential, also active in diastolic depolarization[c,d]

[a–d]See reference 11a–11d.
Ca^{2+} blockers, calcium channel blocking drugs.

fibers have a high resting potassium conductance, so that the outward potassium current more than neutralizes the inward current carried by I_f. When the Purkinje fibers, however, are damaged, as may occur in ischemia, the resting voltage range moves into that appropriate for firing of I_f, with the risk of spontaneous depolarization and ectopic beats (Chapter 20).

The His bundle has a dual blood supply, from both the left anterior and posterior descending coronary arteries, so that ischemic damage is unusual. In contrast, the bundle branches run to the ventricles where coronary artery disease is common and can cause ischemia of the bundles with the risk of bundle branch block.

THE ELECTROCARDIOGRAM

There is a large gap from the origin of the heartbeat in the specialized cells of the sinus node to the contraction of the ventricular myofibril. That gap is bridged first by the rapid conduction of the electrical impulse through the atria, so as to fire the AV node, which in turn sends another impulse down the specialized His bundle and Purkinje fibers. The terminal branches (*arborization* of the Purkinje system) spread the impulse throughout the ventricles, eventually traveling along the sarcolemma of the myocytes, from where the process of *excitation–contraction coupling* links the wave of depolarization on the cell surface to the contractile system. This whole sequence can be monitored relatively simply by measuring voltage changes on the body surface with the ECG (Fig. 5-9).

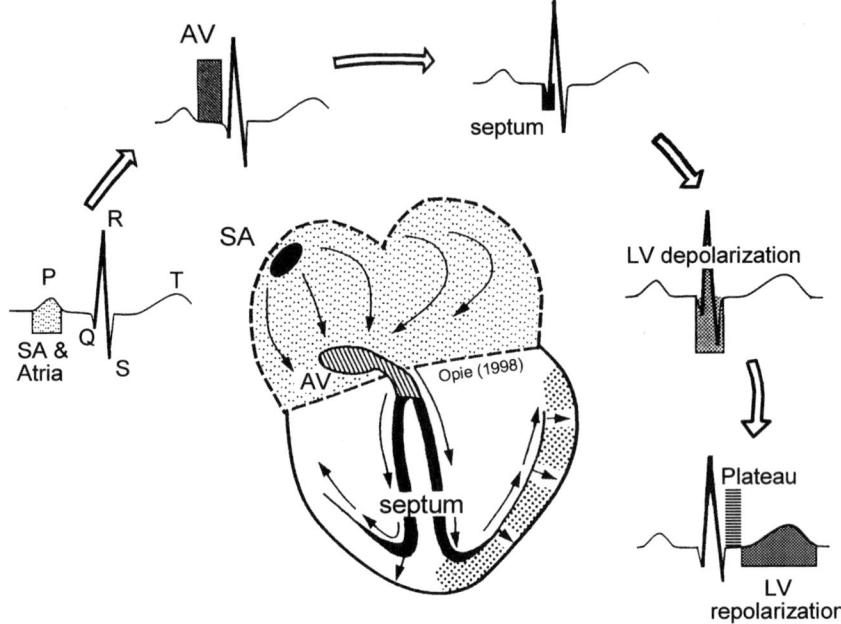

FIG. 5-9. Cardiac impulse and electrocardiographic patterns. From the pacemaker situated in the sinoatrial (*SA*) node, the wave of electrical depolarization spreads throughout both atria, causing the greater part of the P wave of the electrocardiogram (*ECG*). Conduction slows down considerably through the atrioventricular (*AV node*), causing the interval between the P and Q waves. Then conduction accelerates through the His–Purkinje system and immediately reaches the cardiac septum where it causes the small Q wave. Later, it reaches the left ventricle to cause the QRS deflection in the bottom ECG. Thereafter, ventricular repolarization follows, causing the T wave. The ECG pattern is that found in V_6.

The normal ECG complex consists of the P wave, the PR interval, the QRS complex, the ST segment, and the T wave (Fig. 5-10). The *P wave* of the normal electrocardiographic trace reflects the spread of the impulse through the atria (Fig. 5-9). Although activity is confined to the AV node, little voltage is seen on the body surface. The period of inactivity between the P wave and the start of the QRS complex is termed the *PR interval* and reflects the slower rate of conduction through the AV node (strictly speaking, it should be the PQ interval). Next, the small Q wave shows that the ventricular impulse is spreading through the septum in the direction opposite the placing of the body surface electrode.

The start of the *Q wave* corresponds to phase 0 of the ventricular action potential (Fig. 4-2). The large *R wave* represents fast depolarization with rapid conduction toward the electrode (hence, a positive wave), followed by a stage at which the whole ventricle is fully depolarized, corresponding to the plateau phase of the ventricular action potential. Because there is no current flowing at that stage, the body surface registers this absence of flow as an isoelectric (Greek, *iso*, the same) state.

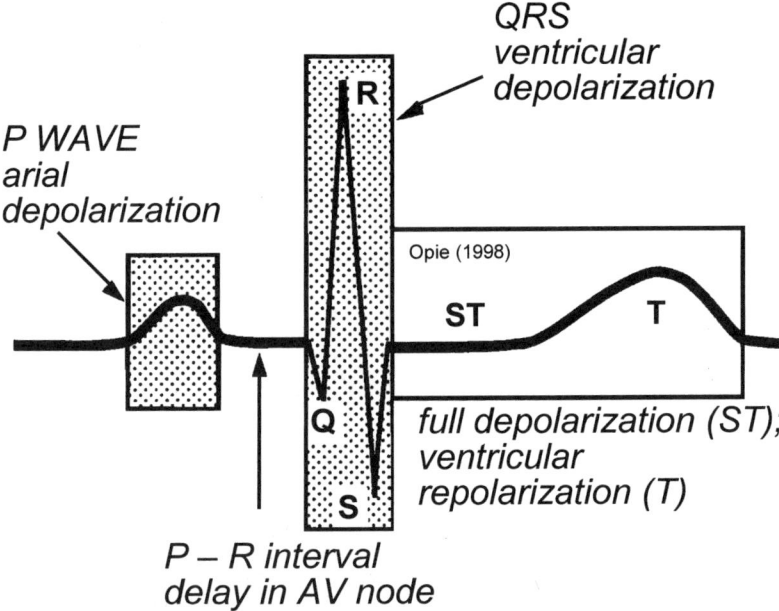

FIG. 5-10. Normal electrocardiogram. This shows the normal electrocardiographic pattern of a limb lead such as lead II, and the basic events that each component represents. See also Figure 5-9.

Thus, after the *S wave*, the heart returns to an isoelectric state (the *ST segment*) for the duration of the plateau phase. Note that the term segments refers to voltage and the term intervals refers to time. Finally, the myocardium repolarizes, and the ensuing *T wave* is in the same direction as the QRS wave. Hence, the surface ECG makes it possible to follow the wave of conduction from the SA node, through the atria, to the AV node, and ultimately to the ventricles.

Size and Direction of the QRS Complex and T Wave

Polarized cells are positively charged on the outside (Fig. 4-1), whereas depolarized tissue tends to be negatively charged. Voltages occur in the ECG only when there is a mixture of polarized and depolarized tissue in the heart. Thus, an electrode facing an approaching wave of depolarization records a positive potential that inscribes an upright deflection in the ECG, positive potentials conventionally being recorded as upward deflections. The greater the mass of tissue that the electrode faces, the greater are the deflection and width of the QRS wave (Fig. 5-11). Confusingly, the term QRS complex is also used when there is no visible Q wave. If the wave of repolarization moves toward the recording electrode, a downward deflection results. This rule makes it difficult to understand why the T wave normally reflects a positive and not

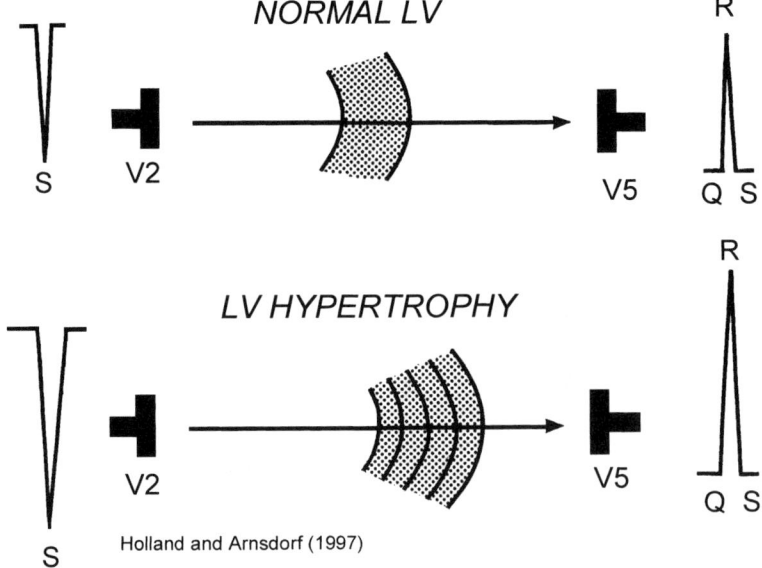

FIG. 5-11. Two fundamental laws. As the electrical impulse approaches the surface electrocardiographic electrode, a positive wave develops (upward deflection on right). Conversely, a negative wave indicates current flow away from the electrocardiographic electrode (downward deflection on left). Second, when the mass of muscle underlying the electrode is thicker and closer to the electrode, the current flow and voltage deflection are greater. The second law is a simplification of the solid angle theory. LV, left ventricular. (Holland RP, Arnsdorf MF. Solid angle theory and the electrocardiogram: physiologic and quantitative interpretations. *Prog Cardiovasc Dis* 1977;19:431–457.)

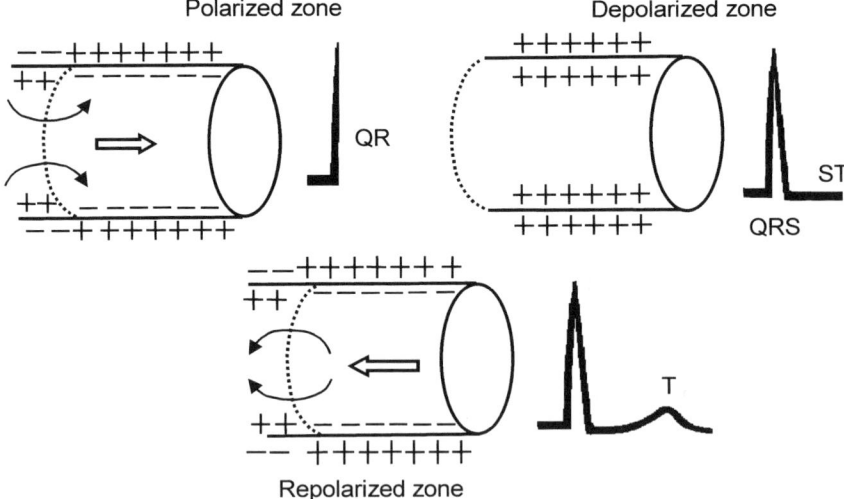

FIG. 5-12. Polarity of QRS and T waves. When the direction of depolarization is toward the recording electrode, then the electrocardiogram deflection is upward **(top left)**, thereby forming QR. The isoelectric line is reached when depolarization is complete, thereby forming the QRS complex and initiating the ST segment. This process corresponds to the impulse traveling from the endocardium to the epicardium in the whole heart. During repolarization, the electrical wave going in the opposite direction should produce a negative T wave. In the whole heart, the direction of repolarization is from the endocardium to the epicardium, not just a reverse process, thus producing the upright T wave.

a negative signal during repolarization because the repolarization would be expected to follow the same path as depolarization. The reason is that the ventricle actually tends to repolarize in the opposite order in which it depolarized, as illustrated in Figure 5-12. The last cell to depolarize is the first cell to repolarize.

Twelve Conventional Electrocardiogram Leads

The rhythmic, repetitive spread of the electrical impulse throughout the heart from the SA node to ventricular myocytes can be monitored by the body surface ECG. The original ECG recorded by Einthoven (Fig. 5-13) had three huge saline-filled immersion electrodes into which were placed the left and right arms

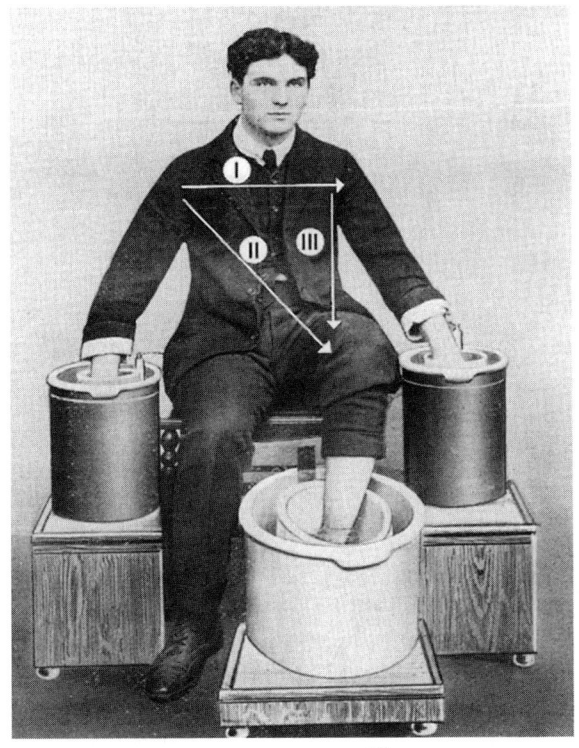

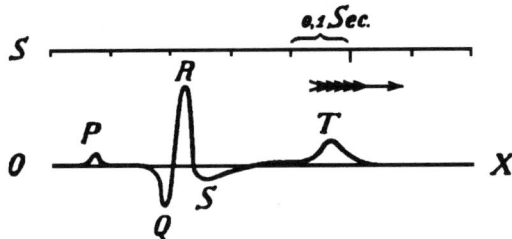

FIG. 5-13. The Einthoven electrocardiogram. The apparatus used to obtain this electrocardiogram in 1913 is taken from *Clinical Electrocardiography* by Sir Thomas Lewis. Note the Einthoven triangle (in white) on the subject's chest.

and the left leg, while the right leg was used as the earth. These electrodes recorded the difference of electrical potential between each of these limbs. The immersion electrodes were perfect, although huge, but the primitive electronics gave traces that were poor and difficult to interpret. With modern suction electrodes and high-fidelity electronic amplifiers, it is possible to achieve excellent recordings of the body surface ECG.

The *bipolar standard leads*, leads I, II, and III, are the same as those used by Einthoven (Fig. 5-14). A unipolar (V) exploring electrode can be constructed by measuring the voltage on that lead relative to a reference lead made by tying the

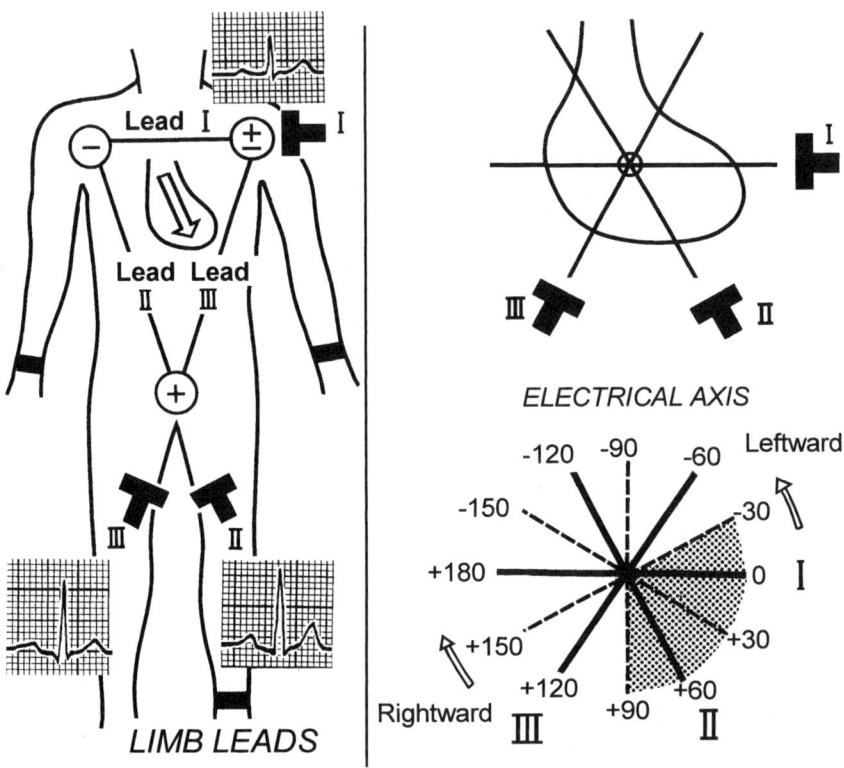

FIG. 5-14. Limb leads and electrical axis. Limb leads I, II, and III of the body surface electrocardiogram. When the axis is normal (between −30 and +90 degrees, *shaded area*), the electrocardiogram deflection is usually positive in all three leads, as shown. To derive the mean electrical axis, the Einthoven triangle (on body at left) is transposed to the frontal plane diagram shown on the right. The peak amplitudes of leads I, II, and III can be plotted on their respective axes as shown in Figure 5-23. The resulting vector for this example is +70 degrees and is in the normal range depicted by the shaded area. An axis situated from −30 to −90 degrees represents left axis deviation and an axis from +90 to +180 degrees represents right axis deviation (the latter is often found in right ventricular hypertrophy).

two arms and the foot together. The unipolar limb leads can record the electrical potential at each of the limbs (Fig. 5-15). The letter *a* for augmented is added to the letter V for unipolar leads. Augmented refers to an increase in the signal obtained by dropping the point of V lead attachment from the reference system, thereby theoretically increasing the signal amplitude by 50%. The unipolar recording from each point is called aVR from the right arm, aVL from the left arm, and aVF from the left foot. Thus, for example, aVR records the voltage from the right arm versus the combined voltage from the left leg and left arm. Leads V_1 to V_6 represent *unipolar precordial chest leads*, working on a similar principle to the augmented limb leads. Each V lead is taken from a specific site on the chest wall (Fig. 5-16). The pattern of the V leads shown in the bottom panel of Fig. 5-16 can be explained by the route that the electrical impulse takes through the ventricles and the overall direction or *vector* of the forces generated (Fig. 5-17).

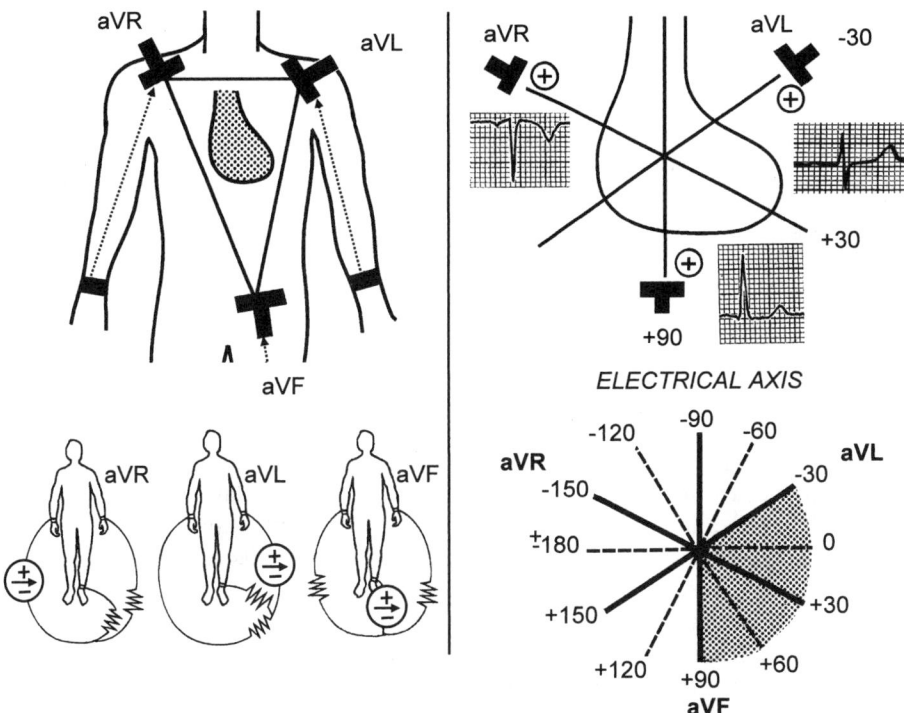

FIG. 5-15. Augmented limb leads. These are for the aVR (right arm), aVL (left arm), and aVF (left foot) with their contributions to the hexaxial system. The axis can also be calculated from these leads. For example, in the traces shown, aVF has a positive deflection of 12 small squares and aVR a negative deflection of 12 small squares. Using the same principles as in Figure 5-23, the axis can be calculated to be +60 degrees, again within normal limits.

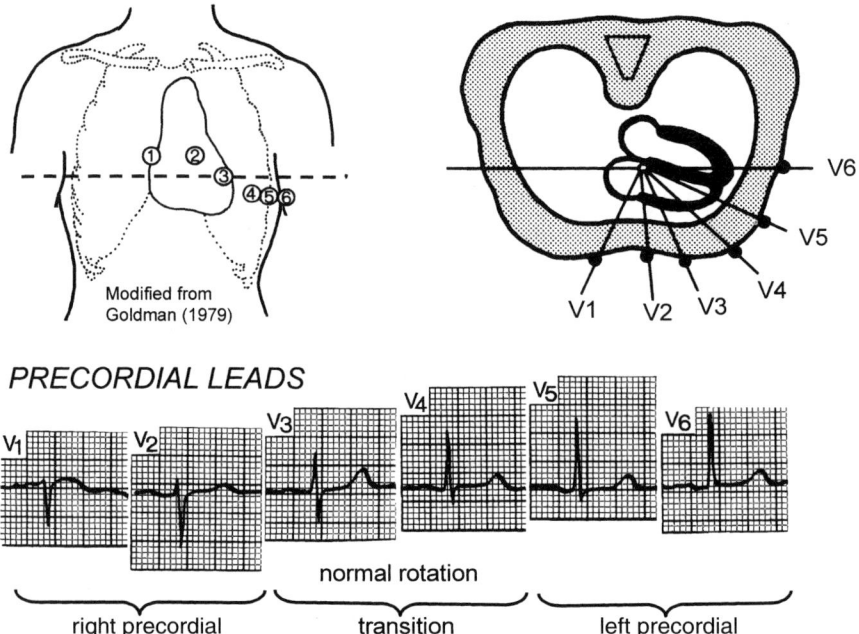

FIG. 5-16. Precordial electrodes. The standard anatomic situation of the precordial electrodes agreed on by the American Heart Association and the British Cardiac Society. The positions are V_1, fourth right intercostal space at the sternal edge; V_2, fourth left intercostal space at the sternal edge; V_3, halfway between V_2 and V_4; V_4, fifth left intercostal space in the midclavicular line; V_5, anterior axillary line, same plane as V_4; V_6, midaxillary line, same plane as V_5. With a normal position of the heart (normal rotation), the electrocardiographic complexes change from an S wave-dominant trave in V_1 to an R wave-dominant trace in V_6.

ELECTRICAL AXIS

As the ventricle depolarizes, it creates an electrical signal in the chest that has both magnitude and direction, a vector. The six frontal plane leads (leads I, II, III, aVR, aVL, and aVF) are arranged at 30-degree intervals around the heart, and each tells a different story about the axis of the electrical activity of the heart. This is called the hexaxial (composed of six axes) reference system. The procedures for obtaining the axis from the limb leads are shown in Figure 5-14. The average orientation of the QRS complex is termed the mean electrical axis. To obtain the axis from any two of the augmented limb leads, follow Figure 5-15. In reality, electrocardiography reports now come with the axis automatically calculated. One of the major reasons for a leftward axis is left bundle branch block, and the major reason for a rightward axis is right ventricular hypertrophy, two conditions discussed later in this chapter.

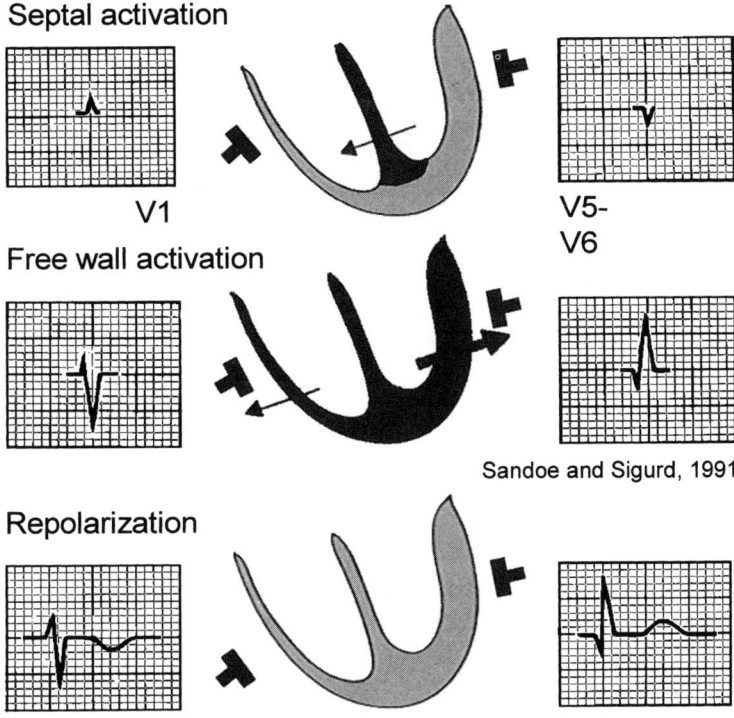

FIG. 5-17. Precordial electrocardiographic patterns. Note how conduction through the interventricular septum and then through the ventricles influences the patterns.

SINOATRIAL RATE

A simple rule to derive the rate of sinus node discharge (heart rate) is to count the number of R-R intervals per 3 seconds of ECG tracing and to multiply by 20. At the standard ECG paper speed of 25 mm per second, every fifteenth large square has a vertical line above it and indicates 3 seconds. Conventionally, if the rate exceeds 100 per minute (R-R less than three large squares) and the beat originates in the sinus node (a P wave is present), that constitutes a sinus tachycardia (Greek, *tachy*, fast; *kardia*, heart). Conversely, if the R-R interval exceeds five large squares, the sinus rate is less than 60 per minute, and there is a sinus bradycardia (*brady*, slow). In the normal subject, the heart rate may vary between a sinus tachycardia (exercise, emotion) and a sinus bradycardia as during sleep.

Sinus Arrhythmia

Normally during inspiration, there is a reflex mechanism that transiently increases the heart rate (Fig. 5-18). In some individuals, this reflex (the *Hering–*

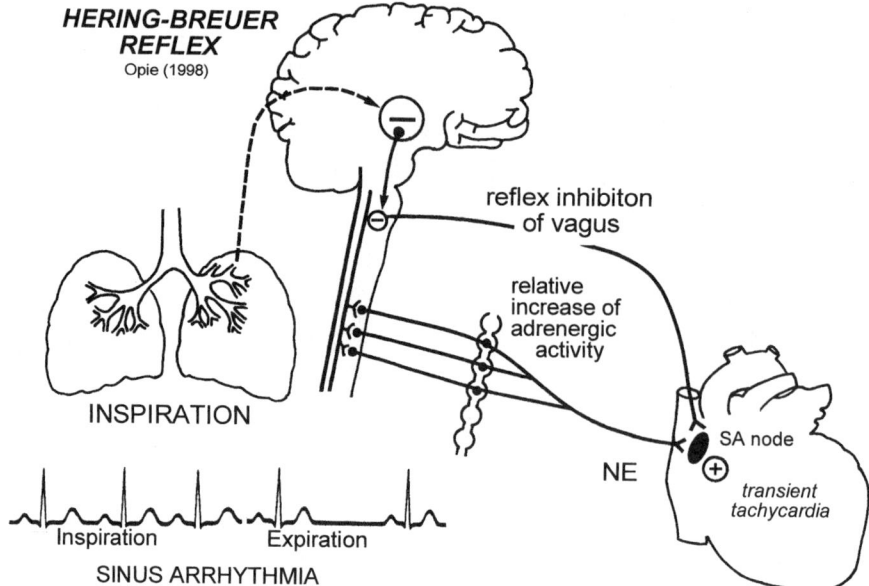

FIG. 5-18. Sinus arrhythmia. This is one of the most common physiologic irregularities of the rhythm. It reflects varying rates of discharge of the sinus node. During inspiration, the Hering–Breuer reflex is stimulated to inhibit the vagal center. The latter normally depresses the sinus rate and its inhibition results in a relative increase of adrenergic activity. Consequently, there is a transient tachycardia. *NE*, norepinephrine; *SA*, sinoatrial.

Breuer reflex) seems highly active, so that the inspiratory-expiratory cycle produces a marked change in heart rate. This physiologic variation is only an apparent irregularity, called sinus arrhythmia (*a* = not; i.e., not normal rhythm). It must be distinguished from serious pathologic arrhythmias; the latter are usually the result of organic heart disease (Chapter 20).

Sinus Tachycardia and Bradycardia

Sinus tachycardia, the most common of the supraventricular tachycardias, physiologically occurs in response to acute exercise or emotional stimuli as a result of increased activity of the adrenergic system (Fig. 5-19). Drugs or diseases such as thyrotoxicosis or heart failure can also cause sinus tachycardia (Table 5-2).

Sinus bradycardia often occurs in athletes because aerobic training increases the parasympathetic tone relative to that of the sympathetic adrenergic system (Table 5-3). The longer diastolic interval of the athlete's heart allows a greater end-diastolic fiber length and a greater stroke volume according to the Starling law (Fig. 12-15), so that the cardiac output is kept normal despite the slower heart rate. Another physiologic cause of bradycardia is

A. Normal sinus rhythm (60-100 /min)

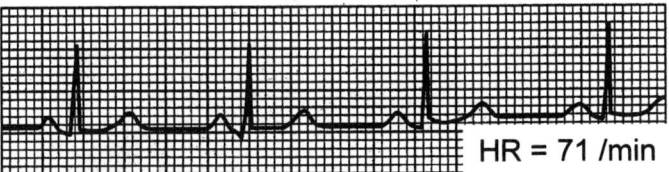

HR = 71 /min

B. Sinus tachycardia (> 100 /min)

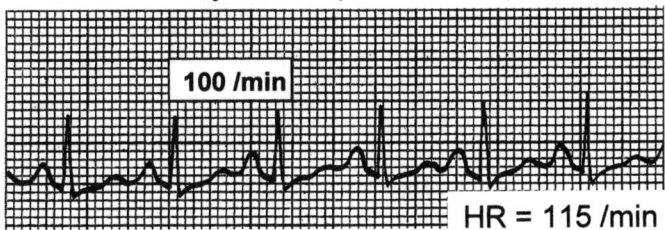

HR = 115 /min

C. Sinus bradycardia (< 60 /min)

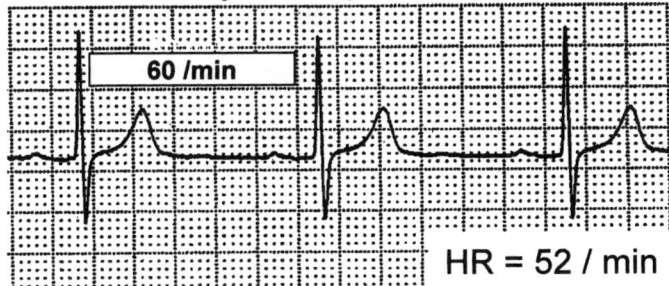

HR = 52 / min

FIG. 5-19. Sinus tachycardia and sinus bradycardia.

TABLE 5-2. *Physiologic or pharmacologic procedures or agents that increase the discharge rate of the sinoatrial node and the heart rate*

Procedure or agent	Presumed mechanism
Acute exercise, emotional stimuli	β-Adrenergic discharge
β-Adrenergic receptor agonists	Increased opening of probability of L-calcium channels via formation of cAMP and L-channel phosphorylation; also increased I_f
Atropine	Competitive inhibition of acetylcholine at muscarinic cholinergic receptors
Congestive heart failure	Compensatory reflex increase in adrenergic tone required to maintain blood pressure

cAMP, cyclic adenosine 3′, 5′-monophosphate.

TABLE 5-3. *Physiologic or pharmacologic procedures or agents that inhibit the sinoatrial node and decrease the heart rate*

Procedure or agent	Presumed mechanism
Athletic training	Increased vagal activity and decreased adrenergic effects
Sleep	Increased vagal and decreased adrenergic effects
Vagal stimulation	Release of acetylcholine increases nitric oxide, inhibits β adrenergic increase of I_f and decreases L-calcium channel activity by inhibition of formation of cAMP; if intense, also increases I_{KACh} with hyperpolarization[a]
β-Adrenergic blockade	Inhibition of formation of cAMP with beta-blockers; hence lower probability of L-calcium channels being in open state; also inhibition of I_f
Calcium channel blockers	Inhibition of L-calcium channel current (verapamil, diltiazem, high-dose dihydropyridines such as nifedipine)
Digitalis	Vagal stimulation
Adenosine	Stimulation of adenosine-operated potassium channel I_{KAdo} resulting in hyperpolarization

[a]Reference 8.
cAMP, cyclic adenosine 3′, 5′-monophosphate.

sleep, when the high vagal tone causes the heart rate to decrease. Pharmacologically, sinus bradycardia is typical of treatment by β-adrenergic antagonist drugs (Table 5-3).

In the *sick sinus syndrome*, the SA node intermittently and progressively fails to fire, with the risk of *sinus arrest*. This disease characteristically occurs in the older age group, frequently a result of coronary artery disease or idiopathic fibrosis (also see Overdrive Suppression, page 127).

ATRIOVENTRICULAR NODAL DISEASE AND HEART BLOCK

First, the physiologic function of the AV node should be recalled. The depolarization of ventricular cells starts approximately 80 milliseconds after the impulse leaves atrial tissue (11). This is the time it takes the impulse to traverse the AV node, His bundle, and bundle branches. Electrocardiographically, this interval forms part of the *PR interval* (the beginning of the P wave to the beginning of the QRS complex with a normal upper limit of 0.20 seconds), which includes delays within the AV node (Fig. 5-20). The importance of this delay is that the atrial booster contraction, occurring with the P wave, has sufficient time to complete the process of completely filling the ventricle before ventricular contraction starts. The delay within the AV node, however, can be excessive when this node is damaged by disease, as in ischemia and myocarditis (an inflammatory disease). In addition, excess AV delay occurs in some overtrained athletes. This condition is termed AV nodal block or often simply heart block (Fig. 5-21).

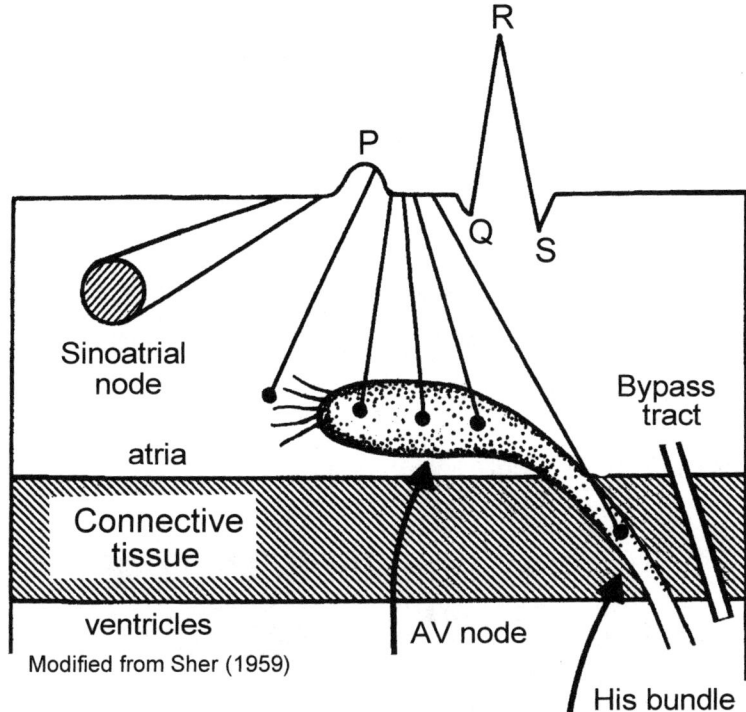

FIG. 5-20. PR interval of an electrocardiogram. Components of the conduction system and their contribution to the PR interval of the electrocardiogram are illustrated. For the significance of the bypass tract in the production of arrhythmias, see Chapter 20. (Modified from Scher AM, Rodriquez MI, Liikane J, et al. The mechanism of atrioventricular conduction. *Circ Res* 1959;7: 54–61.)

When the abnormality on the ECG is the prolonged PR interval, there is *first-degree heart block*. In addition to its occurrence in ischemia, myocarditis, and overtraining, it can also be caused by a variety of drugs inhibiting the AV node. Not surprisingly, the calcium channel blockers verapamil and diltiazem and the β-adrenergic blockers inhibit the AV node. This inhibition reflects the prominent role of the L-type calcium channel in AV nodal conduction (Fig. 5-8). Another inhibitory drug is digitalis, which stimulates the vagus and inhibits the sodium pump (Fig. 4-25).

When the conduction between the atria and ventricles is severely inhibited, usually as a result of disease of the AV node and His bundle, the P wave intermittently fails in its efforts to reach the ventricles (*second-degree heart block*) or there is a total block between the atria and ventricles (*third-degree* or *complete heart block*). In the latter instance, ventricular asystole occurs, and death is inevitable unless a subsidiary pacemaker takes over.

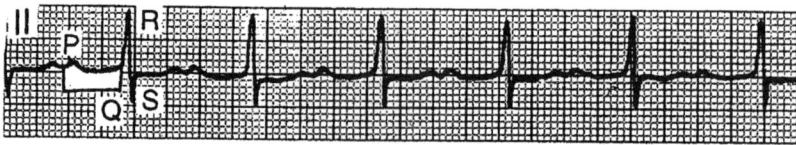

AV BLOCK 1st degree PR = 0.36 sec

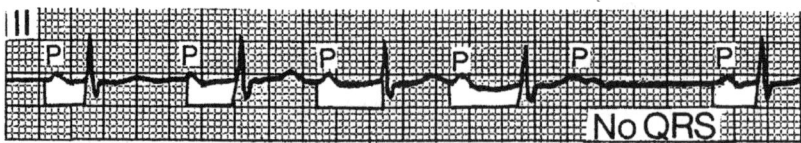

AV BLOCK 2nd degree Wenckebach

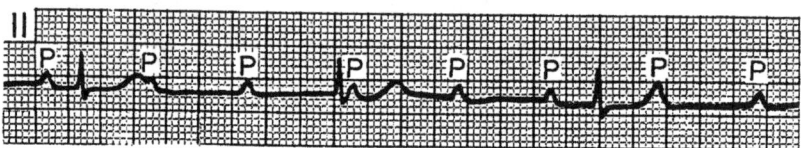

AV BLOCK 3rd degree AV dissociation

FIG. 5-21. Atrioventricular (AV) block. In first-degree AV block **(top)**, the PR interval is prolonged beyond 0.2 seconds. In second-degree AV block **(middle)**, some of the atrial impulses (P) fail to reach the ventricles, so that there are dropped beats (no QRS complexes). In third-degree AV block **(bottom)**, there is complete AV dissociation, so that P and QRS waves bear no relation to each other. Second-degree heart block has many different varieties. The type shown in the middle is also called the Wenckebach phenomenon, where progressive lengthening of the PR interval leads to "dropped" QRS complexes. First- and second-degree block may not be pathologic and can occur physiologically in athletes (Fig. 2-3).

Subsidiary Pacemakers

Physiologically, only the sinus node functions as a pacemaker. When it fails, the AV node can take over at 36 to 60 depolarizations per minute (*nodal rhythm*). When the AV node itself is blocked or injured, a new, even slower pacemaker site may form at the junction of the AV node and the His bundle (*junctional escape rhythm*). When this site is also inhibited, the Purkinje fibers in the His bundle or below may fire at approximately 30 per minute (*idioventricular rhythm*). When there is sudden development of complete heart block, the idioventricular rhythm may take some time to develop. Thus, the heart stops beating. During this period of asystole, there is risk of cerebral ischemia and syncope developing (*Stokes–Adams syndrome*).

Bundle Branch Block

In coronary artery disease, the blood supply to one of the two main divisions of the His bundle may be blocked with characteristic electrocardiographic changes. In *left bundle branch block*, there is typically a bifid- (*bifid* means a double deflection divided by a notch) widened QRS complex in leads facing the left ventricle such as V_4 to V_6 (Fig. 5-22). Note the left axis deviation (Fig. 5-23). In *right bundle branch block*, a similar bifid pattern holds in leads facing the right ventricle, i.e., V_1 and V_2 (Fig. 5-24). Each of the two branches of the left bundle may be independently blocked. It must be emphasized that these are functional not anatomic branches. In *left anterior hemiblock*, also called left anterior fascicular block (Latin, *fascis*, a bundle), there is an electrically silent zone of the heart in the territory of this bundle. The result is that the initial phase of left ventricular depolarization occurs by the posterior rather than the anterior bundle. The result is an initial R wave in the leads facing the left ventricle, such as leads II and V_6. Because of the electrical silence of the territory of the left anterior bundle, the normal full development of the positive deflection of the QRS wave is impaired. Instead, there is a net wave away from the LV leads, i.e., an S wave. As a rough rule, if the S-wave amplitude equals or exceeds the that of the R-wave in lead II, the cause can be left ante-

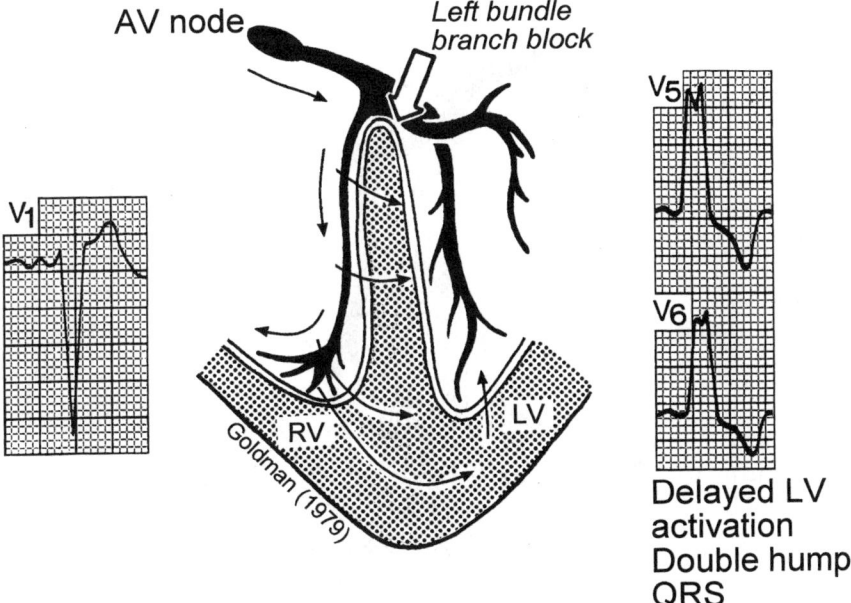

FIG. 5-22. Left bundle branch block. Mechanism and electrocardiographic traces are shown. (Modified from Goldman MJ. *Principles of clinical electrocardiography*, 10th ed. Los Altos, CA: Lange Medical Publications, 1979.)

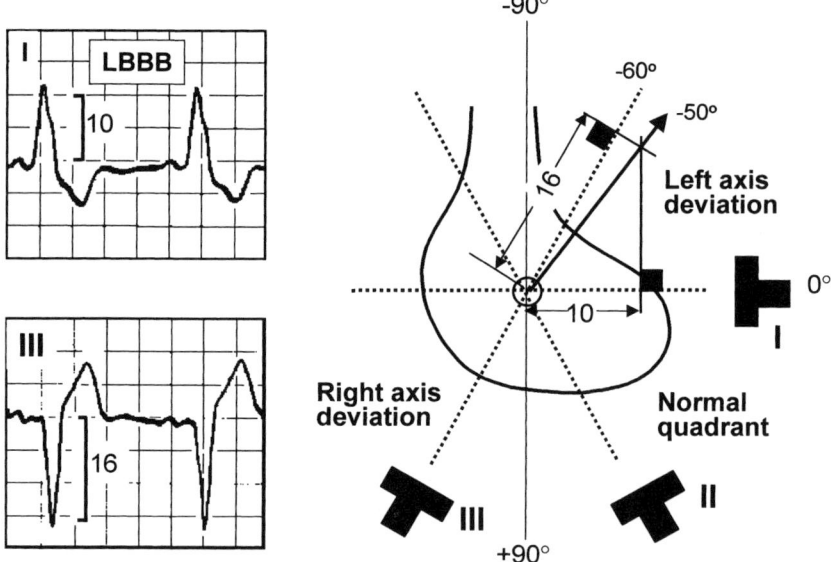

FIG. 5-23. Left axis deviation. In left bundle branch block, the major current flow is toward lead I (10 mm) and away from lead III (16 mm). There is thus left axis deviation of −50 degrees, calculated according to the legend of Figure 5-14. Also note the current flow toward leads V_5 and V_6 that face the left ventricle.

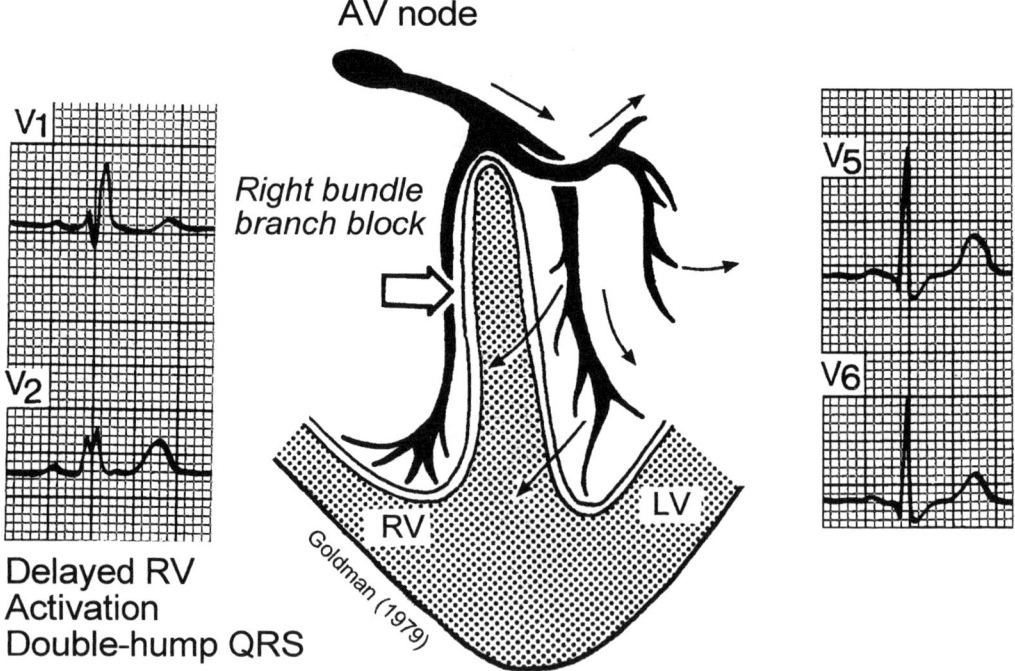

FIG. 5-24. Right bundle branch block. Mechanism and electrocardiographic traces. Modified from Goldman MJ. *Principles of clinical electrocardiography*, 10th ed. Los Altos, CA: Lange Medical Publications, 1979.)

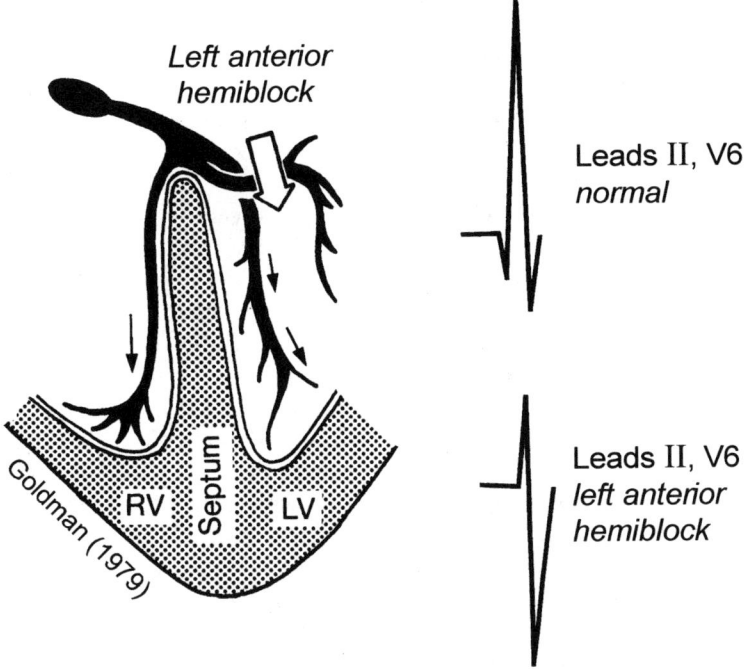

FIG. 5-25. Left anterior hemiblock (left anterior fascicular block). Mechanism and electrocardiographic traces. Hypothetically, there is an electrically "silent" area in the left anterior part of the left ventricle. Leads facing the left ventricle, such as II and V_6 (Figs. 5-16 and 5-26), display a greater amplitude of negative than positive deflection. (Modified from Goldman MJ. *Principles of clinical electrocardiography*, 10th ed. Los Altos, CA: Lange Medical Publications, 1979.)

rior hemiblock (Fig. 5-25). As in other conduction blocks, the QRS interval is increased.

In *left posterior hemiblock*, there is an electrically silent part of the heart in the territory of the left posterior bundle, which serves the left ventricular side of the septum and the posterior wall of the left ventricle. This is a rare condition, apart from acute myocardial infarction. aVL normally showing a positive QRS deflection as the electrical wave moves toward it, now becomes negative as the wave moves away from it, and the QRS has a downward pattern.

One important complication of bundle branch block is in the presence of coronary artery disease. If, for example, in a patient with acute myocardial infarction there is a block of two of the three bundles (*bifascicular block*), then the fear is that extension of the infarction will block all three bundles with complete heart block and threat of cardiac arrest. Hence, a temporary cardiac pacemaker may be inserted until the outlook improves.

VENTRICULAR HYPERTROPHY

When either ventricle grows thicker in response to a sustained increased of the intraventricular pressure, there is a progressive increase of the positive wave that develops as the electrical impulse travels toward the precordial electrode (Fig. 5-26). Thus, in left ventricular hypertrophy, those precordial leads that face the left ventricle, i.e., V_{5-6}, will record an increased positive RR deflection (Fig. 5-26). Conversely, there is greater RS voltage in the right ventricular lead V_1, caused by the electrical impulse traveling away from the right ventricle through the thickened left ventricle. A simple rule is that if the sum of the left ventricle RS height in V_5 or V_6 and the right ventricular RS depth in V_1 exceeds 35 mm (3.5 mV at standard calibration), then left ventricular hypertrophy is strongly suspected. These are the Sokolow–Lyon voltage criteria.

Other changes in left ventricular hypertrophy are (a) increased R voltage in the other leads facing the enlarged left ventricle (I and II, aVL), (b) increased RS duration because the wave of depolarization takes longer to get through the thickened ventricle (this can be seen in the traces in Figure 15-26); and (c) increased RS voltage in V_3 as the enlarged left ventricle rotates the heart and changes the axis of the heart in such a way that V_3 records from the right ventricle instead of from the transitional zone (Fig. 5-16) and "sees" the greater amplitude of the receding RS traveling away from the electrode through the thickened left ventricle. This change in electrical position of the heart is called counterclockwise rotation. The *Cornell voltage-duration product* is the sum of R in aVL and S in V_3, with 6 mm added in women; this needs to exceed 2,440 mm × msec to establish left ventricular hypertrophy (12).

Left ventricular strain refers to an abnormality in repolarization that is associated with the greater left ventricular mass and a greater chance of left ventricular hypertrophy than in the absence of strain (13). Strain is defined as a downsloping convex ST segment with an inverted asymmetric T wave in the opposite direction of the RS in V_5 and/or V_6 (Fig. 5-26).

Right ventricular hypertrophy is diagnosed by modification of the principles applied to left ventricular hypertrophy. For example, those leads that face the thickened right ventricle, V_{1-2} and aVR will reflect an increased positive deflection with tall R waves as the impulse travels "further" toward the sensing electrode through the thickened right ventricle (Fig. 5-26, lower panel). Thus, there is a reversal of the normal R-wave progression from V_1 to V_6, whereby the R wave progresses in height across the precordial leads (Fig. 5-16).

ACUTE MYOCARDIAL INFARCTION AND ISCHEMIA

Acute myocardial infarction results from prolonged total coronary occlusion. The tissue first becomes ischemic, and much will eventually undergo necrosis, causing the clinical condition of myocardial infarction (Chapter 18). In the first hours of occlusion, no cells will be dead, so that compared with the normal pattern (Fig. 5-27A), there is only prominent ST elevation that reflects epicardial

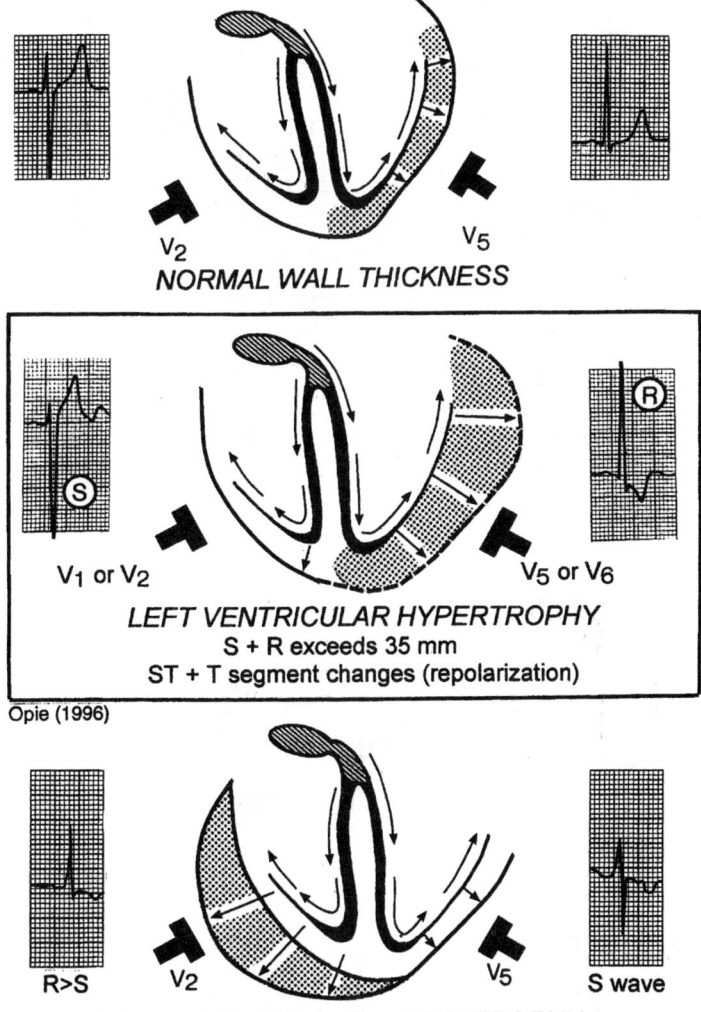

FIG. 5-26. Electrocardiogram shows ventricular hypertrophy. Thickening of the ventricular wall (hypertrophy) changes the electrocardiographic pattern. The normal electrocardiographic deflections in lead V_5, facing the left ventricle, and V_2, "looking" at the left ventricle from the other side, are shown **(top)**. In the presence of left ventricular hypertrophy **(middle)**, there is a greater positive voltage deflection in the electrodes facing the left ventricle, such as leads II, V_5, and V_6, and a greater negative voltage in leads facing from the other direction such as V_2. Hence, the S wave in V_1 and V_2 is increased, as is the R wave in V_5 and V_6. **Bottom:** Similar principles are applied to right ventricular hypertrophy. Left ventricular hypertrophy exists when (a) the sum of RS in V_1 and QR in V_5 or V_6 exceeds 35 mV, (b) there is widening of the QRS (conduction delay), and (c) there are repolarization changes in the ST segment and T wave. Right ventricular hypertrophy exists when QR exceeds RS in V_1 and the limb leads show right axis deviation. Ventricular "strain" is diagnosed by the repolarization changes that cause the abnormal ST-patterns in the middle and lower panels.

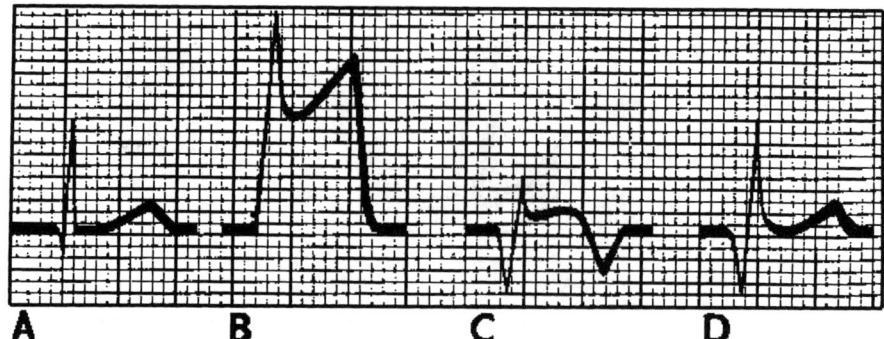

FIG. 5-27. Sequential changes in acute myocardial infarction. A: Normal trace lead V_3. **B:** Early ST elevation in the first hours indicate acute transmural (and hence epicardial) ischemia; followed by the formation of the Q wave with residual ST elevation, reflecting a mixture of dead cells and residual ischemia that lasts for hours to days **(C)**; and finally the permanent persistence of the Q wave with return to baseline of the ST segment **(D)**. (From Schamroth L. In: Schamroth C, ed *An introduction to electrocardiography*, 7th ed. Oxford: Blackwell Scientific, 1990, with permission.)

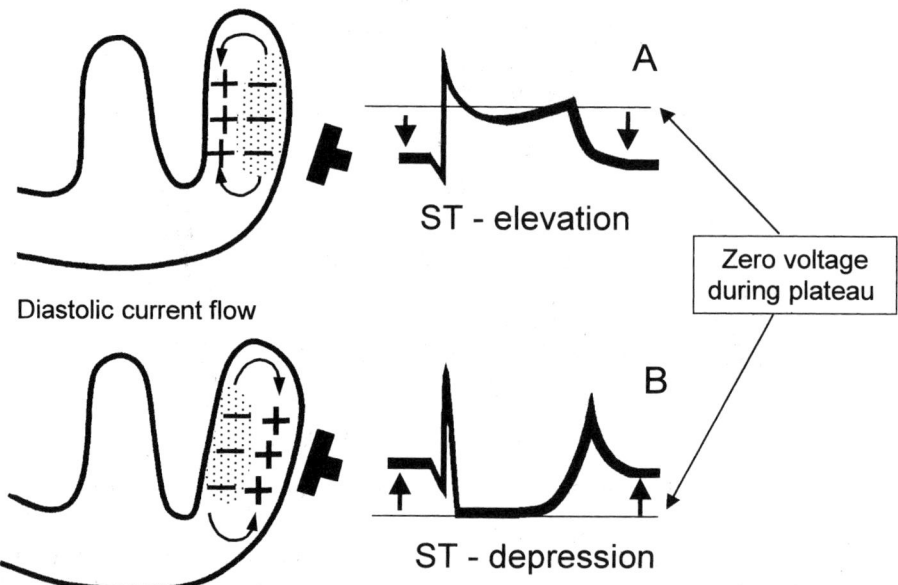

FIG. 5-28. Effects of ischemia on ST segment. With subepicardial ischemia **(top)**, the diastolic flow of current away from the electrode depresses the baseline and gives apparent ST segment elevation. Converse changes are found with subendocardial ischemia **(bottom)**.

ischemia (Fig. 5-27B). Ion pumps in the ischemic tissue fail, so that the cells are depolarized throughout the cardiac cycle. Because normal tissue is positively charged outside the cells and depolarized tissue is negatively charged, a current of injury will flow during diastole from the normal zone to the ischemic zone (Fig. 5-28). Only during the plateau of the action potential will all tissue be depolarized and all currents disappear. This will depress the baseline from any lead on the same side of the heart as the ischemic tissue causing the ST segment to appear elevated (even though it is the true zero voltage).

After 3 to 6 hours of occlusion, prolonged ischemia starts to change to cell death (necrosis). The ST elevation of ischemia drops, and a new series of electrocardiographic changes develops, characterized first by more prominent Q waves (Fig. 5-27C). The electrode "sees" through the dead myocardium to look at the other wall of the ventricle, where the major electrical force is going in the opposite direction from endocardium through the ventricular wall. Thus, the exploring electrode records a negative deflection, i.e., a Q wave when it is over the infarct (Fig. 5-29). Some days later, as the cells initially threatened by ische-

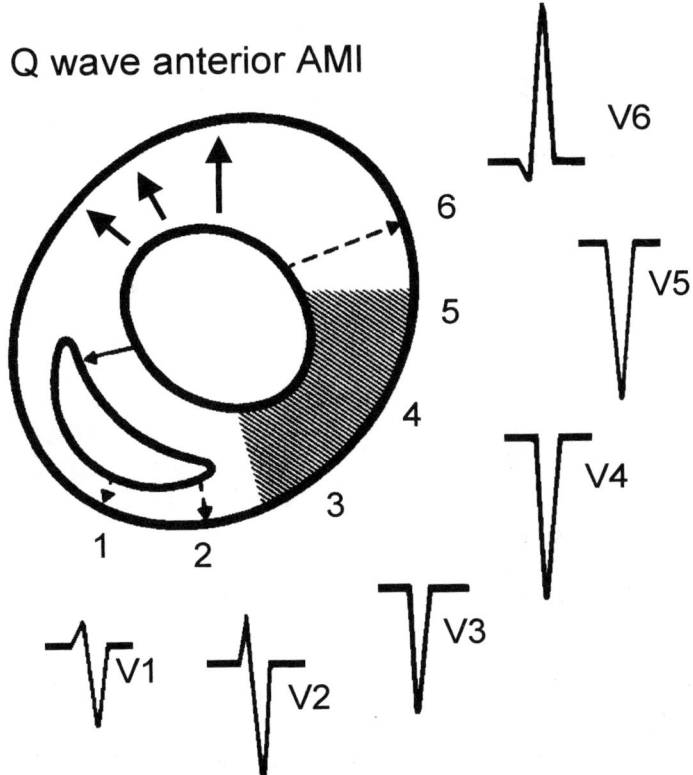

FIG. 5-29. Formation of the Q wave in myocardial infarction. Leads facing the infarct zone (*shaded area*) "see through" the dead cells to record the negative deflection of the impulse traveling away from the electrode.

mia either die or recover, the ST elevation reverts to baseline while the Q wave remains as a sign of an old infarct (Fig. 5-29D).

Patterns of ST-Segment Change

In transient ischemia, the impaired blood supply causes the myocardial cells in that area to become depolarized. The result is that during the ischemic attack, a current will flow from the normal region to the ischemic region during diastole (Fig. 5-27). If the ischemia lies just below the epicardium of the heart (subepicardial), the diastolic baseline is displaced downward in such a way that the ST segment again appears to be elevated, different in pattern from that found in left ventricular hypertrophy (compare Figs. 5-26 and 5-28). Conversely, if the ischemic zone is subendocardial, the changes will appear in such a way that the ST segment appears depressed (in reality, it is the baseline that has changed). Such ischemic changes occur mainly in two situations. First, ST-segment depression typically occurs during an attack of acute chest pain called *angina pectoris*, typically provoked by exercise (Fig. 17-5). Here the tachycardia of exercise increases the oxygen demand of the heart so that the blood supply flowing through the narrowed coronary arteries becomes inadequate. The oxygen demand of the inner layers of the myocardium is high because of mechanical factors. The result is endocardial ischemia (Fig. 5-28). Second, ST-segment elevation occurs very soon after the onset of coronary artery occlusion when initial ischemia has not yet progressed to cell death (necrosis). Because there is epicardial ischemia, the typical early change

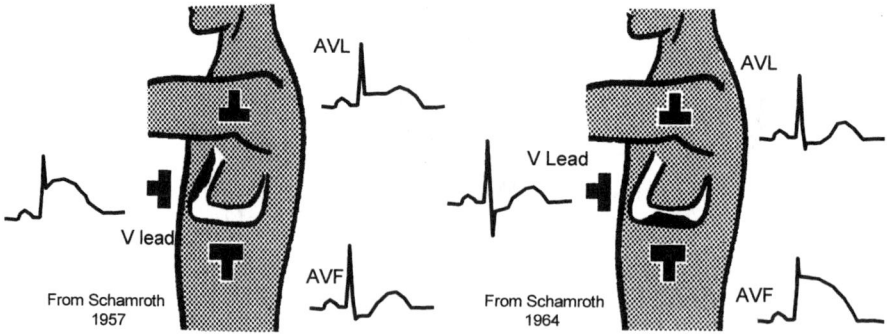

Acute occlusion of the left anterior descending coronary artery

Acute occlusion of the right coronary artery

FIG. 5-30. Electrocardiographic detection of a site of myocardial infarction. In the first hours of anterior wall infarction **(left)**, there is ischemic ST elevation in those leads facing the infarct, the V leads and aVL, with reciprocal depression of the ST segment in opposite lead, aVF. Conversely, in inferior infarcts, aVF shows the ST elevation, with reciprocal depression in the V leads and aVL. (Modified from Schamroth C. *An introduction to electrocardiography*, 7th ed. Oxford: Blackwell Scientific, 1990.)

is ST elevation. Which electrode senses this change best depends on which of the main coronary arteries is occluded (Fig. 5-30).

SUMMARY

1. *The spontaneous heart rate is chiefly governed by the rate of diastolic depolarization of the pacemaker (P) cells of the sinus node,* the mechanism of which is still not completely understood. There are at least three pacemaker currents: the decaying potassium current I_k, the calcium current I_{Ca}, and the inward current I_f. A background inward current is the fourth pacemaking current. These currents respond to adrenergic or cholinergic stimulation to increase or decrease the heart rate, for example, during exercise or at night, respectively.
2. *The electrical impulse travels from the sinus node to the AV node.* Conduction through the AV node is normally slow. Conduction through the His bundle and down the bundle branches to the ventricular endocardium is by Purkinje cells, which in some ways are primitive and in other ways are highly specialized, with a very rapid rate of conduction. The cardiac impulse has now arrived at the sarcolemma of the ventricular myocyte, and the next step is excitation–contraction coupling whereby depolarization leads to the contraction process.
3. *These processes can be monitored by the body surface ECG* in which the P wave represents atrial depolarization, the PR interval includes the delay in the AV node, and the QRS wave represents the phase of rapid ventricular depolarization. The ST segment represents the fully depolarized ventricle, corresponding to the plateau of the action potential. The T wave reflects the process of repolarization. Although it would be expected that the T wave would be negative, it is normally positive, i.e., in the same direction as the QRS wave.
4. *The ECG allows precise determination of the heart rate and rhythm.* There are also characteristic electrocardiographic changes of ventricular hypertrophy, heart block when conduction from the atria to the ventricles is impaired, and ischemia and infarction.

STUDENT QUESTIONS

1. How is the heart rate derived? Define tachycardia and bradycardia.
2. What are the effects of stimulation of the autonomic nervous system on the SA node? Describe the currents involved.
3. Describe the spread of the cardiac impulse from the SA node to the epicardial surface of the contractile myocardium.
4. Describe a typical normal electrocardiographic complex from limb lead I. What basic electrophysiologic events does each component of the ECG complex reflect?
5. What is the Einthoven triangle? How is the electrical axis of the heart calculated?
6. What are the physiologic events that increase the heart rate? What events decrease the heart rate? What is sinus arrhythmia?

CARDIOLOGIST-IN-TRAINING QUESTIONS

1. Describe the action potential of the SA node, including the participation of each of the pacemaker currents.
2. Explain in detail the effects of the autonomic nervous system on the discharge rate of the SA node.
3. Explain the proposed cellular basis of overdrive suppression.
4. How does adenosine inhibits the AV node? Does this differ from the mechanism involved in the inhibitory effects of verapamil and diltiazem?
5. How many types of conduction block do you recognize?
6. Left axis deviation is found in the left bundle branch block. What is it, how does it occur, and how is it calculated?
7. Explain the characteristic electrocardiographic changes of left ventricular hypertrophy.

REFERENCES

1. Irisawa H, et al. Cardiac pacemaking in the sinoatrial node. *Physiol Rev* 1993;73:197–227.
2. Vinogradova T, et al. Sinoatrial node pacemaker activity requires Ca^{2+}/calmodulin-dependent protein kinase II activation. *Circ Res* 2000;87:760–767.
3. Opthof T. The mammalian sinoatrial node. *Cardiovasc Drugs Ther* 1988;1:573–579.
4. Wilders R, et al. Pacemaker activity of the rabbit sinoatrial node. A comparison of mathematical models. *Biophys J* 1991;60:1202–1216.
5. Liu Y, et al. Mitochondrial ATP-dependent potassium channels. Novel effectors of cardioprotection? *Circulation* 1998; 97:2463–2469.
6. Verheijck EE, et al. Contribution of L-type Ca^{2+} current to electrical activity in sinoatrial nodal myocytes of rabbits. *Am J Physiol* 1999;276:H1064–H1077.
7. Lipscombe D. L-type calcium channels. Highs and new lows [Editorial]. *Circ Res* 2002;90:933–935.
8. DiFrancesco D, et al. Cardiac pacemaker currents. In: Sperelakis N, et al., eds. *Heart physiology and pathophysiology*, 4th ed. San Diego: Academic Press, 2001:357–372.
9. Er F, et al. Dominant-negative suppression of HCN channels markedly reduces the native pacemaker current I_f and undermines spontaneous beating of neonatal cardiomyocytes. *Circulation* 2003;107:485–489.
10. Jose AD. Effect of combined sympathetic and parasympathetic blockade on heart rate and cardiac function in man. *Am J Cardiol* 1966;18:476–478.
11. Scher AM, Spah MS. Cardiac depolarization and repolarization and the electrocardiogram. In: Berne RM, ed. *Handbook of physiology. The cardiovascular system. Vol. 1.* Bethesda: American Physiological Society, 1979:357–392.
11a. Irisawa H, Noma A. Pacemaker currents in mammalian nodal cells. *J Mol Cell Cardiol* 1984;16:777.
11b. Brown HF, DiFrancesco D. Voltage-clamp investigations of membrane currents underlying pacemaker activity in rabbit sino-atrial node. *J Physiol* 1980;308:331–351.
11c. Hagiwara N, et al. Contribution of two types of calcium currents to the pacemaker potentials of rabbit sino-atrial node cells. *J Physiol* 1988;395:233.
11d. Verheijck EE, et al. Contribution of L-type Ca^{2+} current to electrical activity in sinoatrial nodal myocytes of rabbits. *Am J Physiol* 1999;276:H1064.
12. Okin PM, et al. For the LIFE Study Investigators. Relation of echocardiographic left ventricular mass and hypertrophy to persistent electrocardiographic left ventricular hypertrophy in hypertensive patients: the LIFE Study. *Am J Hypertens* 2001;14:775–782.
13. Okin PM, et al. Relationship of the electrocardiographic strain pattern to left ventricular structure and function in hypertensive patients: the LIFE Study. *J Am Coll Cardiol* 2001;38:514–520.
14. Yanagihara K, et al. Reconstruction of sino-atrial node pacemaker potential based on the voltage clamp experiments. *Jpn J Physiol* 1980;30:841–857.
15. Goldman MJ. *Principles of clinical electrocardiography*, 10th ed. Los Altos, CA: Lange Medical Publications, 1979.

PART III

Calcium and Contraction: Receptors and Signals

6

Excitation–Contraction Coupling and Calcium

Lionel H. Opie and Donald M. Bers

We must think increasingly in terms of microdomains and local control.
Bers (1)

In the past decade, elucidation of the molecular basis of cardiac excitation-coupling has led to a dramatic increase in our understanding of basic mechanisms that regulate cardiac function.
Marks et al. (2)

The rapid propagation of the cardiac impulse from the pacemaker cells of the sinus node to the ventricular cells is largely dependent on the activity of sodium and calcium channels. When the impulse has reached the ventricular cells, the next event of critical importance is the voltage-induced increased opening of the calcium channels of contractile cells of the ventricles, followed by a series of intracellular movements of calcium ions, leading to myocardial contraction and relaxation (Fig. 6-1). Contraction must be followed by relaxation, which results from uptake of calcium ions into the sarcoplasmic reticulum (SR). Only small amounts of calcium ions actually enter and leave the cell with each cardiac cycle. Most calcium ion movements are from the calcium stores in the SR to the cytosol and back again (Fig. 6-2). The sarcolemma maintains a vast gradient of calcium ion concentration from the extracellular value of approximately 1 mmol/L (10^{-3} mol/L) to intracellular cytosolic values, which increase from diastolic values of approximately 10^{-7} mol/L (0.15 μmol/L (3) to systolic values of approximately 10^{-6} mol/L or possibly more during maximal contraction (Fig. 6-3). The free calcium concentration in the SR is approximately 10^{-3} mol/L (3), reflecting active uptake of calcium into the SR.

This chapter concentrates on those calcium ion fluxes that link the wave of excitation to myocardial contraction by the process of excitation–contraction coupling. The chapters that follow explain the role of the adrenergic system, the

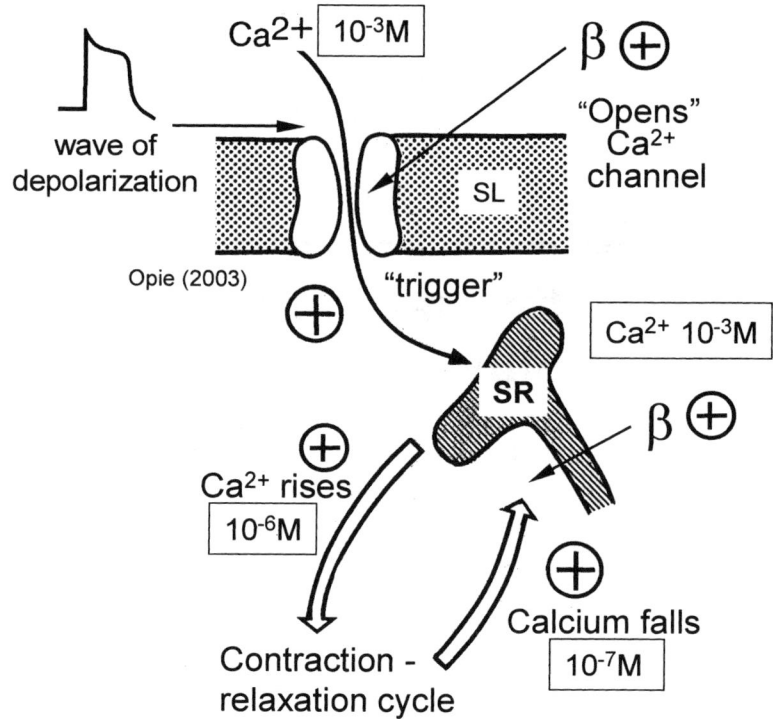

FIG. 6-1. Excitation–contraction coupling simplified. The wave of depolarization travels along the sarcolemma (SL) to "open" the calcium channels. Calcium ions (Ca^{2+}) entering via these channels trigger the release of much more calcium from the sarcoplasmic reticulum (*SR*). The cytosolic calcium ion concentration increases sufficiently to cause contraction. As calcium ions are taken back into the SR, relaxation starts. β-Adrenergic stimulation (*β*) promotes the opening of the calcium channels and accelerates the uptake of calcium ions into the SR. Note the much higher extracellular (10^{-3} mol/L) than cytosolic value of Ca^{2+} (approximately 10^{-7} mol/L in diastole to 10^{-6} mol/L in systole) and a hypothetical SR value of approximately 10^{-3} mol/L.

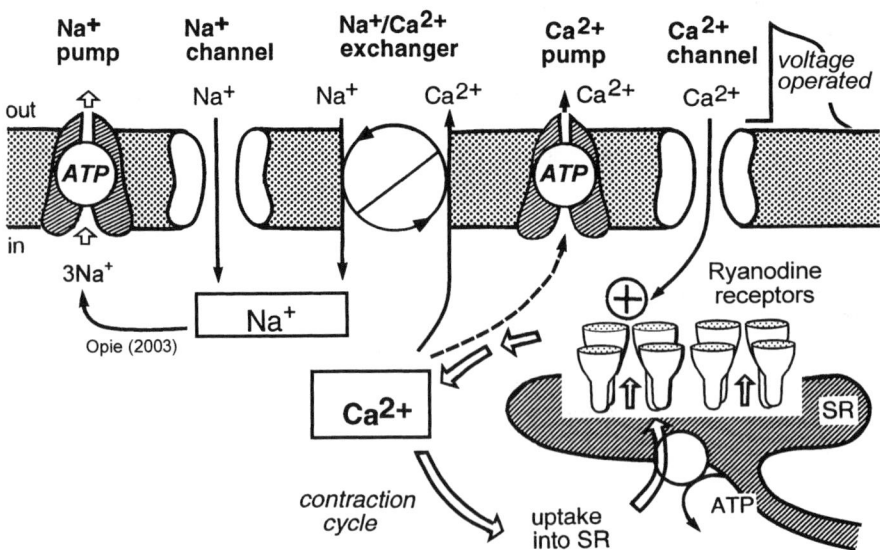

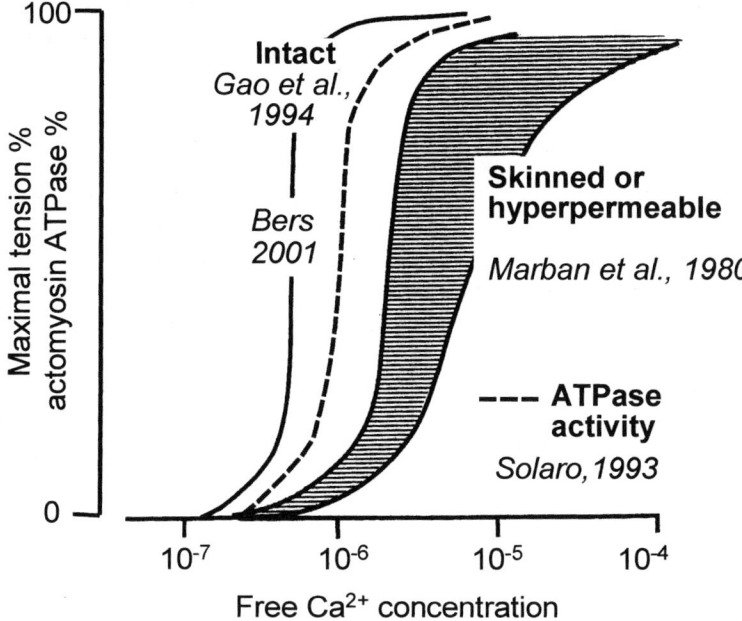

FIG. 6-3. Relation of free ionized calcium concentration to tension development. The resting diastolic value is approximately 0.2 μmol/L, rising to 10^{-6} mol/L at maximal tension development. For details, see Marban et al. *Nature* 1980;286:845; Solaro et al. *Circulation* 1993;87[Suppl VI]: 38; Gao et al. *Circ Res* 1994;76:720; and Bers. *Nature* 2002;415:198.

FIG. 6-2. Calcium ion fluxes in ventricular myocardium. Calcium ions (*Ca*) enter through the open sarcolemmal L-type channels to trigger the release of calcium from the sarcoplasmic reticulum via the ryanodine receptor (*RyR*), accounting in the human for approximately 75% of the increase in cytosolic calcium that promotes the actin–myosin interaction. The remaining (approximately 25%) enters directly via the L channels or by the sodium–calcium exchanger (Na^+/Ca^{2+}). Relaxation is initiated by uptake of calcium into the SR (requiring adenosine 5′-triphosphate), with a smaller amount (approximately 25%) of the cytosolic calcium leaving across the sarcolemma, mostly by the Na^+/Ca^{2+} exchanger now working in the opposite direction. For percentage values, see Table 6-1. Figure 4-3 shows the time course of an action potential, intracellular Ca^{2+} transient, and contraction in a ventricular rabbit myocyte.

162   6. EXCITATION–CONTRACTION COUPLING AND CALCIUM

β-adrenergic receptor and its messengers cyclic adenosine 3′,5′-monophosphate (cAMP) and protein kinase A (PKA) in the control of cellular calcium ion movements and the calcium-dependent contractile mechanism of the myocardium.

CALCIUM ION MOVEMENTS

The overall pattern of calcium ion movements associated with the contraction cycle is reasonably clear (Fig. 6-2). The key event in the generally accepted model is calcium-induced calcium release from the SR (4,5) as follows. The major intracellular calcium store is in the SR. Small but varying amounts of calcium enter the cell during the opening of the L-type calcium channels induced by depolarization. Such calcium triggers the release of relatively large amounts of calcium ions from the SR by opening the calcium release channels of the SR. Cytosolic calcium increases so that there is increasing interaction of calcium ions with the contractile protein troponin C. When the ambient calcium concen-

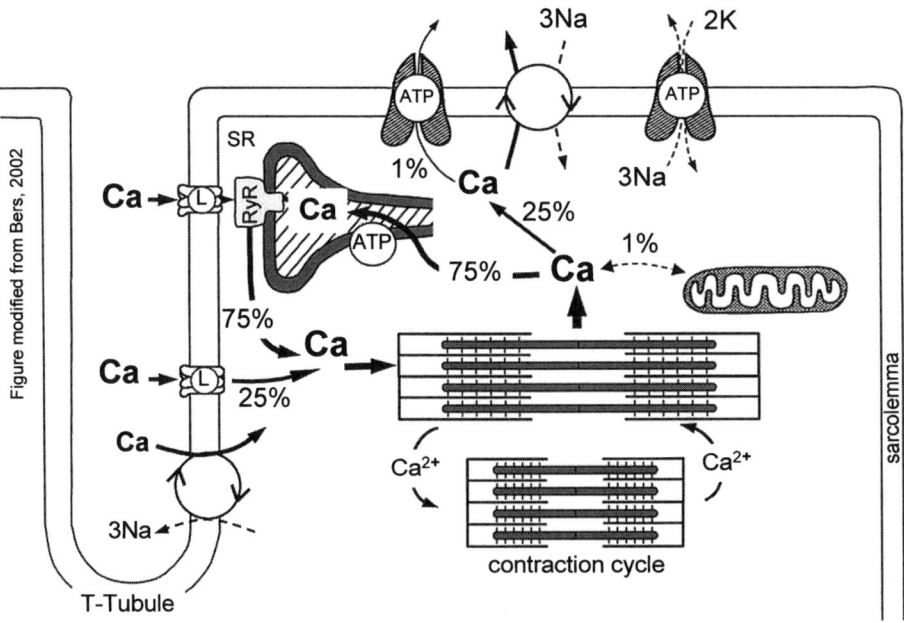

FIG. 6-4. Regulation of calcium balance in the cardiac myocyte. There is a balance between the Ca^{2+} ions entering on depolarization (at right) and those leaving the cell by the Na^+/Ca^{2+} exchange mechanism. A smaller number of Ca^{2+} ions leaves by an adenosine 5′-triphosphate (ATP)–dependent sarcolemmal Ca^{2+} pump (Fig. 6-2). Ion gradients for Na^+ and K^+ are maintained by the operation of the sodium pump (Na^+/K^+-ATPase). An increased internal Ca^{2+} following triggered Ca^{2+} release from the sarcoplasmic reticulum (SR) is reduced by competition among one of three routes: the dominant uptake mechanism being into the SR, followed by the exchanger, followed by the membrane pump. See also Figure 6-2.

TABLE 6-1. Mechanisms for lowering cytosolic Ca^{2+} concentration in myocardial cells

	Percentage of total uptake of calcium from cytosol		
	Rat	Rabbit	Human
Sarcoplasmic reticulum			
Ca^{2+} uptake pump	92	70	75
Sarcolemma			
Na^+-Ca^{2+} exchange	7	28	25
Ca^{2+} pump[a]	0.5	1	(1)
Mitochondria[a]	0.5	1	(1)

[a]Combined as slow systems.
Data from references 1, 5a.

tration is low, troponin C has a molecular structure that allows the inhibitory troponin I to block the interaction between actin and myosin. As the cytosolic calcium increases, troponin I binds more firmly to the troponin C and not to actin. The result is that the interaction of actin and myosin is facilitated and contraction takes place (details described in Chapter 8). When the release of calcium ions from the SR ceases, then the increase in cytosolic calcium comes to an end. To initiate relaxation, the cytosolic calcium is rapidly taken up by the calcium pump of the SR. Calcium ions leave their binding site on troponin C, and troponin I once again blocks the interaction between actin and myosin.

To balance the small amount of calcium entering the heart cell with each depolarization, a similar quantity of calcium ions leave the cell by one of two processes (Fig. 6-4). First, internal calcium can be exchanged for external sodium ions by the Na^+/Ca^{2+} exchanger (Table 6-1). Second, and of less importance, a sarcolemmal calcium pump that uses adenosine 5'-triphosphate (ATP) can transfer calcium outward into the extracellular space against a concentration gradient. The exchange between mitochondrial and cytosolic calcium is relatively slow compared with that between the SR and the cytosol. Hence, mitochondria do not participate in the beat-to-beat control of calcium ion movements. Mitochondrial calcium increases physiologically in response to β-adrenergic stimulation as the cytosolic calcium increases. This increase may stimulate enzymes of the citrate cycle to help to produce more ATP (Chapter 11). Pathologically, during conditions of cellular cytosolic calcium overload (discussed later in this chapter), mitochondria help to protect the cell by storing some of the excess calcium.

CRUCIAL ROLE OF SARCOPLASMIC RETICULUM IN CONTRACTILE CYCLE

Calcium Transients

Calcium transients are the cyclical variations in the concentration of cytosolic calcium ions during systole and diastole (Fig. 6-5). Calcium transients are increased in amplitude by β-adrenergic stimulation. Experimentally, an increase

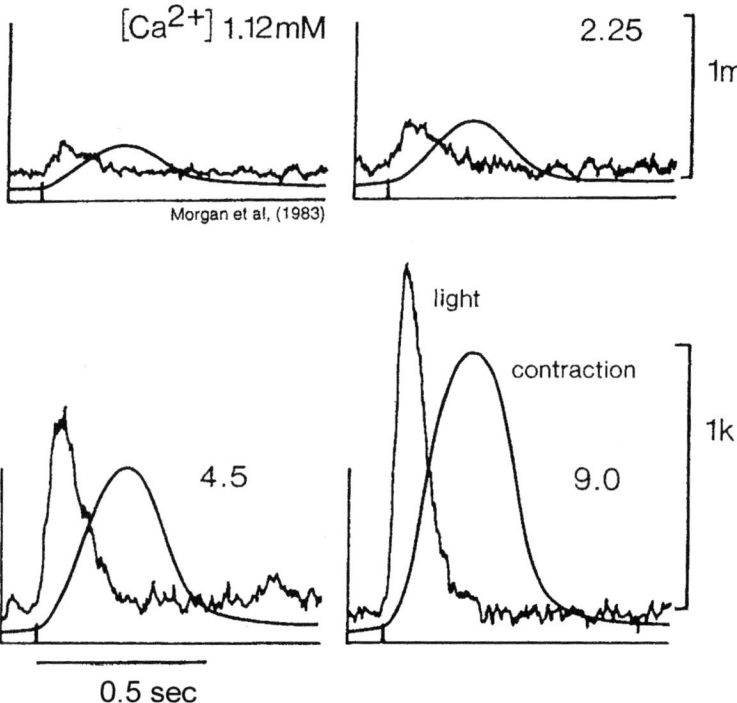

FIG. 6-5. Effect of extracellular calcium on intracellular calcium and tension development. Influence of increasing extracellular calcium ion concentration on the aequorin-measured intracellular calcium signals for papillary muscle (in mN). The external calcium concentrations are given in the individual panels (mM). The symbol k donates thousands of photon counts per second and is a reflection of the calcium ion concentration that activates aequorin. The contractile activity is shown as the smooth continuous line. (Modified from Morgan et al. Circ Res 1983;52[Suppl 1]:47.)

in external calcium ions will also increase internal calcium transients (6). It might be supposed that there would be a simple relationship between the calcium transients and the events of the contraction–relaxation cycle because the contractile proteins are directly sensitive to the prevailing internal calcium concentration (Fig. 8-7). Nonetheless, indirect evidence suggests that there are intracellular gradients for calcium ions, with more marked increases in the concentration in the subsarcolemmal space than in the cytosol as a whole, especially at the mouth of the open calcium channel (7).

Calcium Release from the Sarcoplasmic Reticulum

The cardiac SR plays an indispensable role in regulating the contraction–relaxation sequence (6). First, the close anatomic proximity of the L-type calcium channels of the T tubules and the specialized parts of the SR concerned with calcium release provide the anatomic framework for the links between calcium ions entering via the sarcolemmal channels and the release of calcium from the SR. There is good concordance between the duration of opening of the sarcolemmal L-type calcium channels and release of calcium from the SR (8). The proposal is that one L channel activates a small group, possibly six to 20, of adjacent calcium release channels (1). Alternatively, a cluster of L channels may regulate a cluster of release channels (9). The *calcium release channels* of the SR are part of a complex molecular structure known as the ryanodine receptor, so called because it binds the potent insecticide ryanodine (1). Part of the ryanodine receptor (RyR or, more accurately, RyR2 to indicate the cardiac isoform) extends from the membrane of the SR to the T tubule to constitute the "foot" region (Fig. 6-6). Thus, the SR is effectively joined to the T tubule by such junc-

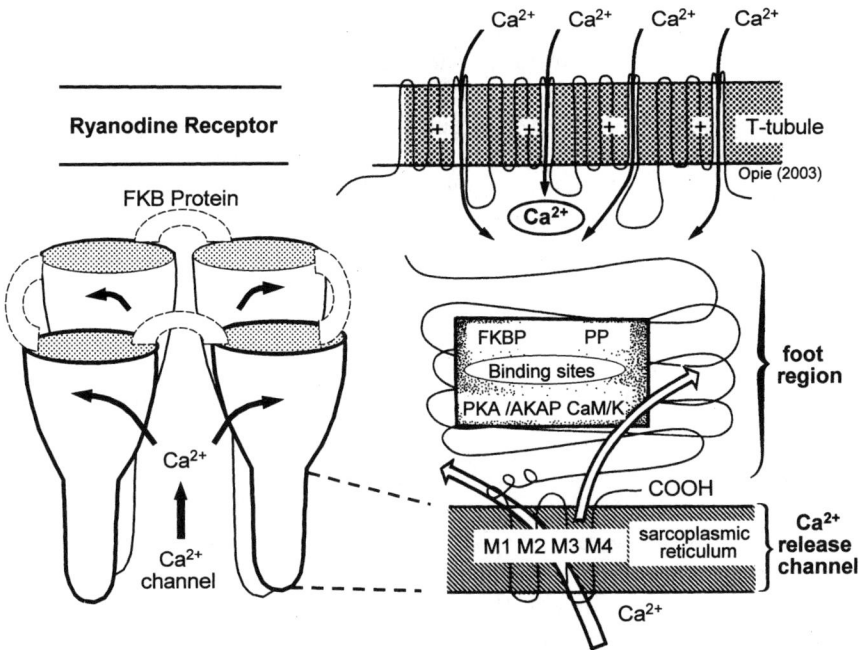

FIG. 6-6. Role of ryanodine receptor (RyR) in calcium-induced calcium release. The RyR protein forms a link between the T tubule and the sarcoplasmic reticulum (SR) and is a scaffolding protein (that binds other proteins such as kinases and phosphatases). This makes a macromolecular complex, also called the foot region. One high-affinity RyR is composed of four RyR monomer proteins. **Right:** The molecular model of one RyR is schematically shown. The four RyR proteins make a single calcium release channel, in a manner similar to the formation of some other ion channels (schematic) **(left).** Depolarization stimulates the L-type calcium channel of the T tubule to allow calcium ion entry. The incoming calcium binds to the RyR to cause molecular conformational changes that result in opening the calcium release channel and calcium release from the SR. *FKBP*, FK-506 binding protein; *PKA*, protein kinase A; *AKAP*, A kinase anchoring protein; *CaM/K*, calmodulin or calmodulin kinase; *PP*, protein phosphatases.

tions, constituting a *junctional calcium release complex* or the *SR calcium release complex* (1). Here the RyRs are packed in large organized arrays of perhaps 50 to 300 RyRs in a typical junction. The arrival of calcium ions from the L-type calcium channels of the adjacent T tubule of the sarcolemma is thought to induce a change in the molecular configuration of the foot, which is the molecular signal that opens the calcium release channel of the RyR. The L-type calcium channel of the T tubule thereby acts as a voltage-responsive sensor that promotes calcium release from the SR.

Calcium Uptake by Sarcoplasmic Reticulum

Relaxation of the contractile proteins occurs in response to a decrease in the cytosolic calcium level, as calcium ions are taken up by the energy-requiring pump located in the membrane of the SR, the ATP-consuming calcium uptake pump. This pump is also called the sarco(endo)plasmic reticulum calcium–ATPase or *SERCA*, which occurs in several isoforms, of which SERCA-2a is the one found in cardiac muscle (10). The high cytosolic calcium concentration reached during the contraction phase stimulates calcium uptake by SERCA. This calcium pump also responds to β-adrenergic stimulation by phosphorylation of a specific regulatory protein, called phospholamban, which is located in the membrane of the SR. The overall effect is that maximal rates of activity of the pump can be achieved either by high cytosolic calcium or by β-adrenergic stimulation, so that the relaxation phase is faster. Thus, the mechanisms of control of the calcium release channel and the uptake pump of the SR are directly relevant to the control of the contractile state.

Excitation–Contraction Coupling: Timing of Events

To summarize the preceding paragraphs, the wave of depolarization during electrical excitation is coupled with contraction by calcium-induced calcium release from the RyR of the SR, by a sequence of events initiated by the entry of calcium ions through the L-type calcium channel (Fig. 6-2).

When one L channel opens, the local subsarcolemmal calcium ion concentration increases by approximately 100-fold to activate several adjacent RyRs (5). The whole process occurs very rapidly. Each L-type channel opens only very briefly, perhaps for 0.2 milliseconds (7). The overall time between the initial stimulus that opens the L channels and the start of the increase in cytosolic calcium is only approximately 4 milliseconds, of which much less (less than 2 milliseconds) is the interval between the time of activation of the calcium channel and the release of calcium from the SR (11). To reach the peak cytosolic calcium concentration takes longer, approximately 40 to 100 milliseconds at a heart rate of 60 beats per minute (1). Approximately 200 milliseconds later, peak contraction is reached. Another 200 milliseconds later, the cytosolic calcium is nearly back to baseline and relaxation is almost complete. Full recovery of cytosolic

6. EXCITATION–CONTRACTION COUPLING AND CALCIUM

calcium and the contractile cycle takes approximately another 300 milliseconds. In all, approximately half of the interval between beats is occupied by the cardiac contraction–relaxation cycle.

Alternate Routes for Calcium Ion Influx

An important question is whether calcium ions entering through the L-type channels are the only trigger for the release of calcium from the SR. Calcium ions also enter the cytosol by a reversal of the exchange mechanism used for calcium efflux (1). Thus, sodium–calcium exchange, which normally operates to expel calcium from the cell, can, at depolarized voltages, reverse transiently to admit calcium, as may happen very shortly after the opening of the sodium channel (Fig. 4-25). The proposal is that sodium ions, having entered by the fast channel, accumulate in a microzone just within the sarcolemma, the "fuzzy zone" (12,13). This localized accumulation of sodium can then, hypothetically, transiently activate the sodium–calcium exchange in the direction of calcium entry (the reverse mode) so that even more calcium ions enter the myocardial cell (Fig. 6-7) to release many more calcium ions from the SR and the contractile process is enhanced.

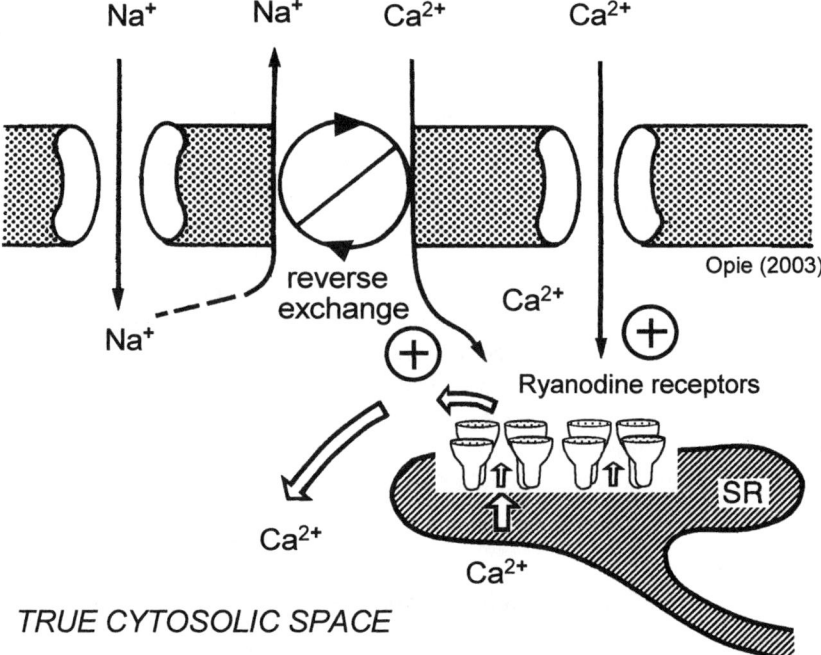

FIG. 6-7. Reverse mode sodium–calcium exchange. A proposal for the role of sodium–calcium exchange in the direction of calcium entry after accumulation of sodium ions in the "fuzzy space" to play a role in the liberation of calcium involved in the cardiac contractile cycle is illustrated.

CALCIUM RELEASE LINKED TO CONTRACTION

The release of calcium from the SR is a graded effect, being greater when the SR is more heavily loaded with calcium or when the concentration of triggering calcium is greater (13). Strong evidence linking the release of calcium from the SR to contraction is found when the cytosolic calcium is increased by the flash-sensitive loading compound nitr-5. This has the unusual property of releasing calcium ions in response to illumination at a particular wavelength. Thus, a flash of light can increase internal calcium in cells so loaded and simultaneously produce a cardiac contraction. Hence, the flash illumination must release calcium from some intracellular store, such as the SR, and that calcium initiates the contractile cycle. Such local release of calcium can be imaged by fast confocal microscopes showing intrasarcomere calcium gradients with local release of calcium during the initial phase of calcium transients (14).

The local control theory of cardiac excitation–contraction coupling proposes the release of calcium from individual junctional RyRs is controlled by the local calcium ion concentration. To achieve a sufficiently high local calcium concentration to open a cluster of RyRs requires the influx of calcium ions from the closely apposed L-type calcium channels. The greater the intensity of the incoming calcium current, the greater the opening of the RyRs with a corresponding increase in calcium release from the SR.

Calcium Sparks and Local Control

Calcium sparks are the very small amounts of calcium that are spontaneously and locally released from the RyRs even in the absence of L channel opening. Such sparks are rare and do not propagate because they do not elevate the local calcium ion concentration at adjacent RyR junctions sufficiently to cause calcium release. With the arrival of the action potential and the opening of neighboring L channels, several thousand calcium sparks can join in space and time to become the whole cell calcium transient (14). Thus, the synchronous activation of a large number of calcium release units leads to the calcium transient that triggers excitation–contraction coupling. Thus, the graded response in calcium release can be explained by both an increased number of RyR channels that are opened and an increased amount of calcium released by each channel (11).

Cessation of Calcium Release from the Sarcoplasmic Reticulum

As already described, the SR has its RyR release channel opened by an increasing concentration of external calcium. However, how are the release channels switched off to allow diastolic refilling of the heart? Three possibilities are (a) inactivation of the release channel, perhaps in response to a continuing increase in the local calcium concentration to supraoptimal levels (4,15), (b) local depletion of SR calcium in response to the discharge of calcium, and (c) stochastic attrition (1). For the latter to happen requires all the L-type calcium channels and RyRs in one microzone to shut down simultaneously, so that the local calcium concentration decreases precipitously. This could happen more easily if many RyRs opened and closed simultaneously according to the "coupled gating" hypothesis (15,16). Probably none of these three possibilities is of itself a sufficient explanation.

CONTROL OF THE RYANODINE RECEPTOR

The RyR (or more correctly RyR2 to indicate the cardiac isoform) is both the calcium release channel of the SR and a scaffolding protein that localizes numerous regulatory proteins to the junction, where the SR lies very close to and "joins" the T tubule via the "feet" of the RyR (Fig. 6-6). The RyR protein is large, comprising more than 5,000 amino acids, with two major components. The larger part of each RyR is the "foot" or scaffolding protein, lying outside the SR, which links it to the neighboring part of the T tubules. The smaller structure is the C terminal channel region, which constitutes the actual calcium-release channel of the RyR. It takes four identical RyR proteins to make the megacomplex that constitutes one release channel of the RyR. This homotetramer has an estimated molecular weight of as much as 2,260 kd (3), making it almost as large as titin (Table 8-1). The scaffolding part of each of the four RyR units also links to one regulatory protein subunit (technical term is FK-506 binding protein), thought to facilitate the concerted opening of neighboring RyR channels (17). The latter process is called *coupled gating*, potentially important in excitation contraction coupling. There are also binding sites for PKA, the essential end messenger of β-adrenergic signaling (Fig. 7-11), linked to the PKA anchoring protein, for calmodulin, and for two phosphatases that oppose the action of PKA. Thus, RyR, already a large molecule, is part of an even larger complex containing all these binding sites and regulatory proteins (18).

Why the name RyR? Ryanodine is a toxic insecticide that interacts with its receptor in a complex biphasic manner (Table 6-2). Each RyR homotetramer has one high-affinity and three low-affinity binding sites (3). At low ryanodine concentrations, when it interacts with the high-affinity binding site, it locks the channel in the semiopen position, with a rapid release of calcium, until the SR becomes calcium depleted. At high concentrations, ryanodine locks the channel in the closed mode.

Response of Ryanodine Receptor to Calcium

The RyR receptor is ligand operated, and the physiologic ligand is calcium. When the subsarcolemmal calcium increases very rapidly, as in response to abrupt opening of an L-type calcium channel, the RyR responds ultrarapidly by

TABLE 6-2. Effects of drugs on sarcoplasmic reticulum

Substance/agent	Ca^{2+} uptake into SR	Ca^{2+} release from SR
Catecholamines, β-adrenergic	Increased. Uptake pump stimulated (increased phosphorylation of phospholamban)	Indirectly increased by greater opening of L-calcium channels, hence greater Ca^{2+} influx
Catecholamines, α-adrenergic	No direct effect	Increased release via second messenger IP_3, which acts on IP_3 receptor of SR
Caffeine, high doses, 5 mmol/L	No direct effect on pump	Opens release channel; sensitizes to Ca^{2+} induced Ca^{2+} release[a,b,c]
Local anesthetic (procaine)	No direct effect	Inhibits[b]
Ruthenium red	No direct effect	Inhibits ryanodine receptor[d]
Ca^{2+} antagonists	No direct effect	Indirect decrease. Less Ca^{2+} entry by the L-Ca^{2+}channel with less Ca^{2+}-induced Ca^{2+} release
Ryanodine (low dose)	No direct effect	Increases by locking release channel in open mode[e]
Ryanodine (high dose)	No direct effect	Decreases by locking channel in closed mode
Thapsigargin[f]	Inhibition	No effect
Cyclopiazonic acid[f]	Inhibition	No effect
Heparin	No direct effect	Inhibits IP_3 receptor and activates ryanodine receptor[g]

SR, sarcoplasmic reticulum; IP_3, inositol triphosphate.
[a-g]See reference 18a–18g.

opening the calcium release channel within 1 to 2 milliseconds (3). How the RyR channel closes is still controversial, as already discussed. Closely related to the calcium response is that to PKA. β-Adrenergic stimulation mediates its effects by a series of signals, leading to activation of PKA. PKA exerts several intracellular effects that increase the rate of increase and decrease in internal calcium (Fig. 7-16). PKA also phosphorylates the RyR; the rate of calcium release by RyR can thereby be enhanced. In addition, PKA phosphorylates phospholamban on the calcium uptake pump (SERCA), which keeps the SR loaded with the calcium that is needed to maintain calcium release by the RyR (19).

Response of Ryanodine Receptor to Caffeine

Caffeine can empty the SR of its calcium. The molecular site of action of caffeine is the RyR. In high concentrations, caffeine considerably increases the opening probability of the sarcoplasmic calcium release channel, to release all the SR calcium. Thus, any net uptake of calcium by the SR does not occur. Therefore, the rapid increase of internal calcium concentration found after caffeine is a measure of the calcium that had been stored in the SR (3,20). The normal calcium load is approximately 100 μmol/L of SR cytosol or approximately twice the amount of calcium required to activate contraction (3,20).

IP$_3$–Induced Release of Calcium from the Sarcoplasmic Reticulum

In addition to the RyR, there is a second receptor, that for inositol 1,4,5-trisphosphate (IP$_3$), which also controls calcium release. IP$_3$ is part of the messenger system for a group of receptors including α_1-adrenergic activity, angiotensin II, and endothelin. Although the physiologic role of these agonists in stimulating the myocardium is still in question, in vascular smooth muscle, they all mediate IP$_3$-dependent vasoconstriction. By contrast, in cardiac muscle, the IP$_3$ receptor probably plays a much lesser role than the RyR, as reflected in the relative scarcity of IP$_3$ cardiac receptors (15). In human heart failure, the RyR is downgraded, whereas the IP$_3$ receptor is upgraded, thereby speculatively providing some measure of alternate support pathway for maintenance of calcium transients (21).

CALCIUM UPTAKE PUMP OF THE SARCOPLASMIC RETICULUM

To allow diastolic relaxation, calcium must be removed from the cytosol (Fig. 6-2). In the rabbit, with electrophysiologic properties similar to the human, approximately 75% of the activator calcium is removed by the calcium uptake pump of the SR, while sodium–calcium exchange removes approximately 25%, with only approximately 1% removed by the calcium pump of the sarcolemma or transport into mitochondria (1). Therefore, the larger fraction of calcium by far released from the SR is returned to its site of origin by the activity of the ATP-consuming pump SERCA (or more precisely SERCA-2A).

SERCA Requires ATP

Studies on isolated fragments of the SR (as tiny vesicles) show that the calcium-accumulating activity of the SR requires ATP. This ATP can be derived either from mitochondrial sources or glycolysis (22). The pump constitutes nearly 40% of the protein component of the SR and is the major mechanism for reducing the cytosolic calcium ion level, thereby initiating diastole. The pump accounts for approximately 15% of the myocardial energy expenditure (23). The pump has a molecular weight of approximately 115 kd and is distributed asymmetrically across the membrane in such a way that part of it actually protrudes into the cytosol (Fig. 6-8). It probably consists of dimers of a single polypeptide. For each mole of ATP that is hydrolyzed by this enzyme, two calcium ions are

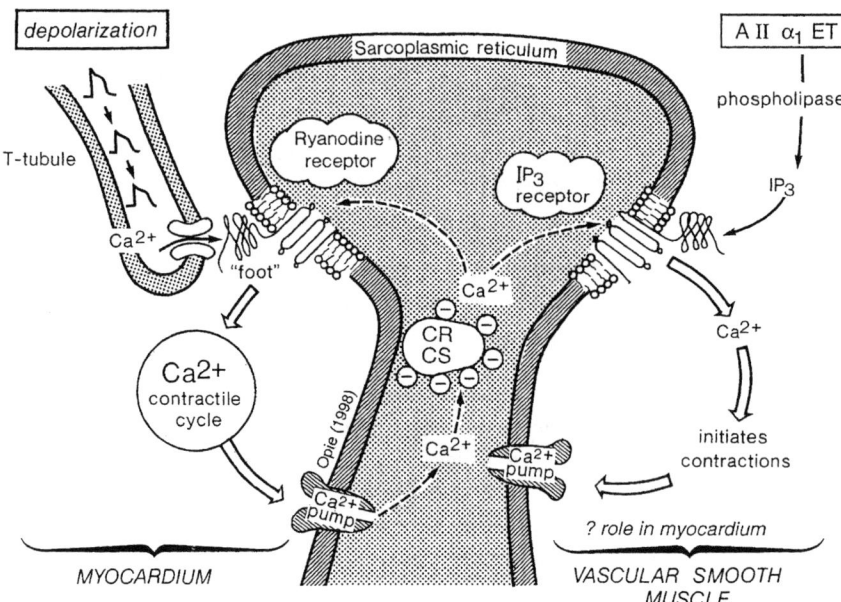

FIG. 6-8. Contrasts between the myocardium and vascular smooth muscle in calcium release mechanisms. In the myocardium (on the left), calcium is released from the sarcoplasmic reticulum (SR) via the calcium release channel (part of the ryanodine receptor), mainly in response to calcium that has entered during voltage depolarization. Calcium is taken up again by the calcium pump of the longitudinal SR to interact with the storage proteins calsequestrin (*CS*) and calreticulin (*CR*), from there to be released again. In contrast, in vascular smooth muscle, stimulation of vasoconstrictor receptors leads to release of inositol 1,4,5-trisphosphate (IP$_3$), which acts on its receptor to release calcium from the SR. Whether the IP$_3$ path for calcium release operates in the normal myocardium is controversial. *A* II, angiotensin II; α_1, α_1-adrenergic activity; *ET*, endothelin.

accumulated within the reticulum. This ATPase of the SR differs in many ways from that of the sarcolemma, despite their common ability to pump calcium. In particular, only the SR pump is modulated by phospholamban, and only this pump is crucial for diastolic relaxation.

Phospholamban Inhibits Calcium Accumulation by SERCA

The activity of the calcium uptake pump of the SR is normally inhibited by phospholamban, which means phosphate receptor (24). Phospholamban is an integral part of the membrane proteins of the longitudinal SR and colocalizes with the metabolic pump that provides the energy for the transport of calcium. Phospholamban exists in at least two molecular forms: the monomer that is strongly inhibitory to SERCA and the less inhibitory pentamer (25). The pen-

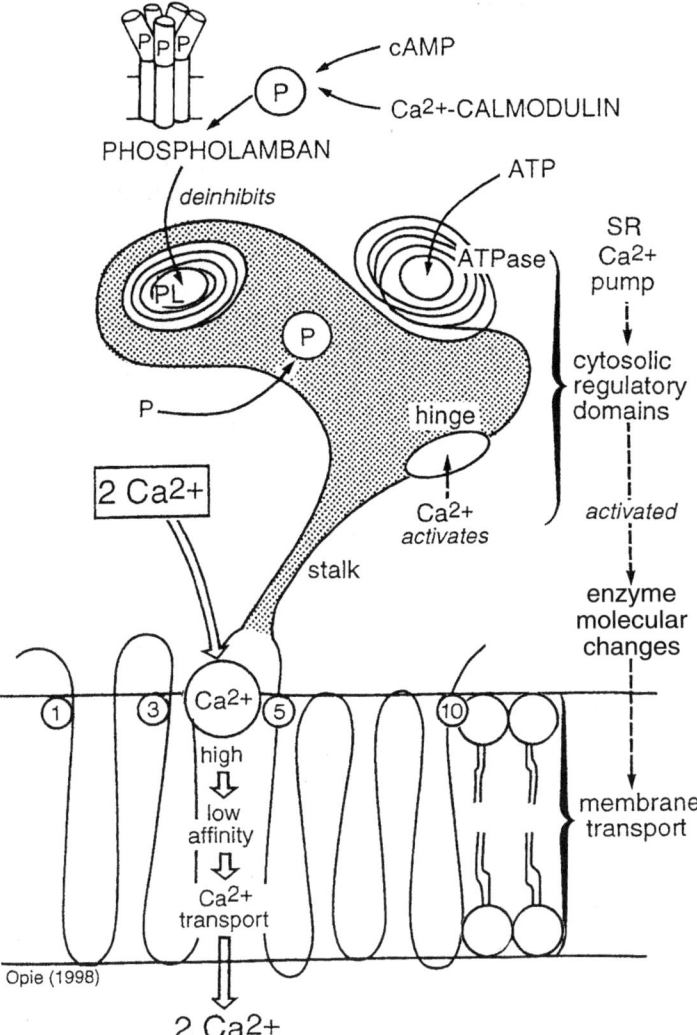

FIG. 6-9. Regulation of calcium uptake pump (SERCA) by phospholamban. The diagram shows the cytosolic regulatory domains of the calcium uptake pump SERCA (cardiac isoform, SERCA-2a), with activation by the removal of the phospholamban inhibitory "brake," and by calcium ions at two sites. There are cytosolic binding sites for adenosine 5′-triphosphate (*ATP*), phospholamban (*PL*), and a nearby phosphorylation site (*P*). ATP has two essential functions: it is required both for energy to drive the pump and for the phosphorylation. *SR*, sarcoplasmic reticulum.

tamer consists of five 52-amino-acid subunits, each of molecular weight 6 kd (Fig. 6-9). Using gene knockout and transgenic mouse models, the levels of expression of phospholamban can be ablated or increased (25). Ablation results in hyperfunction, with much increased rates of contraction and relaxation. Overexpression causes mechanical failure. Heterozygous models show that only approximately 40% of SR calcium pumps are inhibited by phospholamban *in vivo*. β-Adrenergic stimulation acting via cAMP and PKA phosphorylates phospholamban to relieve this inhibition, so that calcium uptake is stimulated. Another important stimulus to phosphorylation of phospholamban is an increased intracellular calcium level, acting via calmodulin and the calmodulin-dependent kinase. Calcium also acts directly on the molecular configuration of the calcium pump to enhance its activity (Fig. 6-9). Thus, calcium, calmodulin kinase, and PKA phosphorylate at two different sites on phospholamban, and calcium also acts directly on the calcium uptake pump, all these changes increasing the pump activity.

Molecular Interaction between Phospholamban and SERCA

One proposal is that, from a large pool of pentamers, the highly inhibitory monomers form and preferentially bind to SERCA (10,25). When phosphorylated, these monomers no longer can bind as tightly to SERCA, so that the inhibition they exert on SERCA is lessened and calcium uptake by the SR proceeds. Another model depicts phosphorylation shifting the equilibrium from monomers to oligomers, thereby lessening the monomer inhibition (26). An earlier and currently less favored model suggests that five phosphorylated phospholamban molecules form a calcium-permeable ion pore (27). There are additional modes of phosphorylation of phospholamban, of little physiologic importance in heart muscle, i.e., by protein kinase C or cyclic guanosine 3′,5′-monophosphate. The latter path may be more important in blood vessels to explain part of the vasodilatory effects of cyclic guanosine 3′,5′-monophosphate produced, for example, by the action of nitric oxide.

Response to β-Adrenergic Stimulation

This acts via cAMP and PKA to phosphorylate phospholamban and to relieve its normal inhibition of the calcium uptake pump of the SR. The pump takes up more calcium so that the SR is "loaded" to release more calcium during subsequent depolarizations. Consequently, the increased cytosolic calcium further phosphorylates phospholamban at a second site so that there is an added stimulation of the calcium uptake pump. There is a further increase in the rate of relaxation, and thus the SR is even more loaded with more calcium to allow a greater release from the SR in response to the next wave of depolarization. Hence, phosphorylation of phospholamban promotes the rate of relaxation (lusitropic effect) and indirectly the positive inotropic response, as shown in studies with transgenic mice deficient in phospholamban (28,29). Thus, with justification, phospholamban is called a "critical repressor of myocardial contractility" (27). In response to β-adrenergic stimulation, as in the "fight-or-flight" response, the phospholamban "brake" is released, with a rapid increase in both contraction and relaxation (27).

CALCIUM STORAGE AND ITS CONTROL

Calsequestrin and Calreticulin

The calcium taken up into the SR by the calcium uptake pump needs to be stored in anticipation of further release by the next wave of depolarization. Such storage occurs at the highly charged storage protein calsequestrin. This is a 55-kd protein not found in the network component of the SR but in the other parts including the cisternal component that lies near the T tubules. Such calcium stored in association with calsequestrin can then be released when the calcium release channel of the SR is stimulated to open by the next wave of depolarization. It is estimated that there are 175 to 350 µmol of calcium binding sites per liter of cytosol or 5 to 10 mmol/L SR (3), more than enough to cope with the maximal expected SR calcium content of approximately 100 µmol/L cytosol (3). When calsequestrin is overexpressed in mouse hearts, the SR calcium content increases markedly and heart failure develops (3). Calreticulin is another storage protein, similar in structure and function to calsequestrin.

Store-Regulated Uptake and Release of Calcium by the Sarcoplasmic Reticulum

How does the SR "know" when to take up calcium from the cytoplasm and when to release it? The mechanism of such fine coordination is still a challenge. The calcium content of the SR is "set" in such a way that an increase in the SR content of calcium results in greater release by the RyR, which in turn "unloads" the cell calcium by lessening the calcium entry into the cell and promoting greater calcium efflux from the cell. Decreased SR calcium sets in motion opposite events, but which are the molecular controls? The concept is that the level of the calcium store acts to regulate itself (30). The mechanism of such autoregulation is at both the sites of uptake and release of calcium by the SR. It has been proposed that depletion of the SR calcium stores prompts more rapid refilling (31). This involves activation of the calcium uptake pump SERCA. Another mechanism for storage regulation is at the release channel RyR. A high calcium load of the SR can "dramatically increase the fraction of the SR calcium that is released for a given trigger" (3). Thus, the level of stored calcium is autoregulated.

CALCIUM ION EFFLUX FROM CELLS

To avoid the myocardial cells from becoming overloaded with calcium requires the ejection of a small number of calcium ions, equivalent to those entering with each wave of depolarization. There are two exit pathways. The major route for calcium ion efflux is the sarcolemmal sodium–calcium exchange mechanism (Fig. 6-2), which is designed to eject calcium ions whenever the cytosolic calcium ion concentration increases and when the voltage conditions are favorable (Fig. 4-25), as probably occurs in the latter part of the action potential plateau. Anatomically, this exchanger is located mainly in the T-tubules, but not near the cisternae of the SR, so that it plays a lesser role in bringing in calcium that can act on the calcium release channel of the SR. It also acts in the other direction to eject excess calcium ions when the subsarcolemmal space is overloaded with calcium, as when the action potential is over.

The sarcolemmal calcium pump is a backup calcium ejection system that uses ATP and pumps calcium ions outward. The chief function of the calcium pump may be as follows. The pump is just active enough to respond to the low cytosolic calcium ion concentration normally found in diastole (0.15×10^{-6} mol/L) (Fig. 6-3). Thus, the pump responds to any higher value to help to maintain the diastolic cytosolic calcium concentration. The protein of this calcium pump can be stimulated directly by calcium-calmodulin (CaM) or by phosphorylation by cAMP-dependent PKA. When the calcium level is high or during catecholamine stimulation, the pump is switched on to function more actively, without being fast enough to cope with all the calcium ions requiring removal from the cytosol in diastole.

CALMODULIN

The previous sections describe how calcium acts as a molecular switch to turn on the contractile proteins. In addition, calcium ions may self-regulate their concentration in the cytosol, an important concept because when self-regulation fails, calcium overload ensues, and lethal cellular damage can follow. The calcium regulator protein calmodulin is thought to play a role in such self-regulation. Calmodulin is a small but ubiquitously distributed protein of 16,700 d that is activated when calcium binds to high-affinity binding sites to become CaM (32). Some "calcium-lowering" effects are mediated directly by CaM, such as inactivation of the inward calcium current I_{Ca} (32). CaM also acts via the calmodulin-dependent protein kinase calmodulin-kinase II, which phosphorylates phospholamban to increase the uptake of calcium from the cytosol into the SR (29). Thus, potentially calmodulin and/or calmodulin-kinase II help to regulate calcium ion fluxes and could do so on a beat-to-beat basis (32).

Calcineurin and Growth

As part of the very complex myocardial response to sustained mechanical stress, several signals such as increased calcium influx (Fig. 6-10) converge to

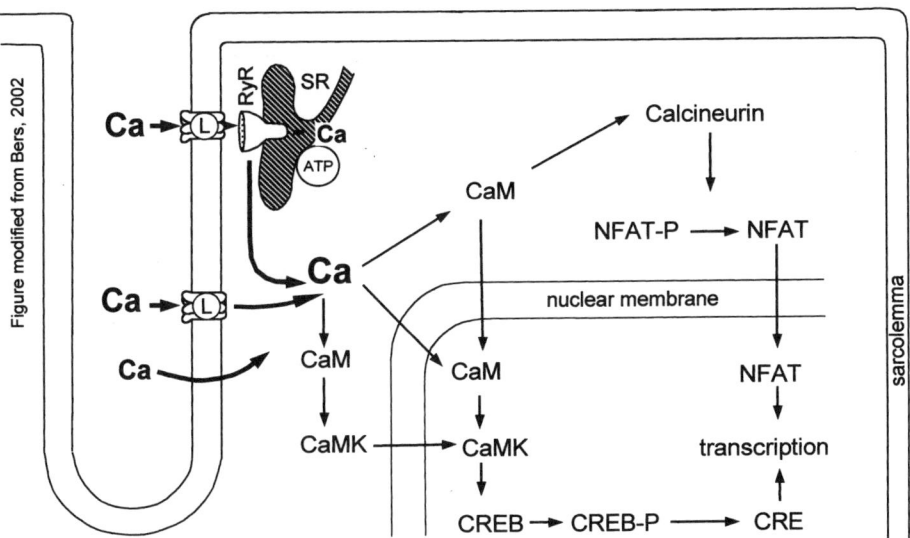

FIG. 6-10. Proposed role of calcium influx in growth induced by load and mechanical stress. The increased calcium entry is mediated both by the L-type calcium channels (*L*) and by stretch-activated channels (33). Cytosolic calcium also increases in response to angiotensin II, an important growth factor (not shown). *SAC*, stretch-activated channels; *CaM*, calmodulin; *CaMK*, calmodulin kinase; *CREB*, cyclic adenosine 3′,5′-monophosphate response element binding protein; *NFAT*, nuclear factor of activated T cells.

give a sustained increase in cytosolic calcium and hence to promote hypertrophy (33). CaM II influences myocardial hypertrophy by interacting with *calcineurin*, the CaM-activated growth factor. Calcineurin is a phosphatase that dephosphorylates and activates NFAT (nuclear factor of activated T cells) that in turn promotes nuclear transcription. This process potentially links increased cytosolic calcium levels to nuclear transcription and involves calcium-dependent paths similar to those in excitation–transcription coupling (32).

POSITIVE INOTROPIC AND RELAXANT EFFECTS OF β-ADRENERGIC STIMULATION

β-Adrenergic stimulation enhances the force of contraction (positive inotropic effect) and the rate of relaxation (relaxant or lusitropic effect; Greek, *lusi*, relaxation), thereby altering the pattern of contraction and relaxation (Fig. 6-11). The cardiac inotropic state is governed largely by the amount of calcium ions entering the cytosol during the process of activation. β-Adrenergic stimulation increases the inotropic state by an increase in cAMP-mediated activation of PKA that in turn increases the inward calcium current (I_{Ca}), causing a greater rate of release of calcium ions from the RyR. β-Adrenergic stimulation also accelerates reuptake of

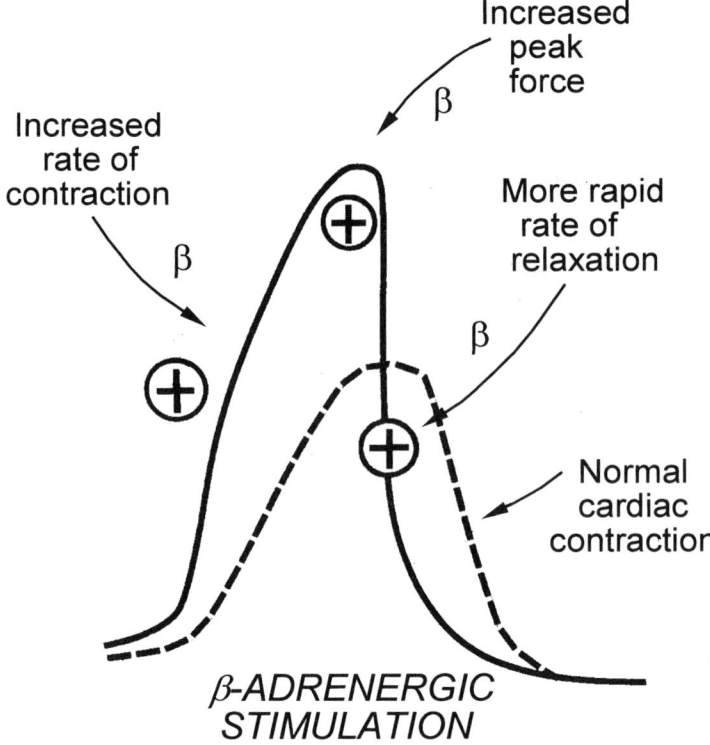

FIG. 6-11. Proposed effects of β-adrenergic stimulation on the pattern of cardiac contraction. Increased release of calcium from the sarcoplasmic reticulum (SR) causes the increased rate of contraction and increased peak force. An increased rate of calcium uptake into the SR enhances the rate of relaxation.

calcium into the SR; therefore, preloading the SR with more calcium will indirectly enhance the amount of calcium released in response to any given amount of trigger calcium, so the contraction phase of the contractile cycle will be further stimulated (6). Whether there is PKA-mediated, increased open probability of the RyR channels remains controversial. To accelerate relaxation, the phosphorylation of phospholamban (28) is much more important than that of troponin I (29). Thus, an increased rate of both contraction and relaxation is ultimately achieved in response to β-adrenergic stimulation, and the increased peak cytosolic calcium transient ensures that the force of contraction is likewise increased (Fig. 7-15).

CALCIUM OVERLOAD AND ARRHYTHMIAS

An important concept in cardiac pathology is that of calcium overload, first emphasized by Fleckenstein in the early 1970s. He proposed that calcium overload could damage myocardial cells, as now is thought to occur by several mechanisms in response to myocardial ischemia, reperfusion, and excess catecholamine stimulation. First, as the mitochondria attempt to buffer the cytosolic calcium, they become overloaded with calcium and waste ATP in the process, thereby demanding more oxygen and extending the severity of ischemia. Second, excess calcium may stimulate the phospholipase enzymes that break down cell membranes. Third, calcium overload may cause the development of contracture, which is a state of sustained excess contraction. Fourth, excess calcium cycling in and out of the SR may explain some arrhythmias.

Increased calcium sparks may help to "unload" a calcium-overloaded SR (14a). The danger is that such unloading sparks can lead to propagated calcium waves with the risk of serious arrhythmias or impaired contractile activity. When the SR has a high calcium load, that directly increases the amount of calcium available for release yet it greatly enhances the fraction of the SR calcium that is released in response to any specific amount of trigger calcium. The reason for this is in part owing to the stimulatory effect of high intra-SR free calcium on the RyR release channels.

Some arrhythmias of ischemia and reperfusion are calcium based. Calcium-dependent inward currents give rise to excess afterdepolarizations or oscillatory aftercontractions, which involve recycling of calcium through the SR. These are caused by calcium-dependent inward currents, mainly through the sodium–calcium exchangers. Increased internal calcium cycling is also involved because ventricular arrhythmias dependent on such oscillations are stopped by agents that inhibit calcium release from the SR (high concentrations of ryanodine) or by inhibitors of the calcium uptake pump SERCA-2a, such as thapsigargin. Mutations of the RyR may cause defective functioning of the RyR channel, an example of a channelopathy (Chapter 20). Thus, "leaky feet" of the RyR may lead to serious arrhythmias and sudden death (18).

Diastolic Calcium Overload

Because of the phasic nature of the increase and decrease in internal calcium in response to the initial wave of depolarization, a situation may arise in which calcium does not return rapidly to a static diastolic level at the end of relaxation. Rather, there could be spontaneous oscillations as the cytosolic calcium gradually decreased to the normal low diastolic level (34). Internal calcium may increase focally within calcium-overloaded cells rather than uniformly (35). This process in turn stimulates the sodium–calcium exchange mechanism with an increase of the transient inward current (Fig. 20-8). Abnormal inward currents may form at irregular sites throughout the calcium overloaded cell with risk of arrhythmias, a good example of "calcium mismanagement" (3). As ischemia proceeds, there is eventually an increase of internal calcium (36) occurring concurrently with the development of ischemic contracture, often an irreversible event. In the hypertrophied, pressure-overloaded heart, diastolic dysfunction is an early abnormality (Chapter 13). This can be linked to decreased transcription of the SERCA-2 gene (37), thus lessening the rate of uptake of calcium by the SR and hence impairing diastolic relaxation.

SARCOPLASMIC RETICULUM IN HEART FAILURE

In heart failure, the force of cardiac contraction is reduced and there is an abnormal delayed pattern of cardiac relaxation. Because the SR is so intimately involved in both phases of the contractile cycle, it is not surprising that abnormalities at this organelle may play a fundamental role in heart failure.

Deficient Activity of SERCA-2a

The activity of the calcium uptake pump SERCA is reduced and sodium–calcium exchange is enhanced, so that in diastole relatively more calcium is extruded across the sarcolemma and relatively less taken up by the SR. Furthermore, the RyRs may be hyperphosphorylated (see later), promoting calcium leaks from the SR. The depleted SR stores are one important factor in the decreased contractile strength of the failing heart (38). In end-stage human heart failure, the messenger RNA levels of proteins regulating calcium uptake and release are decreased. Specifically, the messenger RNAs for the RyR, the calcium uptake pump SERCA-2a, and phospholamban are all abnormally low (39). Because defective SERCA-2a activity is a basic problem in heart failure, the gene replacement of SERCA-2a should help contractile function, as it does in a rat heart failure model (23).

Excess Inhibition by Phospholamban

A second hypothesis relates decreased contractility of the failing heart to enhanced inhibition of SERCA-2a by phospholamban (40,41). Thus, phospholamban is underphosphorylated with excess "braking" of SERCA-2a and deficient calcium cycling. To remedy this defect in a mouse model of cardiomyopathic heart failure, Chien's group (42) transferred a pseudophosphorylated mutant of phospholamban that was able to relieve the inhibited calcium uptake pump and to lessen the rate of decline of cardiac function. An alternate approach is the genetic transfer of antisense of the phospholamban gene, with improved contractile performance of cells isolated from failing human hearts (43). Antisense techniques reduce expression of any given gene, the opposite aim of the gene-enhancing "sense strategy."

Hyperphosphorylation of the Ryanodine Receptor

A third hypothesis emphasizes that activity of the RyR is altered in human heart failure. The proposal is that hyperphosphorylation of the RyR (Fig. 6-12)

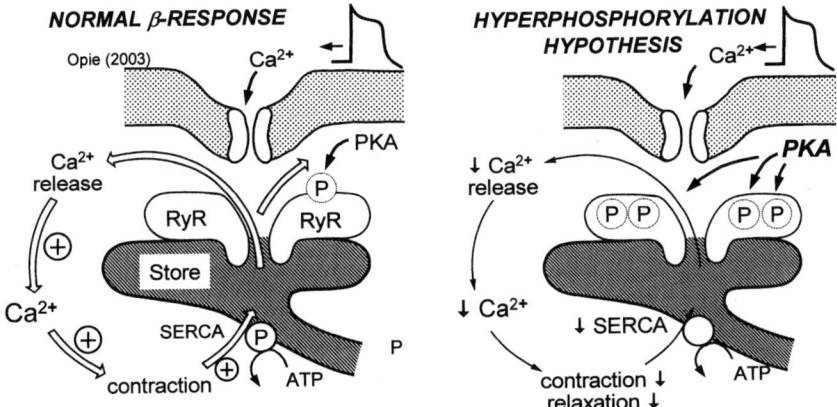

FIG. 6-12. Molecular model for proposed role of ryanodine receptor (RyR) in calcium cycling in heart failure. Hypothetically and controversially, phosphorylation of the RyR by protein kinase A promotes opening of the calcium release channel. In heart failure, the hyperadrenergic state leads to hyperphosphorylation with uncoupling of the RyR monomers from each other and decreased calcium release from the sarcoplasmic reticulum. This contributes to the decreased force of contraction. See Marks et al. (2) for alternate views; see text.

results from the hyperadrenergic state that characterizes heart failure (2). The suggested consequences include a diastolic calcium leak from the SR contributing to diastolic cytosolic calcium overload and reducing calcium stores in the SR and reduced triggered release of calcium with decreased cytosolic calcium transients and a lower rate of rise of force development (2). Of relevance to the therapy of heart failure, prior β-blockade reduces hyperphosphorylation (2) and improves cardiac function. Equally interesting, after giving patients a left ventricular assist device, hyperphosphorylation decreases and cardiac function improves (17). These proposals are questioned by others who find no abnormalities in the RyRs in heart failure (44). Rather, the alternate view emphasizes that the basic abnormality is depressed activity of SERCA with decreased calcium uptake by the SR, thereby decreasing the SR calcium stores and thus lessening the release of calcium from the SR.

Heart Rate in Heart Failure

Normally, increasing the stimulation rate of heart cells increases the SR calcium load owing to more frequent calcium influx and less time for calcium extrusion by the sodium–calcium exchanger, with less time for the RyR to recover and to be ready for the next beat (3). Crucial to achieving the greater loaded state is that the activity of the SR calcium uptake pump, SERCA-2a, must be normal (40). The loaded SR means greater calcium transients, so that the force–frequency relationship of the normal human heart is positive (Fig. 12-9).

However, in the failing human heart, where the activity of SERCA-2a is decreased, the SR is calcium depleted, and the force–frequency relationship is flat (Fig. 12-9) or negative (38). Of interest, in myocytes from normal rats and mice, there is actually a negative force–frequency relationship. They start with a highly loaded SR, so that no heart rate–induced increase is possible. As the heart rate increases, more calcium enters, and there is insufficient time for the RyR to fully recover, thereby reducing the amount of calcium release and hence the uptake of calcium by the SR. A similar situation may occur in large animal hearts when they are constantly driven by fast heart rate pacing until heart failure develops.

SUMMARY

1. *Cardiac contraction and relaxation are explained by an intracellular calcium cycle.* During depolarization, the small amount of calcium that enters the heart cell triggers the release of more calcium from the SR by the process of calcium-induced calcium release.
2. *The wave of depolarization is the initiating event.* It sweeps along the T tubule to open the calcium channel of the tubular membrane to allow calcium ions to penetrate. The latter trigger the release of much more calcium from the calcium channel of the RyR that lies at the junction of the T tubule and the SR. The cytosolic calcium increases and myocardial contraction occurs.
3. *Relaxation is initiated when the cytosolic calcium starts to decrease.* The activity of the ATP-dependent calcium uptake pump of the SR is crucial. This pump is also called SERCA and the cardiac isoform is called SERCA-2a. Activity of this pump is increased by the increase in cytosolic calcium and can be further stimulated by phosphorylation of the regulatory protein phospholamban. Calcium uptake into the SR is thereby promoted, and myocardial relaxation occurs after a short delay. The sodium-calcium exchanger also contributes to relaxation, removing as much calcium as entered via the tubular calcium channels.
4. *β-Adrenergic stimulation via the formation of cAMP* and activation of PKA increases the entry of calcium ions into myocardial cells through the calcium channels of the SR, thereby stimulating cardiac contraction (positive inotropic effect). β-Adrenergic stimulation also stimulates the rate of uptake of calcium ions back into the SR by phosphorylating phospholamban. Thus, cytosolic calcium decreases at a greater rate, so that diastolic relaxation is enhanced.
5. *Clinically important events* such as enhanced myocyte necrosis, shortening of the action potential duration, and potentially fatal arrhythmias can occur when the control mechanisms regulating the cytosolic calcium concentration fail, and cytosolic calcium overload develops.

6. *In heart failure, calcium cycling in and out of the SR is impaired.* Uptake of calcium by the calcium uptake pump (SERCA) is suppressed, and there is a leak through the RyR. The latter is hypothetically thought to reflect the hyperadrenergic state that characterizes heart failure. Such changes may contribute to the impaired contractility found in these conditions. Gene transfer techniques to upregulate the defective calcium uptake pump are under intense study and may be ready for clinical testing within a few years.

STUDENT QUESTIONS

1. How does cytosolic calcium increase at the start of systole?
2. How does cytosolic calcium decrease to initiate diastole?
3. What is the function of phospholamban?
4. Describe the physiologic role of the RyR and its calcium channel.
5. What is calmodulin? How does it influence the contractile process?

CARDIOLOGIST-IN-TRAINING QUESTIONS

1. Describe the sequence of events involved in excitation–contraction coupling.
2. What is the RyR? How does it respond to β-adrenergic stimulation?
3. Phospholamban is described as a prominent regulator of myocardial contractility. How is it related to a positive lusitropic effect?
4. What is SERCA? What is its proposed role in heart failure?
5. How is cytosolic calcium overload normally avoided? What are some clinically applied consequences of calcium overload?

REFERENCES

1. Bers DM. Cardiac excitation-contraction coupling. *Nature* 2002;415:198–205.
2. Marks AR, Reiken S, Marx SO. Progression of heart failure. Is protein kinase a hyperphosphorylation of the ryanodine receptor a contributing factor. *Circulation* 2002;105:272–275.
3. Bers DM. *Excitation-contraction coupling and cardiac contractile force.* Boston: Kluwer Academic Publishers, 2001.
4. Fabiato A. Calcium-induced release of calcium from the sarcoplasmic reticulum. *J Gen Physiol* 1985; 85:189–320.
5. Santana LF, et al. Relation between sarcolemmal Ca^{2+} current and Ca^{2+} sparks and local theories for cardiac excitation-contraction coupling. *Circ Res* 1996;78:166–171.
5a. Piacentino V 3rd, Weber CR, Chen X, et al. Cellular basis of abnormal calcium transients of failing human ventricular myocytes. *Circ Res* 2003;92:651–658.
6. Trafford AW, et al. Coordinated control of cell Ca^{2+} loading and triggered release from the sarcoplasmic reticulum underlies the rapid inotropic response to increased L-type Ca^{2+} current. *Circ Res* 2001;2001:195–201.
7. Wier WG, Egan TM, Lopez-Lopez JR, et al. Local control of excitation-contraction coupling in rat heart cells. *J Physiol* 1994;474:463–471.
8. Bouchard RA, Clark RB, Giles WR. Effects of action potential duration on excitation-contraction coupling in rat ventricular myocytes. *Circ Res* 1995;76:790–801.

184   6. EXCITATION–CONTRACTION COUPLING AND CALCIUM

9. Inoue M, et al. Ca^{2+} sparks in rabbit ventricular myocytes evoked by action potentials. *Circ Res* 2003; 92:532–538.
10. Kimura Y, et al. Phospholamban inhibitory function is activated by depolymerization. *J Biol Chem* 1997;272:15061–15064.
11. Cheng H, Cannell MB, Lederer WJ. Propagation of excitation-contraction coupling into ventricular myocytes. *Pflugers Arch* 1994;428:415–417.
12. Lederer WJ, Niggli E, Hadley RW. Sodium-calcium exchange in excitable cells: fuzzy space. *Science* 1990;248:283.
13. Callewaert G. Excitation-coupling in mammalian cardiac cells. *Cardiovasc Res* 1992;26:923–932.
14. Wier WG, et al. Ca^{2+} release mechanisms, Ca^{2+} sparks, and local control of excitation-contraction coupling in normal heart muscle. *Circ Res* 1999;85:770–776.
15. Marks AR. Cardiac intracellular calcium release channels. Role in heart failure. *Circ Res* 2000; 87:8–11.
16. Bers DM, et al. Coordinated feet and the dance of ryanodine receptors. *Science* 1998;281:790–791.
17. Marx SO, et al. PKA phosphorylation dissociates FKBP12.6 from the calcium release channel (ryanodine receptor): Defective regulation in failing hearts. *Cell* 2000;101:365–376.
18. Allen P. Leaky "feet" and sudden death [Editorial]. *Circ Res* 2002;91:181–182.
18a. Rasmussen CA, Jr., et al. Effects of ryanodine and caffeine on contractility, membrane voltage, and calcium exchange in cultured heart cells. *Circ Res* 1987;60:495.
18b. Hunter DR. et al. Cellular calcium turnover in the perfused rat heart: modulation by caffeine and procaine. *Circ Res* 1982;51:363.
18c. Sitsapesan R, Williams AJ. Mechanisms of caffeine activation of single calcium release channels of sheep cardiac sarcoplasmic reticulum. *J Physiol* 1990;423:425–439.
18d. Ruwhof C, et al. Mechanical stress stimulates phospholipase C activity and intracellular calcium ion levels in neonatal rat cardiomyocytes. *Cell Calcium* 2001;29:73.
18e. Rousseau E, Smith JS, Meissner G. Ryanodine modifies conductance and gating behavior of single Ca^{2+} release channel. *Am J Physiol* 1987;253:C364–C368.
18f. Du Toit EF, Opie LH. Inhibitors of Ca^{2+}-ATPase pump of sarcoplasmic reticulum attenuate reperfusion stunning in isolated rat heart. *J Cardiovasc Pharmacol* 1994;24:674–678.
18g. Ehrlich BE, et al. The pharmacology of intracellular Ca^{2+}-release channels. *Trends Pharmacol Sci* 1994;15:145.
19. Li Y, et al. Protein kinase A phosphorylation of the ryanodine receptor does not affect calcium sparks in mouse ventricular myocytes. *Circ Res* 2002;90:309–316.
20. Bers DM. Calcium fluxes involved in control of cardiac myocyte contraction. *Circ Res* 2000;87: 275–281.
21. Go LO, et al. Differential regulation of two types of intracellular calcium release channels during endstage heart failure. *J Clin Invest* 1995;95:888–894.
22. Boehm E, et al. Glycolysis supports calcium uptake by the sarcoplasmic reticulum in skinned ventricular fibers of mice deficient in mitochondrial and cytosolic creatinine kinase. *J Mol Cell Cardiol* 2000;32:891–902.
23. del Monte F, et al. Improvement in survival and cardiac metabolism after gene transfer of sarcoplasmic reticulum Ca^{2+}-ATPase in a rat model of heart failure. *Circulation* 2001;104:1424–1429.
24. Tada M, Katz AM. Phosphorylation of the sarcoplasmic reticulum and sarcolemma. *Annu Rev Physiol* 1982;44:401–423.
25. Brittsan AG, et al. Phospholamban and cardiac contractile function. *J Mol Cell Cardiol* 2000;32: 2131–2139.
26. Cornea R, et al. Mutation and phosphorylation change the oligomeric structure of phospholamban in lipid bilayers. *Biochemistry* 1997;36:2960–2967.
27. Koss KL, Kranias EG. Phospholamban: a prominent regulator of myocardial contractility. *Circ Res* 1996;79:1059–1063.
28. Luo W, Grupp IL, Harrer J, et al. Targeted ablation of the phospholamban gene is associated with markedly enhanced myocardial contractility and loss of beta-agonist stimulation. *Circ Res* 1994;75: 401–409.
29. Li L, et al. Phosphorylation of phospholamban and troponin I in β-adrenergic-induced acceleration of cardiac relaxation. *Am J Physiol* 2000;278:H769–H779.
30. Eisner DA, et al. Integrative analysis of calcium cycling in cardiac muscle. *Circ Res* 2000;87: 1087–1094.
31. Bhogal MS, et al. Depletion of Ca^{2+} from the sarcoplasmic reticulum of cardiac muscle prompts

phosphorylation of phospholamban to stimulate store refilling. *Proc Natl Acad Sci U S A* 1998;95: 1484–1489.
32. Maier LS, et al. Calcium, calmodulin, and calcium-calmodulin kinase II: heartbeat to heartbeat and beyond. *J Mol Cell Cardiol* 2002;14:919–939.
33. Sussman MA, et al. Dance band on the *Titanic*. Biomechanical signaling in cardiac hypertrophy. *Circ Res* 2002;91:888–898.
34. Meissner A, et al. Contractile dysfunction and abnormal Ca^{2+} modulation during postischemic reperfusion in rat heart. *Am J Physiol* 1995;268:H100–H111.
35. Berlin JR, Cannell MB, Lederer WJ. Cellular origins of the transient inward current in cardiac myocytes. Role of fluctuations and waves of elevated intracellular calcium. *Circ Res* 1989;65: 115–126.
36. Steenbergen C, Murphy E, Watts JA, et al. Correlation between cytosolic free calcium, contracture, ATP, and irreversible ischemic injury in perfused rat heart. *Circ Res* 1990;66:135–146.
37. Takizawa T, et al. Transcription of the SERCA2 gene is decreased in pressure-overloaded hearts: a study using *in vivo* direct gene transfer into living myocardium. *J Mol Cell Cardiol* 1999;31: 2167–2174.
38. Pieske B, et al. Ca^{2+} handling and sarcoplasmic reticulum Ca^{2+} content in isolated failing and non-failing human myocardium. *Circ Res* 1999;85:38–46.
39. Arai M, Suzuki T, Nagai R. Sarcoplasmic reticulum gene expression in cardiac hypertrophy and heart failure. *Circ Res* 1994;74:555–564.
40. Münch G, et al. SERCA2a activity correlates with the force-frequency relationship in human myocardium. *Am J Physiol* 2000;278:H1924–H1932.
41. Minamisawa S, et al. Chronic phospholamban-sarcoplasmic reticulum calcium ATPase interaction is the critical calcium cycling defect in dilated cardiomyopathy. *Cell* 1999;99:313–322.
42. Hoshijima M, et al. Chronic suppression of heart-failure progression by a pseudophosphorylated mutant of phospholamban via in vivo cardiac rAAV gene delivery. *Nat Med* 2002;8:864–871.
43. del Monte F, et al. Targeting phospholamban by gene transfer in human heart failure. *Circulation* 2002;105:904–907.
44. Jiang M, et al. Abnormal Ca^{2+} release, but normal ryanodine receptors, in canine and human heart failure. *Circ Res* 2002;91:1015–1022.

7

Receptors and Signal Transduction

Adrenergic receptors do not simply generate second messengers but rather activate a host of signaling proteins and pathways that control cardiac function, myocyte growth and cell death.

Rockman et al. (1)

The calcium cycles described in the preceding chapters are crucial for the regulation of cardiac contraction and the heart rate. These two key physiologic activities are stimulated by exercise and emotional stimulation and are decreased during sleep. The relevant calcium cycles need to respond to control by the autonomic nervous system that emits stimulatory adrenergic or inhibitory cholinergic messages. These do not communicate directly with cell calcium but require an intermediary system of cellular signals. When the primary autonomic messenger (e.g., epinephrine/norepinephrine or acetylcholine) binds to the adrenergic or cholinergic receptor on the sarcolemma, it initiates a series of molecular signals that eventually results in a corresponding increase or decrease in cell calcium. Such signals cause the heart rate and force of contraction to either increase or decrease. *Signal transduction can be defined as the sum total of those processes converting an extracellular stimulus to an intracellular regulator such as calcium, usually starting with an agonist binding to a receptor site and ending in a physiologic event such a contraction* (Fig. 7-1).

The *first* of the four major types of signal systems that regulate cardiovascular function leads from β-adrenergic stimulation to an increase in cell calcium (frontispiece; Fig. 7-2). Adrenergic stimulation releases of the first messenger (epinephrine from the adrenal gland or norepinephrine from the adrenergic nerve terminals) that occupies the β-adrenergic receptor. Then the sarcolemmal G proteins pass on the signal from the receptor to the next step to activate an enzyme called adenylyl cyclase that produces the second messenger, cyclic adenosine 3′,5′-monophosphate (cAMP). The latter unleashes a further series of intracellular signals that acts via the third messenger, protein kinase A (PKA), thereby increasing cytosolic calcium transients, so that the heart rate and the force of myocardial contraction increase. The coupling proteins belong to the super family of G proteins (G, guanine nucleotide binding), specific members of which

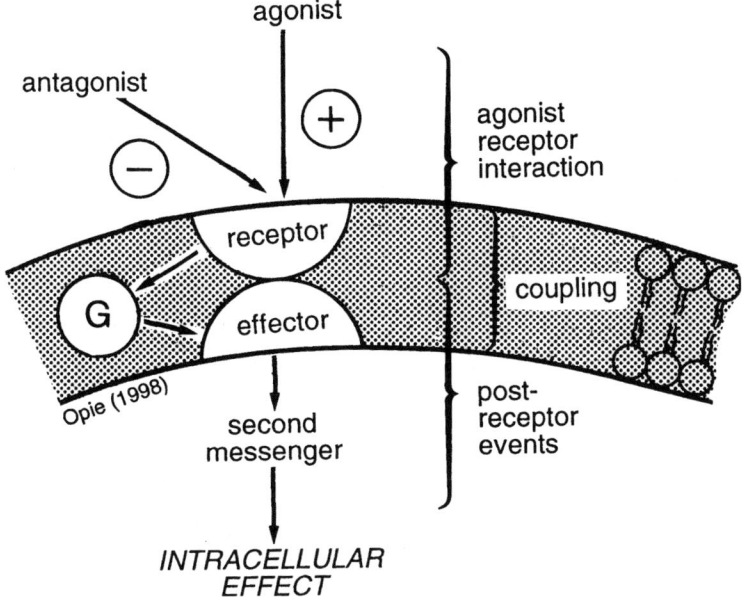

FIG. 7-1. General receptor pattern for interaction of hormone or other agonist with membrane-bound receptor.

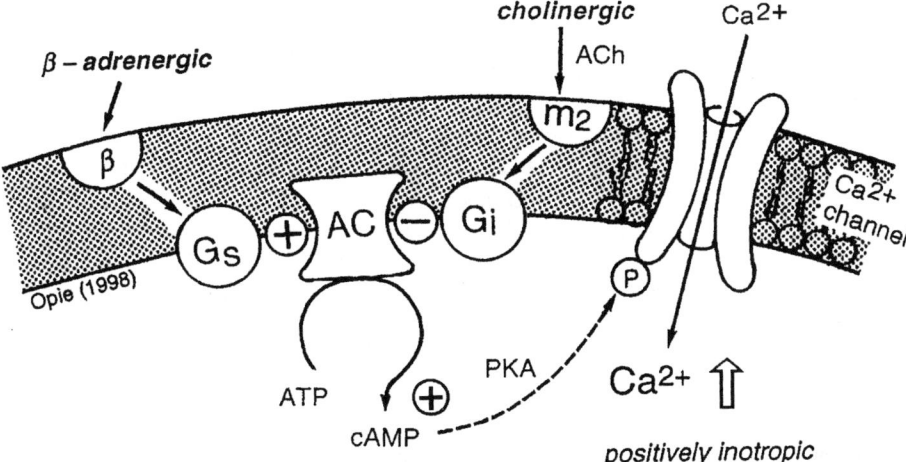

FIG. 7-2. Two major receptors. These are the β-adrenergic receptor and the cholinergic muscarinic (m_2) receptor, the latter for acetylcholine (*ACh*). The β-adrenergic receptor is coupled to adenylyl cyclase (*AC*) via the activated stimulatory G protein G_s (Fig. 7-8). Consequent formation of cyclic adenosine 3',5'-monophosphate (*cAMP*) activates protein kinase A (*PKA*) to phosphorylate the calcium channel to increase calcium entry. Activity of adenylyl cyclase can be decreased by the inhibitory subunits of the acetylcholine-associated inhibitory G protein G_i. ATP, adenosine 5'-triphosphate.

can either stimulate (G_s) or inhibit (G_i) adenylyl cyclase. For example, cholinergic stimulation of the muscarinic receptor by coupling to G_i rather than to G_s exerts inhibitory influences on the heart, at least in part by decreasing the rate of formation of cAMP.

The *second* signal system leads from α-adrenergic stimulation to increased cytosolic calcium in vascular smooth muscle. Release of norepinephrine from the adrenergic nerve terminals in the blood vessels is followed by occupation of the α-adrenergic receptors that link to another G protein–coupled enzyme. The latter activates the sarcolemmal enzyme phospholipase C to produce two messengers, inositol 1,4,5-trisphosphate (IP_3) and diacylglycerol (DAG), both of which, via different mechanisms, increase cytosolic calcium in vascular smooth muscle cells to cause vascular contraction (vasoconstriction). The DAG acts via the third messenger, protein kinase C (PKC), which, through a further series of messages, provides sustained vasoconstriction. The result is that both the peripheral vascular resistance and the blood pressure increase.

The *third* signal system causes vasodilation. Nitric oxide (NO), the messenger of this system, is formed in the inner endothelial layers of the blood vessels in response to several stimuli, including an increase in blood flow as occurs in exercise. NO then diffuses to the vascular smooth muscle cells to stimulate the formation of the second messenger, cyclic guanosine 3′,5′-monophosphate (cGMP), which lowers the calcium level and causes relaxation. These two opposing messenger systems in vascular smooth muscle, by promoting vasoconstriction (α-adrenergic) and vasodilation (NO), are able to regulate the peripheral vascular resistance and hence the blood pressure and the load against which the heart works. Similar signal systems also occur in the myocardium to increase or decrease the force of contraction but are probably less important than the β-adrenergic and cholinergic systems.

The fourth group of signaling systems is in contrast to the above three signal sequences that link neurotransmitters and hormones to cell calcium and hence to contraction. This fourth system ultimately regulates cell growth. Growth stimuli such as insulin and insulin growth factors act on tyrosine kinases to initiate a signaling system in which a key role is played by protein kinase B, or Akt, which in turn guides the stimulus to activators of nuclear transcription thereby promoting growth (Fig. 9-1).

PROPERTIES OF RECEPTORS

In 1905, Langley made the fundamental proposal that agents released at the nerve endings did not interact directly with the adjacent muscle cells. Rather, receptors were involved, as described by Ehrlich in 1913, to designate the hypothetical specific chemical groupings of the cell that reacted with chemotherapeutic drugs. This concept of receptors is fundamental to modern cardiovascular pharmacology and hence to clinical cardiology (Table 7-1). Ahlquist (2) pro-

TABLE 7-1. *Classification of cardiac receptors, including vascular and myocardial sites*

Broad types and agonists	Subtypes	Comments
Classic neurotransmitters		
Adrenergic	α_1, α_2	Chiefly vascular
	β_1	Chiefly cardiac (also vascular)
	β_2	Chiefly vascular, also cardiac
Cholinergic (muscarinic)	M_2	Heart and coronary arteries
	M_3	Endothelial, NO linked
Adrenergic-related receptors		
Histamine	H_1	Chiefly vascular
	H_2	Chiefly myocardial
Glucagon	—	Adenylate cyclase linked
Dopamine[a]	DA_1	Postsynaptic; cyclase linked; vasodilatory
Dopamine	DA_2	Presynaptic; inhibits NE release
Adenosine	A_1	Inhibits myocardial cAMP; role in preconditioning
Vascular receptors (other than adrenergic-cholinergic)		
Adenosine[b]	A_2	Vascular cAMP↑
Angiotensin II	AT_1	Phospholipase C linked
Endothelin[c]	ET_A	Phospholipase C linked
Thromboxane	—	Vascular Ca^{2+} influx↑
Prostacyclin	—	Vascular cAMP↑
Purinergic	P_1	Adenosine sensitive
	P_2	ATP sensitive, vascular
Peptidergic including	—	Vasoactive
Neuropeptide Y[d]	—	Inactive on coronary artery
Vasoactive intestinal peptide[e]	—	Coreleased with ACh
CGRP[d]	—	Vascular cAMP↑
Substance P[d]	—	Endothelial, NO linked
Enzymes		
Digitalis	—	Sodium-potassium pump
Other hormonal receptors		
Insulin	—	Tyrosine kinase linked
Steroid	—	—

NO, nitric oxide; NE, norepinephrine; cAMP, cyclic adenosine 3′, 5′-monophosphate; ↑, increased; ATP, adenosine 3′-triphosphate; ACh, acetylcholine; CGRP, calcitonin gene related peptide.
[a–e]See reference 1a–1e.

posed that sympathetic adrenergic stimulation interacted with two types of adrenergic receptors, α-adrenergic and β-adrenergic.

The term receptor *refers to a molecule (or molecular complex) that is capable of recognizing and selectively interacting with the agonist agent and, after binding it, is capable of generating some signal that initiates the chain of events leading to the biologic response (3).*

The biologic response is generated by a functionally separate *effector unit* (Fig. 7-1). Generally, the receptor is a specialized part of the external layer of the sarcolemma, sometimes extending through the sarcolemma, whereas the effector is a specialized part of the internal layer. Communication between the two is called coupling. Structurally, many receptors appear to be integral membrane proteins that require strong detergents to break the hydrophobic bonds holding them to the membrane. Sometimes, as in the case of thyroid hormone, the receptors are located within the cell so that the hormone has to cross the sarcolemma to reach the receptor. Especially in the case of drugs, the receptors are ill defined and possibly rather nonspecific. Thus, the term receptor is not always as definite as might be imagined. In other cases, techniques of molecular biology have revealed highly specific details of the receptor molecule, often pinning down the actual receptor site to a small number of amino acids. Such a close molecular fit can be compared with a "lock-and-key" pattern in which the agonist molecule is the key and the receptor molecule the lock. The key turns the lock to produce an intracellular effect mediated by a second messenger.

The interaction between receptor sites and antagonists may be reversible or irreversible. Reversible agonists and antagonists compete for the same receptor site, and the degree of effectiveness of each depends on the concentration at the receptor site. Irreversible agonists and antagonists bind irreversibly, and no amount of increased concentration of an agonist can overcome the blockade of the receptor site by the antagonist.

Dose–Response Curves

The classic way of relating the concentration of a drug or hormone to its effect is by a dose–response curve (Fig. 7-3). The dose causing 50% of the maximal effect is known as the ED_{50} (effective dose). When the effect is inhibition, the concentration of the agent causing 50% of the maximal inhibition is the IC_{50} (inhibitory concentration). Determination of the ED_{50} or IC_{50} can show whether a drug or hormone is active in producing its effect (low ED_{50} or IC_{50}) or not as active (high ED_{50} or IC_{50}). When a low concentration of a drug initiates a marked response, it has high intrinsic activity because the drug is assumed to bind to its receptor in such a way that a maximal signal is elicited. For example, the circulating concentrations of the catecholamines are normally very low, approximately 10^{-10} or 10^{-9} mol/L. The concentration actually reaching the receptors in the space between the terminal neurons and the receptors (the synaptic clefts) must be higher, possibly by 10-fold, because norepinephrine is released into that space.

In the presence of the β-adrenergic receptor blocking agent *propranolol*, the dose–response curve is shifted to the right, and a much higher concentration of the artificial catecholamine isoproterenol is required to increase the heart rate (Fig. 7-3). With excess propranolol (*β-blockade toxicity*), a suprapharmacologic concentration of isoproterenol is required to increase the heart rate. These are the characteristics of competitive antagonism.

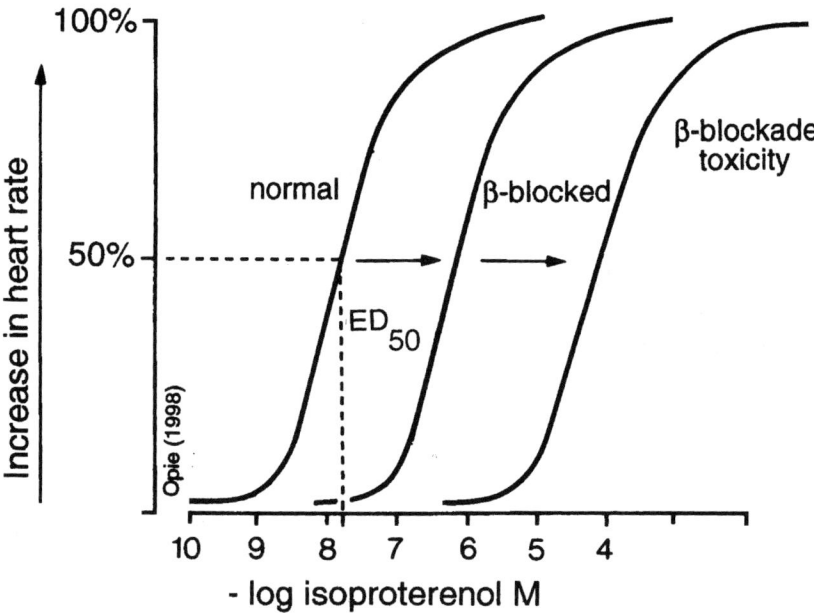

FIG. 7-3. Competitive antagonism between the pharmacologic β-adrenergic agonist isoproterenol and a β-adrenergic receptor antagonist, propranolol. These estimates are based on (a) a high plasma catecholamine concentration of 10^{-9} mol/L, (b) an agonist concentration of 10^{-7} mol/L might be needed to displace propranolol from the β-adrenergic receptor, and (c) the much higher doses of propranolol required for toxicity. Thus, β-blockade moves the ED_{50} to the right.

The receptor concept allows understanding of two important characteristics of effective drug–tissue interaction: high affinity and marked specificity. High affinity explains why a low concentration of a drug can be so effective, and marked specificity explains why only a small change in molecular structure can decisively change the properties of that drug.

β-ADRENERGIC RECEPTORS

There are two major receptor subtypes. Cardiac β-adrenergic receptors are mainly the *β₁-adrenergic receptor subtype*, whereas most noncardiac receptors are β₂ (4). Evidence of the existence of different receptors rests on molecular and immunologic studies that allow an exact differentiation of the distribution of β-adrenergic receptor subtypes, varying from 100% β₁-adrenergic receptors in the dog ventricle to 100% β₂-adrenergic receptors in the liver. In humans, there is a substantial population of *β₂-receptors in the atria*, with perhaps approximately 20% β₂-receptors in the left ventricle (5). Both receptor subtypes can coexist in the same ventricular cell, and both are involved in positive inotropic responses,

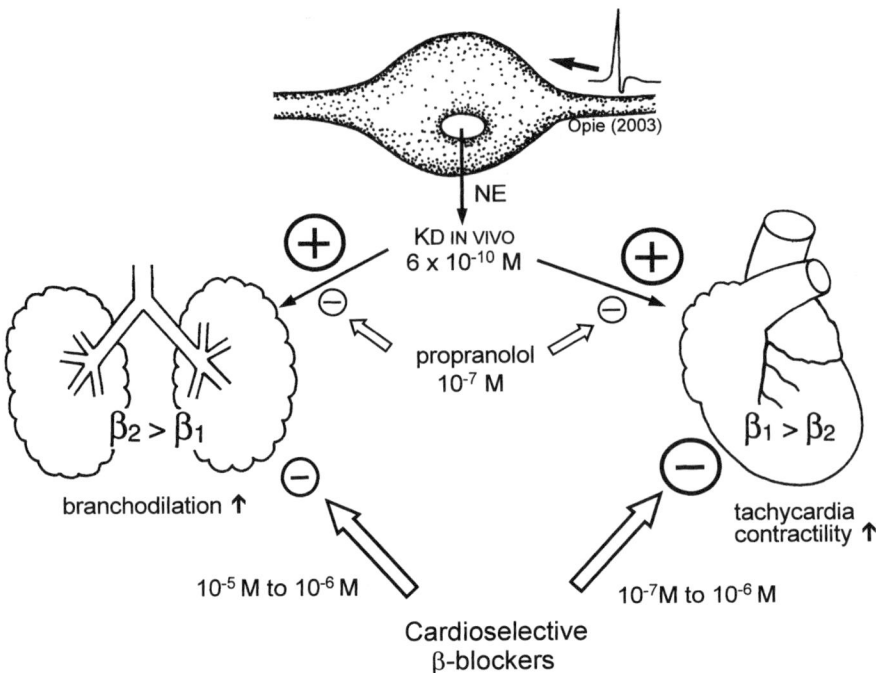

FIG. 7-4. Concept of cardioselectivity shows the role of comparative density of β_1 and β_2 receptors in the normal heart (80% β_1) and bronchi (mainly β_2). Note the low concentration of norepinephrine (*NE*) released in the synaptic cleft, which may, however, be concentrated by several orders of magnitude if the norepinephrine stays in the limited space of the cleft. The nonselective beta-blocker propranolol inhibits both β_1- and β_2-receptors. The cardioselective beta-blockers are more selective for the heart but at higher concentrations have an effect on the bronchi. K_D, apparent dissociation constant.

although the signal systems may differ (see Physiologic β-Adrenergic Effects section). The major clinical significance of the subtype difference is in relation to cardioselective *β_1-adrenergic blocking agents* (Fig. 7-4). There is a greater density of β_1-adrenergic receptors in the ventricular myocardium and β-adrenergic receptors in the lung, so that these drugs are preferred if there is lung disease. It must be emphasized that the β_1- and β_2-adrenergic receptors still have some molecular similarity despite their functional differences, so that β_1-blockers are only relatively selective, and at high doses, selectivity is lost. Molecular proof of differences in receptor subtypes is now available (6).

β_1-Adrenergic receptor density varies throughout the heart, and the sinus node has approximately seven to eight times more receptors than has the surrounding atrial muscle or atrioventricular node. The next highest concentration of receptors is found in the ventricles. It seems likely that differences in β-adrenergic receptor density are one factor determining the magnitude of the tissue response to β-adrenergic stimulation. To explain why some $β_1$-agonist drugs, such as dobutamine, have a more marked inotropic than chronotropic effect, it should be recalled that the ventricles contain mainly $β_1$-adrenergic receptors, whereas the sinus nodal tissue contains both subtypes. Hence, $β_2$ stimulants also cause tachycardia as well as an inotropic response, whereas $β_1$-agonists, such as dobutamine, may have an apparently dominant inotropic selectivity.

$β_2$- and $β_3$-Adrenergic Receptors

Whereas the postreceptor signaling sequence of the $β_1$-receptor is well understood, that of the cardiac $β_2$-receptor is still not fully clarified. $β_2$-Receptors link efficiently via G_s to adenyl cyclase. They may also couple to the inhibitory G_i proteins, a pathway that is functionally latent because of subcellular compartmentation of cAMP (7). In humans, the positive inotropic response to $β_2$ stimulation by salbutamol occurs at least in part via $β_2$-receptors on the terminal neurons of the cardiac sympathetic nerves, thereby releasing norepinephrine that in turns exerts dominant $β_1$ effects (8). Thus, the overall evidence is that $β_2$-receptor stimulation in humans has inotropic and lusitropic effects similar to those of $β_1$-receptor stimulation, even though the precise mechanisms and signal systems may differ. In heart failure, however, the percentage of $β_2$-receptors may double from the 20% found in the normal ventricle as the $β_1$-receptors become more severely downregulated. Based on animal work, the proposal is that the inhibitory G_i pathway couples to an antiapoptotic mechanism, thereby exerting beneficial effects (Fig. 16-18) (9).

$β_3$-Adrenergic receptors have also been cloned. Although their chief function is in adipose tissue, where they help to regulate the rate of breakdown of fat, they also occur in the heart. Unexpectedly, they mediate a negative inotropic response that might contribute to the poor mechanical function of the failing heart (Chapter 16).

Molecular Structure of the β-Adrenergic Receptor

The β-adrenergic receptor site is highly stereospecific, and the best fit among catecholamines is obtained with the pharmacologic agent isoproterenol rather than with the naturally occurring catecholamines norepinephrine, and epinephrine. The $β_2$-adrenergic receptor has been cloned. The $β_2$-adrenergic receptor and the cholinergic receptor share substantial structural similarities (homology), with the highest homology residing in the membrane-spanning domains. The transmembrane domains appear to be the site of agonist and antagonist binding, whereas the cytoplasmic domain is where G protein interacts and the terminal COOH tail is the location of one of the phosphorylation sites (Fig. 7-5). Phosphorylation is involved in the process of desensitization (next section).

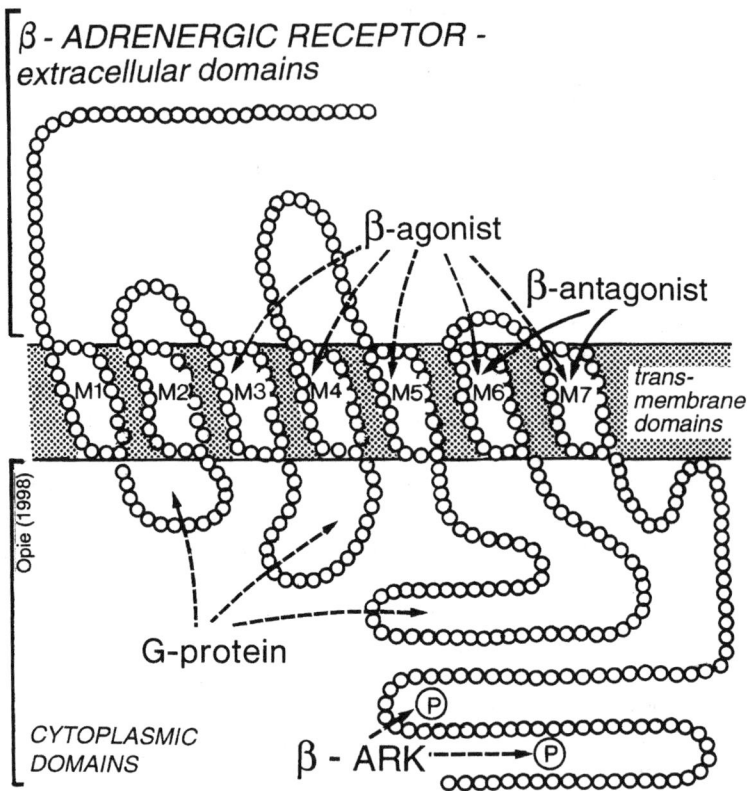

FIG. 7-5. Molecular structure of a G protein–coupled receptor, also called heptahelical or 7-transmembrane receptor. Example of β_2-adrenergic receptor. Note the three domains. The transmembrane domains act as a ligand-binding pocket, with domains M6 and M7 more specific for β-antagonists. β-Agonist binding is more diffuse but must also involve M6 and M7. Cytoplasmic domains can interact with G proteins and kinases, such as β-adrenergic receptor kinase (β-ARK). The latter can phosphorylate and desensitize the receptor by decreasing the interaction with G proteins (Fig. 7-6). Note that there are structural differences between β_1- and β_2- receptors (7). (Modified from Raymond JR, Hnatowich M, Lefkowitz RJ, et al. Adrenergic receptors. Models for regulation of signal transduction processes. *Hypertension* 1990;15:119–131.)

PHYSIOLOGIC SWITCH OFF, β-AGONIST RECEPTOR KINASE, AND ARRESTIN

Short-Term Inhibitory Mechanisms

Bearing in mind that β-adrenergic stimulation of the heart speeds up both the heart rate and force of contraction and increases the blood pressure, it is easy to imagine that excess stimulation could be harmful. To smooth the effects of overstimulation, there are potent feedback mechanisms, both short term and long term, whereby the degree of postreceptor response to a given degree of β-adrenergic receptor stimulation can be muted (Fig. 7-6). The physiologically decreased response whereby the β-receptor signal is terminated within minutes to seconds is called desensitization of the β-receptor. The key event is that sustained β-agonist stimulation rapidly induces the activity of the β-agonist receptor kinase (β-ARK), which is involved in the transfer of the phosphate group to the phosphorylation site on the terminal COOH tail of the receptor. This functionally uncouples both the β_1- and β_2-receptors from the stimulatory G protein G_s. Next, β-ARK (more correctly, β-ARK1 or G protein–coupled receptor kinase) increases the affinity of the β-receptors for another protein family, the arrestins. Hypothetically, arrestins change the molecular configuration of the receptor in such a way that the G proteins cannot interact optimally with it. This disconnection of receptor stimulation from the activity of adenyl cyclase is called uncoupling. Further desensitization is provided by PKA, activated by cAMP, which phosphorylates the β-receptor within minutes and acts independently, whether or not the receptor is occupied. This

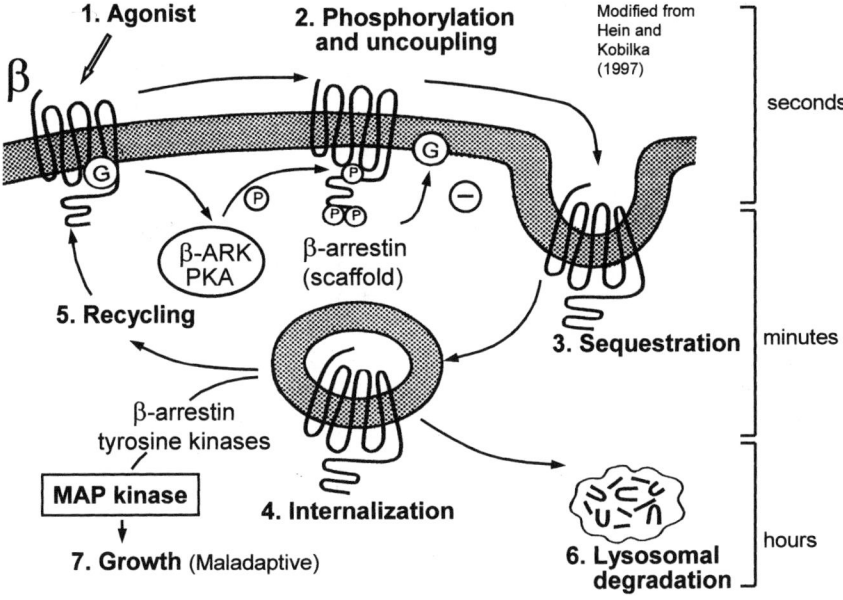

FIG. 7-6. Mechanisms of β-adrenergic receptor desensitization and internalization. Uncoupling is initiated by β-receptor stimulation, which leads to activation of the β-adrenergic receptor kinase (β-ARK). This kinase phosphorylates both β_1- and β_2-adrenergic receptors to functionally uncouple them from G_s. The receptor can become resensitized by the activity of a phosphatase, which splits off the phosphate group. Alternatively, the receptor can become internalized through one of two processes. In sequestration, an internal vesicle forms that can be reincorporated into the cell membrane. In true down-regulation, the receptor numbers decrease because there is degradation of the receptor, possibly by a lysosomal pathway. Down-regulation results from exposure to high concentrations of agonist. Note the links between the internalized receptor complex and growth stimulation via mitogen-activated protein kinase. PKA, protein kinase A. (Modified from Hein and Kobilka, Trends Cardiovasc Med. 1997; 7:137.) Also see Choi (48).

mechanism provides a feedback inhibitory mechanism to prevent the adverse effects of excess cAMP elevation and PKA activation. Resensitization of the receptor occurs when the phosphate groups are split off the β-receptor by a phosphatase, so that the receptor may then again readily be linked to G_s. Such resensitization, like desensitization, occurs rapidly. Such short-term changes probably occur whenever there is an emotional crisis or a burst of exercise to fine tune the effects of β-adrenergic stimulation and to prevent the risks of excess such as severe and potentially lethal arrhythmias.

Long-Term Inhibitory Mechanisms

Prolonged desensitization during sustained excess β-adrenergic receptor stimulation, as during long infusions of sympathomimetic agents, may be explained by receptor sequestration, *internalization*, and even lysosomal degradation. In addition, the internalized receptor can participate in growth signaling because arrestin forms a complex with the β-receptor and with tyrosine kinases, thereby ultimately linking to the mitogen-activated protein kinase complex (10). Thus, prolonged β-receptor stimulation may have growth as a result, while losing physiologic effects such as positive inotropic and lusitropic stimulation.

Overall Picture

There is a reciprocal effect of β-adrenergic receptor stimulation by the catecholamine β-agonists, soon followed by self-desensitization of the β-receptor by the β-ARK–arrestin and PKA mechanisms (11). β-ARK expression and activity in the heart are therefore major negative regulators of cardiac contractile function. Long-term stimulation of the β-adrenergic receptor increases the mRNA for β-ARK, whereas β-blockade decreases the expression of β-ARK to enhance receptor signaling. In addition, arrestin formation and receptor internalization may promote increased cardiac growth. Although the β-ARK-arrestin effects are best described for the $β_2$-receptor, they also occur to a lesser extent with the $β_1$-receptor. These changes in postreceptor signaling help to explain pathologic alterations in the β-receptor signaling system in heart failure, which is a chronic hyperadrenergic state with decreased contractile activity and increased growth of the ventricles (Fig. 16-18).

Drug Therapy and β-receptor Down- or Up-regulation

In the case of some cardiac drugs that act as positive inotropic agents via β-receptor stimulation, such as dobutamine, continued use may lead to a decrease in clinical response, an example of drug tolerance. The presumed molecular mechanism is by β-adrenergic receptor desensitization. Although the time scale involved is not well delineated, there appears to be an initial rapid component measured in minutes, perhaps corresponding to uncoupling and/or sequestration.

Then follows a delayed decrease in clinical response, measured in hours or days, probably corresponding to true receptor down-regulation. When a β-receptor antagonist is used in the long-term therapy of heart failure, down-regulation of β-ARK improves β-adrenergic signaling, which in turn may help to explain the therapeutic benefits of beta-blocker therapy in heart failure (11). Future heart failure therapy may include inhibition of β-ARK.

SCAFFOLDING AND ANCHORING PROTEINS

In a freely diffusible system, signaling initiated by heptahelical G protein–coupled receptors would depend on the random collision of the interacting proteins. In reality, the components of the signaling system are organized into microdomains by scaffolding and anchoring proteins. Scaffolding proteins bind to multiple molecules to enhance the efficiency and/or specificity of cellular signaling pathways (12). They bring together willing partners for intimate interaction. An example is β-arrestin that links to one of the G protein–coupled receptor protein's cytosolic loops to inhibit receptor function (Fig. 7-7). β-Arrestin also links to other signaling molecules such as tyrosine kinases and members of the mitogen-activated protein kinase family to facilitate receptor-mediated growth pathways (12). Furthermore, β-arrestin scaffolds for several other G protein–coupled receptors, providing one explanation for cross-talk.

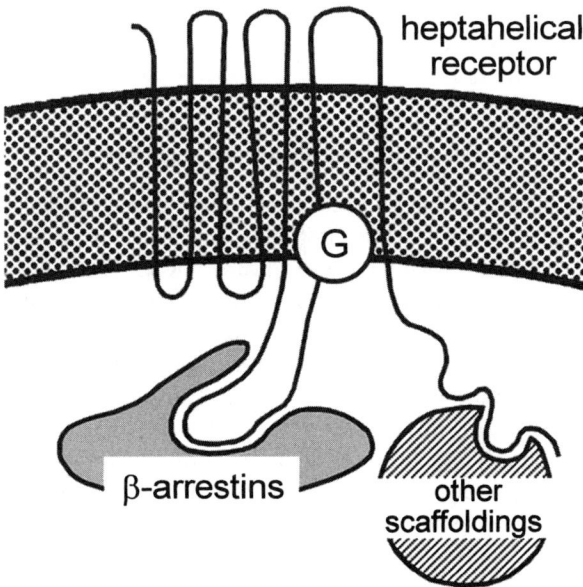

FIG. 7-7. Scaffolding proteins. These bring together molecules into a microdomain where they can better interact.

Anchoring proteins tether their molecular targets to specific subcellular structures, thereby facilitating interaction (Fig. 7-7). An example is, the A-kinase anchoring protein (AKAP), which has a targeting domain that anchors PKA during β-adrenergic stimulation and thereby permits the PKA to phosphorylate those proteins that regulate calcium cycling and increase cardiac contractility (13). The distinction between scaffolding and anchoring proteins may be artificial because scaffolding proteins largely work by simple tethering (14).

ADENYLYL CYCLASE AND G PROTEINS

To reiterate, the β-adrenergic receptor is situated on the outer surface of the sarcolemma and is coupled to adenylyl (adenyl or adenylate) cyclase by the stimulatory G protein G_s. Adenylyl cyclase is the only enzyme system producing cAMP and specifically requires low concentrations of adenosine 5'-triphosphate (ATP) (and magnesium) as substrate. The concentration of cAMP in the cell is approximately 1,000 times lower than the overall cell content of ATP. Thus, activity of adenylyl cyclase is unlikely to be limited by decreases in the cell ATP level (even in ischemia or hypoxia), nor is the conversion of ATP to cAMP by adenylyl cyclase an important route of ATP use in the cell. Adenylyl cyclase in broken cell preparations generally responds to the same hormones that are effective in the intact heart, and this evidence is particularly good for catecholamine stimulation. Only recently has the structure of adenylyl cyclase yielded to cloning technology. Surprisingly, the proposed molecular structure (typography) resembles some channel proteins, such as that of the calcium channel. Most of the protein is, however, located on the cytoplasmic side (15), the presumed site of interaction with the G protein.

G Proteins and Signal Transduction

G proteins are a family of GTP binding proteins, crucial in linking the primary event, receptor occupancy by the first messenger, to the activity of adenylyl cyclase, which is increased by G_s and inhibited by G_i. These G proteins act as on-off switches to adenylyl cyclase (16). In the resting state, guanosine 5'-diphosphate is tightly bound to the α subunit, in the "off" position. The arrival of the β-adrenergic first messenger at its receptor activates the system by displacing guanosine 5'-diphosphate by GTP. The stimulatory α subunit of G_s ($α_s$) now combines with GTP and then separates from the other two subunits to promote activity of adenylyl cyclase and formation of cAMP (Fig. 7-8). The whole GTP complex also includes the β and γ subunits that appear to be linked in structure and function. The $α_s$ subunit may also directly activate the calcium channel. Between these effects, it is possible to explain both positive inotropic and the relaxant (lusitropic) effects of catecholamines on contractile cells (Fig. 7-9).

In contrast, a second GTP binding protein, G_i, is responsible for inhibition of adenylyl cyclase. During cholinergic signaling, the muscarinic receptor is stimulated and GTP binds to the inhibitory α subunit, $α_i$. The latter then dissociates

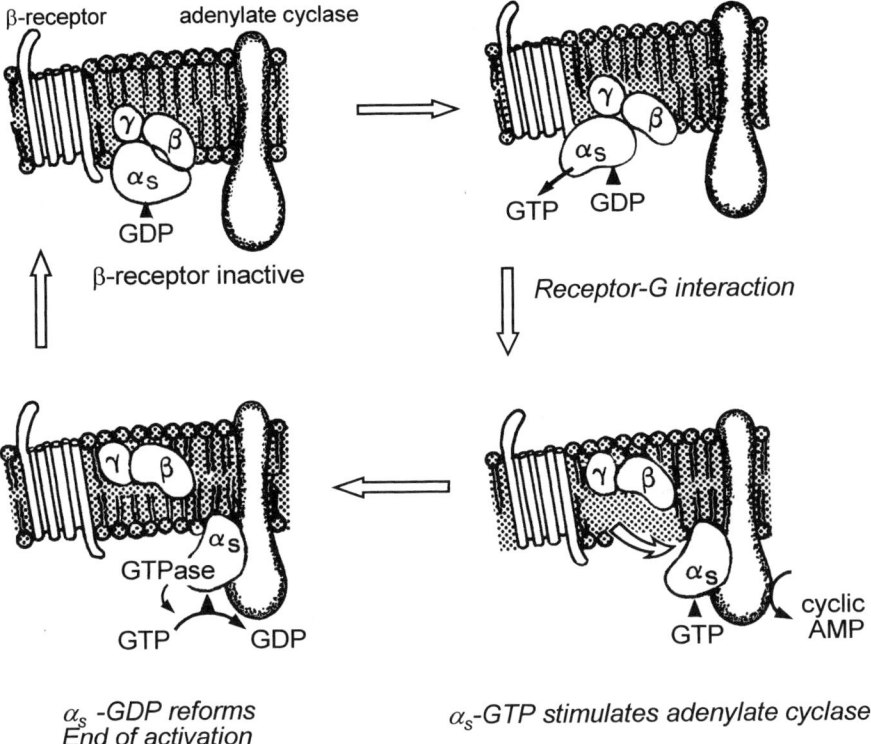

FIG. 7-8. G-protein cycle during activation by β-adrenergic receptor stimulation. In the unliganded state (receptor unoccupied), the G protein consists of three associated units: α, β, and γ. The latter two act as one functional subunit. The α subunit can either stimulate (α_s) or inhibit (α_i) the effector corresponding to the G proteins G_s and G_i. The subunit α_s stimulates adenylyl cyclase when it is activated by binding with guanosine 5′-triphosphate (*GTP*) at the time of β-agonist occupation of its receptor site. α_s-GTP then interacts with adenylyl cyclase, which produces cyclic adenosine 3′,5′-monophosphate. The inherent GTPase activity of the α_i subunit breaks down GTP to guanosine 5′-diphosphate (*GDP*), and the initial resting (nonliganded) state re-forms.

from the other two components of the G-protein complex, which are the β-γ subunits. The latter seem to play an important role (Fig. 7-9): By stimulating GTPase, they break down the active α_s subunit (α_s-GTP), so that the activity of adenylyl cyclase in response to a β-agonist decreases (Fig. 7-9). In addition, the α_i subunit activates the potassium channel (17) via an unknown mechanism. The latter event contributes to the reduction in heart rate on cholinergic stimulation.

Two G proteins, the newly described G_h and G_q, link myocardial α-adrenergic receptors to the membrane-associated enzyme phospholipase C (18). It is not clear which G protein works and when (19).

Other G proteins help to gate ion channels. For example, β-adrenergic stimulation may increase calcium channel activity independently of the formation of cAMP, presumably by direct stimulation of this channel by a G protein.

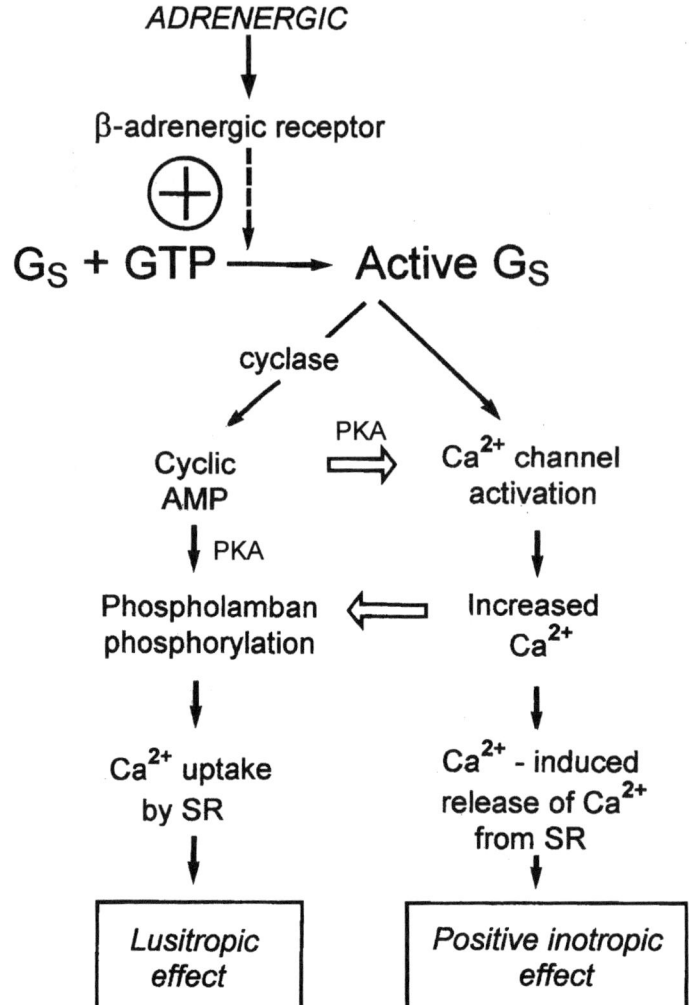

FIG. 7-9. β-Adrenergic signal system, with the proposed role of G_s protein. Ultimately, there is a calcium-dependent effect in increasing contractile activity (positive inotropic effect) and a phospholamban-dependent increase in the rate of relaxation (lusitropic effect). *AKAP*, A-kinase anchoring protein. For further details of inotropic and lusitropic changes, see frontispiece.

At present, the G proteins are subject to intense investigation for their role in cardiovascular responses and in disease states. For example, in dilated, poorly contracting and failing hearts, an increase in G_i and a decrease in G_h are found (18). The mechanism and significance of such changes are not currently clear (for details, see Chapter 16).

THE SECOND AND THIRD MESSENGER CONCEPT

The general hypothesis that the two major messenger systems, the adrenergic and cholinergic, have opposing effects on cAMP (Figs. 7-9 and 7-10), formed from ATP under the influence of activated adenylyl cyclase (Fig. 7-11). Another concept is that calcium is the third messenger of β stimulation, brought into play by several intermediate steps (Fig. 7-9). Cholinergic activity, acting on a different receptor, inhibits the formation of cAMP (Fig. 7-10). Another cyclic nucleotide, cGMP, acts as a second messenger for some aspects of vagal activity in heart muscle. In vascular smooth muscle, cGMP is the second messenger of the NO vasodilatory system (Fig. 9-12).

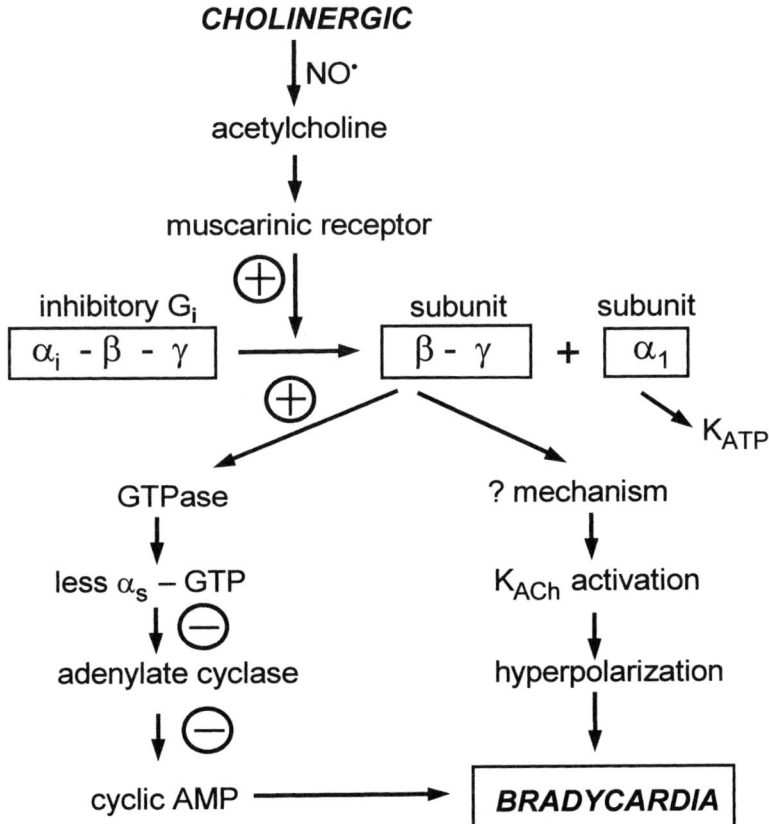

FIG. 7-10. Cholinergic signal system. The proposed role of G protein (α_i-β-γ) in the inhibitory effects of cholinergic stimulation on the heart. In response to the occupancy of the muscarinic (M₂) receptor by acetylcholine, guanosine 5′-triphosphate (GTP) binds to the inhibitory α subunit (α_i), which dissociates from the rest of the G-protein complex (β-γ). The latter unit has at least two identified functions: to stimulate GTPase to break down GTP, thereby decreasing adenylyl cyclase activity and to help open the acetylcholine-operated potassium channel. In addition, α_i-GTP may also open the ATP–dependent potassium channel.

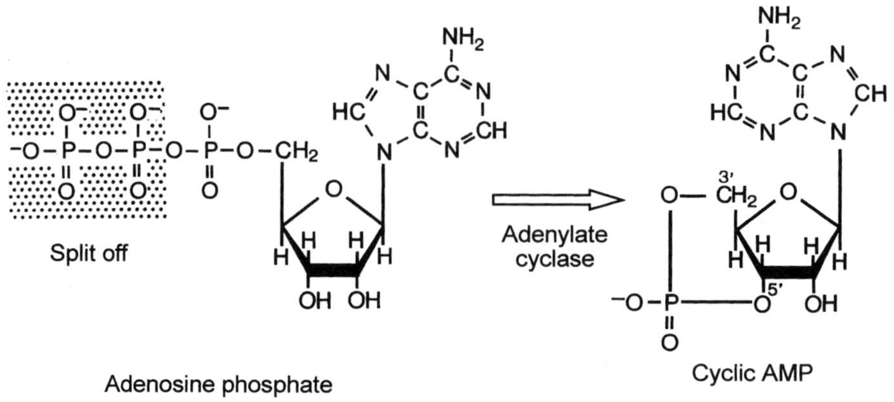

FIG. 7-11. Cyclic adenosine 3′,5′-monophosphate, the second messenger of β-adrenergic stimulation, is formed from adenosine 5′-triphosphate by the activity of activated adenylyl cyclase.

All these messenger chemicals are present in the heart cell in minute concentrations, approximately 10^{-10} mol/L for cAMP and approximately 10^{-11} mol/L for cGMP. The real concentrations in the cytosol are somewhat higher because 80% of the cell is water. A basic feature of the concept of cAMP as a second messenger is its very rapid turnover as a result of a constant dynamic balance between its formation by adenylyl cyclase and removal by another enzyme, phosphodiesterase. In general, changes in the tissue content of cAMP can be related to the effects of catecholamines in stimulating the contractile activity of the heart (Tables 7-2 and 7-3).

TABLE 7-2. *Effects of elevated intracellular levels of cAMP on the heart*

Target	Effect
Sinus node	Accelerated discharge
Atrioventricular node	Accelerated conduction
Purkinje fibers	Accelerated conduction
Normal action potential	Increased slow channel activity (increased Ca^{2+})
Blocked action potential	Provocation of slow responses
Troponin I	Decreased sensitivity of ATPase to Ca^{2+}
Sarcoplasmic reticulum	Phosphorylation of phospholamban with increased activity of calcium pump
Sarcolemma	Phosphorylation of L channel with increased entry of calcium
Glycogen	Synthase kinase stimulated; glycogen synthase *b* formed; less glycogen synthesis. Phosphorylase kinase stimulated; increased conversion of phosphorylase *b* to *a*; increased glycogenolysis
Lipases	Stimulation of lipolysis with provision of energy

TABLE 7-3. *Pharmacologically active agents that alter myocardial levels of cAMP and contractile activity of the heart*

Agent	Mechanism	Effect on cyclic nucleotide	Effect on contractile activity
Epinephrine, norepinephrine	Stimulate adenylate cyclase via β-receptor	↑ cAMP	↑
Glucagon, histamine	Stimulate adenylate cyclase via non–β-receptor	↑ cAMP	↑
Forskolin	Directly stimulates adenylate cyclase	↑ cAMP	↑
β-Adrenergic blocking agents	Antagonize effects of β-stimulating catecholamines	↓ cAMP	↓
Adenosine	Inhibits adenylate cyclase	↓ cAMP	↓

↑, increased; cAMP, cyclic adenosine 3′, 5′-monophosphate; ↓, decreased.

cAMP Compartmentation

There is more involved in responses to adrenergic stimulation than changes in the overall tissue levels of cAMP. When catecholamines are bound covalently to glass beads, which severely limits the amount of contact that the catecholamines have with the cell surface, maximal contraction of papillary muscles can be achieved without a measurable change in tissue cAMP concentrations (20). This may be an example of β-agonist activity in only a very small percentage of receptors, according to the spare receptor concept. Second, at any given level of cAMP, it is the degree of stimulation of various protein kinases by cAMP that is of ultimate importance. Theoretically, changes in the activity of specific protein kinases could occur in response to very small localized changes in compartmentalized cAMP. Conversely, some agents stimulating adenylyl cyclase, such as forskolin, can achieve large increases in myocardial cAMP levels without corresponding changes in the inotropic state. Such noticeable exceptions between the degree of increase of cAMP and the expected consequences show that it is very likely that there is some degree of compartmentation of cAMP in the heart, with only a specific compartment available to increase contractile activity (21).

cAMP in Vascular Smooth Muscle

Whereas cAMP increases the contractile activity of the heart, it causes relaxation of vascular smooth muscle (Chapter 9). Hence, β-adrenergic stimulation will both increase cardiac contraction and cause vasodilation (Fig. 2-4).

Other Agents Stimulating Formation of cAMP

Glucagon is a naturally occurring hormone secreted by the pancreas when the blood sugar is low. It stimulates the formation of cAMP in liver cells to break down liver glycogen, thereby replenishing the blood sugar. In the heart, its receptor is coupled by G_s to adenylyl cyclase with formation of cAMP. Glucagon therefore increases the heart rate and contractile activity. These stimulatory effects bypass the β-receptor (Fig. 7-12), and glucagon is used in the therapy of overdoses of β-blocking agents.

Thyroid hormone can also activate adenylyl cyclase independently of the β-adrenergic receptor. A membrane-bound thyroid receptor is by no means the only receptor involved in the explanation of thyroid effects. Formation of cAMP is not likely to be the sole or even the main effect of thyroid hormone on the heart. The basic site of thyroid action is probably the nuclear receptor for triiodothyronine, which stimulates the formation of a diversity of messenger RNA complexes in the presence of this hormone.

Adenosine, formed by the breakdown of ATP (e.g., in hypoxia) couples to G_i, inhibiting contraction and heart rate. In addition, adenosine also opens the potassium channel to cause hyperpolarization, thereby directly inhibiting calcium ion entry.

Prostacyclin is a vasodilatory prostaglandin released from the vascular endothelium. It couples to adenylyl cyclase via G_s to promote the formation of cAMP. Whereas the vasodilatory effect is thought to have physiologic significance, the positive effects on contraction and heart rate appear to be more of a laboratory phenomenon.

Calcitonin gene related peptide is a vasoactive neurotransmitter. It is found in the nervous system, blood vessels, and heart. It is coupled by its receptor to G_s

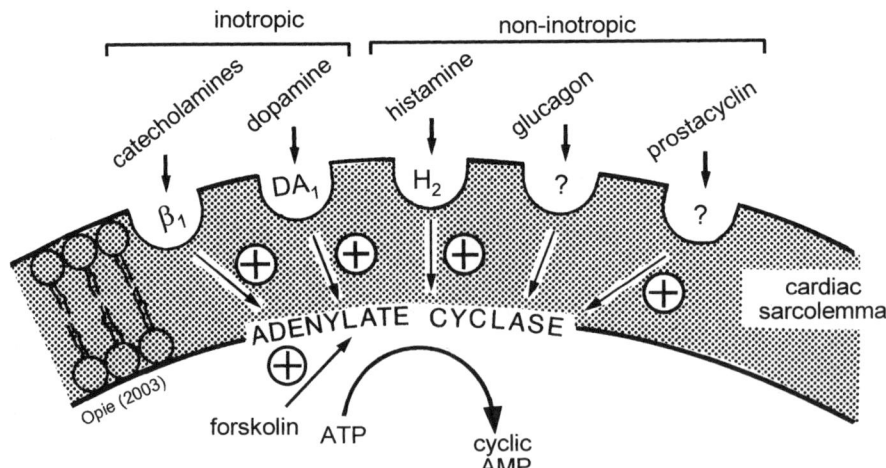

FIG. 7-12. Other receptors linked to cAMP. In addition to the β-adrenergic receptor, there are several other receptors potentially coupled to adenylyl (adenylate) cyclase, hence promoting the formation of cAMP. Only some of these have effects similar to those of β-adrenergic stimulation, probably because the cAMP–protein kinase A is not produced in the appropriate microdomains. For bypass of cAMP–protein kinase A, see Zhu et al. (42).

and hence activates adenylyl cyclase to form cAMP, which is vasodilatory. Experimentally, it also stimulates the contractile activity of the atria but not of the ventricles. The physiologic role of this peptide is still unknown.

Forskolin directly stimulates cardiac adenylyl cyclase. Forskolin is a diterpene isolated from the roots of *Coleus forskohlii*. Even a low concentration of forskolin increases the formation of cAMP and stimulates contractile activity. To explain why forskolin can increase cAMP formation so substantially and yet not have the expected end-organ results, it is now postulated that it is the formation of compartmentalized cAMP that is stimulated by forskolin (22).

Dopamine is a natural catecholamine neurotransmitter, also used pharmacologically. It stimulates both pre- and postsynaptic dopamine receptors to vasodilate and to increase contractile activity.

Phosphodiesterase inhibitors are pharmacologic agents that increase cAMP by inhibiting its breakdown. The net effect is similar to that of β-stimulation: increased contractile activity, increased rate of relaxation, and an increased heart rate.

Organelles Influenced by cAMP

To reiterate, cAMP itself is unable to alter the cytosolic level of calcium, the third messenger. The intermediate step is activation of the enzyme moving (kinase) a phosphate group from ATP to a specific target protein that is then said to be phosphorylated (Fig. 7-13). Thus, contraction and relaxation are both

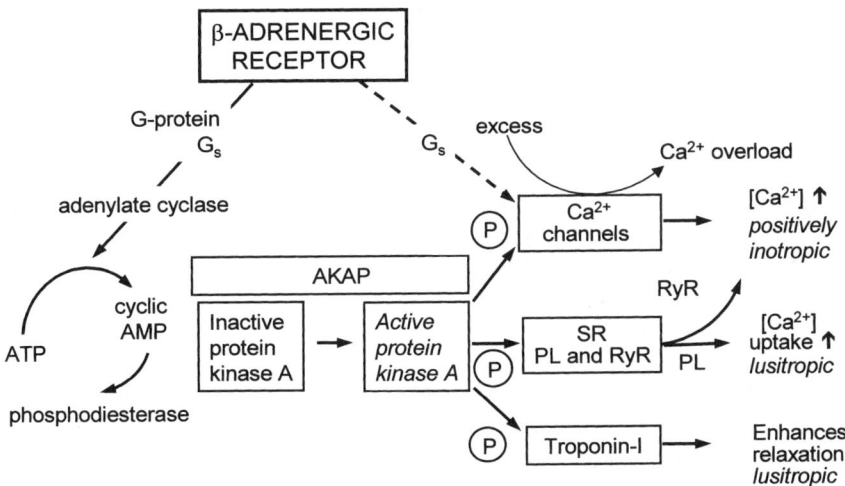

FIG. 7-13. Role of protein kinase A. The major intracellular effects of β-agonist catecholamines are by formation of cAMP, which increases the activity of the cAMP-dependent protein kinase A. The latter phosphorylates various proteins involved in contraction. For bypass of this path see Zhu et al. (42). *SR*, sarcoplasmic reticulum; *AKAP*, A-kinase anchoring protein. For inotropic and lusitropic, see frontispiece.

enhanced by phosphorylation of a sarcolemmal protein of the calcium channel, of phospholamban of the sarcoplasmic reticulum, and of troponin I. Of these effects, that on the calcium channel of the sarcolemma and on phospholamban in the sarcoplasmic reticulum have already been discussed in detail. Phosphorylation of the inhibitory subunit of troponin I decreases the sensitivity of the contractile system to calcium and promotes the rate of crossbridge detachment (23), thereby enhancing cardiac relaxation.

Protein Kinases: Next in the Signal System

At a subcellular level, most, if not all, of the effects of cAMP are ultimately mediated by protein kinases that phosphorylate various important proteins and enzymes. Each protein kinase is composed of two subunits, regulatory (R) and catalytic (C). When cAMP interacts with protein kinases, it binds to the R subunit to liberate the C subunit. The inactive kinase, composed of both R and C subunits, is split by cAMP so that active kinase (C) forms $(R_2 + C_2) + 2cAMP \rightarrow 2RcAMP + 2C$.

The ratio of the active protein kinase to the inactive form is called the *protein kinase activity ratio*. The activity ratio increases in direct relation to the increase of the intracellular cAMP level during stimulation by a variety of agents increasing cAMP, such as epinephrine, glucagon, and phosphodiesterase inhibition. The activated kinase in turn acts as the trigger for a variety of physiologic effects because it switches on or off several different enzymes concerned with the regulation of calcium ion movements and the breakdown of glycogen and lipid. There are at least eight phosphorylations mediated by the active form of the cAMP-dependent protein kinase. Phosphorylation, the donation of a phosphate group to the enzyme concerned, is therefore a fundamental metabolic switch that can function as a cascade to produce extensive amplification of a signal.

At a molecular level, the basic action of the cAMP-dependent protein kinase is to catalyze the transfer of the terminal phosphate of ATP to serine and threonine residues of the protein substrates, leading to a modification of the properties of the proteins concerned. This then leads to further key reactions.

Protein kinase A, activated by cAMP, with its many diverse intracellular substrates, occurs in different cells in two forms, with different but similar regulator subunits. The type called protein kinase II predominates in cardiac cells. The aim of current work is to determine the order of phosphorylation of the various proteins that occurs in response to a given cAMP signal within heart cells because this pecking order may determine the order of the ultimate physiologic response.

Protein kinase B (or Akt) is a key regulator of the insulin growth path (Fig. 9-1).

Protein kinase C is of major importance in explaining how α-adrenergic stimulation, endothelin, and angiotensin II increase contractile activity in arterioles

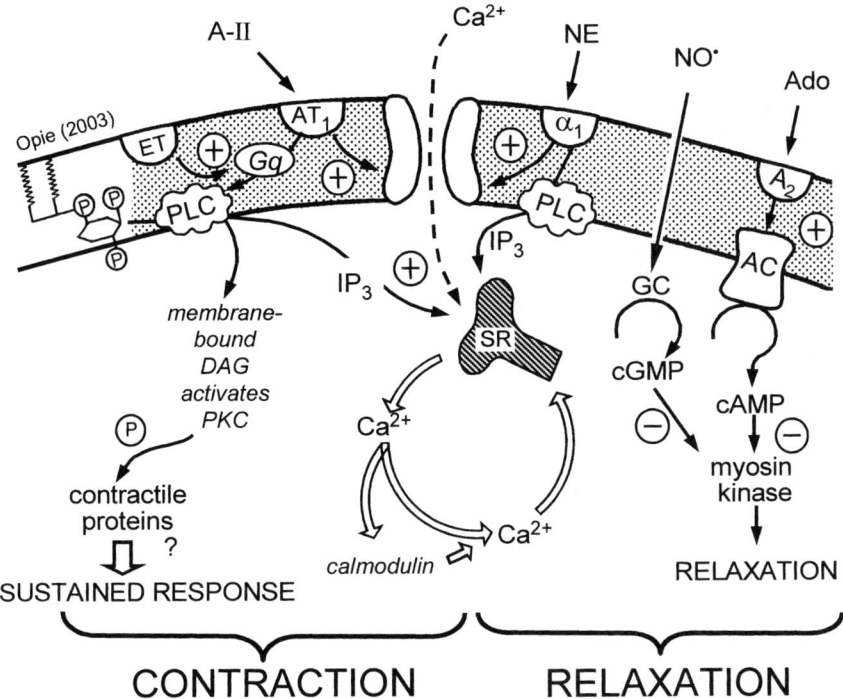

FIG. 7-14. Protein kinase C (*PKC*)-linked receptors in vascular smooth muscle. For example, the α_1-agonist signaling system is coupled via a G protein to phospholipase C (*PLC*), which breaks down phosphatidylinositol 4,5-bisphosphate (*PIP₂*) to 1,2-diacylglycerol (*DAG*) and IP₃ (inositol 1,4,5-trisphosphate). DAG is thought to translocate protein kinase C from cytosol to the sarcolemma, thereby activating protein kinase C. Signals beyond protein kinase C are not clear. It may phosphorylate ion channels and be concerned with growth regulation. Inositol 1,4,5-triphosphate (IP₃) releases calcium from the sarcoplasmic reticulum to initiate contraction in vascular smooth muscle. Other vasoconstrictors such as angiotensin II and endothelin act by the same signal system. In the myocardium, a complementary inotropic system operates via the α_1-receptors to stimulate formation of IP₃ with a relatively small contractile response.

(Fig. 7-14). This kinase also occurs in the myocardium, where it has several isoforms and is crucial in the protective signaling that results in preconditioning (Chapter 19).

Protein kinase G responds to cGMP much as PKA responds to cAMP.

If phosphorylation of various critical cellular proteins by kinases is so important in the regulation of heart cell function, it follows that the phosphoprotein *phosphatase* enzymes catalyzing the breakdown of the phosphorylated proteins are equally important in regulation. Similar principles govern glycogen synthesis and breakdown (see Fig. 11–13). For example, in vascular smooth muscle, a specific phosphatase dephosphorylates the P light chain of myosin to decrease actin–myosin interaction and to cause vascular relaxation.

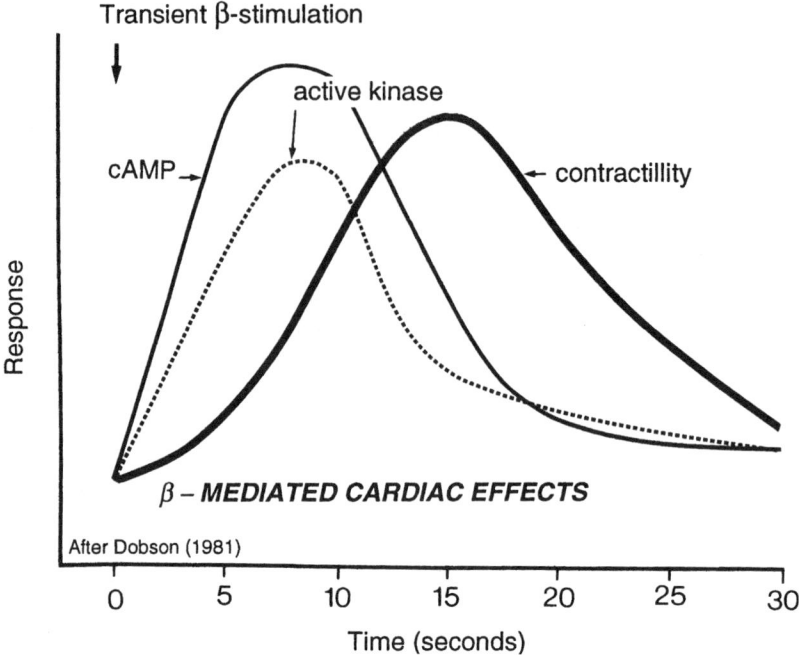

FIG. 7-15. β-Adrenergic–mediated cardiac effects. After stimulation of the heart by a bolus injection of epinephrine at zero time, cyclic adenosine 3′,5′-monophosphate increases before protein kinase is activated. Thereafter, an index of contractility (dP/dt) increases. Only thereafter is there a metabolic response (phosphorylase breaks down glycogen). (From Dobson. In: Delius W, Gerlach E, Grobecker H, et al., eds. *Catecholamines and the heart.* Berlin: Springer-Verlag, 1981:128, with permission.)

PHYSIOLOGIC β-ADRENERGIC EFFECTS

The sequence of molecular signals already described results in particular responses that can be traced out in the whole heart. Thus, β_1-adrenergic stimulation is followed by an increase of tissue cAMP, then the active PKA increases, and thereafter there is increased contractility, the whole sequence taking approximately 15 seconds (Fig. 7-15). The overall effect of β_1-adrenergic stimulation on the heart includes the positive inotropic effect, the relaxant effect, the chronotropic effect, and the dromotropic effect. Each is now considered in turn.

1. *Positive inotropic effect.* When β_1-adrenergic stimulation increases the rate of contraction and the force developed, then it is said to induce a positive inotropic response, also called increased contractility. The definition of these terms is given in Chapter 13. At present, the probable sequence of events describing the inotropic effects of catecholamines (Fig. 7-13) is

Catecholamine stimulation → β-receptor → molecular changes → binding of G_s to GTP → catalytic subunit of adenylyl cyclase → formation of cAMP from ATP → activation of PKA and anchoring to AKAP → phosphorylation of a sarcolemmal protein → increased entry of calcium ion through the cell membrane → calcium-induced calcium release → increase of intracellular free calcium ion concentration → increased splitting of ATP by myosin ATPase to increase the rate of development of contractile force and increased deinhibition of actin and myosin by interaction of calcium with troponin C to increase total force developed.

An interesting aspect of the catecholamine-induced inotropic response is that it passes off rapidly, within minutes, even though the catecholamine stimulation is maintained. One reason for this turn off of the inotropic response is that the tissue level of cAMP increases much more initially than later. When cAMP increases in the myocardial cell, the enhanced cytosolic calcium concentration activates calmodulin, which in turn enhances the activity of phosphodiesterase, so that the rate of cAMP breakdown is increased. In addition, the intense stimulation of the β-adrenergic receptor leads to activation of β-ARK and down-regulation (Fig. 7-6).

2. *Relaxant or lusitropic effect.* This effect, which Katz (24) called the lusitropic response (Greek, *lusi*, relaxation), can be explained at a subcellular level by increased activity of the calcium pump of the sarcoplasmic reticulum in response to phosphorylation of phospholamban by cAMP and the effect of an increased internal calcium, as a result of cAMP-induced calcium channel phosphorylation, with the increased calcium also leading to enhanced phosphorylation of phospholamban (Fig. 6-9). In addition, PKA also phosphorylates troponin I to increase the rate of crossbridge detachment (23).

3. *Chronotropic effect.* Besides an increased rate of contraction and relaxation characteristic of the positive inotropic effect, the beating rate of the heart also increases during catecholamine stimulation. This positive chronotropic (Greek, *chrono*, time) effect results from the stimulation of the pacemaker (Fig. 5-4).

4. *Dromotropic effect.* Not only does β_1 stimulation cause the positive inotropic and chronotropic effects, but the impulse is conducted more rapidly down the atrioventricular node, His bundle, and Purkinje fibers. This is the positive dromotropic (Greek, *dromo*, running) effect. Conduction velocity through the atrioventricular node is enhanced, probably as a result of stimulation of the slow calcium channel in atrioventricular nodal cells. Clinically, the result is shortening of the PR interval on the electrocardiogram (Chapter 5).

β_2-Adrenergic Effects

It is controversial whether these receptors are linked, like their β_1 brothers, to the adenylyl cyclase–cAMP–PKA signal system. One current view is that these receptors are linked to both the stimulatory G protein G_s and the inhibitory G_i, so that pathway "bifurcates at the very first post-receptor step" (7). Physiologically, the former dominates, whereas in heart failure, the inhibitor effect appears to dominate (Fig. 16-18).

α-ADRENERGIC RECEPTORS

α-Adrenergic receptors may help to mediate the influx of calcium in cardiac and especially in vascular smooth muscle. In general, the cardiac effects are usually not prominent, whereas those on the arterioles are substantial (Table 7-4). Pharmacologically, an α-adrenergic receptor mediates the response in which the effects resemble those of the pharmacologic agent phenylephrine. Among catecholamines, the α-agonist potencies are norepinephrine > epinephrine > isoproterenol (2). Physiologically, norepinephrine is liberated from nerve terminals, which is the chief stimulus to vascular α-adrenergic activity. The antagonist properties are mediated by α-blocking agents, such as phentolamine, at low concentrations. Subdivisions of the α-adrenergic receptor are complex. The basic division is into the postsynaptic $α_1$-adrenergic receptor (inhibited by prazosin) and the presynaptic $α_2$-adrenergic receptors (inhibited by yohimbine). In the heart, postsynaptic $α_1$-receptors, when stimulated, usually cause a modest inotropic effect by increased cytosolic calcium. Although several $α_1$-adrenergic receptor subtypes exist, their differentiation is still incomplete (19).

Coupling of $α_1$-Receptor by G Proteins

When an agonist occupies the $α_1$-receptor, one of the G protein family, G_h, couples the receptor to the activity of the sarcolemmal enzyme system, phospholipase C (18). The exact steps involved are not as well understood as coupling of the β-receptor to adenylyl cyclase (25). Another G protein, G_q, may also link to the $α_1$-receptor (19).

Phosphatidyl Inositol System

After activation of phospholipase C by the G protein, the compound phosphatidylinositol, part of the membrane phospholipid system (lipid compounds containing phosphate groups) is split into two components, IP_3 and DAG (Fig. 7-14). IP_3 is one of the second messengers of this system and stimulates the release

TABLE 7-4. *Comparative cardiovascular effects of α- and β-adrenergic receptor stimulation*

	α-Mediated	β-Mediated
Electrophysiologic effects	±	++ Conduction, pacemaker, heart rate
Myocardial mechanics	±	++ Contractility, stroke volume, cardiac output
Myocardial metabolism	+ Glycolysis	++ O_2 uptake, ATP
Coronary arterioles	++ Constriction	+ Direct dilation, +++ indirect dilation (metabolic)
Peripheral arterioles	+++ Constriction, PVR, blood pressure	+ Dilation

ATP, adenosine 5′-triphosphate; PVR, peripheral vascular resistance.

of calcium from the sarcoplasmic reticulum, which explains why α-receptor stimulation can cause vascular smooth muscle to contract without any entry of calcium from the outside. Berridge (26) proposed a general role for inositol phosphates in regulating oscillations of cytosolic calcium. Whereas IP_3 travels to the sarcoplasmic reticulum to liberate calcium, DAG stays in the cell membrane, being highly lipophilic. It stimulates another protein kinase into activity, protein kinase C, by promoting its translocation from cytosol to sarcolemma.

The experimental agents, the phorbol esters, are able directly to stimulate protein kinase C and, therefore, to mimic some of the effects of $α_1$-adrenergic stimulation. In the myocardium, phorbol ester stimulation increases the contractile force.

Positive Inotropic Effect of $α_1$-Stimulation

This effect is not thought to be of major importance in the normal myocardium, when the prime regulation of contraction is through the β-adrenergic system. Nonetheless, there is a small positive inotropic effect associated with the formation of IP_3 (27). In advanced heart failure, when the β-adrenergic receptor system undergoes desensitization and down-regulation, it might be that the α-adrenergic system could come into play as a supportive positive inotropic mechanism. However, components of its coupling system are also downgraded (18).

Other Inositol Phosphates

In addition to IP_3, at least two other similar compounds, IP_4 and IP_5, may form in response to α-adrenergic stimulation. These compounds presumably are messengers whose full function is still unknown. A current hypothesis for skeletal muscle is that IP_4 can increase calcium influx across the sarcolemma. Such calcium is then able, together with IP_3, to release calcium from the sarcoplasmic reticulum.

Non–α-adrenergic Receptors Coupled to Phospholipase C

Several other receptors couple to phospholipase C. Angiotensin II receptors in the myocardium and in vascular smooth muscle are thus coupled to the phospholipase C system (28). Formation of protein kinase C may explain the growth-stimulating properties of angiotensin II. In blood vessels, angiotensin II is strongly vasoconstrictive, acting via IP_3 to release calcium from the sarcoplasmic reticulum. The newly identified endothelium-derived vasoconstrictor peptide endothelin is also coupled to the phospholipase C system in the myocardium and in vascular smooth muscle. Endothelin may contribute to the release of atrial natriuretic peptide (Fig. 16-12).

Negative Inotropic Effects of Phospholipase C

Unexpectedly, a number of inhibitory effects on cardiac contraction have been found as a result of agonists linked to phospholipase C. For example, $α_1$ stimulation may have negative rather than positive inotropic effects at high levels of internal calcium (29). In some species, but not in humans, angiotensin II also has a negative rather than a positive inotropic effect. The mechanism of these negative effects is not understood.

CHOLINERGIC RECEPTORS AND PARASYMPATHETIC VAGAL EFFECTS

Turning now from the adrenergic system and its messengers to the parasympathetic system, the latter has signal systems that oppose those of the adrenergic system (Fig. 7-16). There is again an extracellular first messenger (the neurotransmitter acetylcholine), a receptor system (the muscarinic receptor), and an intracellular signaling system (the G-protein system). In the vagal nerve terminals, acetylcholine is repacked into vesicles from which it is released in response to vagal nerve stimulation and influx of calcium ions, thereby releasing the acetylcholine. There are two types of cholinergic receptors, the nicotinic receptors at the autonomic ganglia and the muscarinic receptors at the effector tissue.

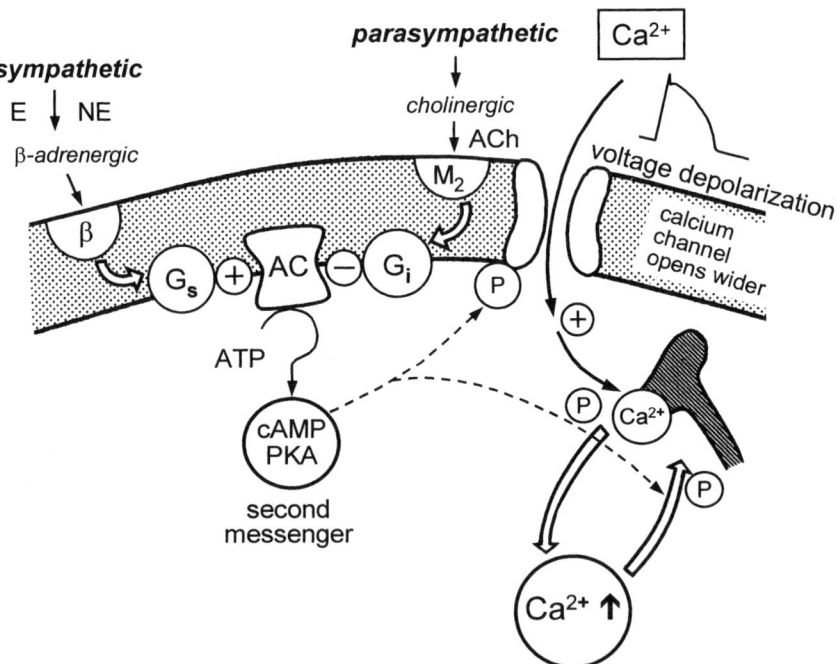

FIG. 7-16. **Interaction between parasympathetic and sympathetic systems** at a cellular level may involve two opposing cyclic nucleotides, cyclic adenosine 3',5'-monophosphate (cAMP) and cyclic guanosine 3',5'-monophosphate. Many effects of vagal stimulation could best be explained by the inhibitory effect on the formulation of cAMP, including formation of the inhibitory G protein G_i in response to M_2-receptor stimulation.

The myocardial muscarinic receptor (M_2) is associated specifically with the activity of the vagal nerve endings and has as its characteristics the production of a negative inotropic response and inhibition by atropine. The nicotinic receptor by definition responds to nicotine and is inhibited by ganglion-blocking agents, such as hexamethonium. This differentiation between the nicotinic ganglionic receptor sites and the tissue muscarinic sites is broadly correct, although some nicotinic receptors have also been found at the nerve endings.

The major effects of parasympathetic vagal stimulation on the heart have already been described, including bradycardia and a negative inotropic effect. The chief function of muscarinic cholinergic receptors is seen as the inhibitory modulation of the effects of sympathetic stimulation, known as accentuated antagonism, by several mechanisms including less formation of cAMP in response to β-adrenergic stimulation (Fig. 7-16). In addition, the NO messenger system may contribute by the formation of inhibitory cGMP and/or by increasing the release of acetylcholine from vagal nerve endings (next section). Overall, cGMP may act as a second messenger to vagal stimulation just as cAMP does to β-adrenergic stimulation.

In more detail, stimulation of the muscarinic receptor leads to breakdown (hydrolysis) of GTP, with the result that the binding between GTP and the α_s subunit of G_s cannot occur. The β-γ component of the G protein dissociates from the rest (α_i) to stimulate the GTPase and hence indirectly to decreased formation of cAMP (Fig. 7-10). Thus, the extent of adenylyl cyclase activation in response to a given degree of β-adrenergic stimulation is decreased. (Readers should be careful to distinguish between α_1-adrenergic receptors and the inhibitory α component of the G protein α_i).

In nodal tissue, opening of the G-dependent potassium channels inhibits the rate of spontaneous depolarization and slows the sinus node (Fig. 4-19). *In the myocardium,* the ventricles are less responsive to muscarinic agonists than are the atria, despite similar receptor densities (30), so that there must be postreceptor differences, probably in the degree of G-protein coupling. Nonetheless, there is a negative inotropic effect of vagal stimulation, now confirmed in humans (31). The triple mechanism is (a) heart rate slowing, mediated by NO (Fig. 7-17) with a negative Treppe effect (Fig. 12-8); (b) inhibition of the formation of cAMP; and (c) the negative inotropic effect of cGMP, formed as result of activity of guanyl (guanylyl) cyclase and closely interacting with NO.

Nitric Oxide Augments and Mediates Cholinergic Messenger

Besides inhibiting the formation of cAMP, increasing evidence suggests that cholinergic receptor stimulation can be linked to the enzyme complex guanylate cyclase, much as β-adrenergic stimulation is linked to adenylyl cyclase. cGMP, produced by guanylate cyclase, in general, has opposite effects to those of cAMP on the myocardium. For example, calcium channel opening is promoted by cAMP but is inhibited by cGMP, which activates a cGMP-dependent kinase that induces an inhibitory phosphorylation. cGMP is also the second messenger of the NO messenger system (Fig. 9-12).

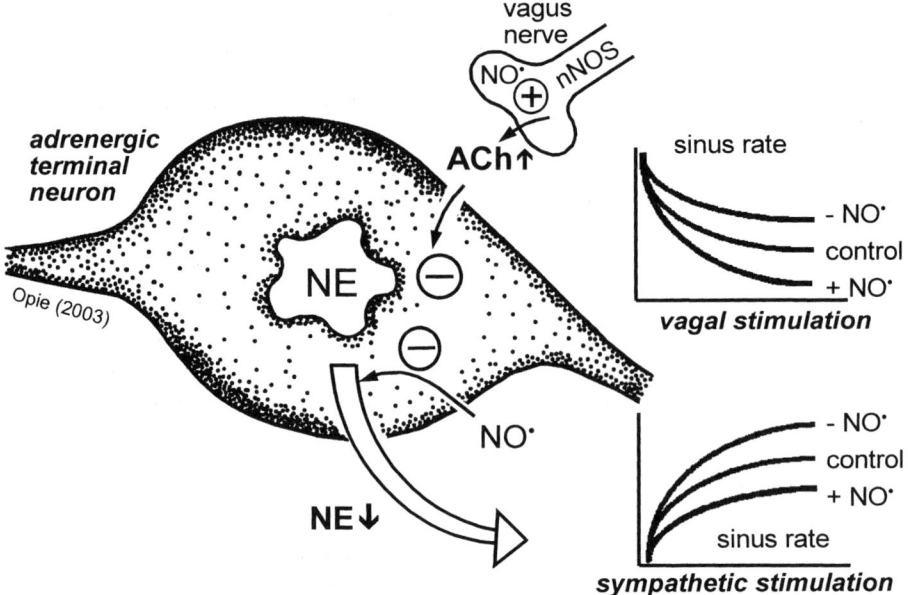

FIG. 7-17. Nitric oxide mediates the release of acetylcholine from vagal nerve terminals. Nitric oxide, produced in the terminal vagal nerve endings, increases the release of acetylcholine (*ACh*) and decreases that of norepinephrine (*NE*). Thus, the sinus rate response to either vagal or sympathetic stimulation is changed accordingly. *nNOS*, neuronal nitric oxide synthase. For the concept, see Paterson, *Exp Physiol*, 2001;86:1.

Nitric Oxide Signal Transduction in Cholinergic Stimulation

There are two apparently conflicting proposals for the inhibitory effects of NO on heart rate and cardiac contraction, both supported by data from different knockout mice models. Historically, the first, cholinergic activation of the M_2-receptor may stimulate endothelial NO synthase (eNOS) to form NO that in turn promotes formation of cGMP (32). The latter opposes the effects of β-adrenergic activity by stimulating the phosphodiesterase that breaks down cAMP and by activating protein kinase G that inhibits calcium entry via the calcium channel (32). A different and more recent proposal is that neuronal NOS (nNOS, NOS1) stimulates the release of acetylcholine from the vagal nerve terminals (Fig. 7-17) (33). When the vagus is excited, calcium is increased in the nerve terminal as a result of the opening of voltage-gated N-type calcium channels; this leads to calcium-dependent activation of nNOS. nNOS itself can be increased by exercise training (Chapter 15).

Thus, *in the sinus node,* NO mediates cholinergic stimulation to decrease the tachycardia mediated by adrenergic stimulation. In the myocardium, NO decreases the β-adrenergic–induced increases in contractility, either acting as a cholinergic messenger (32) or inhibiting calcium cycling at the level of the sarcoplasmic reticulum (34). There may be a feedback loop whereby increased cytosolic calcium, as in calcium overload, stimulates the synthesis of nNOS in the sarcoplasmic reticulum that in turn inhibits cytosolic calcium levels (35). This leads to the suggestion of a NO feedback loop whereby increased cytosolic calcium, as in calcium overload, stimulates the synthesis of nNOS in the sarcoplasmic reticulum that in turn inhibits cytosolic calcium levels (35). Thus, the NO system plays a physiologic role in promoting vagal bradycardia and in lessening the effects of β-adrenergic activity such as tachycardia and increased contractility.

In vascular smooth muscle, guanylate cyclase responds to stimulation by NO, released by the vascular endothelium or formed during therapy with the vasodilator nitrate drugs, by formation of vasodilatory cGMP. The latter inhibits myosin kinase, causing vasodilation (Fig. 8-5).

Cross-talk between Receptors

Thus, the picture emerges of a host of important cardiovascular receptors, with subtypes, signaling systems, and second messengers. There are "bustling communication networks within and between clans of signaling proteins" (36). Eventually, these receptors and signaling systems almost all control cytosolic calcium in different ways. To avoid too many conflicting signals, the activity of the receptors needs to be integrated. There are two major ways to achieve integration. First, the process of switching on or off the adrenergic or cholinergic autonomic systems causes a coordinated series of cell changes calculated to mediate the overall adrenergic effects, in general stimulatory, or the inhibitory effects of cholinergic stimulation. Second, excess receptor stimulation can be muted by receptor down-regulation or by self-regulation of internal calcium. Cytosolic calcium that is too high may stimulate formation of NO with a negative inotropic effect. Third, and most novel, is the concept of cross-talk whereby receptors can send interactive regulatory messages to each other. For example, enhanced cholinergic M_2 stimulation leads to an increase in the inhibitory G_i protein, and to increased formation of cGMP, thereby limiting the effects of β-adrenergic stimulation.

SIGNALS AND RECEPTORS IN DISEASE STATES

Physiologically, there is a brisk adrenergic response to fight or flight, with numerous controls at various levels to avoid the potentially harmful effects of excess adrenergic stimulation. Pathologically, these controls often fail with excess β-adrenergic stimulation and potentially harmful results.

In myocardial ischemia, there is a brisk activation of the β-adrenergic–cAMP system in the first 15 to 30 minutes of severe ischemia, which may be linked to an increased propensity to ventricular tachycardia and fibrillation at the onset of a heart attack (37). At this stage, there is the combination of intense release of norepinephrine from the nerve endings in the ischemic area and an increased density of $β_1$-adrenergic receptor, the latter change being a response to the rapid up-regulation of the messenger RNA levels for this receptor (38). Thereafter, despite continued adrenergic stimulation and persistence of the increased receptor density, the activity of adenylyl cyclase decreases (39). The proposed explanation is that the β-ARK is activated in response to intense adrenergic stimulation to down-regulate the receptor (Fig. 7-6).

Prolonged excess catecholamine stimulation, as in experimental overexpression of the G_s protein, first enhances β-adrenergic signaling and then leads to myocardial damage with a calcium overload type of myocardial damage with cell necrosis and replacement fibrosis (40). The human counterpart is the cardiomyopathy of pheochromocytoma.

In severe heart failure, there is a hyperadrenergic state resulting from baroreflex stimulation of the adrenergic system by the low blood pressure (Fig. 16-14). The excess catecholamines lead to myocardial damage (preceding section). One hypothesis is that various mechanisms come into play to down-regulate the myocardial β-adrenergic–cAMP system, thus desensitizing the myocardium and thereby protecting it from the excess β-adrenergic stimulation. The major changes are (a) defective functioning of adenylyl cyclase; (b) reduced targeting of PKA by AKAP (41); (c) $β_1$-receptor downgrading; and (d) relative upgrading of the $β_2$-receptors. In addition to loss of receptor density, there may be loss of function because levels of the inhibitory kinase β-ARK are much increased (Fig. 16-18). A new approach focuses on the ryanodine receptor. According to this hypothesis, the receptor undergoes hyperphosphorylation in response to excess β-adrenergic stimulation and develops a calcium leak (Fig. 6-12). A third proposal is that there is a β-adrenergic path bypassing the adenylyl cyclase–cAMP–PKA sequence, whereby G_s directly overactivates the L calcium channels, thereby leading to calcium overload and possible cell death by apoptosis (42). Taken together, these abnormalities explain the slow increase and decrease of cytosolic calcium levels in heart failure with excess resting levels (Fig. 16-9). Thus, myocardial contraction and relaxation, already defective because of the heart failure, are further impaired.

Excess Nitric Oxide in Dilated Cardiomyopathy and Septic Shock

In severe dilated human heart failure (dilated cardiomyopathy), the inducible form of NOS (iNOS) is stimulated so that excess NO is made in the myocardium (43). The negative inotropic effect of the NO contributes to the severity of the heart failure. The hypothesis is that stimuli from the failing and dilated heart set off the production of cytokines such as tumor necrosis factor that induce iNOS. This hypothesis can be extended to other types of heart failure including septic shock in which there is increased formation of tumor necrosis factor and other cytokines (44,45).

Exercise in Cardiac Transplant Recipients

An interesting clinical problem has been how to understand the mechanism by which the transplanted denervated heart continues to respond to exercise with a tachycardia. The answer is that cardiac β$_2$-receptors respond to circulating catecholamines, even in the absence of neuronally released norepinephrine (46).

SUMMARY

1. *General model.* Neurotransmitters and regulatory peptides activate intracellular processes by initial occupation of a receptor, followed by coupling via one of the G-protein family to an effector molecule, which produces an intracellular second messenger. This messenger activates protein kinases that, in turn, regulate cytosolic calcium levels by altering the activity of crucial organelles such as channels or the sarcoplasmic reticulum. When cytosolic calcium increases, cell processes are in general switched on, including the sinus node discharge rate and the force of cardiac contraction.
2. *β-Adrenergic stimulation.* Occupancy of the β-receptor stimulates the reaction between the stimulatory G$_s$ protein and GTP to increase adenylyl cyclase activity. Adenylyl cyclase converts ATP to cAMP, the second messenger that activates PKA. This kinase phosphorylates a subunit of the calcium channel to admit more calcium ions. cAMP also phosphorylates phospholamban on the sarcoplasmic reticulum to enhance uptake of calcium by the sarcoplasmic reticulum. Thus, both the rates of contraction and the relaxation are enhanced, explaining the positive inotropic and lusitropic effects.
3. *Vagal stimulation.* Activity of the parasympathetic nervous system releases the messenger acetylcholine. The latter decreases the heart rate and force of contraction by several mechanisms including a decreased rate of release of norepinephrine from the terminal neurons by the process of neuromodulation and activation of the inhibitory G protein G$_i$. In addition, cGMP may be the direct second messenger of acetylcholine, and it inhibits the calcium channel. All these changes will decrease the heart rate and thereby the force of contraction (negative Treppe effect).
4. *NO as part of the vagal inhibitory system.* NO has inhibitory effects on heart rate and on contractility. It intimately interacts with the vagal system and aids self-protection against the adverse effects of excess adrenergic stimulation. An attractive hypothesis is that NO is essential for the release of acetylcholine from the vagal nerve terminals. NO also stimulates guanylate cyclase to produce cGMP that decreases cytosolic calcium and thereby has negative inotropic effects. In blood vessels, NO formed in the vascular endothelium permeates to the vascular smooth muscle to result in vasodilation.
5. *α$_1$-Adrenergic stimulation.* In general, the α-adrenergic system acts mainly on vascular smooth muscle and has a relatively minor role in the control of the contractile activity of the myocardium. Its receptor is linked by another G protein (G$_q$) to its effector, phospholipase C, with hydrolysis

of phosphatidylinositol. Two changes result. First, the formation of the intracellular messenger IP_3 stimulates the release of calcium from the sarcoplasmic reticulum leading to vasoconstriction. Second, protein kinase C is activated by its translocation from the resting cytosolic state to the active membrane-located state. Activated protein kinase C may regulate the activity of ion channels, for example, allowing an enhanced influx of calcium ions to sustain the vascular contraction initiated by IP_3. In the myocardium, protein kinase C is also important in the growth response and the self-protective phenomenon of preconditioning.

STUDENT QUESTIONS

1. What is the full messenger system involved in translating β-adrenergic receptor stimulation into a positive inotropic contractile effect?
2. What is receptor desensitization?
3. How does vagal stimulation decrease the heart rate?
4. How does $α_1$-adrenergic stimulation cause vasoconstriction?
5. Describe the role of the G-protein family in signal transduction with special reference to the interaction between the β-adrenergic system and the cholinergic system.

CARDIOLOGIST-IN-TRAINING QUESTIONS

1. How do the two major subtypes of cardiac β-adrenergic receptors differ in their function? How are these receptor subtypes changed in severe heart failure?
2. A patient with severe acute heart failure is given the positively inotropic drug dobutamine. An initial improvement in cardiac function rapidly falls off unless the dose is increased. Why? Describe the possible molecular mechanisms.
3. There are 10 steps that follow initial β-adrenergic catecholamine stimulation, leading to a positive inotropic effect. How many can you itemize?
4. Describe the α-adrenergic signal system. Why is it of greater importance in the control of vascular than of myocardial contraction?
5. How does NO interact with the adrenergic and cholinergic systems?

REFERENCES

1. Rockman HA, et al. Seven-transmembrane-spanning receptors and heart function. *Nature* 2002;415: 206–212.
1a. Murphy, Vaughan. In: Messerli FH, ed. *Cardiovascular drug therapy*. Philadelphia: WB Saunders, 1996:1162.
1b. Jenkins JR, Belarindelli L. Atrioventricular nodal accommodation in isolated guinea pig hearts: physiological significance and role of adenosine. *Circ Res* 1988;63:97.
1c. Rosendorff C. Endothelin, vascular hypertrophy and hypertension. *Cardiovasc Drug Ther* 1996;10: 795–807.

1d. Gulbenkian S, Saetrun Opgaard O, Ekman R, et al. Peptidergic innervation of human epicardial coronary arteries. *Circ Res* 1993;73:579–588.
1e. Chang F, Yu H, Cohen IS. Actions of vasoactive intestinal peptide and neuropeptide Y in the pacemaker current in canine Purkinje fibers. *Circ Res* 1994;74:157–162.
2. Ahlquist RP. A study of the adrenotropic receptors. *Am J Physiol* 1948;153:586–600.
3. Kahn CR. Membrane receptors for hormones and neurotransmitters. *J Cell Biol* 1976;70:261–286.
4. Lands AM, Arnold A, McAuliff JP, et al. Differentiation of receptor systems activated by sympathomimetic amines. *Nature* 1967;214:597–598.
5. del Monte F, Kaumann AJ, Poole-Wilson PA, et al. Coexistence of functioning β_1- and β_2-adrenoreceptors in single myocytes from human ventricle. *Circulation* 1993;88:854–863.
6. Kobilka B. Molecular and cellular biology of adrenergic receptors. *Trends Cardiovasc Med* 1991;1:189–194.
7. Xiao RP, et al. Recent advances in cardiac β_2-adrenergic signal transduction. *Circ Res* 1999;85:1092–1100.
8. Newton GE, et al. Inotropic and sympathetic responses to the intracoronary infusion of a β_2-receptor agonist. A human in vivo study. *Circulation* 1999;99:2402–2407.
9. Tevaearai HT, et al. Myocardial gene transfer and overexpression of β_2-adrenergic receptors potentiates the functional recovery of unloaded failing hearts. *Circulation* 2002;106:124–129.
10. Luttrell LM, et al. β-Arrestin-dependent formation of β_2 adrenergic receptor-Src protein kinase complexes. *Science* 1999;283:655–661.
11. Iaccarino G, et al. Reciprocal in vivo regulation of myocardial G protein-coupled receptor kinase expression by β-adrenergic receptor stimulation and blockade. *Circulation* 1998;98:1783–1789.
12. Hall RA, et al. Regulation of G protein-coupled receptor signaling by scaffold proteins. *Circ Res* 2002;91:672–680.
13. Fink M, et al. AKAP-mediated targeting of protein kinase A regulates contractility in cardiac myocytes. *Circ Res* 2001;88:291–297.
14. Park S-H, et al. Rewiring MAP kinase pathways using alternative scaffold assembly mechanisms. *Science* 2003;299:1061–1064.
15. Schofield PR, Abbott A. Molecular pharmacology and drug action: structural information casts light on ligand binding. *Trends Pharmacol Sci* 1989;10:207–212.
16. Lefkowitz RJ. Clinical implications of basic research. G proteins in medicine. *N Engl J Med* 1995;332:186–187.
17. Kim D, Lewis DL, Graziadei L, et al. G-protein beta-gamma subunits activate the cardiac muscarinic K^+-channel via phospholipase A2. *Nature* 1989;337:557–560.
18. Hwang K-C, Gray CD, Sweet WE, et al. α_1-Adrenergic receptor coupling with G_h in the failing human heart. *Circulation* 1996;94:718–726.
19. Graham RM, Perez DM, Hwa J, et al. α-Adrenergic receptor subtypes. Molecular structure, function and signalling. *Circ Res* 1996;78:737–749.
20. Venter JC, Ross J, Kaplan NO. Lack of detectable change in cyclic AMP during the cardiac inotropic response to isoproterenol immobilized on glass beads. *Proc Natl Acad Sci U S A* 1975;72:824–828.
21. Hohl CM, Li Q. Compartmentation of cAMP in adult canine ventricular myocytes. Relation to single cell free Ca^{2+} transients. *Circ Res* 1991;69:1369–1379.
22. Worthington M, et al. Contrasting effects of cyclic AMP release caused by β-adrenergic stimulation or by adenylate cyclase activation on ventricular fibrillation threshold of isolated rat heart. *J Cardiovasc Pharmacol* 1992;20:595–600.
23. Strang KT, Sweitzer NK, Greaser ML, et al. β-Adrenergic receptor stimulation increases unloaded shortening velocity of skinned single ventricular myocytes from rats. *Circ Res* 1994;74:542–549.
24. Katz AM. Role of the basic sciences in the practice of cardiology. *J Mol Cell Cardiol* 1987;19:3–17.
25. Deckmyn H, et al. Dual regulation of phospholipase C activity by G-proteins. *News Physiol Sci* 1993;8:61–63.
26. Berridge MJ. Inositol triphosphate and calcium signalling. *Nature* 1993;361:315–325.
27. Otani H, Otani H, Das DK. Alpha-adrenoceptor-mediated phosphoinositide breakdown and inotropic response in rat left ventricular papillary muscles. *Circ Res* 1988; 62:8–17.
28. Allen IS, Neri M, Cohen RS, et al. Angiotensin-II increases spontaneous contractile frequency and stimulates calcium current in cultured neonatal rat heart myocytes: insights into the underlying biochemical mechanisms. *Circ Res* 1988;62:524–534.
29. Capogrossi MC, Kachadorian WA, Gambassi G, et al. Ca^{2+} dependence of a-adrenergic defects on the contractile properties and Ca^{2+} homeostasis of cardiac myocytes. *Circ Res* 1991;69:540–550.

30. Lindemann JP, Watanabe AM. Mechanisms of adrenergic and cholinergic regulation of myocardial contractility. In: Sperelakis N, ed. *Physiology and pathophysiology of the heart*, 3rd ed. Boston: Kluwer Academic Publishers, 1995:467–494.
31. Lewis ME, et al. Vagus nerve stimulation decreases left ventricular contractility *in vivo* in the human and pig heart. *J Physiol* 2001;534:547–552.
32. Balligand J-L. Regulation of cardiac β-adrenergic response by nitric oxide. *Cardiovasc Res* 1999;43: 607–620.
33. Mohan RM, et al. Neuronal nitric oxide synthase gene transfer promotes cardiac vagal gain of function. *Circ Res* 2002;91:1089–1091.
34. Ashley EA, et al. Cardiac nitric oxide synthase 1 regulates basal and β-adrenergic contractility in murine ventricular myocytes. *Circulation* 2002;105:3011–3016.
35. Sears CE, et al. Cardiac neuronal nitric oxide synthase isoform regulates myocardial contraction and calcium handling. *Circ Res* 2003;92:e57–e59.
36. Bourne HR. Team blue sees red. *Nature* 1995;376:727–729.
37. Lubbe WH, Podzuweit T, Opie LH. Potential arrhythmogenic role of cyclic adenosine monophosphate (AMP) and cytosolic calcium overload: implications for prophylactic effects of beta-blockers in myocardial infarction and proarrhythmic effects of phosphodiesterase inhibitors. *J Am Coll Cardiol* 1992;19:1622–1633.
38. Ihl-Vahl R, Marquetant R, Bremerich MJ, et al. Regulation of β-adrenergic receptors in acute myocardial ischemia: subtype-selective increase of mRNA specific for β_1-adrenergic receptors. *J Mol Cell Cardiol* 1995;27:437–452.
39. Ungerer M, Kessbohm K, Kronsbein K, et al. Activation of β-adrenergic receptor kinase during myocardial ischemia. *Circ Res* 1996;79:455–460.
40. Iwase M, Bishop SP, Uechi M, et al. Adverse effects of chronic endogenous sympathetic drive induced by cardiac G_{sa} overexpression. *Circ Res* 1996;78:517–524.
41. Zakhary DR, et al. Regulation of PKA binding to AKAPs in the heart. *Circulation* 2000;101: 1459–1464.
42. Zhu W-Z, et al. Linkage of β_1-adrenergic stimulation to apoptotic heart cell death through protein kinase A-independent activation of Ca^{2+}/calmodulin kinase II. *J Clin Invest* 2003;111:617–625.
43. Habib FM, Springall DR, Davies GJ, et al. Tumour necrosis factor and inducible nitric synthase in dilated cardiomyopathy. *Lancet* 1996;347:1151–1155.
44. Schulz R, Pana DL, Catena R, et al. The role of nitric oxide in cardiac depression induced by interleukin-1β and tumour necrosis factor-α. *Br J Pharmacol* 1995;114:27–34.
45. Kelly RA, Balligand J-L, Smith TW. Nitric oxide and cardiac function. *Circ Res* 1996;79:363–380.
46. Leenen FHH, Davies RA, Fourney A. Role of cardiac β-receptors in cardiac responses to exercise in cardiac transplant patients. *Circulation* 1995;91:685–690.
47. Raymond JR, Hnatowich M, Lefkowitz RJ, et al. Adrenergic receptors. Models for regulation of signal transduction processes. *Hypertension* 1990;15:119–131.
48. Choi D-J, et al. Mechanism of β-adrenergic receptor desensitization in cardiac hypertrophy is increased β-adrenergic receptor kinase. *J Biol Chem* 1997;272:17223–17229.

8

Myocardial Contraction and Relaxation

Lionel H. Opie and R. John Solaro

The critical component of the remarkable biological machine that gives heart muscle its ability to work is myosin, a molecular motor.

Solaro (1)

The triggered release of calcium from the sarcoplasmic reticulum (SR) abruptly increases cytosolic calcium to sufficiently initiate systole as a result of the interaction of the thick and thin filaments of the heart's contractile machinery (Color Plate 1). Contraction results when the heads of the thick myosin filament interact with the thin actin filament. In the absence of calcium ions, such interaction is inhibited by components of the thin filaments, the troponins and tropomyosin. By far the greater percentage of myofibrillar protein is that involved in contraction, with approximately 10% involved in its regulation and another 10% involved in maintenance of the structure of the myofibril (Table 8-1). In living muscle, contraction will not occur unless adenosine 5′-triphosphate (ATP) and calcium are present. According to the generally accepted sliding filament model (2), in the presence of calcium ions, inhibitions on contraction are removed and the thin actin filaments slide between the thicker myosin filaments as a result of repetitive movements of the myosin heads (Color Plate 2). The concept of the power stroke of the myosin head, previously not fully proven, is now established (3,4). The linkage between the myosin head and the actin filament is the cross-bridge. The cross-bridge cycle is the repetitive attachment and detachment of myosin heads to and from actin filaments. The third and newly emphasized filament is titin, noncontractile but elastic (Color Plate 3).

MOLECULAR EVENTS IN CONTRACTILE CYCLE

The transformation of chemical energy into mechanical work involves a series of reactions that center on the splitting of ATP by hydrolysis (Color Plate 2). The

TABLE 8-1. *The proteins of skeletal myofibrils*

Function	Location	Percentage of myofibrillar protein	Molecular weight (kDa)
Contractile			
Myosin	Thick filament	44	460
2 heavy chains		46–50	220×2
4 light chains		10	20
Actin	Thin filament	25	42
Regulatory			
Tropomyosin	Thin filament	5	67
Troponin I	Thin filament		24
Troponin C	Thin filament	7	18
Troponin T	Thin filament		38
Structural			
Titin	From Z to M lines	8–10	2.7×10^3
C protein[a]	Thick filament		140
α-actinin[b]	Z lines		400
β-actin	Thin filament	8–13	400
Dystrophin[c]	Cytoskeleton		427
M-line proteins	M lines		750 (about)

Data in part from references 1a, 1b.
[a]Binds to myosin neck and to actin (Color Plate 8-10) and may limit myosin flexion.
[b]Anti-α-actinin antibodies alter Z-line properties (1c).
[c]Color Plate 8-11; has role in cardiomyopathy (1d).

term hydrolysis describes a reaction in which a compound is split (lysis) by the addition of water (Greek, *hydor*, water). In the case of muscle, the enzyme that is involved is an integral part of the myosin molecule; hence, the enzyme is known as the myosin ATPase. For this function, the important part of ATP is the terminal pyrophosphate (P-O-P) linkage. It is customary to refer to this as a high-energy bond (a concept that was introduced by Fritz Lipmann in 1941) because when the bond is split off, useful energy is released. Thus, in general terms, all the energy needed to cause muscle contraction is obtained by splitting the terminal phosphate bond in ATP, as follows:

$$ATP + H_2O \rightarrow ADP + P_i + H^+ + energy$$

where ADP is adenosine 5′-diphosphate and P_i is inorganic phosphate. To be exact, it is $MgATP^{2-}$, not ATP that is split (Chapter 11). A little more than 30 kJ of energy are released for each mole (500 g) of ATP that is hydrolyzed (or split up). The heart contains approximately 3 mg of ATP/g of fresh weight or approximately 5 μmol/g or 5×10^{-6} mol/L/g of ATP or 10 mmol/L of ATP per liter of cytosol. Together with the approximately threefold greater pool of creatine phosphate, this represents an energy reserve sufficient for only 50 to 75 beats in an adult heart. Thus, continuous production of ATP by mitochondrial metabolism is required to sustain the contractile cycle.

In the heart, the myosin ATPase actually splits ATP in the relaxation phase of the cycle (cross-bridges off), and the power stroke occurs when the products of hydrolysis (first P_i and then ADP) are released. Cyclic interaction of the two contractile proteins of the cross-bridges is controlled in a Ca^{2+}-dependent manner by thin filament regulatory proteins, consisting of the troponin complex [troponin C (TnC), troponin I, and troponin T] together with tropomyosin (to be described).

Microanatomy of Contraction

To explain the contraction cycle requires first a brief review of the microanatomy of the two contractile elements that are the thin actin fibers lying between the much thicker myosin components (Color Plate 1). A third noncontractile element, titin, tethers the myosin molecule to the Z line and provides elasticity (5).

Actin and the Troponin Complex

The thin filaments of actin (approximately 1 μm long and only 5 to 7 nm wide) contain two helical chains that intertwine in a helical pattern (Color Plate 4). Each actin filament is carried on a twisting "backbone" of the heavier *tropomyosin* molecule. Crucial to the interaction between actin and myosin are the *troponin complexes* that occur at regular intervals of 38.5 nm along the tropomyosin. Troponin C (C for calcium) is that component that responds to the calcium ions released from the SR to start the cross-bridge cycle. Troponin C, once activated by calcium ions as in systole, binds to the inhibitory molecule *troponin I* (I for inhibitor) that otherwise restricts the interaction between actin and the myosin heads (Fig. 8-1). However, when calcium levels are low, as in diastole, troponin I binds to actin to inhibit myosin binding. *Troponin T* is involved in distributing the inhibitory effect of the Tn complex, via tropomyosin, to seven actin monomers with which it interacts in the absence of Ca^{2+} (6). In contrast, in the presence of Ca^{2+}, troponin T removes these

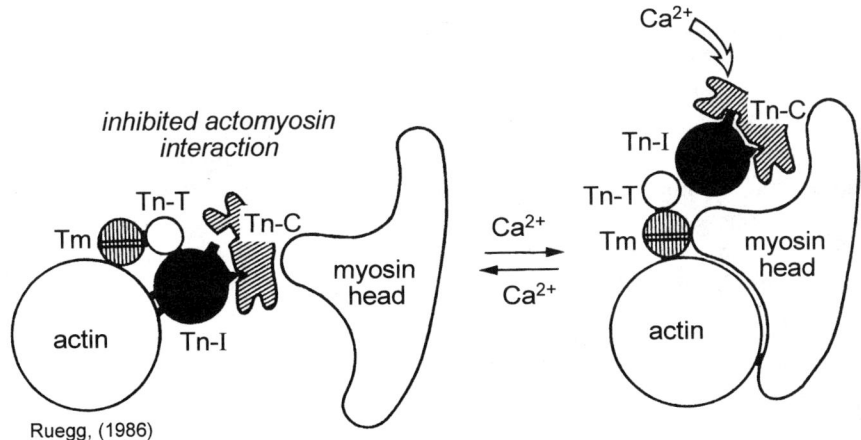

FIG. 8-1. How calcium promotes actin–myosin interaction. When cytosolic calcium concentration is low (on left), then troponin C (*Tn-C*) only has a weak molecular interaction with troponin I (*Tn-I*), which "blocks" the access of myosin to actin. When cytosolic calcium is high (on right) then TnC interacts with troponin I at a molecular level, thereby "moving" the troponin I and "unblocking" the access of myosin to actin. For details, see Ruegg (17).

inhibitions and activates the actomyosin ATPase. Tropomodulin is another regulatory protein that caps the free, pointed ends of the thin actin filaments to prevent their excess elongation during growth.

Myosin Filament

Each myosin thick filament (approximately 1.5 μm or 1,500 nm long and 10 to 15 nm wide) is composed of approximately 300 individual myosin molecules, each molecule being very large and ending in a myosin head that is bilobed (Color Plate 4). Half of these heads are orientated toward one end of the sarcomere and half to the other, leaving a bare area in the middle of the thick filament. The bilobed head of each myosin molecule is connected to the thick filament by an elongated base or "neck," which merges into the remaining "body" of the molecule, consisting of two helical bodies twisting around each other. These are permanently built into the thick myosin filament by side-to-side aggregation with other helices. The pattern in which myosin heads emerge from the body of the thick filaments is still controversial, but in a commonly accepted version, the heads appear in groups of three, each group located 14.3 nm from the next (7). This means that approximately 50 such sets occur on each half of a single thick filament. The heads come out in a spiral fashion, so that one myosin head will reappear in the same line as another every 43 nm. Myosin is composed of two types of chains with different molecular weights (Color Plate 4).

Myosin Heavy Chains

These consist of two long strands twisted together, the one end of each chain embedded in the myosin filament and the other ending in the head. The two strands each terminate in two heads that are closely linked and hence described as bilobed. The myosin molecule is often described as having two functional domains, the body or filament being the light meromyosin in contrast to the heavy meromyosin that represents the cross-bridge including the head. The latter, in turn, can be subdivided into the S1 subfragment that contains the myosin head and the S2 subfragment or neck that connects the head to the body or filament. Previously, it was thought that the flexion and extension of the head at the S1-S2 junction accounted for myosin head movements, but in the revised molecular model, the neck and head are both involved in the myosin motor functions (Color Plate 5).

Myosin Heads

A combination of current molecular techniques has been used to define the microanatomy of the myosin head (Table 8-2). Attachment of ATP to its pocket (*the ATP- or nucleotide-binding pocket*) can cause a series of configurational changes in the myosin head that initiate the cross-bridge cycle (Color Plate 4).

TABLE 8-2. Microanatomy of myosin head[a]

Number of heads per molecule	Two
Shape of head	Pear shaped
Size of head	16.5 nm (with neck) by 6.5 nm (widest)
Molecular weight of each head	
Heavy chain components	95 kDa
2 light chain components	35 kDa
Total	130 kDa
Binding sites on head	Actin
	ATP (nucleotide)
Light chains	
Regulatory	Applied to base of α-helix
Essential	Applied to helix close to neck–head junction

For structure, see Figure 8-5.
[a]Reference 8; ATP, adenosine 5′-triphosphate.

This ATP site is physically distinct from the actin site, also situated on the myosin head (8). Extending from the base of the nucleotide pocket to the actin-binding face is a narrow *cleft* that splits the central 50-kd segment of the myosin head. The proposal is that binding of either ATP or its breakdown products to the nucleotide pocket causes different changes in the physical properties of the cleft in the myosin head and hence in the physical configuration of the head (9). ATP is split by the crucial *myosin ATPase activity*, located near the ATP binding site.

Each myosin head binds to one actin molecule with a secondary binding site on the neighboring actin molecule one turn down on the actin helix (Color Plate 6). There are several strengths of interaction between actin and myosin, so that both the association and dissociation of cross-bridges are progressive molecular interactions rather than on/off in nature. With each successive step in the actin–myosin interaction, the area of the binding site on actin for myosin increases as does the binding constant.

Myosin Light Chains

Aligned to the elongated base or "neck" of each myosin head, there are two myosin light chains (MLCs), each of a different type (MLC-1 and MLC-2), making four light chains per bilobed head (Color Plate 4). The *essential MLC* (MLC-1) is an integral part of the structure of the myosin head, and it appears to interact with actin in such a way that the contractile process is inhibited (10). The other *regulatory MLC* (MLC-2) helps to enhance the contractile response to β-adrenergic stimulation (see later).

Myosin Binding Protein C

Myosin-binding protein C runs at approximately right angles to the myosin molecules to act as a tethering structure that lies around the myosin S2 subfragment of the myosin head. Its proposed function is to stabilize the S2 subfragment as the myosin head itself flexes and extends at the level of the light chains. It may be involved in some types of hypertrophic or dilated cardiomyopathies (see page 239).

Titin

Titin, the largest molecule yet described, is both extraordinarily large (approximately 3 million Da) and very long, approximately 1,000 nm or half of the sarcomere length when the latter is stretched to 2 μm (Color Plate 3). Cardiac titin, flexible and relatively slender, is composed of a folded elastic segment 200 nm in length and an inelastic anchoring segment 800 nm long (11). Titin acts as a third filament (the other two being actin and myosin) with a triple function. First, it tethers the end of the myosin molecule to the Z line, thereby stabilizing the myosin filaments. Second, titin functions as a "molecular spring" that modulates both systole and diastole. As the sarcomere stretches in diastole, the elastic segment of titin expands and then contracts in systole. This process could enhance systolic contraction in response to stretch or deformation (Color Plate 3), thus contributing to the Frank–Starling mechanism (12). Another force, the restoring force (11), is built up when the heart contracts and then releases in early diastole to aid "suction" (Fig. 12-21) and ventricular filling. Thus, titin stretch enhances both systole and early diastole. Third, titin may play a key role in transducing a sustained stretch signal into growth, interacting with two proteins of the Z disk (Fig. 3-11), the MLP protein and the T-cap protein (13).

THE BASIC CROSS-BRIDGE CYCLE

The cross-bridge cycle consists of the repetitive attachment and detachment of myosin heads to and from actin filaments. At the start of systole, muscle contraction is triggered by the arrival of calcium ions from the sarcoplasmic reticulum, in response to the process of calcium-induced calcium release (Color Plates 1 and 5). The calcium ions set in motion a series of molecular changes that result in the thin actin filaments sliding past the thick myosin filaments in such a way that the Z lines come closer together. Crucial to this interaction is the role of the cross-bridges, which extend from the myosin filament toward the actin filament. Such cross-bridges are the myosin heads attached to a binding site on the actin molecule. Each cross-bridge cycle produces a power stroke that drives the actin filament along the thick filament. This interaction between the myosin heads and actin filaments is tightly controlled by the cytosolic calcium ion concentration and its crucial interaction with TnC. To understand the importance of TnC requires a brief review of how the internal calcium concentration changes during the contractile cycle.

The overall concept is that a single contraction of a heart cell is set in motion by a brief period (approximately 600 milliseconds at an average heart rate in humans) during which the cytosolic calcium concentration increases to a peak (approximately 200 milliseconds) and decreases (approximately 400 milliseconds). When cytosolic calcium is high, calcium ions bind increasingly to TnC molecules, turning on more of the actin sites on the thin filament for interaction with any adjacent myosin heads (Color Plate 5). Repetitive cross-bridge cycling occurs, and more and more cross-bridges become activated as long as the calcium concentration increases (physiologic systole). Throughout systole, there are numerous cycles of cross-bridge attachment and detachment. During the detachment phase of one cycle, tension is maintained by other cross-bridges attached at that time. As soon as the calcium concentration begins to decrease, however, increasing numbers of actin sites on thin filaments become unavailable to waiting myosin heads, and the number of cross-bridges interacting per unit time diminishes until ultimately the beat is over when the possibility of interactions has declined to near zero (physiologic diastole).

Models of Contraction

Current concepts can be traced back to the earlier four-step model, still useful although now superseded. According to this model (14), there are two major cross-bridge states, the *actin-attached* and *actin-detached states*. These could equally well be called the myosin-attached and myosin-detached states (Color Plate 2). Each exists in two stages, with the whole sequence as follows:

1. Myosin attaches to actin to form a state that is potentially force generating and "ready to go."
2. The power stroke follows as the head flexes and the rigor state ensues, so that the myosin head stays attached to actin unless "liberated" by ATP.
3. When ATP binds to the myosin head, the rigor state is terminated, and the head detaches from actin.
4. ATP is hydrolyzed by the enzymatic activity of the myosin head, and the products of this hydrolysis "energize" the head, which then reattaches to another actin unit, thereby regaining the first stage.

The key events underlying the cross-bridge cycle can be explained by changes in the molecular configuration of the myosin head that alternates between two major molecular configurations (Fig. 8-2). When ATP is bound to the head, there is a *weak-binding conformation*, and when ADP and P_i (the products of ATP hydrolysis) are released, there is a *strong-binding conformation*, which explains why the power stroke is initiated. The overall concept of weak and strong binding states now has a molecular basis (8).

What determines the *cross-bridge cycling rate*? Brenner (15) provided the following useful concept. The cycling rate is dependent on two apparent rate con-

8. MYOCARDIAL CONTRACTION AND RELAXATION

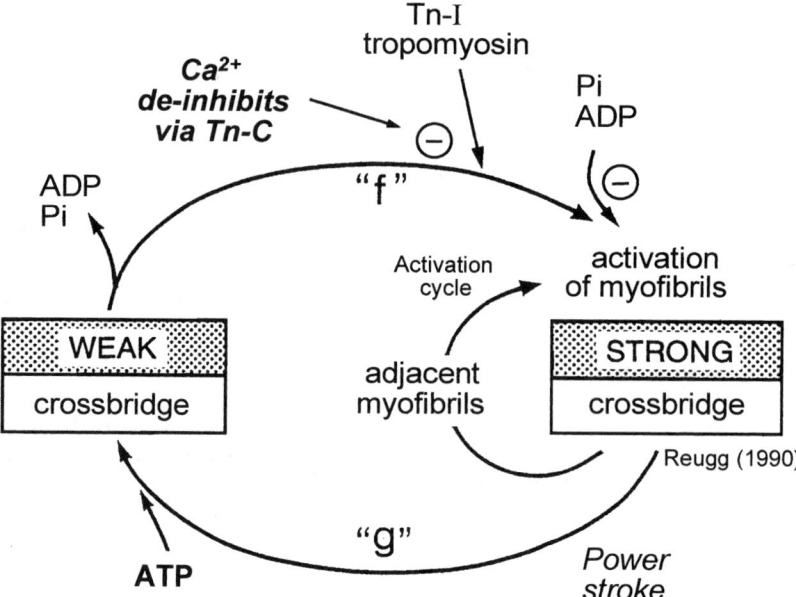

FIG. 8-2. Weak and strong binding states in the cross-bridge cycle. During force generation, the molecular force generators (myosin cross-bridges) cycle between weak and strong states with apparent rate constants, forward (*f*) and reverse (*g*). Calcium, by activating troponin C, increases the probability of forming strong, force-generating cross-bridges. The responsiveness to calcium depends on the relative values of g and f, as well as on the calcium affinity for troponin C. (Modified from the concepts of Prof. J. C. Ruegg, Heidelberg, Germany.)

stants: the f constant that controls the rate at which cross-bridges enter the attached state and the g constant that controls the rate of cross-bridge detachment. Assuming that one molecule of ATP is split in each cross-bridge cycle, the cross-bridge cycling rate will correspond to the ATP splitting rate.

In technical terms, the ATP splitting rate corresponds to the molecular turnover number of the actin-activated myosin ATPase activity, which is proportional to fg/f + g (15).

The Rayment Five-Step Molecular Model

This currently favored five-step model has a clearly identified molecular basis (8,16). The five steps are shown in Color Plates 5 and 6. Color Plate 5 gives the overall picture and the effects of calcium arrival and departure, whereas Color Plate 6 shows the molecular processes in greater detail. One of the salient features is that the molecular motor that powers the cross-bridge cycle acts so that extension and flexion occur at the elongated base of the head (the "neck," Color Plate 4). Starting with the rigor state at the end of the power stroke, this state is broken (Color Plate 6A) by the binding of ATP to the myosin head in two stages. First, there is binding to the pocket of most of the ATP molecules including the terminal γ phosphate, which opens the narrow nucleotide pocket. The resultant change in molecular configuration transforms the strong binding state into the weak binding state and myosin detaches from actin (Color Plate 6B). Next, the ATP binding pocket closes around its base, and there is a further molecular change in the myosin head, so that the flexible domain (or "neck" of the head) extends on the body and the myosin head comes to lie opposite a new actin unit (Color Plate 6C) to which it binds weakly.

Thereupon, ATP undergoes hydrolysis to ADP and P_i by the myosin ATPase activity that is located near the nucleotide pocket (Color Plate 4). The result is that ADP is now bound to the site previously occupied by ATP and P_i is extruded from the cleft (Color Plate 6D). The resultant molecular changes partially close the nucleotide pocket and the strong binding state ensues so that the power stroke occurs as the head straightens at the "neck" and flexes on the body. Thus, the actin molecule is moved by 5 to 10 nm (Color Plate 6E). Thereafter, ADP is released (Color Plate 6A) to expose an empty nucleotide binding pocket where ATP can rebind, thus terminating the rigor state (Color Plate 6A, B).

CONTROL OF CONTRACTILE CYCLE BY CALCIUM IONS

In basal physiologic states, the sarcomeres only generate approximately 25% of the possible peak force (1). Increased force development can result from one of three processes: (a) increased activation of the cross-bridges by calcium ions; (b) phosphorylation or dephosphorylation of the contractile proteins, thereby altering the cross-bridge response to calcium; and (c) length effects that increase the force of contraction even when the calcium level does not change (the Frank–Starling relationship). These will now be examined in sequence. Once calcium is bound to TnC, a molecular signal is generated within the thin filament that eventually leads to an increased rate of cross-bridge attachment. How and where does calcium act?

When calcium occupies TnC, the binding of TnC to troponin I is strengthened, thereby decreasing the negative interaction of troponin I with actin and causing a molecular change in tropomyosin, which becomes less inhibitory to the actin–myosin interaction (17). Cardiac troponin C (Color Plate 4) has only one important receptor site for calcium in the case of cardiac troponin (18). When this site is occupied by calcium, it produces conformational changes in the distant regions of the TnC molecule.

Calcium Regulatory System

When calcium levels are low, there is a weak interaction between TnC and the inhibitory peptide of troponin I. The result is that troponin I inhibits the actin–myosin interaction (Fig. 8-1). In addition, when calcium is low, the

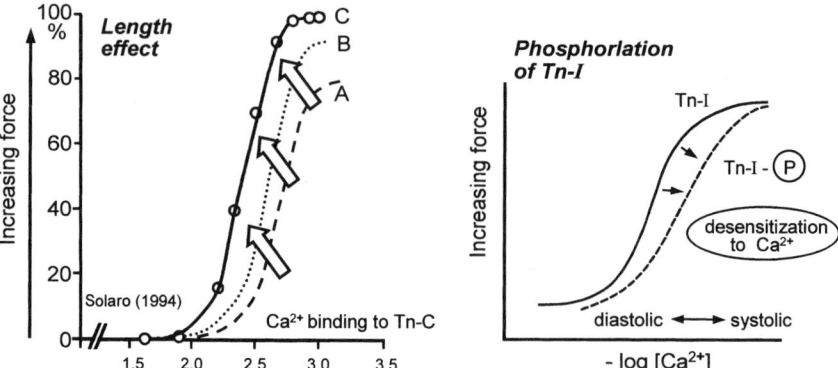

FIG. 8-3. Sensitization and desensitization to calcium. Left: When the fiber is stretched and the sarcomere length increased, for any given number of Ca^{2+} ions binding to troponin C (TnC), there is a greater force development, so that TnC has become sensitized to Ca^{2+}. (Modified from Solaro RJ, et al. Regulatory proteins and diastolic relaxation. In: Lorell BH, et al., eds. *Diastolic relaxation of the heart*. Boston: Kluwer Academic Publishers, 1994:43–53.) **Right:** Phosphorylation of troponin I (*Tn-I-P*) leads to a greatly accelerated dissociation of calcium from the TnC–calcium complex. By inference, there is accelerated relaxation, as occurs during β-adrenergic stimulation.

tropomyosin molecule is twisted in such a way that the myosin heads cannot interact with actin. Then, when TnC interacts with calcium, its interaction with troponin I is strengthened, whereas that between troponin I and actin is weakened. As a result, the tropomyosin molecule "moves out of the way" to permit strong interaction between actin and myosin, allowing cross-bridges to attach and produce force. This effect is cooperative inasmuch as any attachment of cross-bridges enhances the binding of calcium to TnC. Hence, the relationship between the free calcium concentration and force production is steep (Fig. 8-3).

Binding Sites of Calcium on Troponin C

Each molecule of cardiac TnC has only one calcium-specific binding site. Thus, the amount of calcium-TnC formed depends on the calcium affinity and the calcium ion concentration, according to the law of mass action:IQ4

$$TnC.Ca \underset{(k^{+1})}{\overset{(k^{-1})}{\rightleftarrows}} TnC + Ca^{2+}$$

$$(TnC.Ca) = K(TnC)(Ca^{2+})$$

where K is the calcium affinity of TnC or simply the quotient of the on-rate k^{+1} and the off-rate k^{-1}. Its reciprocal value is the dissociation constant of the calcium–troponin complex (approximately 10^{-6} mol/L) and specifies the calcium ion concentration giving 50% calcium occupancy of TnC and hence half-maximal activation of the contractile proteins. Interestingly, approximately 10^{-6} mol/L Ca^{2+} is also the calcium level normally reached during systole (Fig. 6-3).

Mechanism of Control by Calcium

Do these effects of calcium ions control the apparent rate constants f and g for cross-bridge attachment and detachment? According to Brenner (15), the cross-bridge attachment rate constant is predominantly affected by calcium. Thus, any increase in the free calcium ion concentration in the cytoplasm would enhance the calcium occupancy of TnC, normally only approximately 25% occupied, which in turn would increase the probability of cross-bridge attachment (Fig. 8-1). The first effect of calcium ions would be to increase steady-state force development. Additionally, indices of contractility, such as the rate of force increase or the rate of pressure change in the intact heart (dP/dt), would also be altered by calcium acting in this manner.

In contrast, Hancock et al. (19) propose that calcium ions, interacting with TnC increase the availability of the myosin binding sites on the actin rather than altering the rates of transition between cross-bridge states. Hancock et al. believe that Brenner's proposals, based on data obtained from skeletal muscle fibers, may not apply to the heart.

In reality, these two apparently opposing views may not be that different because calcium promotes binding of myosin to actin, an effect that will also change the molecular configuration of the myosin head (8) and thereby the degree of interaction of myosin with actin.

β-Adrenergic Effects and Calcium

Normally, the calcium ion concentration in the cardiac cytosol during systole is such that the contractile sites are approximately half activated. Therefore, the heart has a considerable contractile reserve that might be exploited by increasing the calcium occupancy of TnC. Force development would ultimately depend on the amount of calcium released from the SR and delivered to TnC, which would explain the increased force development during catecholamine stimulation (Fig. 8-4). β-Adrenergic stimulation acts either indirectly through cyclic adenosine 3',5'-monophosphate (cAMP) and protein kinase A or more directly to increase cytosolic calcium levels. An increased rate of cross-bridge attachment increases the rate of increase in tension, dP/dt (where P is pressure and t is time). This is the positive inotropic effect. The rate of relaxation (–dP/dt) will also be augmented. This lusitropic effect is explained by two factors. First, phosphorylation of phospholamban activates the calcium transport into the SR, so that the cytosolic free calcium will be lowered more rapidly in the presence of catecholamines. Second, the lowering of free calcium ion concentration causes

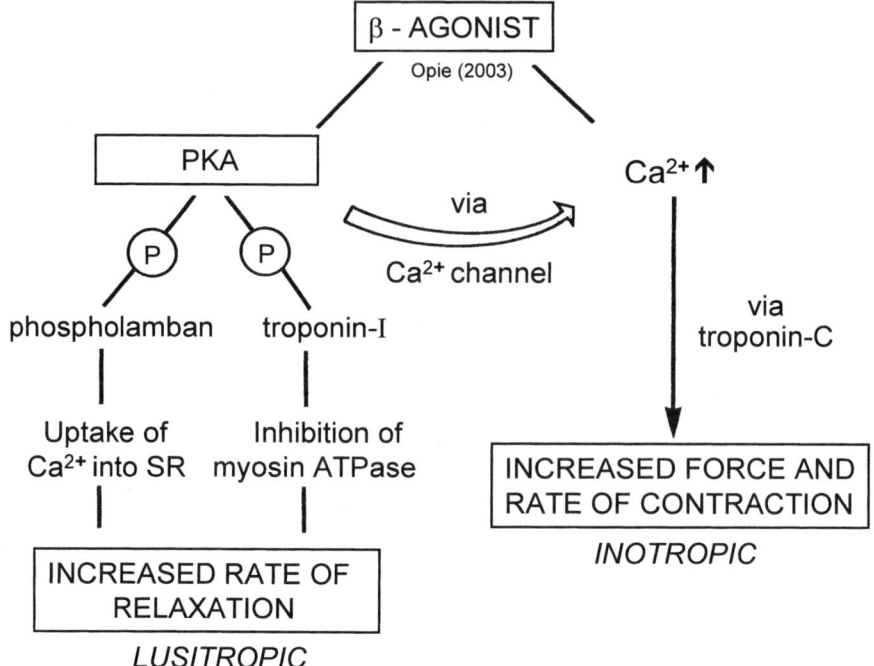

FIG. 8-4. Catecholamine regulation of contraction and relaxation. Proposed links between β-adrenergic agonist stimulation by catecholamines and calcium-dependent changes in rates of contraction and relaxation of heart muscle. *P*, phosphorylation mediated by protein kinase A; *SR*, sarcoplasmic reticulum.

the dissociation of the TnC calcium complex and hence the detachment of cross-bridges and the decrease in force. Additionally, phosphorylation of the regulatory proteins is involved (1,20).

PHOSPHORYLATION OF CONTRACTILE PROTEINS

Troponin I

During β-adrenergic stimulation, contraction is faster and more powerful, but relaxation must also be enhanced to allow diastolic coronary perfusion even when the heart rate has increased (Fig. 7-16). The rate of dissociation of the TnC–calcium complex is greatly enhanced when troponin I is phosphorylated by a cAMP-dependent protein kinase. The reduction in calcium affinity of troponin C (Fig. 8-3) causes a rightward shift in the direction of a higher calcium ion concentration in the relationship between force and calcium ion concentration. Thus, enhanced relaxation with β-adrenergic stimulation has a triple basis (1). Besides faster release of calcium ions from TnC, there are enhanced cross-bridge cycling and an increased rate of uptake of calcium ions by the SR. Enhancing the rate of relaxation increases the overall rate of the cross-bridge cycle.

Myosin Light Chain Phosphorylation

Myosin phosphorylation is increased by cAMP in response to β-adrenergic stimulation. It is phosphorylated in the serine-13 residue of the regulatory light chains (MLC-2) by the enzyme MLC kinase, which is activated by calcium in conjunction with calmodulin, the ubiquitous calcium binding protein. Such an increased phosphorylation may enhance the responsiveness of the cardiac contractile proteins to calcium (21), perhaps by slowing the transition from strong to weak cross-bridges (Fig. 8-2) (1). This mechanism could explain why epinephrine increases the rate of cross-bridge cycling independently of the degree of activation of the contractile proteins by calcium. However, the real role of MLC-2 phosphorylation in cardiac muscle remains ill defined (1), in contrast to the very clear function in vascular smooth muscle.

In vascular smooth muscle the regulation of contraction is also calcium dependent but by a different molecular mechanism (Fig. 8-5). Calcium-calmodulin activates the MLC kinase that phosphorylates MLC-2. This process is essen-

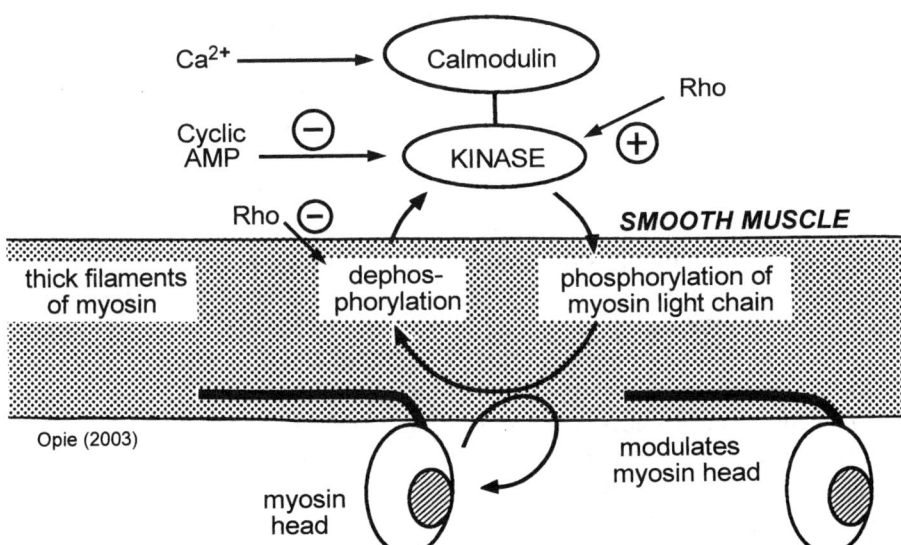

FIG. 8-5. Myosin light chain kinase in vascular smooth muscle, where this enzyme plays an essential role. Although phosphorylation of myosin light chains may also occur in the heart, the kinase (myosin light chain kinase) is not inhibited by cyclic adenosine 3′,5′-monophosphate (cAMP), an important difference from vascular smooth muscle. Thus, β-adrenergic stimulation, via cAMP (and protein kinase A) is vasorelaxing as opposed to the stimulatory effects in the heart (Fig. 8-4).

tial for vascular contraction to take place. Another stimulator of MLC kinase is the small G protein Rho, a member of the Ras family that acts through Rho kinase (22). Rho also inhibits the dephosphorylation of MLC kinase, thereby further increasing vascular contraction. Increased Rho-kinase activity may therefore cause cardiac vascular spasm in patients (23).

Other Phosphorylations and Dephosphorylations

Other contractile proteins that undergo phosphorylation include troponin T and myosin binding protein C. One proposal is that phosphorylation of myosin binding protein C could enhance cross-bridge cycling rate (20). Furthermore, for every phosphorylation, there must also be the possibility of dephosphorylation. Kinases must be balanced by phosphatases or else the contractile mechanism would seize up. Intense research now underway may help to clarify these issues, thereby helping us to understand better the finer regulation of cardiac contraction and relaxation (1).

SARCOMERE LENGTH AND THE STARLING LAW

The left ventricle increases the cardiac output as the venous return increases (Starling law, Fig. 12-3). The mechanism does not involve increased calcium levels or phosphorylation, but nonetheless there are increased rate and force of contraction (Frank data, Fig. 12-6). As the sarcomere length of papillary muscle increases from short lengths of approximately 1.7 μm to long lengths of approximately 2.2 to 2.3 μm, so does the tension increase to a maximum (Fig. 12-5). Thus, there is no doubt that contractile performance is length dependent. However, the mechanism of the Frank–Starling relationship remains imperfectly understood.

Ascending Limb of the Starling Curve

The steeply ascending tension–length relationship of the myocardium cannot be explained by changes in the extent of actin–myosin overlap. In contrast, in skeletal muscle, pure geometric factors such as the degree of actin–myosin overlap can explain the slowly ascending limb of the force–tension line. To explain the pattern in the heart, there is good evidence of *length-dependent activation.* Thus, in intact papillary muscles, stretching causes a large increase in force, whereas the amplitude of the intracellular free calcium transient does not increase (Fig. 8-6). The mechanism for this increase in calcium sensitivity in response to stretching eludes detection. One favored explanation is that with stretch, the volume of the cardiac cell remains constant so that the diameter decreases to lessen the "filament lattice spacing" (Color Plate 7, left) so that thick and thin filaments lie closer to each other and are more likely to interact (12). Additionally or alternatively, the giant molecule titin is the length sensor (24). As it is stretched, radial forces come into play, pulling the myosin heads toward actin (Color Plate 7, right). Then, it is proposed, even more cross-bridges could be recruited into action by the phenomenon of cross-bridge–induced acti-

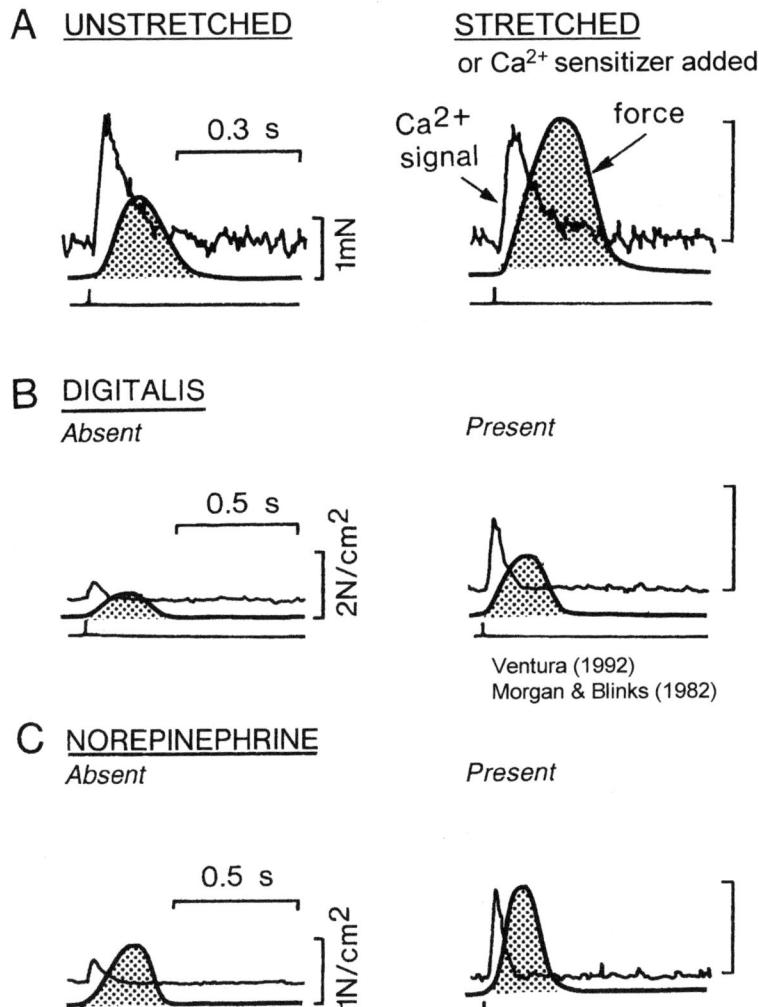

FIG. 8-6. Intracellular calcium and contraction. Contrasts between stretch effect **(A)** and two positive inotropic interventions **(B, C)**. Increase in force by stretching is not associated with any increase in free calcium, so that stretch is a calcium-sensitizing procedure. The increase in force obtained by digitalis **(B)** or norepinephrine **(C)** is due to an increase in the intracellular free calcium, so that inotropic interventions increase calcium transients. A calcium-sensitizing drug, such as stretch, permits a greater force of contraction in the absence of any change in cytosolic calcium. *Continuous lines*, force; *noisy tracings*, aequorin luminescence of electrically stimulated cat papillary muscle. Calibration bars: force (N) or tension (N/cm²). Lmax, maximal luminescence signal. (Data from Ventura et al. *Circ Res* 1992;70:1081 and Morgan, Blinks. *Can J Physiol Pharmacol* 1982;60:520–528.)

vation of near-neighbor cross-bridges (Fig. 8-2). Not only do more cross-bridges interact in response to stretch, but the myosin ATPase activity also increases (25). The result is that in response to a volume load (Color Plate 8, left), the myofibrils are more stretched at the end of diastole, and there is a more powerful contraction that generates a greater end-systolic pressure. This is the Starling effect. After some minutes, the systolic pressure generated at any given end-diastolic pressure increases, probably because of increased entry of calcium ions in response to mechanosensors (Fig. 13-5). The increased cytosolic calcium augments the length effect (Color Plate 8, right).

This rather satisfactory lattice-dependent explanation of the Frank–Starling relationship has been dealt a setback by the careful x-ray diffraction studies of Konhilas et al. (26). They ingeniously reduced sarcomere lattice spacing by osmotic compression, which failed to influence calcium sensitivity. Thus, lattice spacing is only part of the answer.

Descending Limb of the Starling Curve

Starling found that increasing the venous pressure beyond a particular point led to a decrease rather than an increase in the cardiac output. This is the descending limb of the Starling curve. The explanation has often erroneously been ascribed to decreased actin–myosin overlap as the sarcomere stretches. In the case of skeletal muscle, the relationship between sarcomere length and force development is more or less bell shaped, the optimal force being developed at a sarcomere length of approximately 2.2 μm (Fig. 12-6). At greater sarcomere lengths, force decreases because of the decreased overlap of actin and myosin. This sequence is unlikely in the failing whole heart. First, in the heart, the sarcomere length rarely exceeds 2.2 to 2.4 μm, even in the dilated state (Fig. 16-2). The pericellular collagen and connecting filaments such as titin give heart muscle a high degree of resting stiffness that opposes myofibril stretching. Rather, the explanation of the descending limb of the failing heart probably lies in diastolic ventricular interaction whereby the dilated right ventricle compresses the left to impair its function (Chapter 12).

Titin also plays a role, especially in isolated cardiac myocytes, which are deprived of the stretch-limiting effects of extracellular collagen. In these cells, optimal force development also occurs at sarcomere lengths between 2.2 and 2.4 μm. Further stretch gives a descending limb that declines to zero force development at 2.8 μm (27). Bearing in mind that the resting tension of cardiac titin increases rapidly beyond 2.2 μm (Color Plate 3), the only way that the cardiac myocyte can become longer is by structural damage as titin progressively detaches from the myosin thick filament (27). By contrast, in skeletal muscle a substantial increase in resting tensions only occurs when stretched more than approximately 3.0 μm (5), so that the descending limb found in skeletal muscle between 2.2 and 3.0 μm (Fig. 12-5) is genuine and is correctly explained by a decreasing overlap of actin and myosin.

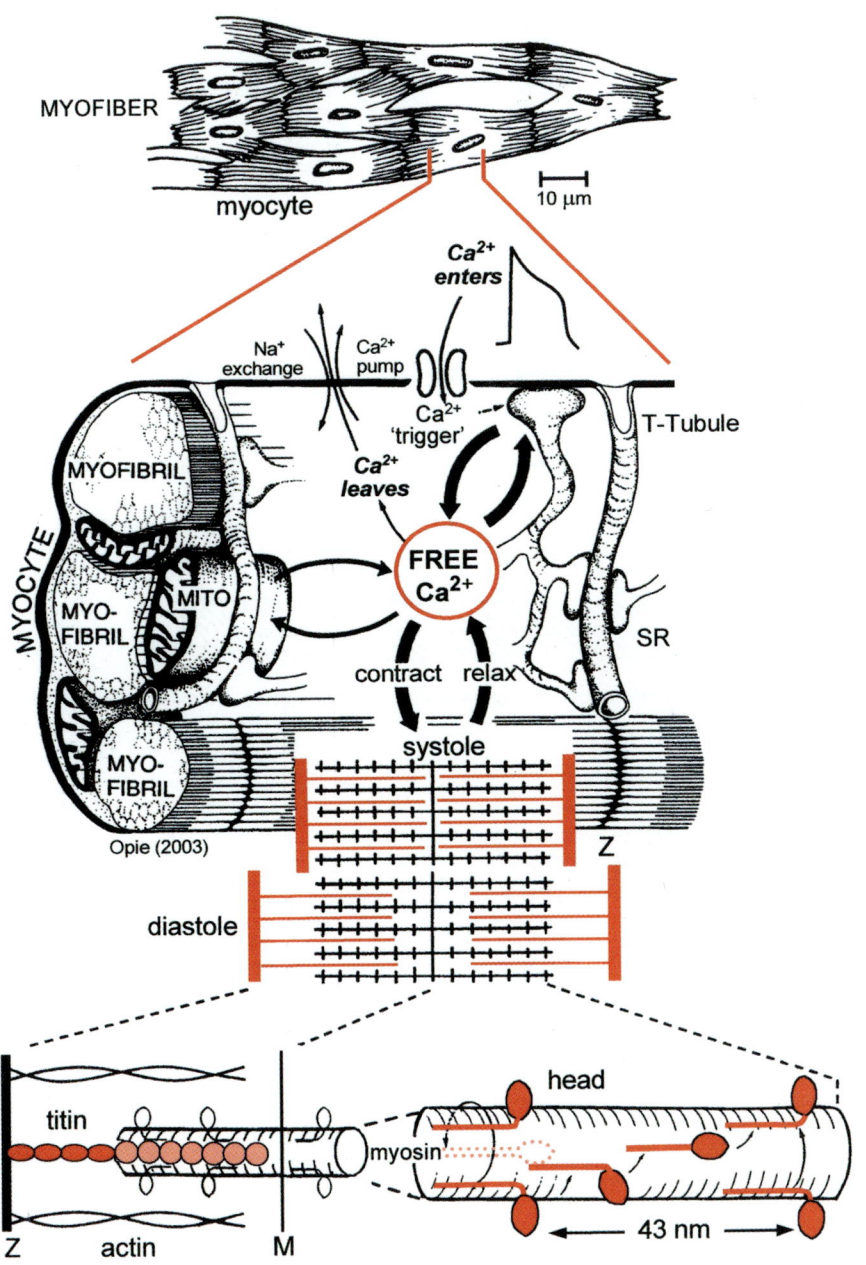

COLOR PLATE 1. Map of the myocyte. The crux of the contractile process lies in the changing concentrations of Ca^{2+} ions in the myocardial cytosol. Ca^{2+} ions "trigger" the release of more calcium from the sarcoplasmic reticulum (*SR*) and thereby initiate a contraction–relaxation cycle, which is terminated by the uptake of calcium by the sarcolemmal pump. Contraction is driven by the interaction of actin and myosin. The myosin heads, projecting from the thick myosin bodies, provide the power stroke that moves the thin actin filaments. Titin is the giant molecule that both supports the myosin molecules by attaching to the Z lines and provides elasticity. (Upper panel from Braunwald et al. *Mechanisms of contraction of the normal and failing heart*, 2nd ed. Boston: Little Brown, 1976, with permission. Other panels from L. H. Opie.)

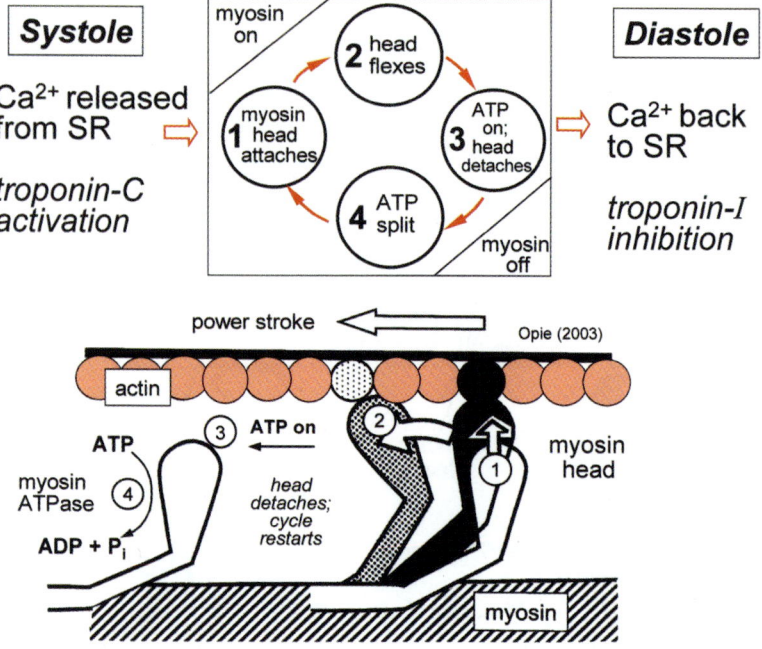

COLOR PLATE 2. Simplified model of contraction–relaxation cycle. Note relationship of systole and diastole.

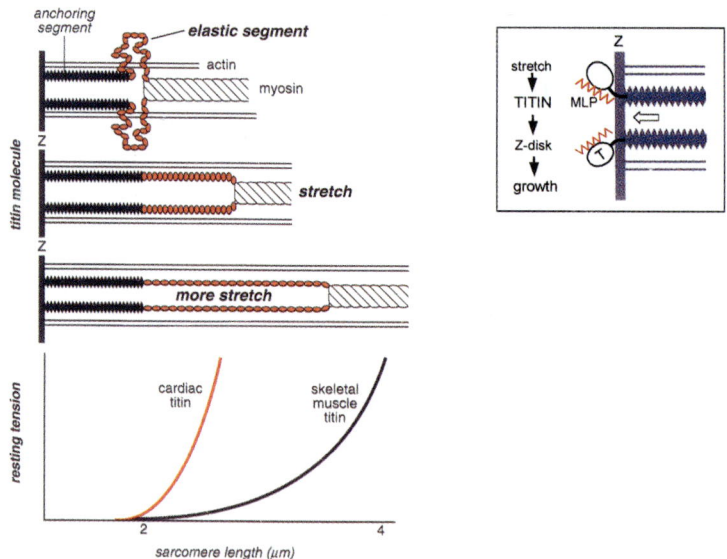

COLOR PLATE 3. Titin, the elastic giant molecule. It links myosin to the Z line and unfolds when stretched. When titin relaxes in diastole, restoring forces develop. The *box* focuses on titin binding to the Z disk, with its terminal end capped by the T-cap protein close to the muscle LIM protein (*MLP*). With sustained stretch, growth signals are sent downstream. (Top panel modified from Helmes M, et al. Titin develops restoring force in rat cardiac myocytes. *Circ Res* 1996;79:619–626; bottom panel from Trombitas K, et al. The mechanically active domain of titin in cardiac muscle. *Circ Res* 1995;77:856–861.)

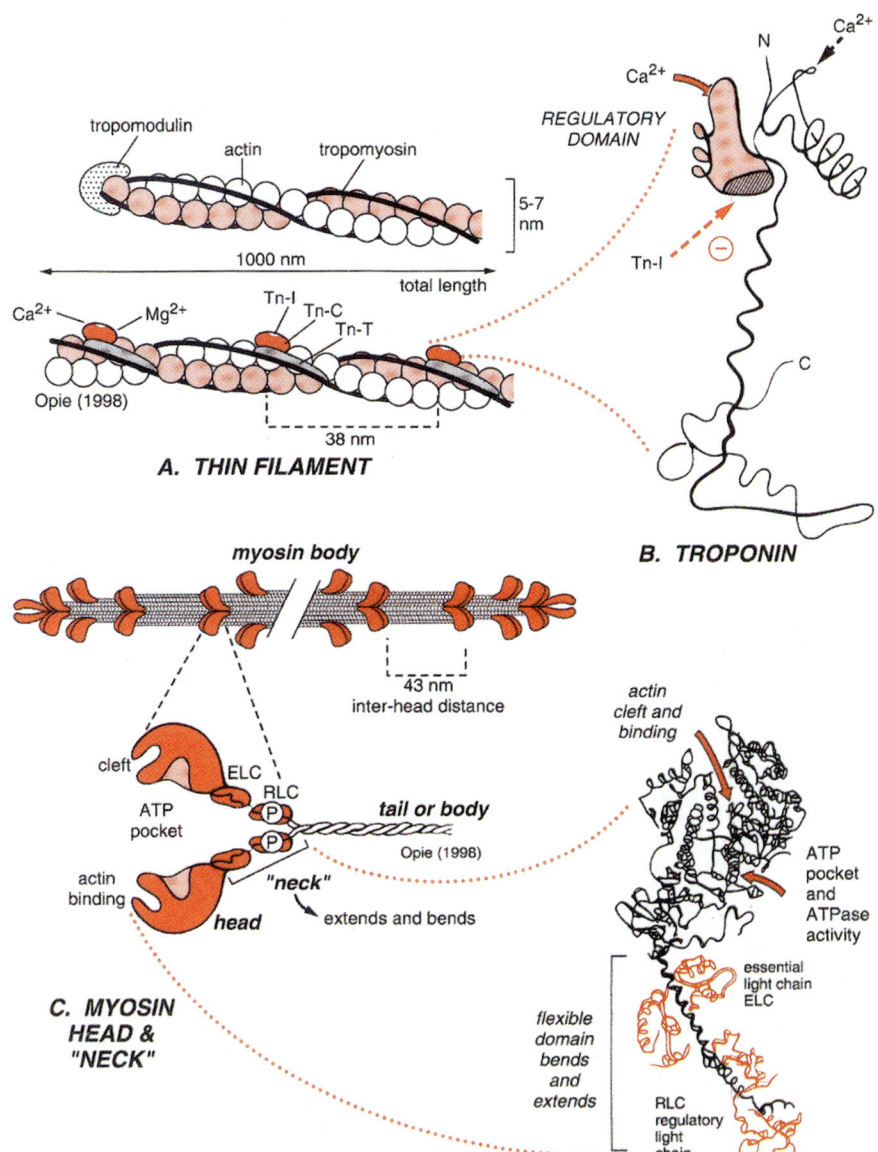

COLOR PLATE 4. The major molecules of the contractile system. **Top:** The thin actin filament is shown, which contains troponin C (*Tn-C*). Note the Ca^{2+} binding sites in the regulatory domain of TnC, with another site for interaction with troponin I (*Tn-I*). When TnC is not activated by Ca^{2+}, then troponin I inhibits the actin–myosin interaction. The role of troponin T (*Tn-T*) is less well defined. **Bottom:** The whole myosin molecule and the myosin head. Each myosin molecule is composed of two intertwining heavy chains and four associated light chains. The myosin heads are attached by a flexible neck to the myosin tails, also called bodies. Myosin light chains lie in apposition to the neck of the myosin heads. The essential light chain (*ELC*) is part of the structure. The other regulatory light chain (*RLC*) influences the extent of the actin–myosin interaction. At right is shown the myosin head molecular structure, based on Rayment et al. (8). The head is composed of heavy and light chains. The heavy head chain in turn has two major domains: one of 70 kd (i.e., 70,000 molecular weight) that interacts with actin at the actin cleft and has an ATP binding pocket. The other domain of 20 kd is elongated, extends, and bends and has the two light chains attached to it.

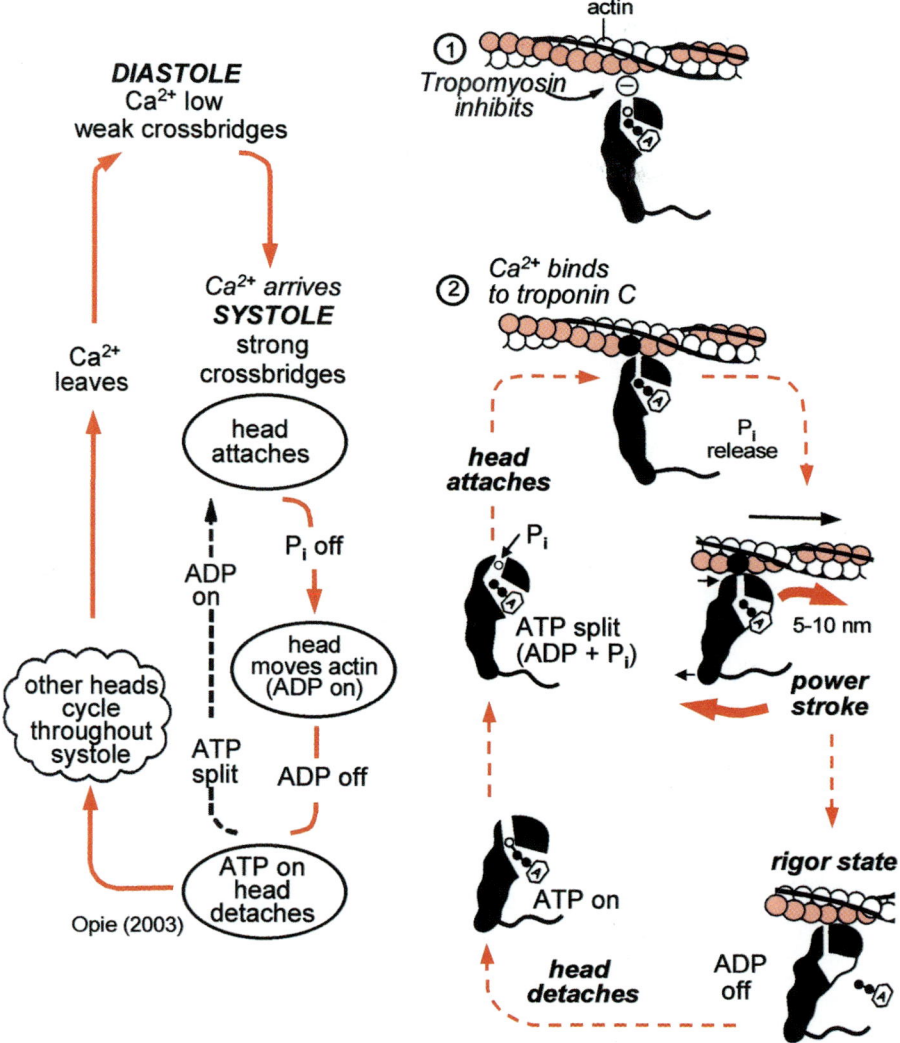

COLOR PLATE 5. A simplified molecular model of calcium activation of the contractile cycle. The contraction phase of the cycle is initiated when the cytosolic calcium increases as calcium is released from the sarcoplasmic reticulum. The calcium interacts with a specialized component of the thin actin filament in such a way that the myosin heads are now able to interact with actin. The result is a power stroke that moves the thin actin filament 10 nm. As energy in the form of adenosine 5′-triphosphate reaches the myosin head, it extends again. In the meantime, the whole cycle is being repeated at other sites so that there are repetitive microcycles with flexion and extension of the myosin heads. When calcium leaves the cytosol to be sucked back into the sarcoplasmic reticulum, diastole starts.

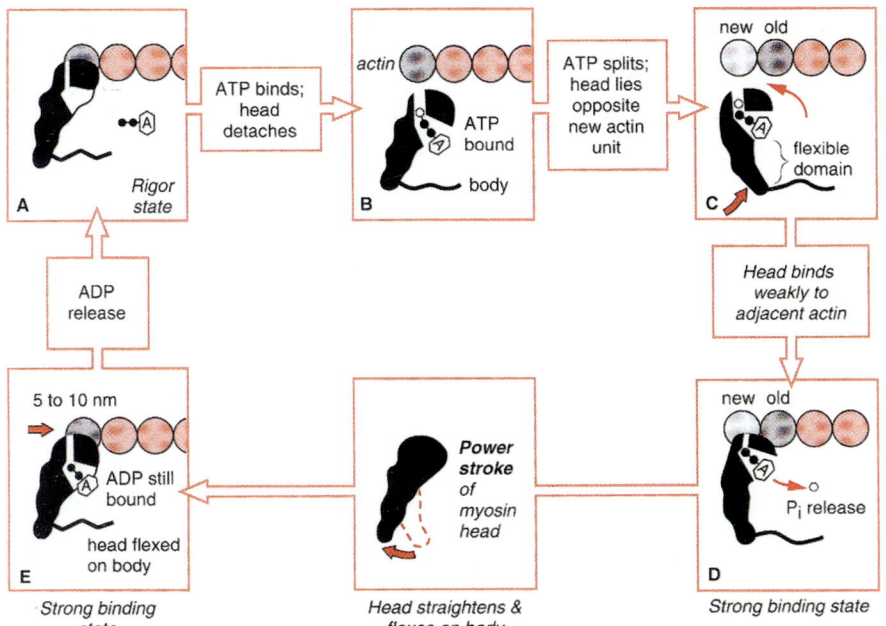

COLOR PLATE 6. Cross-bridge cycling model, modified from Rayment et al. (8). Starting with the rigor state (*A*), binding of ATP to the pocket opens the cleft (*B*) and the strong binding state becomes weak. Next, the binding pocket closes around its base to further close the cleft; ATP is split into ADP and P_i (*C*). Myosin binds strongly to actin and P_i is released (*D*), causing a molecular change in the myosin head and power stroke (*E*). Finally, ADP is released, the binding pocket becomes vacant (*A*) and the cycle can restart.

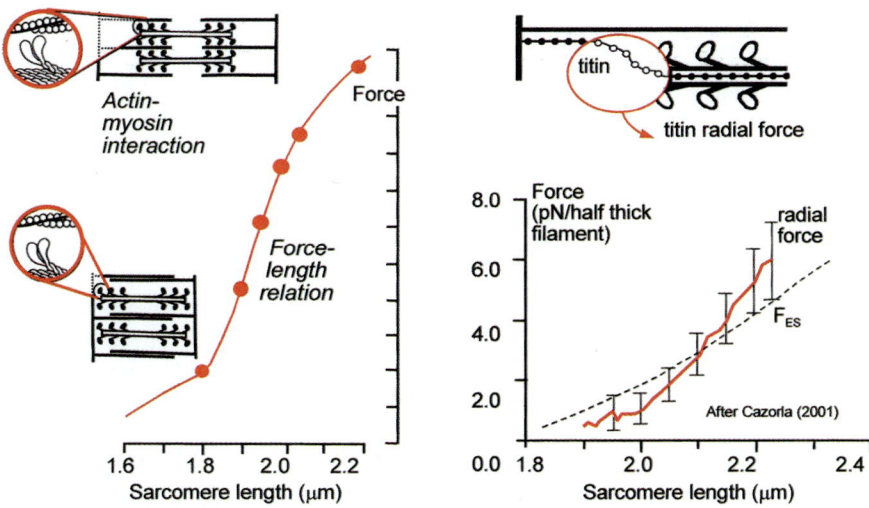

COLOR PLATE 7. The force–length relationship of the cardiac sarcomere **(left)**. This is explained, at least in part, by the closer proximity of the myosin leads to actin. **Right:** The role of radial forces generated by titin stretch that increasingly come into play as the sarcomere lengthens (24).

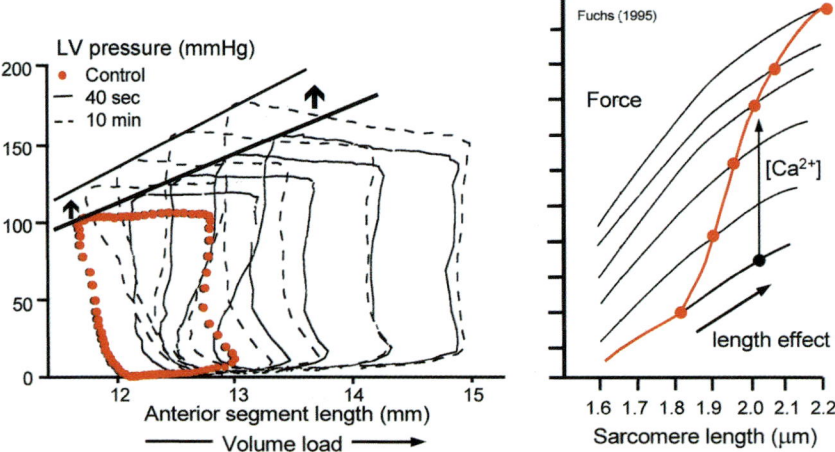

COLOR PLATE 8. Interaction between the Starling length effect and calcium. **Left:** This shows the abrupt early Starling effect in response to an acute volume load, followed by a delayed effect, probably mediated by calcium ions. During an acute volume load, the left ventricular segment length increases, as does the developed pressure, as shown by the solid lines of the pressure–volume loop. After a few minutes (*dotted and broken lines*), there is a further increase in left ventricular developed pressure at any given segment length and hence not the Starling effect. The probable mechanism is increased entry of calcium ions by the action of mechanosensors (Fig. 13-4). (Modified from Lew WYW. Time-dependent increase in left ventricular contractility following acute volume loading in the dog. *Circ Res* 1988;63:635–647.) **Right:** Illustration of how the steep ascending limb of the cardiac force–length curve is explained by an interaction between sarcomere length and calcium ions. Changes in end-diastolic fiber length at any given free Ca^{2+} concentration increase force by the Starling effect and cause cooperative interactions within the thin filament that lead to a greater binding of Ca^{2+} to the thin filament with greater force. (Modified from Fuchs F. Mechanical modulation of the Ca2+ regulatory protein complex in cardiac muscle. *News Physiol Sci* 1995;10:6–12.)

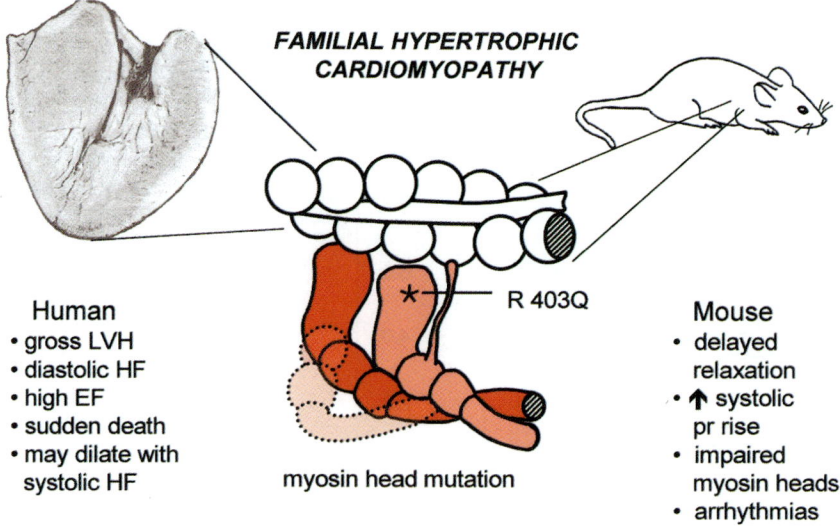

COLOR PLATE 9. Proposed myosin head mutation in one type of familial hypertrophic cardiomyopathy. **Left:** An example of the grossly enlarged left ventricle in the human disease. The myosin mutant R403Q ($Arg^{403} \rightarrow Gln$), when found, is associated with a particularly lethal form of the disease. **Right:** Illustration shows that in the R403Q mutant mouse, typical features of the human disease develop. [Based on the concepts of Tyska et al. (42).]

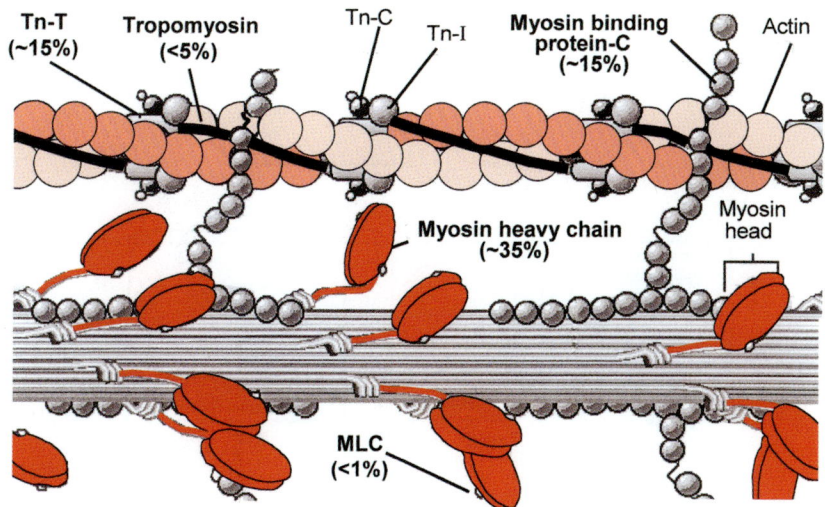

COLOR PLATE 10. Hypertrophic cardiomyopathy mutations. Note the greatest frequency of myosin heavy chain mutations. (Modified from Spirito P, et al. The management of hypertrophic cardiomyopathy. *N Engl J Med* 1997;336:775–785.)

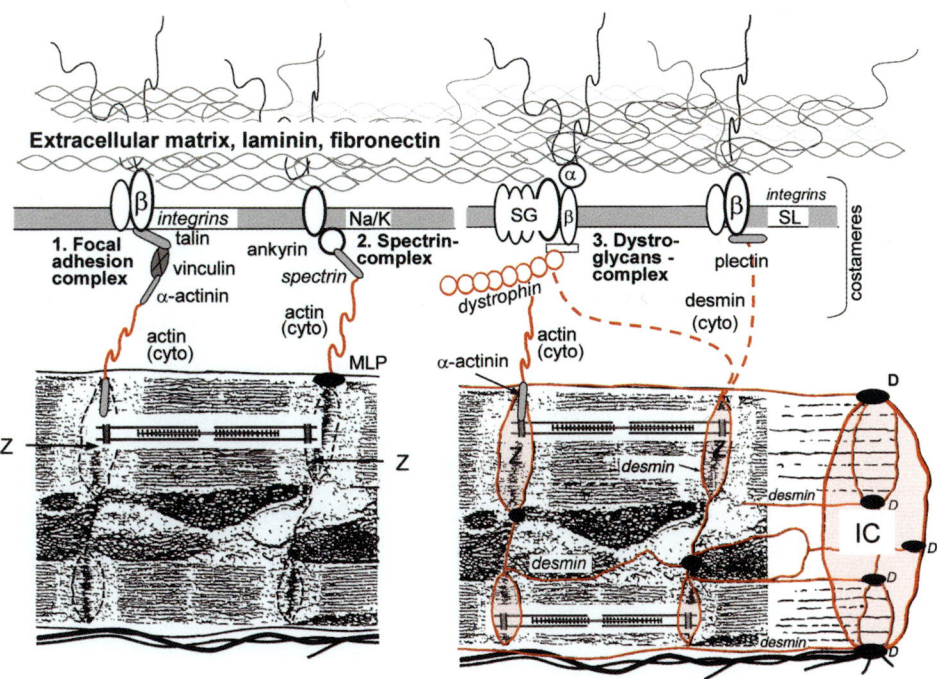

COLOR PLATE 11. Cytoskeletal proteins and costameres. The latter are protein networks that link the Z and M lines to the extracellular matrix and to each other. The three main costameres are the focal adhesion complex, the spectrin complex, and the dystroglycan complex. Dystrophin is a large intracellular protein that links the Z lines by means of actin to the sarcolemma and T tubule and thence to the extracellular matrix. Dystrophin is cleaved in enterovirus myocarditis. *D*, desmosomes; *MLP*, muscle LIM protein, here schematically linked to the Z disk; *IC*, intercalated disk; *SL*, sarcolemma; *SG*, sarcoglycans; *Na/K*, sodium–potassium pump; *cyto*, cytoplasmic.

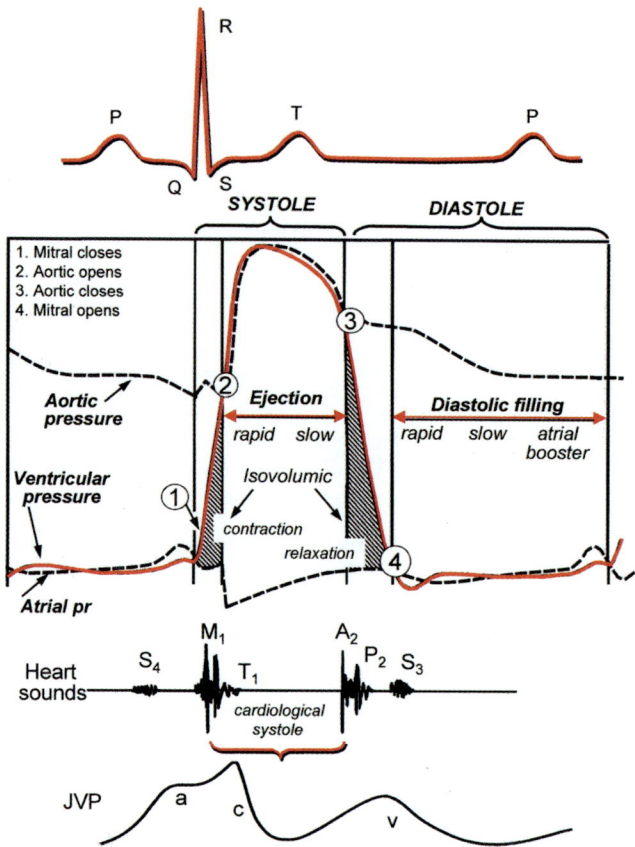

COLOR PLATE 12. The cardiac cycle, first assembled by Lewis in 1920, although conceived by Wiggers (44). Note that mitral valve closure occurs after the crossover point of atrial and ventricular pressures at the start of systole. View in conjunction with Fig. 12-1. PQRST, components of the electrocardiogram. Heart valves: *1*, mitral valve closure; *2*, aortic valve opening, normally inaudible; *3*, aortic valve closure; *4*, mitral valve opening, sometimes audible in mitral stenosis as the opening snap. Heart sounds: M_1, mitral component of the first sound at time of mitral valve closure; T_1, tricuspid valve closure, second component of first heart sound; A_2, aortic valve closure, first component of second sound; P_2, pulmonary component of second sound, pulmonary valve closure; S_3, third heart sound, rapid ventricular filling; S_4, fourth heart sound, atrial contraction. JVP, jugular venous pressure: *a*, wave produced by right atrial contraction; *c*, carotid wave artifact during rapid left ventricular ejection phase; *v*, venous return wave that causes venous pressure to increase while tricuspid valve is closed. Cycle length of 800 milliseconds for 75 beats per minute.

REGULATION OF MYOSIN ATPASE

To review, there are three short-term adjustments to the immediate need to increase cardiac force of contraction, and these are mediated by calcium, phosphorylations of contractile proteins, and length-induced changes (Starling law). The interaction of calcium ions with TnC initiates a cascade of alterations to the regulatory proteins of the thin filament (troponin I and tropomyosin). The result is that myosin heads interact with binding sites on the actin filament in such a way that muscle shortening occurs. The greater the availability of calcium is, the greater the force generated (within limits). Calcium has multiple effects on the cross-bridge cycle. First, calcium initiates the contractile cycle by "turning on" TnC (Fig. 8-1). The subsequent cross-bridge attachment serves as a positive feedback mechanism to increase the calcium sensitivity of TnC (Fig. 8-2) (28).

In addition, increasing the calcium concentration can enhance the myosin ATPase activity (25). The mechanism of this effect is still speculative, although much can be explained by the interaction of calcium with TnC. The latter proposal is consonant with the work of Brenner (15). He studied an isometric model in which the sarcomere length was carefully kept constant. The kinetics of the rate of force redevelopment after an isotonic period allowed the conclusion that even at a constant number of cross-bridges participating in cycling, an increased calcium level could increase myosin ATPase activity and force. A further proposal still under evaluation is that calcium can indirectly promote MLC phosphorylation and thereby convert the weakly attached cross-bridges into the strongly attached force-generating state (1).

Isoenzymes of Myosin Heavy-Chain ATPase

When the cytosolic calcium contraction increases, so does the ATPase activity of cardiac myosin. This is a short-term response. In addition, long-term gene-based changes in the actual activity of myosin ATPase also occur, as is shown by the effect of thyrotoxicosis in increasing both cardiac myosin heavy-chain ATPase activity and the velocity of contraction. The explanation is the reemergence of the fetal isoform of myosin ATPase (Fig. 8-6). Such enzymes with similar function (breaking down ATP, myosin ATPase) but with alterations in their molecular structure are called myosin isoenzymes or *myosin isoforms* (Table 8-3). There are two types of molecular myosin heavy chains: α and β. These can give rise to three types of combinations, α-α and β-β (homodimers), and α-β (heterodimer), and these correspond to V_1 (α-α), V_2 (α-β), and V_3 (β-β) isomyosins. The α-isoform, predominant in the rodent ventricle but also found in smaller amounts in humans (Fig. 13-10), has two to three times more actin-activated ATPase activity and shortening velocity (29). Exercise training in rats leads to dominant α-myosin ATPase with faster contraction, whereas pressure overload produces a dominant β-isoform so that contraction is slower, which is also energetically more efficient. Thus, the rat heart can "change gear" when loaded (Fig. 8-7).

TABLE 8-3. Contractile protein isoforms with effects of mechanical overload

	Fetus and neonate	Normal adult	Mechanical overload, heart failure
Myosin			
Ventricular heavy chain[a]	β, α ($\beta = V_3$, $\alpha = V_1$)	$\alpha > \beta$ (rat) $\beta > \alpha$ (human)	β, α (rat) Unchanged (human)[b]
Atrial heavy chain[c]	α	α (human)	$\alpha\downarrow$ (human)
LC 1 in ventricles[d]	A and V forms	V form	A and V forms
LC 2 in ventricles[e]	No data	LC2/LC1 ratio 1:1	Ratio reduced
Troponin I in ventricles[f]	TnIc TnIs	TnIc	TnIc
Troponin T in ventricles[g]	TnT_1 TnT_{2-4}	TnT_1 TnT_2 (4%)	Increased TnT_2 (12%)
Actin in ventricles[h]	Skeletal and smooth muscle α-actin	Decreased fetal form (rat)	Increased fetal form (rat)

[a–h]See reference 28a–28h.
V, ventricular; LC, light chain; A, atrial.

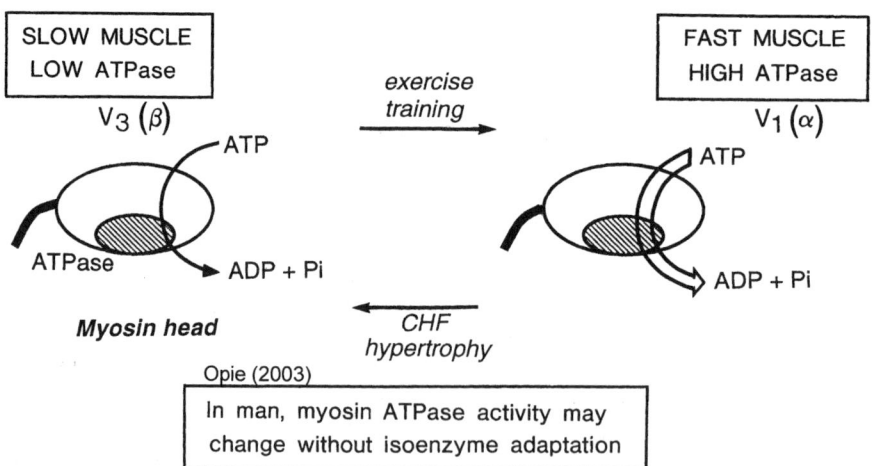

FIG. 8-7. Myosin isoenzyme hypothesis. When myosin ATPase activity is high (V1 or α form), there is a more rapid rate of breakdown of adenosine 5′-triphosphate (*ATP*) to adenosine 5′-diphosphate (*ADP*) and inorganic phosphate (P_i), and cross-cycle bridging is enhanced. In rats, the transition from slow (β) V3 to faster V1 can be achieved by vigorous exercise. Conversely, experimental congestive heart failure (*CHF*) or myocardial hypertrophy decreases the percentage of V1 and increases that of V3. For further details, see Table 8-3 and Figure 13-10.

In human ventricles, the dominant isoform is the β type, with little α type, so that the heart is already in low gear. However, an even lower gear emerges in heart failure when the normally low amount of α-myosin is further reduced (Fig. 13-10). Of note, even small changes in the amount of α-myosin can markedly influence power output (29). Thus, the decreased contractility of the failing human heart may, at least in part, be related to isoform changes. The time scale for these changes is over hours and days, in contrast to the acute changes in force development within a few beats in response to positive inotropic agents or to the Starling effect with an increased end-diastolic fiber length (Fig. 8-8).

SARCOMERE GENE MUTATIONS AND CARDIOMYOPATHY

Mutant Contractile Proteins and Hypertrophic Cardiomyopathy

The three salient features of this type of cardiomyopathy are unexplained myocardial hypertrophy, histologic myofibrillar disarray (which gives an abnor-

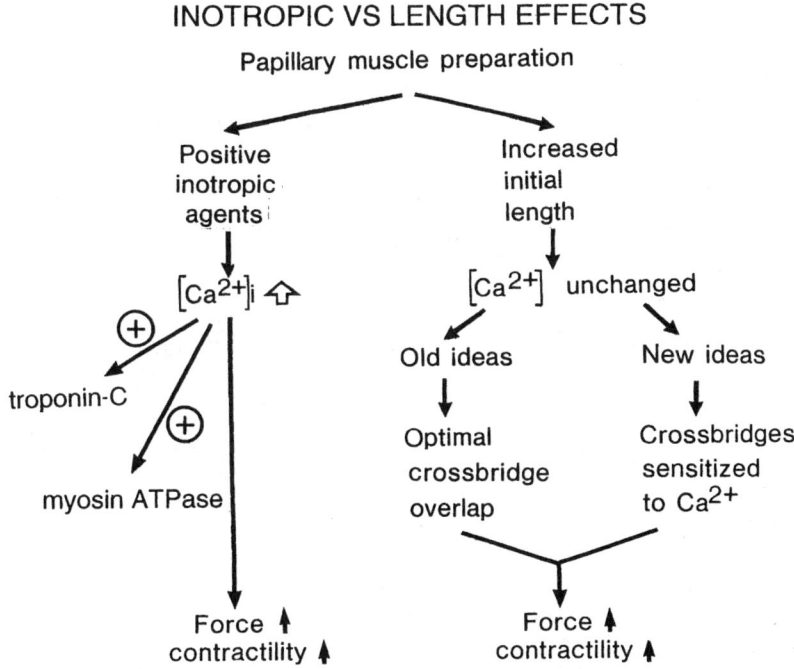

FIG. 8-8. Inotropic versus length effects on contractile apparatus. Positively inotropic agents act by increasing cytosolic calcium, whereas length effects act at a constant calcium level. The old ideas of optimal cross-bridge overlap are now set aside. Rather, the initial fiber length helps to sensitize the cross-bridges to calcium, thus explaining the increased force and contractility in response to fiber stretching.

mal sarcomere pattern), and a defined genetic basis (Chapter 6). "Most HCM-causing mutations are relatively subtle, typically missense changes in just one DNA nucleotide and resulting in the substitution of just one amino acid in the particular protein" (6). In all, nine abnormal genes have been found, encoding for different contractile proteins such as β-myosin heavy chain or α-tropomyosin or cardiac troponin T (30). Human data are often in accord with mouse genetic models (Color Plate 9). In most human cases, there are mutations in the myosin heavy chain or in troponin T or in myosin binding protein C (Color Plate 10). In some with the familial disease, there are links to mutations in the genes for AMP-activated protein kinase, a key enzyme in the control of ATP levels in the heart (Fig. 16-3). Thus, one current hypothesis is that the mutations all impair the contractile response, with less force generated per ATP spent (30). The result is energy depletion in the affected fibers that hypothetically promotes compensatory hypertrophy in the remaining fibers.

Dilated Cardiomyopathy

The hallmark of dilated cardiomyopathy is left ventricular enlargement with poor systolic function and decreased values for ejection fraction and cardiac output. There must be no clear-cut acquired causative condition, such as metabolic disease (Fig. 16-4), coronary artery disease hypertension, or valve disease. Paradoxically, suspected preceding viral infection of the myocardium is still included in dilated cardiomyopathy because it can act on the same cytoskeletal protein as the genetic variety, dystrophin (31). Dystrophin is a large intracellular molecule that links actin to the sarcolemma and thence to the extracellular matrix, thereby stabilizing the sarcomeres (Color Plate 11). Other cytoskeleton proteins that may be associated with dilated cardiomyopathy are (a) *desmin*, which links the Z lines and intercalated disks and their attachments to the sarcolemma; (b) the *MLP protein*, which is part of the Z disk–titin complex (13); and (c) the $\alpha\beta$ crystallin protein, a chaperone molecule that guards protein folding (32). Disruption of cytoskeletal integrity could be a common feature to both hereditary and acquired forms of dilated cardiomyopathy. More recently and more confusingly, defects in the sarcomere proteins, such as those in myosin heavy chain and troponin, have also been found in dilated cardiomyopathy, so that the molecular distinction between this entity and hypertrophic cardiomyopathy seems to be blurring (33).

Restrictive Cardiomyopathy

In this disease, the myocardium is "stiff," thus impairing diastolic relaxation and ventricular filling. The genotype is still under study. Unexpectedly, a single mutation of troponin I could, in the same family, cause either restrictive or hypertrophic cardiomyopathy, another example of overlap of clinical phenotypes associated with the same molecular genotype (33).

Nonspecific Protein Defects in Advanced Heart Failure

Defective functioning of the contractile proteins and their regulatory companions have long been proposed as part of the overall changes that impair systolic function in advanced heart failure, whatever its origin (34). The slower thin filament sliding found in end-stage human heart failure (35) may be the result of phosphorylations of troponin T or I in response to protein kinase C (34). Protein kinase C is part of the angiotensin II messenger system (Fig. 9-3) that is activated in severe heart failure.

ISCHEMIA AND MYOFILAMENTS

The myofilaments become desensitized to calcium when the coronary flow becomes too low, as in ischemia. Several factors are involved (Table 8-4), yet two of the most important are the increased concentrations of hydrogen ions and of P_i (36).

Rigor State and Ischemic Contracture

Hearts subjected to long periods of ischemia can become stiff and develop ischemic contracture. This change is because at the low ATP concentration and high cytosolic calcium levels characteristic of the ischemic state, the crossbridges are no longer occupied by ATP and become permanently attached, thereby forming so-called rigor bridges. In other words, the dominant form of the myosin head is in the strongly binding attached rigor state, in flexion (Color Plate 6A). These bridges exert a cooperative effect on the thin filaments, increasing the calcium sensitivity. Thus, force development may go far beyond that caused by an increase in only the calcium ion concentration (37). The high force development may then cause hypercontracture, which exerts

TABLE 8-4. *Modulation of calcium sensitivity in cardiac muscle[a]*

Modulator[b]	Effect[b]
Increase in sarcomere length	+
Phosphorylation of regulatory myosin light chain	+
Phosphorylation of troponin I or troponin T	−
Ischemia	
Acidosis	−
Inorganic phosphate	−
New cardiotonic drugs (calcium sensitizers)	
Pimobendan and others	+

[a]Reference 17 and Table 7-2.
[b]Increase (+) or decrease (−) in calcium sensitivity of cardiac myofilaments as determined in skinned cardiac muscle preparations or *in vivo*. Ca^{2+} sensitivity as used here is defined as the pCa (negative log of the Ca^{2+} concentration) inducing half-maximal activation of skinned fiber preparation.

excess tension on the sarcolemma to cause microlesions that leak so that extracellular calcium can invade the cell. Internal calcium can, however, increase during ischemia long before sarcolemmal rupture. For example, within minutes, lack of energy supplying the calcium uptake pump of the SR directly increases cytosolic calcium. The sodium–potassium pump, also energy requiring, becomes inhibited somewhat later and causes the intracellular sodium levels to increase, after which sodium–calcium exchange brings in calcium. In addition, under partially depolarized conditions, calcium channels may remain open. The term *stone heart* describes severe irreversible hypercontracture.

Creatine Kinase and Myosin ATPase

The ATP made in the mitochondria is normally delivered to the myosin ATPase indirectly by a shuttle involving phosphocreatine (Fig. 11-15). The enzyme creatine kinase, which converts phosphocreatine back to ATP, is located in relation to the A band of the sarcomere, which contains myosin ATPase. Hence, the proposal is that this enzyme delivers ATP to the myosin ATPase. In ischemia, the creatine kinase isoenzyme concerned (A band creatine kinase) diffuses from the A to the I band and then to outside the cell (38) so that energy transfer within the cell is impaired. These events are associated with irreversible ischemic injury.

Release of Troponin T and Troponin I in Myocardial Infarction

These proteins are released when the cell membranes are severely damaged, as in myocardial infarction (Fig. 18-10). The troponins increase rapidly in the blood, are specific for the myocardium, and the increase is even able to detect microinfarcts such as those that occur in some cases of acute coronary syndromes.

SUMMARY

1. *The cross-bridge cycle.* The energy that is needed to sustain the contractile activity of the heart comes from the hydrolysis of ATP by an ATPase located in the myosin head. In diastole, the force-generating interaction between actin and myosin is suppressed because of an inhibitory effect exerted by troponin I, which forms part of the troponin complex. When calcium is supplied to TnC during systole, the inhibitory effect of troponin I is overcome, and actin and myosin can then associate. The physical nature of the actin–myosin interaction involves steps in which the attached myosin heads pull the thin filaments a very small distance toward the center of the sarcomeres in which they are located. This is the power stroke. Then the myosin heads detach from actin and reattach further along the thin filament to repeat the cross-bridge cycle.

2. *Role of ATP.* Detachment of the myosin head from the actin filament is achieved when ATP binds to a special pocket on the head. Thereafter, ATP is hydrolyzed to ADP and P_i, and the shape of this pocket changes. When ADP and P_i come off the head, there is a further change in the molecular configuration of the myosin head, and the power stroke is initiated.
3. *Systole and diastole.* During a single heart beat, tension develops by recruitment of more cross-bridge cycles as the cytosolic calcium concentration increases to a peak, to be followed by relaxation as the cross-bridge cycling activity diminishes in response to a decreasing calcium concentration. During the detachment stage of an individual cross-bridge cycle, tension is maintained by other cross-bridges that are attached during that time.
4. *Cross-bridge interaction is enhanced by β-adrenergic receptor stimulation.* First, there is more calcium ion entry by the L channels with increased release of more calcium from the SR to interact with more TnC. In addition, the cross-bridges react at a faster rate, partially the result of a direct effect of the increased quantity and rate of increase of cytosolic calcium on cross-bridge kinetics and partially an indirect effect of the associated increase of cAMP on the MLCs that help to regulate myosin ATPase activity. cAMP also mediates phosphorylation of troponin I to increase the rate of relaxation.
5. *Sarcomere length and force generation.* In the myocardium, there is no simple relationship between these factors. The previous concept of optimal or inadequate overlap of actin and myosin filaments was incorrectly based on skeletal muscle models and has now been replaced by the concept of stretch activation. It is proposed that stretch sensitizes the myofibrils to the prevailing calcium ion concentration, acting through changes in the lateral distance between actin and myosin.
6. *Gene mutations and cardiomyopathy.* In general, mutations in the sarcomere contractile proteins explain hypertrophic cardiomyopathy, whereas cytoskeleton protein changes explain dilated cardiomyopathy. Current research shows substantial molecular overlap between these clinically dissimilar conditions.
7. *Permanent rigor bonds.* During severe and prolonged ischemia, the total ATP level decreases. There is insufficient ATP to break the rigor bonds between the myosin heads and actin, with the development of stone heart.

STUDENT QUESTIONS

1. Describe the basic cross-bridge cycle.
2. Outline the properties of the major cardiac contractile proteins.
3. Why is ATP important for cardiac contraction if the power stroke can occur without using any ATP?
4. Describe various mechanisms whereby calcium ions can increase the force of cardiac contraction.
5. What is myosin ATPase? What are its isoenzymes? What is their proposed importance?

CARDIOLOGIST-IN-TRAINING QUESTIONS

1. How does an increase in cytosolic calcium ion concentration trigger the contractile cycle? Which are the major contractile proteins involved?
2. How is ATP split during the contractile cycle? How does the binding of ATP to the myosin head influence the molecular shape of myosin?
3. What is titin and what are its functions?
4. Explain the ascending limb of the Starling curve in terms of myocardial contractile proteins.
5. Which molecular abnormalities can be linked to which type of cardiomyopathy?

REFERENCES

1. Solaro RJ. Modulation of cardiac myofilament activity by protein phosphorylation. In: Page E, et al., eds. *Handbook of physiology, section 2: the cardiovascular system*. New York: Oxford University Press, 2002:264–300.
1a. Perry SV. The regulation of contractile activity in muscle. *Biochem Soc Trans* 1979;7:593–617.
1b. Swynghedauw B. Developmental and functional adaptation of contractile proteins in cardiac and skeletal muscles. *Physiol Rev* 1986;66:710–771.
1c. Linke WA, et al. Spontaneous sarcomeric oscillations at intermediate activation levels in single isolated cardiac myofibrils. *Circ Res* 1993;73:724–734.
1d. Kaprielian RR, et al. Distinct patterns of dystrophin organization in myocyte sarcolemma and transverse tubules of normal and diseased human myocardium. *Circulation* 2000;101:2586–2594.
2. Huxley HE. Sliding filaments and molecular motile systems. *J Biol Chem* 1990;265:8347–8350.
3. Irving M, et al. Myosin head movements are synchronous with the elementary force-generating process in muscle. *Nature* 1992;357:156–158.
4. Geeves M. Stretching the lever-arm theory. *Nature* 2002;415:129–130.
5. Trombitas K, et al. The mechanically active domain of titin in cardiac muscle. *Circ Res* 1995;77:856–861.
6. Redwood CS, et al. Properties of mutant contractile proteins that cause hypertrophic cardiomyopathy. *Cardiovasc Res* 1999;44:20–36.
7. Squire JM. *The structural basis of muscular contraction*. New York, Plenum Press, 1981.
8. Rayment I, Holden HM, Whittaker M. Structure of the actin-myosin complex and its implications for muscle contraction. *Science* 1993;261:58–65.
9. Fisher AJ, et al. Structural studies of myosin: a revised model for the molecular basis of muscle contraction. *Biophys J* 1995;68:19s–26s.
10. Morano I, et al. Myosin light chain-actin interaction regulates cardiac contractility. *Circ Res* 1995;76:720–725.
11. Helmes M, et al. Titin develops restoring force in rat cardiac myocytes. *Circ Res* 1996;79:619–626.
12. Sutko JL, et al. An elastic link between length and active force production in myocardium. *Circulation* 2001;104:1585–1587.
13. Knoll R, et al. The cardiac mechanical stretch sensor machinery involves a Z disc complex that is defective in a subset of human dilated cardiomyopathy. *Cell* 2002;111:943–955.
14. Lymn RW, Taylor EW. Mechanism of adenosine triphosphate hydrolysis by actomyosin. *Biochemistry* 1971;10:4617–4624.
15. Brenner B. Effect of Ca^{2+} crossbridge turnover kinetics in skinned single rabbit psoas fibers. *Proc Natl Acad Sci U S A* 1988;85:3265–3269.
16. Rayment I, et al. The three-dimensional structure of a molecular motor. *Trends Biochem Sci* 1994;19:129–134.
17. Ruegg JC. *Calcium in muscle activation. A comparative approach*. Berlin: Springer-Verlag, 1986.
18. Babu A, et al. The control of myocardial contraction with skeletal fast muscle troponin-C. *J Biol Chem* 1987;262:5815–5822.
19. Hancock WO, et al. Ca^{2+} and segment length dependence of isometric force kinetics in intact ferret cardiac muscle. *Circ Res* 1993;73:603–611.

20. Herron T, et al. Power output is increased after phosphorylation of myofibrillar proteins in rat skinned cardiac myocytes. *Circ Res* 2001;89:1184–1190.
21. Morano I, et al. The influence of P-light chain phosphorylation by myosin light chain kinase on the calcium sensitivity of chemically skinned heart fibers. *FEBS Lett* 1985;189:221–224.
22. Sato M, et al. Involvement of Rho-kinase-mediated phosphorylation of myosin light chain in enhancement of cerebral vasospasm. *Circ Res* 2002;87:195–200.
23. Mohri M, et al. Rho-kinase inhibition with intracoronary fasudil prevents myocardial ischemia in patients with coronary microvascular spasm. *J Am Coll Cardiol* 2003;41:15–19.
24. Cazorla O, et al. Titin-based modulation of calcium sensitivity of active tension in mouse skinned cardiac myocytes. *Circ Res* 2001;88:1028–1035.
25. Kuhn HJ, et al. Stretch-induced increase in the Ca^{2+} sensitivity of myofibrillar ATPase activity in skinned fibres from pig ventricles. *Pflugers Arch* 1990;415:741–746.
26. Konhilas JP, et al. Myofilament calcium sensitivity in skinned rat cardiac trabeculae. Role of interfilament spacing. *Circ Res* 2002;90:59–65.
27. Weiwad WKK, et al. Sarcomere length-tension relationship of rat cardiac myocytes at lengths greater than optimum. *J Mol Cell Cardiol* 2000;32:247–259.
28. Hannon JD, et al. Effects of cycling and rigor crossbridges on the conformation of cardiac troponin C. *Circ Res* 1992;71:984–991.
28a. Mercadier JJ, et al. Myosin isoenzymes in normal and hypertrophied human ventricular myocardium. *Circ Res* 1983;53:52–62.
28b. Mercadier JJ, et al. Alpha-myosin heavy chain isoform and atrial size in patients with various types of mitral valve dysfunction: a quantitative study. *J Am Coll Cardiol* 1987;9:1024–1030.
28c. Nakao K, et al. Increased expression and regional differences of atrial myosin light chain 1 in human ventricles with old myocardial infarction. *Circulation* 1992;86:1727–1737.
28d. Margossian SS, et al. Light chain 2 profile and activity of human ventricular myosin during dilated cardiomyopathy. Identification of a causal agent for impaired myocardial function. *Circulation* 1992;85:1720–1733.
28e. Sasse S, et al. Troponin I gene expression during human cardiac development and in end-stage heart failure. *Circ Res* 1993;72:932–938.
28f. Anderson PA, et al. Troponin T isoform expression in humans. A comparison among normal and failing adult heart, fetal heart, and adult and fetal skeletal muscle. *Circ Res* 1991;69:1226–1233.
28g. Schwartz K, et al. Alpha-skeletal muscle actin mRNA's accumulate in hypertrophied adult rat hearts. *Circ Res* 1986;59:551–555.
28h Lowes BD, et al. Changes in gene expression in the intact human heart. Downregulation of alpha-myosin heavy chain in hypertrophied, failing ventricular myocardium. *J Clin Invest* 1997;100:2315–2324.
29. Herron T, et al. Small amounts of α-myosin heavy chain isoform expression significantly increase power output of rat cardiac myocyte fragments. *Circ Res* 2002;90:1150–1152.
30. Blair E, et al. Mutations of the g_2 subunit of AMP-activated protein kinase cause familial hypertrophic cardiomyopathy: evidence for the central role of energy compromise in disease pathogenesis. *Hum Mol Genet* 2001;10:1215–1220.
31. Vatta M, et al. Molecular remodelling of dystrophin in patients with end-stage cardiomyopathies and reversal in patients on assistance-device therapy. *Lancet* 2002;359:936—941.
32. Marian AJ. On genetics of dilated cardiomyopathy and transgenic models. All is not crystal clear in myopathic hearts. *Circ Res* 2001;89:3–5.
33. Chien KR. Genotype, phenotype: upstairs, downstairs in the family of cardiomyopathies. *J Clin Invest* 2003;111:175–178.
34. Solaro RJ, et al. Functional defects in troponin and the systems biology of heart failure [Editorial]. *J Mol Cell Cardiol* 2002;34:689–693.
35. Knott A, et al. In vitro Motility analysis of thin filaments from failing and non-failing human heart: Troponin from failing human hearts induces slower filament sliding and higher Ca^{2+} sensitivity. *J Mol Cell Cardiol* 2002;34:469–482.
36. Allen DG, et al. Myocardial contractile function during ischemia and hypoxia. *Circ Res* 1987;60:153–168.
37. Allen DG, et al. Factors influencing free intracellular calcium concentration in quiescent ferret ventricular muscle. *J Physiol (Lond)* 1984;350:615–630.
38. Otsu N, et al. Changes in creatine kinase M localization in acute ischemic myocardial cells. *Circ Res* 1993;73:935–942.

39. Eisenberg E, et al. Muscle contraction and free energy transduction in biological systems. *Science* 1985;227:999–1006.
40. Lew WYW. Time-dependent increase in left ventricular contractility following acute volume loading in the dog. *Circ Res* 1988;63:635–647.
41. Fuchs F. Mechanical modulation of the Ca2+ regulatory protein complex in cardiac muscle. *News Physiol Sci* 1995;10:6–12.
42. Tyska MJ, et al. Single-molecule mechanics of R403Q cardiac myosin isolated from the mouse model of familial hypertrophic cardiomyopathy. *Circ Res* 2000;86:737–744.
43. Spirito P, et al. The management of hypertrophic cardiomyopathy. *N Engl J Med* 1997;336:775–785.
44. Wiggers CJ. *Modern aspects of circulation in health and disease*. Philadelphia: Lea and Febiger, 1915.
45. Solaro RJ, et al. Regulatory proteins and diastolic relaxation. In: Lorell BH, et al., eds. *Diastolic relaxation of the heart*. Boston: Kluwer Academic Publishers, 1994:43–53.

9

Signal Systems: Coordinating Life and Death

Lionel H. Opie and Michael M. Sack

Have you ever got lost in a signaling cascade?
Anonymous quotation in *Nature Reviews*, 2001

In nature, there is a constant struggle between life and death, nowhere more evident than in the large animals that roam Africa. Likewise, in the heart there is a struggle between cell signals that promote cell growth and survival (prosurvival) and those that promote programmed cell death (apoptosis). The growth pathways are largely those that also govern fetal and neonatal growth, but in adult life, this prosurvival signaling dominates in response to the complex stimuli induced by pressure or volume overload (Chapter 13). The pathways promoting apoptosis are also similar to those that limit cell growth in neonatal life but are now activated by disease states such as lack of blood flow or its return (ischemia–reperfusion, Chapter 18). Confusion arises when the same signal systems seem to transmit both beneficial and harmful signals, as seems to be the case with the key enzyme complex mitogen-activated protein kinase (MAP kinase).

Further complexities arise when signals originating in nonmyocytes actually regulate myocyte growth or activity. For example, nitric oxide (NO) arising in the vascular endothelium acts as a paracrine signaling molecule to modulate myocyte function. Moreover, damaged endothelium modulates NO production, which in turn regulates vascular and hence cardiac function in disease. Recently, circulating fuel substrates have been recognized to modulate metabolism in the heart via the direct regulation of metabolic enzyme encoding genes. This metabolic control of gene activity has been termed *metacrine* signaling, for example, when serum (and intracellular) fatty acid levels activate the nuclear regulatory peptide peroxisome proliferator–activated receptor (PPAR) (1). PPARα, in turn, transactivates genes that direct fatty acid oxidation. Finally, the temporal and extent of signal pathway activation can result in divergent effects that span from the promotion of cell survival to apoptosis. An example of this temporal and dose effect is illustrated by signaling activated by the pleiotropic cytokine tumor necrosis factor-α (TNF-α). TNF-α originates in myocardial cells with concentration-dependent protective physiologic and pathologic disease–enhancing effects (2,3). Signaling by reactive oxygen species (ROS) appears to mirror TNF-α with both harmful effects and as integral regulatory molecules in cell survival and metabolic signaling events (4).

This chapter outlines these complex signal systems and their role in cell growth and destruction, showing the dual nature of many signals (Fig. 9-1). Furthermore, growth may be desirable in one context, such as early hypertrophy in adaptation to mechanical overload, but undesirable in another, such as when the heart is failing and excess growth and cell death by apoptosis occur together (4a). An equally radical idea follows. Suppose that human cardiac myocytes can actually divide and hence grow by hyperplasia, as proposed by Anversa's group

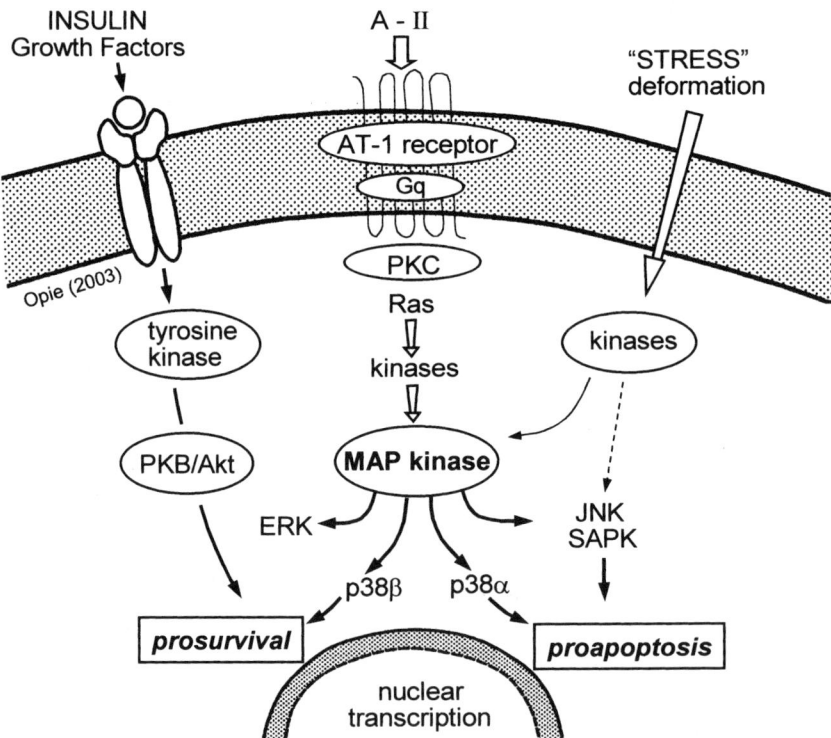

FIG. 9-1. **Signals to survival or to cell death by apoptosis.** Signal paths are not necessarily clear-cut in their sequences. There may be additional intermediate steps, feedback loops, and signaling cross-talk. Furthermore, studies using genetic manipulation (over- or underexpression of key genes) may show conflicting results according to the mouse strain harboring the genetic alternation. Nonetheless, the pattern shown here reflects the overall patterns currently proposed. Note that stimulation of the mitogen-activated protein kinase pathway by angiotensin II (*A-II*) can lead to either keel survival or cell death. For abbreviations, see text.

(4b). This novel concept supports the hypothesis that a homeostatic balance exists between physiologic cell maintenance and survival signaling versus the apoptotic programs. For example, in hypertensive patients with left ventricular hypertrophy, there is evidence of both growth and apoptosis (4c). Thus, left ventricular hypertrophy could represent a state in which more cells undergo hypertrophy than are lost by apoptosis.

This chapter starts by tracing the paths leading from the receptor stimulation by angiotensin II to cardiac hypertrophy, followed by those signals that are mainly prosurvival (such as insulin), then those that are mainly proapoptotic. Cytokine signals can lead either way. Free radicals include ROS that are part of physiologic cell signaling but when in excess are harmful. NO is an example of a free radical with a major physiologic role, promoting vasodilation and inhibiting mitochondrial metabolism. A final group of signals directly regulates nuclear transcription, i.e., the peroxisome proliferator receptors. What emerges illustrates the complexity and cross-talk between signaling pathways and the capacity of the same initial signal to lead to apparently contradictory events such as simultaneous stimulation of prosurvival and proapoptotic paths (5).

GROWTH SIGNALING

Renin–Angiotensin System and Angiotensin II

The renin–angiotensin system (RAS) evolved to help primitive primates withstand difficult living conditions with salt and water deprivation with threat of excessive hypotension. Angiotensin II (A-II), the end product of the RAS, has powerful physiologic and pathologic effects. It carries these out by complex and sometimes contradictory pathways that are an archetype of the multiplicity and diversity of signaling systems. Physiologically, A-II is a potent vasoconstrictor, as its name indicates (Greek, *angeion*, vessel; Latin, *tensio*, stretch), thereby helping to maintain the blood pressure when it decreases too much. A-II also promotes salt reabsorption in the kidneys. Pathologically, A-II is formed in excess in overload left ventricular hypertrophy, in heart failure, and in some types of hypertension. Pharmacologically, inhibition of its action, whether by inhibitors of its formation or of its receptor, is used to treat important diseases such as left ventricular hypertrophy, heart failure, and hypertension.

Origin of Angiotensin II

The octapeptide A-II is formed when its decapeptide precursor, angiotensin I, is cleaved by the activity of the angiotensin-converting enzyme either in the circulation or in tissues such as the heart. Angiotensin-converting enzyme normally resides in the vascular inner layer (endothelium) of the lungs and in the coronary arteries, where it converts angiotensin I as it is formed to A-II. Angiotensin I originates from angiotensinogen (Fig. 9-2) under the influence of the enzyme

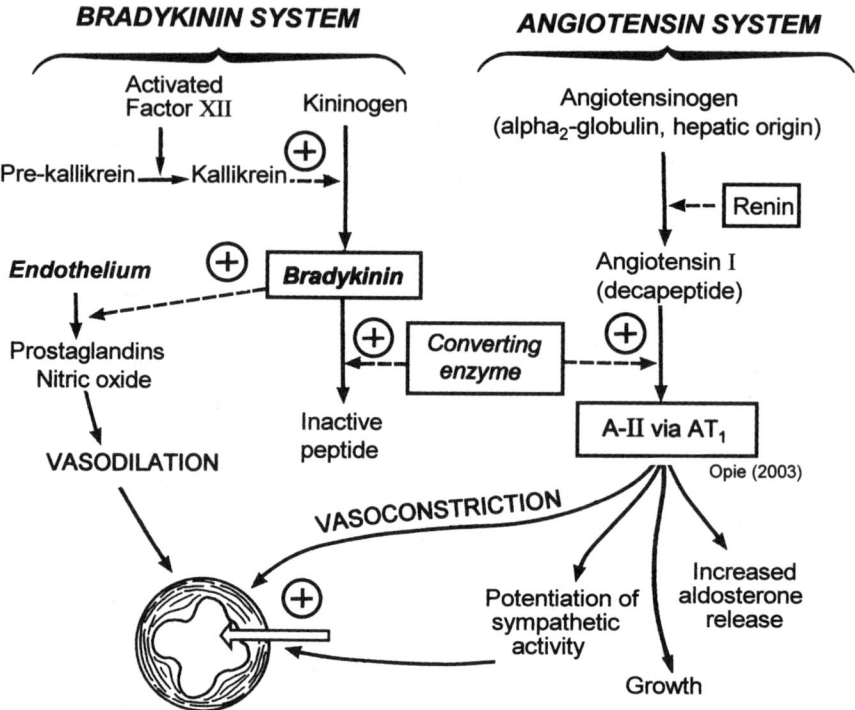

FIG. 9-2. Renin–angiotensin system and the bradykinin system. Angiotensin–bradykinin pathways. Note opposing effects on arterioles to produce vasoconstriction and vasodilation, respectively. Angiotensin II is also a powerful stimulator of growth (Fig. 9-1).

renin. Renin in turn is released into renal arteriolar blood from the juxtaglomerular cells of the kidneys in response to (a) impaired renal blood flow as in ischemia or hypotension; (b) salt depletion or sodium diuresis; and (c) β-adrenergic stimulation as in the fight-or-flight reaction. A-II also stimulates the formation and release of the sodium-retaining hormone aldosterone from the adrenal cortex. In heart failure, the low blood pressure and poor blood flow to the kidneys stimulate the RAS, so that there is excess formation of A-II and hence of aldosterone. This accounts for the abnormal retention of sodium and water as edema fluid (Fig. 16-16).

In hypertension (Fig. 14-1), excess vasoconstriction is partially mediated by A-II. In addition, the enlarged heart often found in hypertension results or is worsened by the effects of A-II on growth. This A-II is largely formed in the heart itself, by a tissue RAS that is activated by the mechanical deformity associated with the excess pressure within the left ventricle, as found in sustained hypertension. Whether the newly described second type of angiotensin-converting enzyme (6) plays a role in human disease remains to be verified.

Angiotensin II and Signaling via AT-1 and AT-2 Receptors

There are two A-II tissue receptor subtypes: AT-1 and AT-2. The AT-1 receptor mediates the adverse effects of A-II on the diseased heart and failing circulation. The results include (a) increased constriction of the peripheral arteries that requires the failing heart to pump harder, (b) excess growth and death rates of the heart cells that further weaken the myocardium, and (c) increased sodium retention. Dzau and others postulate that the AT_2 receptors may reduce some of the adverse effects of AT-1 receptor stimulation by a "yin-yang" effect (7). Although the AT-2 receptors may generate beneficial effects to protect the vascular endothelium, there are additional progrowth and proapoptotic effects prescribed to AT-2 receptor signaling (8). Although less well characterized than AT-1 signaling, the composite of AT-1 and AT-2 signaling provides another example of apparently contradictory signaling from a single receptor ligand, in this case A-II (8).

Angiotensin II Receptors Linked to G_q and Phospholipase C

Occupation of the heptahelical A-II receptor by A-II leads to growth by a signaling system that starts with the guanosine 5′-triphosphate (GTP) binding protein G_q and leads to MAP kinase (Fig. 9-1). Just as G_s links the β-adrenergic receptor to adenyl cyclase, G_q links the A-II receptor to the enzyme phospholipase C (Fig. 9-3). Just as G_s consists of three subunits, so does G_q (α, β, and γ),

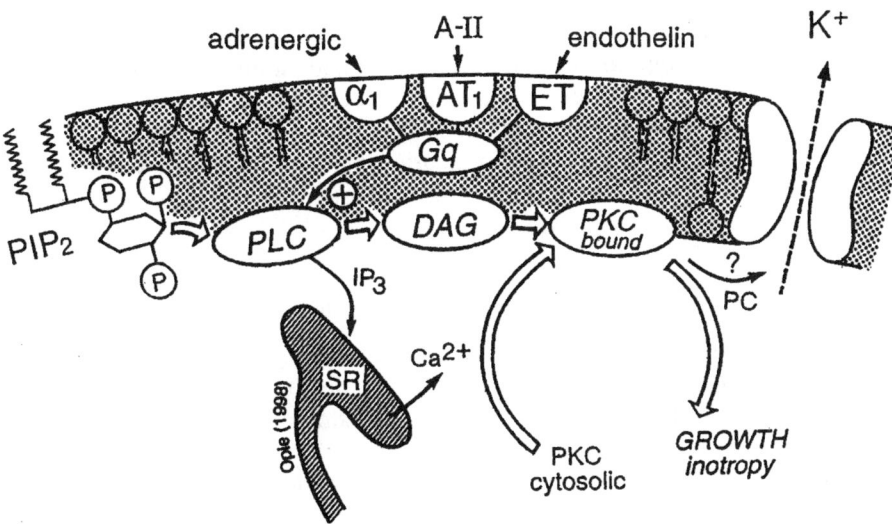

FIG. 9-3. **Angiotensin II signaling.** Angiotensin II interaction with the AT-1 receptor activates the G protein G_q that stimulates the phosphodiesterase phospholipase C to split phosphatidylinositol into two messengers: inositol 1,4,5-trisphosphate (*IP$_3$*) and 1,2-diacylglycerol (*DAG*). IP$_3$ promotes the release of calcium from the sarcoplasmic reticulum (*SR*). Calcium translocates cytosolic protein kinase C (*PKC*) to the sarcolemma where it is activated by 1,2-diacylglycerol. PKC in turn activates the mitogen-activated protein kinase pathway (Fig. 9-4).

and the α-subunit $G_{\alpha q}$ activates phospholipase C. When G_q is genetically overexpressed in mice, the heart grows excessively and fails (9).

Phospholipase C is a membrane-bound enzyme that breaks down phosphatidylinositol to form inositol 1,4,5-trisphosphate (IP_3), which diffuses to the intracellular sarcoplasmic reticulum from which it liberates calcium ions that help to promote calcium-dependent growth paths. To activate phospholipase C requires tyrosine phosphorylation by the poorly understood *Src-tyrosine kinase* family (10). Diacylglycerol is also formed when phosphatidylinositol is split by phospholipase C (Fig. 7-15). Diacylglycerol stimulates the activity of protein kinase C (PKC), a key regulator in signal transduction, by promoting translocation of PKC from the cytosol to the sarcolemma, where it binds to its membrane receptor RACK (receptor for activated C kinase) to become active (11).

Protein Kinase C

PKCs are a family of serine–threonine signaling kinases. There are four major groups, and as many as 11 isoforms (also called isozymes) have been identified, which have putative distinct signaling effects. In general, PKC probably plays a major role in the regulation of cell growth, both in the myocardium and in vascular smooth muscle. Situated in the cytosol when inactive, PKC responds to diacylglycerol by translocation to the sarcolemma, thereby becoming active (Fig. 9-3). It then initiates a signal sequence that involves a complex transduction path, leading to MAP kinase, which explains its role in growth regulation and in preconditioning (Chapter 19). Different PKC isoforms respond to different physiologic and pathologic stimuli. Classical isoforms respond to calcium and diacylglycerol (α-, β-, and γ-isoforms); a second group of novel isoforms includes PKC-ε and is insensitive to calcium, and a third subgroup has atypical regulation and includes PKC-ζ. Low-level overexpression of both the β- and ε-isoforms gives protection against ischemia–reperfusion injury (12,13).

Activation by Angiotensin II

A-II has a broad range of effects on PKC, including translocation and hence activation of all the calcium-sensitive isoforms, plus the ε- (PKC-ε) and ζ-isoforms (13,14). Of these, a major growth-stimulating effect of A-II is mediated by PKC-β, whereas overload hypertrophy proceeds through PKC-ε (15). The subsequent downstream signaling sequence leads to MAP kinase activation via the small signaling molecule Ras (Fig. 9-1).

Degree of Activation of Protein Kinase C-ε

There are important distinct signaling effects mediated by the degree of activation of PKC-ε. First, low-level activation of PKC-ε gives long-term cardioprotection without hypertrophy (13,15). When carrying out this function, PKC-ε is physically linked in a protective signaling module with the extracellular signal-regulated kinase (ERK) components of the MAP kinase complex (13). This signaling module also associates with the mitochondria, and this spatial configuration is postulated to inhibit mitochondria-driven apoptosis as part of its protective function (13). Second, medium degrees of activation of PKC-ε lead to hypertrophy without failure. Third, high-level overexpression of PKC-ε leads to hypertrophy with fibrosis and heart failure (15). Highly activated PKC-ε may act mainly on "bad" components of MAP kinase such as c-Jun N terminal kinase (JNK) (Fig. 9-1) or by stimulation of poorly defined paths leading to formation of TNF-α (16). A third possibility is that PKC-ε, once bound to RACK, proceeds to interact with and to promote the activity of PKC-β, which in turn helps to create the hypertrophic failing phenotype (15).

Vascular Effects of Angiotensin II: Vasoconstriction and Atherogenesis

A-II promotes vasoconstriction in three ways. First, there is a direct calcium-promoted vasoconstrictor action of A-II on the vascular AT-1 receptor. Second, A-II promotes the release of norepinephrine from the terminal neurons into the synaptic space. Norepinephrine in turn acts on the postsynaptic vasoconstrictor α_1-receptors. Third, A-II stimulates the vascular endothelium to form and release endothelin, another powerful vasoconstrictor. This explains why excess A-II, as found in renal disease and in models of overexpression of A-II, causes hypertension (Chapter 15). It also explains why increased formation of A-II produces excessive vasoconstriction and the increased afterload that is disadvantageous for the failing heart (Chapter 16).

A-II also promotes growth of the vascular matrix and in particular formation of collagen, by stimulating the vascular enzyme nicotinamide adenine dinucleotide phosphate (reduced form) oxidase, ROS, and adhesion factors such as vascular cell adhesion molecule. These promote the leukocyte adhesion to the vascular endothelium, an early step in atherogenesis.

Mitogen-Activated Protein Kinase Cascade

MAP kinase is a part of a signaling cascade (Fig. 9-4) that functions as a "central integration module in signal processing" (17). The MAP kinase cascade can be set in motion in response to at least three different extracellular stimuli: A-II and other G-linked receptor agonists, growth factors such as insulin, and stress stimuli. The cascade consists of a series of kinases that, when activated, phosphorylates ("cascades onto") the kinase at the next level down. Thus, extracellular stimuli inaugurate messages that reach all the way to the nucleus, using the sequential components of the MAP kinase signaling cascade. To facilitate signaling, signaling modules and microcellular scaffolding create close contact between the interacting molecules.

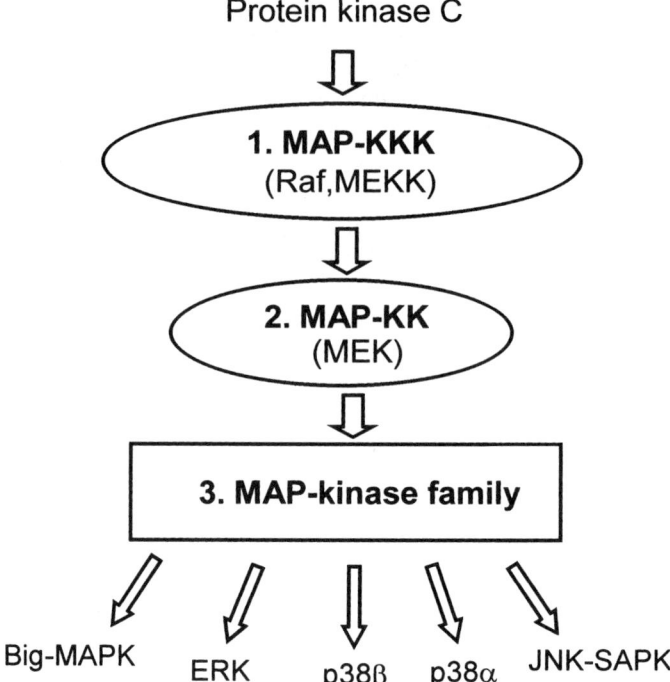

FIG. 9-4. The three tiers of mitogen-activated protein kinase (MAP kinase) activation. The first tier responds to Ras, activated by guanosine 5′-triphosphate and switched off by guanosine 5′-diphosphate (see text). *MAP-KKK*, MAP kinase kinase kinase; *MEKK*, mitogen ERK (extracellular signal-regulated kinase) kinase kinase; *Raf*, a kinase activated by Ras (see text) by recruitment to the cell membrane.

Ras-Raf Signaling

The exact paths from PKC to the MAP kinase are not clear. In many studies, there is a crucial role for *Ras*, a small GTP binding protein that functions as a molecular switch. When GTP is bound to Ras as Ras-GTP, it is in the "on" position and transmits the growth signal, but when in the "off" position, transmission fails (18). "Exchange of GDP for GTP and the rate of GTP hydrolysis are key regulators steps" in the function of Ras (18). Thus, Ras activates the first tier of the three-tier MAP kinase system.

The first tier kinase, activated by Ras, is MAPKKK (MAP kinase kinase kinase), also called ERK kinase kinase 1 (MEKK1) and also known as Raf-1. Note that each of the kinases in the cascade also has an alternate name, thus adding confusion to an already complex signal system. MAPKKK is activated at the sarcolemmal level, setting the cascade in motion, with the next kinase being MAPKK, also called MEK (MAP kinase–ERK kinase). The "bottom" tier is MAP kinase complex. The latter is activated in the cytosol and then phosphorylates target proteins in both cytosol and nucleus.

Mitogen-Activated Protein Kinase Family

MAP kinase is a family name and refers to a complex of enzymes including ERK, p38 MAP kinase, and JNK. The latter is also called stress-activated protein kinase (SAPK). A fourth component, recently added but poorly understood, is "big" MAP kinase (19). There are as many as seven MAP kinase kinases in total, mostly with different substrate specificities. For example, MAP kinase kinase 1 and 2 react with ERK (19).

According to whether they promote survival and growth or cell death by apoptosis, these can be divided into the "good" and the "bad" (20). Ideally and for simplicity, each of these "moral" alternatives would be stimulated by a specific and different set of kinases. Thus, the kinases that activate ERK should lead to "good" outcomes because ERK itself is prosurvival and a "good guy." Indeed, genetic overexpression of the MEK1-ERK signaling pathway promotes concentric hypertrophy in mice without any signs of heart failure or fatality for at least 12 months, a long time for a mouse (21). Furthermore, PKC-ε is linked to ERK when in its protective signaling module. Conversely, JNK-SAPK is one of the proposed "bad guys" of the MAP kinase family, and its activation may lead to a dilated, failing hypertrophic heart (20).

However, any clear division of the MAP kinase family and its activators into good and bad seems simplistic. We know from human nature that the same guy can sometimes be good, but sometimes bad, depending on circumstances. Thus, the third component of MAP kinase, p38 MAP kinase, hovers between bad and good, perhaps because different isoforms are proapoptotic (p38α, next section) or prosurvival (p38β) (22).

It Is Not a One-Way Ticket: Phosphatases

In evaluating another signaling path, Thielmann et al. (23) warn that a simplistic monocausal sequence of mediators is unlikely. Rather, there may be crossover paths and feedback loops. To change the analogy, there are often thought to be upstream sites of control such as Ras that then influence the amount of signal flowing to downstream sites. However, some of the flow may be deviated if side channels open. If the protein kinases sequentially phosphorylate and activate other kinases, then logically there should be control by decreasing the degree of phosphorylation, i.e., by the cleavage of phosphate bonds from the activate kinases. This is achieved by the activity of phosphatases (24). Whether there is one major site at which several phosphatases work or whether the different phosphatases regulate multiple upstream sites is still not known. The complexity of this "reverse regulatory system" will probably turn out to be as exquisite as kinase signaling.

From Kinase Cascade to Nucleus via Transcription Factors

Transcription factors are regulatory peptides that bind to genes in the cell nucleus to activate or repress gene regulation and hence regulate peptide production. These transcription factors can be activated by phosphorylation, which occurs in response to cytosolic pathways, such as those of the MAP kinase cascade that link extracellular stimuli to RNA synthesis in the nucleus (25). MAP kinases phosphorylate and hence activate transcription factors that regulate the expression of a specific gene. For example, the myocyte enhancer factor 2 proteins promote the activity of those myocardial genes required for myocardial hypertrophy in response to aortic banding (25). Another transcription factor, GATA-4, binds to the NFAT3 region of genes (the latter being a transcription factor response element situated in the regulatory region of genes), which is in part involved in calcineurin-mediated hypertrophy (Fig. 13-5). It is likely, although not yet proven, that different transcription factors are activated by different MAP kinase family members (p38 MAP kinase, ERK, JNK-SAPK).

Insulin and Insulin-like Growth Factor

Abnormalities of insulin secretion from the pancreas and abnormal circulating levels of insulin play major roles in the genesis of diabetes mellitus, a common and serious disease that in turn promotes coronary disease and hypertension. Although insulin is best known for it major role in controlling hyperglycemia, it is also a major growth factor (Fig. 9-1), an effect that is enhanced by the cardiac production of insulin-like growth factor I. The latter is a growth-promoting peptide generated by cardiomyocytes under the influence of insulin, mechanical stress, or growth hormone stimulation. Insulin binds to specific insulin receptors, consisting of an external α subunit and an internal β subunit. When insulin occupies the external subunit, there is a rapid self-phosphorylation of the β subunit (26). This *autophosphorylation* greatly amplifies the effect of insulin and in turn activates peptide kinases to phosphorylate tyrosine. Thereafter, the downstream events are complex. A brief summary of one current view is as follows. Tyrosine phosphorylation increases the activity of the insulin receptor substrate 1, an important docking site for several kinases and phosphatases. For example, phosphatidylinositol-3-phosphate (PI-3) kinase, one of the pivotal kinases in insulin and insulinlike growth factor I signaling, binds to insulin receptor substrate 1 when activated.

Akt and Beyond

An important downstream target of PI-3 kinase is protein kinase B, more commonly known as *Akt*. The name is derived from the causative oncogenic agent in the cancer-producing retrovirus AKT. Akt is a serine–tryosine protein kinase that leads to phosphorylation of the mammalian target of rapamycin and the phosphorylation of the signaling kinase p70 s6 kinase (27). From here to improved survival involves the phosphorylation and inactivation of the proapoptotic pep-

9. SIGNAL SYSTEMS: COORDINATING LIFE AND DEATH   257

tide BAD (next section). Of interest, rapamycin is the active component of the stent technically called "sirolimus eluting" that keeps stenosed coronary arteries patent. The rapamycin inhibits the growth pathway that otherwise leads to coronary restenosis. Also of interest, activated Akt is protective against ischemia (28), probably by its antiapoptotic function. Interestingly, Akt has also been shown to be activated by estrogens, which offer a hypothesis as to why survival after myocardial infarction is better in females than in males ("Akt like a woman") (29).

Cross-talk between Pathways

Insulin and insulin-like growth factor I both interact with tyrosine kinase–linked receptors that activate Ras that becomes active Ras-GTP that in turn promotes the activation of Raf-1. This means that they can also activate the growth-promoting components of the MAP kinase cascade. Growth can also follow activation by the enzyme glycogen synthase that synthesizes more than glycogen.

Growth and Protein Synthesis

Transcription Factors and Promoters

Ultimately, all the growth paths stimulate nuclear transcription factors. Transcription is the copying process whereby one RNA strand is synthesized on and copied from one of the two strands of DNA: the template or coding strand ("blueprint"). Initiation of this process requires a promoter, RNA polymerase, and the activity of transcription factors (Fig. 9-5). The promoter includes the *TATA box* (TATA because the nucleotide sequence at this point is thymidine-adenine-thymidine-adenine) and the CAAT box (cytosine-adenine-adenine-thymidine) that bind the RNA polymerase at the start site. Upstream or downstream of this basal transcriptional site lie enhancer elements that respond to signals such as cyclic adenosine 3′,5′-monophosphate and hormones such as thyroxine. Here too is located the peroxisome proliferator response element (Fig. 9-5), which has been alluded to with respect to metacrine signaling earlier this chapter. TATA binding proteins bind the RNA polymerase to the TATA box at the promoter site. Transcription factors bind to the enhancer regions of the gene to moderate basal transcriptional regulation in response to the composite of signaling mediated events described above. Once all these elements are in place, the double helix of the DNA forms an open loop and transcription can start. The enzyme *RNA polymerase* incorporates the correct nucleosides into the growing messenger RNA (mRNA) molecule, while shedding two of the phosphate units (as pyrophosphate). Thus, each nucleoside is incorporated in the precise sequence dictated by the genetic code. A few TATA-less genes also exist. These are also highly regulated and

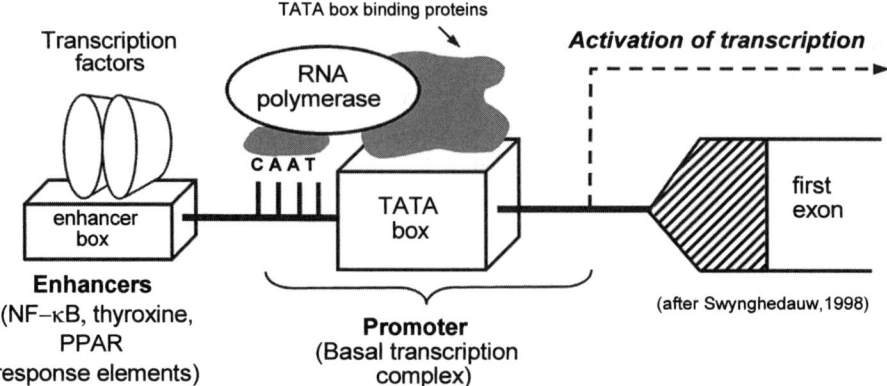

FIG. 9-5. Promoter and enhancer regions of a DNA gene. Note roles of TATA (thymidine-adenine-thymidine-adenine) and CAAT (cytosine-adenine-adenine-thymidine) boxes, enhancers, and transcription factors. (Adapted from Swynghedauw B. *Molecular cardiology for the cardiologist,* 2nd ed. Boston: Kluwer Academic Publishers, 1998.)

include genes that were initially thought to be "housekeeping genes," such as those encoding numerous metabolic enzymes.

Four-Letter Language

The DNA molecules have the well-known regular double-helix structure. When DNA forms the RNA that conveys its genetic signal to the ribosomes (sites of protein assembly), then part of the DNA molecule is unfolded so that one of the strands of the helix is used as a template (blueprint) on which mRNA is newly synthesized from many molecules of the appropriate nucleoside triphosphates (Fig. 9-6). The nucleoside concerned may be adenosine (A), cytidine (C), guanosine (G), or uridine (U). That these are the four nucleoside triphosphates involved in the synthesis of mRNA may seem confusing when considering the four nucleosides that constitute the "four-letter language" of the DNA molecule: they are A, G, C, and T, the latter standing for thymidine. However, uridine differs from thymidine only in the absence of a methyl group, and it forms the same type of hydrogen bonds. Thus, in essence, DNA and RNA speak the same four-letter language.

Ribosomes

The RNA copies made during transcription are chemically modified and shortened (edited during mRNA splicing) to form mRNAs that emerge from the cell nucleus and are used to dictate the sequences of proteins being synthesized on cytoplasmic ribosomes; the latter may be free (the majority in heart cells) or bound to internal cellular membranes. Most individual mRNAs, their coded

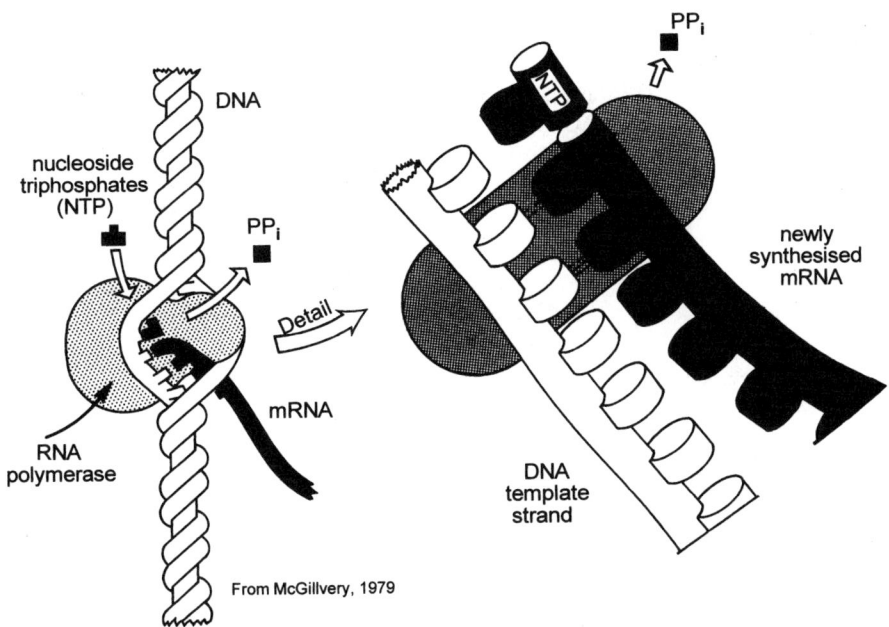

FIG. 9-6. Synthesis of new messenger RNA (premessenger) on the DNA template. (Modified from McGilvery, 1979.)

information written in triplets of succeeding bases called codons, are simultaneously bound and translated by several ribosomes, forming *polysomes*.

The mRNA merely instructs the ribosome how to make the peptide bonds required for protein synthesis, the peptides having been transported to the ribosomes by transfer RNA. To get the process of protein synthesis started in the ribosomes requires *initiation factors*, which are themselves proteins. *Elongation factors* help the chain to grow. At the ribosome, the mRNA translates the genetic message to the growing peptide chains. *Posttranslational events* include the assembly, storage, translocation, and stability of the newly made proteins. Thus, the hemodynamic load, a physical stimulus, can undergo *transduction* to a biochemical signal that has enhanced the rate of gene expression and protein synthesis, resulting in hypertrophy.

New Versus Larger Myocytes in the Adult Heart

When the heart responds to a hemodynamic overload through an acute increase in protein synthesis, there are increases in RNA transcription, nuclear export, and the proportion of actively translating heart ribosomes and a decrease in the relative rate of protein degradation (Fig. 9-7). An important question is whether there are specific new mRNAs invoked by the hypertrophy process or

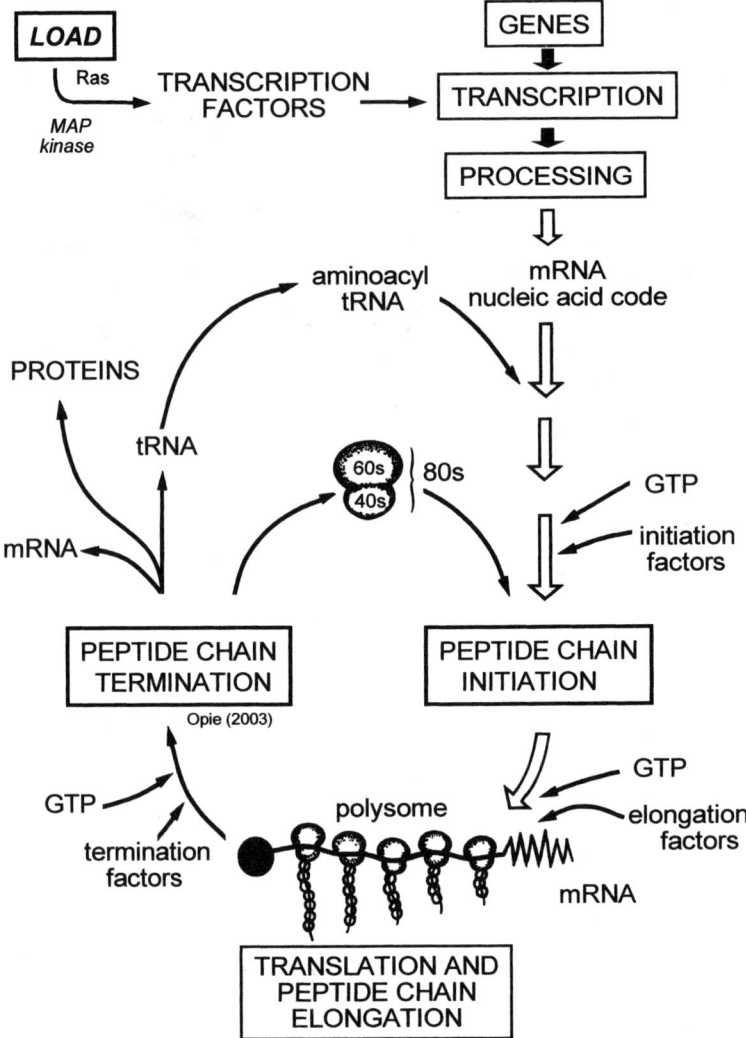

FIG. 9-7. Overall patterns of protein synthesis. (Adapted from Morgan et al., 1979.)

whether there is simply an amplification of the existing mechanisms. At least part of the basic response during hypertrophy consists of an increased rate of turnover of the existing regulatory mechanisms. However, induction of the fetal gene program (see last section of this chapter) during heart failure implies major alterations at the level of transcription. In addition, the capacity to synthesize DNA and hence to make new myocytes, is not completely lost, even in the adult.

In some species, notably primates (including humans), DNA can replicate so that myocytes can contain more than two sets of chromosomes (*polyploid nuclei*), without necessarily being associated with cell division. Compensatory growth is accompanied by a marked shift to nuclei with a high degree of ploidy. Linzbach (29a) proposed that cardiac enlargement above a particular critical size could be supplemented by the addition of new cells, involving the splitting of polyploid nuclei. That stage is reached when the heart has approximately doubled its weight to reach 500 g. At approximately that weight, the cell diameter reaches a peak and then declines because of myocyte division. Cell length, conversely, keeps increasing. Thus, in extremely large hearts, there is both hyperplasia and hypertrophy. More recently, Anversa et al. (30) challenged the common concept that ventricular myocytes are, for practical purposes, terminally differentiated. Rather, myocyte hyperplasia also occurs in the failing ventricle independently of any increase of cell size or myocardial mass. If myocyte regeneration could be therapeutically promoted, that would have important potential after myocardial infarction and in heart failure.

APOPTOSIS AND ITS SIGNAL SYSTEMS

Heart cells die in several different ways. Permanent occlusion of a coronary artery leads to myocardial necrosis and infarction (Chapter 17). During necrosis, cells are deprived of energy and literally explode. In contrast, apoptosis or programmed cell death is a controlled, energy-requiring process that equates to cellular suicide (Fig. 9-8). Literally, the term denotes the dropping of leaves from trees in the fall, reflecting the sporadic and gradual loss of cells in the myocardium and other tissues (31). Today, despite volumes of research, the exact role of apoptosis in cardiovascular pathology still remains to be fully defined. Nonetheless, apoptosis is increasingly implicated in heart failure, pressure-overload hypertrophy, and ischemia–reperfusion injury. Apoptosis is a tightly regulated cell program that can be activated in two ways. First, proapoptotic factors act on either the sarcolemmal death receptor or the mitochondria via the release cytochrome c (Fig. 9-6). The common result of both of these pathways is activation of self-destructive enzymes called caspases and, more specifically, inactive procaspase-3 becoming active caspase-3 that cleaves polypeptides. Conversely, apoptosis can be inhibited by antiapoptotic signals such as those mediated by insulin and other growth factors.

Death Receptor Pathway

There are no fewer than six "death receptors" that lead to apoptosis (31). The best known receptors are those for TNF-α receptor 1 and Fas ligand receptor. Fas, also called APO-1, is a circulating member of the TNF family that binds to Fas ligand and hence to the death receptor. The activated death receptor then conveys signals to the Fas-associated death domain protein, which in turn activates caspase-8 and hence caspase-3. Circulating levels of both TNF-α and the Fas ligand are increased in severe heart failure and in animal experiments promote apoptosis of the heart cells.

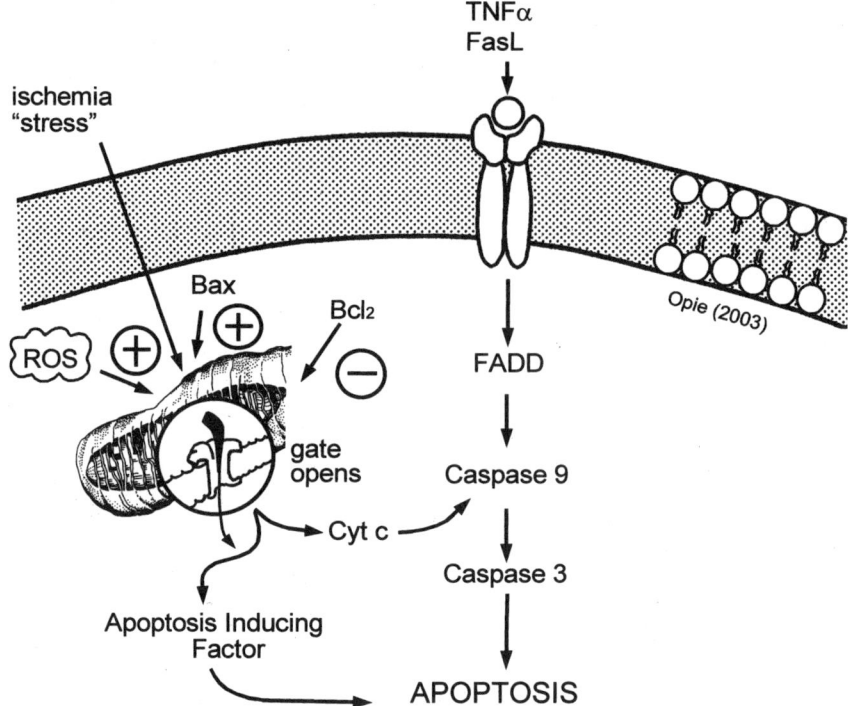

FIG. 9-8. Apoptosis paths. Note the mitochondrial path on the left and the death receptor pathway on the right. *ROS*, reactive oxygen species; *TNF*, tumor necrosis factor; *FasL*, Fas ligand; *cyt C*, cytochrome c; *FADD*, Fas-associated death domain protein. For Bcl-2 and Bax, see text.

Mitochondrial Pathway

Cytochrome c "floods out of the mitochondria during apoptosis" (32) and, together with apoptosis-activating factor, activates the caspase-9 that in turn activates caspase-3. The mitochondria also release apoptosis-inducing factor that neutralizes a set of caspase inhibitors called inhibitors of apoptosis, "thereby freeing the caspases to do their work" (32). The outer mitochondrial membrane associated Bcl-2 family of proteins probably regulate the release of cytochrome c. The first family member identified was called *Bcl-2* because a mutation in this gene promoted the development of lymphomas (B-cell lymphoma 2 gene). The release of cytochrome c is stimulated when a related family member, *Bax*, inserts into the outer mitochondrial membrane (33). This process is, in turn, inhibited by Bcl-2 itself, which is therefore antiapoptotic. *BAD* is a proapoptotic cytosolic peptide that sequesters the protective Bcl. BAD is inhibited when phosphorylated, which occurs in response to the low-level activation of the PKC-ε isoform, thus explaining some of the cardioprotective effects of PKC-ε and in response to Akt activation (13).

Why It Is Not Simple

By now, it is self-evident that apoptosis and its control are no simple matter. It might be supposed that all that is necessary to study the contribution of apoptosis to, say, the genesis or progression of heart failure, would be a suitable model, i.e., an inhibitor of caspase-3 (Fig. 9-8) and the measurement of apoptosis. There are problems all along the way. The choice of model of, for example, heart failure, might differ critically from the human disease. Apoptosis can also be independent of capsase-3, resulting from the activity of apoptosis-inducing factor that is released from damaged mitochondria (31). The best way to measure apoptosis is still not decided. The gold standard for the diagnosis of caspase-3 is tedious microscopic evaluation of the pathologic changes (Fig. 18-6), followed by various ways of evaluating DNA fragmentation. These technical difficulties and the constant discovery of new signals that contribute to either proapoptotic or antiapoptotic signaling or even to both explain why the true role of apoptosis in cardiovascular diseases remains controversial.

CYTOKINES: BOTH PROSURVIVAL AND PROAPOPTOTIC

Tumor Necrosis Factor-α

The cytokine signaling system leads to both prosurvival and apoptotic end points (Fig. 9-9). TNF-α is part of the general immune response, along with members of the interleukin family such as cardiotrophin-1 and interleukin-6. It is produced both by the heart to act on the heart in a local homeostatic way, for which the technical term is an *autocoid* effect, and by circulating macrophages. There are two surface membrane receptors, TNF receptor 1 and TNF receptor 2, of which the former is dominant in the heart. Previously, it was thought that the origin of TNF-α and interleukin-6 produced by the heart was solely in the immune system in cells such as macrophages, which are also found in the heart. Now, it seems certain that there is also production by cardiomyocytes during ischemic–reperfusion injury or other stressors (3). In addition to its better known role in apoptosis (Fig. 9-9), TNF-α also has protective qualities, especially found when the stimulus evokes low levels of TNF-α and is of short duration. Proof of protection is that genetic ablation of both TNF receptors leads to more extensive ischemic cardiac damage (3). These complex and potentially contradictory effects of TNF-α justify the descriptive term *pleiotropic*, with many and varied results.

Some of the *adaptive and protective paths of TNF-α* involve a complex lipid called ceramide, and others involve the transcription factor nuclear factor κB

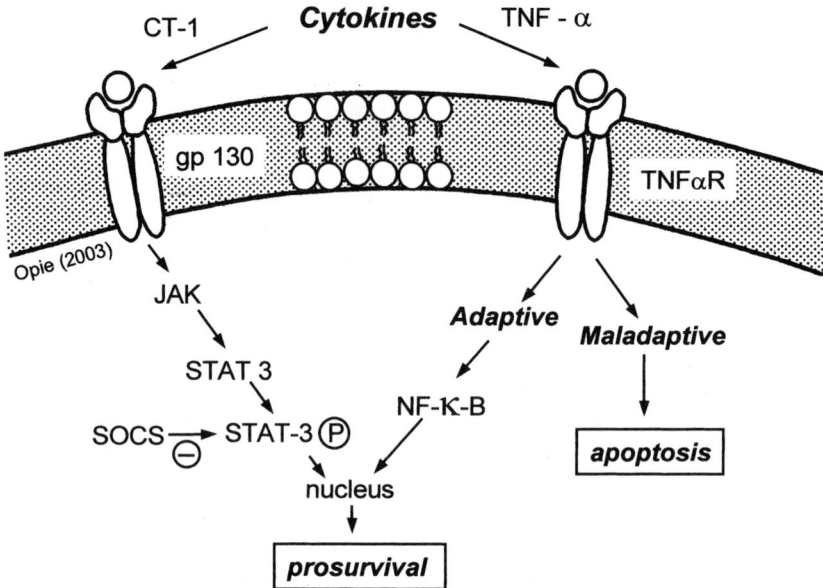

FIG. 9-9. Cytokine signaling. Note contrast between prosurvival protective pathways and maladaptive paths leading to apoptosis. *CT-1*, cardiotrophin-1; *JAK*, Janus kinases; *STAT*, signal transducer and activator of transcription; *SOCS*, suppressor of cytokine signaling, preventing phosphorylation (*P*) of STAT3. See Kile BT, Schulman BA, Alexander WS, et al. *Trends Biochem Sci* 2002;27:235–241. For nuclear factor κB, see Figure 9-11.

(NF-κB) (Fig. 9-10). The latter has multiple functions (see next section). For example, it can promote the expression of cytoprotective genes, such as manganese superoxide dismutase, that break down ROS (next section). An interesting recent hypothesis is that TNF-α depresses cardiac mechanical function and myocardial oxygen demand directly and indirectly. The latter mechanism follows induction of the enzyme inducible NO synthase (iNOS) that produces excess inhibitory nitric oxide (34). The myocardial oxygen requirement is thereby reduced so that viability of the hibernating heart can be sustained even in the face of reduced blood flow (Chapter 19).

In contrast, potentially *maladaptive and harmful paths of TNF-α* include promotion of apoptosis both directly (Fig. 9-8) and indirectly by increased activity of the proapoptotic stress-activated signal JNK-SAPK (Fig. 9-1). In the failing myocardium, increased TNF-α expression may promote cardiac dilation (35) and progressive cardiac dysfunction (23). At least some of the excess TNF-α in heart failure is in response to increased stimulation by A-II and PKC (16).

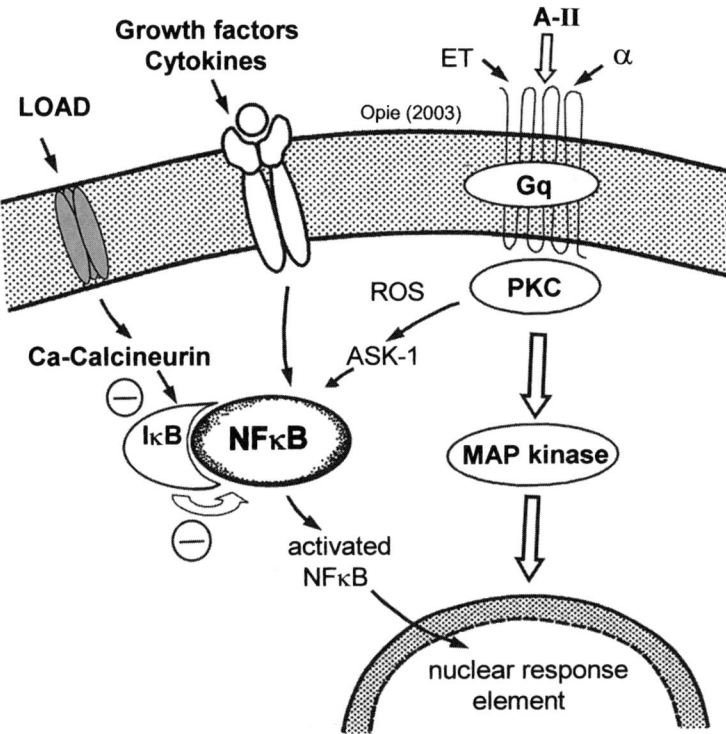

FIG. 9-10. Role of nuclear factor kB (NF-kB) in regulating growth. Calcineurin, activated by calcium and calcium-calmodulin (Fig. 6-10), stimulates growth by phosphorylating and inhibiting inhibitor of NF-κB (*I-κB*), which normally inhibits NF-κB. *ASK-1,* apoptosis signal-regulating kinase, activated by reactive oxygen species.

Cytokines and the Janus Kinase–Signal Transducer and Activator of Transcription Path

The gp-130 receptor responds to stimulation by the cytokines interleukin-6, cardiotrophin-1, leptin, and others. Janus kinases (JAKs) rapidly phosphorylate this receptor, which in turn activates several signal transducing pathways including that of signal transducer and activator of transcription (STAT). STAT transmits the signal from the membrane to the nucleus. STAT3 promotes hypertrophic growth signals, whereas STAT1 paradoxically promotes proapoptotic signaling. JAKs also promote hypertrophy by activating two other pathways, the one leading from Ras to ERK and the insulin growth pathway via PI-3 kinase–Akt (36).

Cytoskeletal Signaling

How does an increased mechanical load on the heart communicate with the signaling systems that promote cardiac growth? The cytoskeleton, previously thought to be a metabolically dormant support system, is now known to be an active communicator that transforms load-induced external mechanical stress into a growth signal (Fig. 9-11). Thus, the cytoskeleton acts as a *mechanotransducer*. Consequently, the pathways regulated both by A-II and the cytokines become active. When isolated rat hearts are subject to increased stretch, TNF-α is induced within 10 minutes (37). Whether this is a direct effect of stretch or whether stretch acts to release A-II, which then induces the synthesis of TNF-α (16) is not yet clear. Another cytokine, *transforming growth factor β_1* (TGF-β_1), is also involved in the growth-inducing effects of A-II (38). TGF-β_1 is so called because, when in excess, it activates ("transforms") fibroblasts to make collagen. Nonetheless, in the A-II–mediated hypertrophic response, TGF-β_1 is implicated in overall growth rather than in specific stimulation of fibroblasts (38).

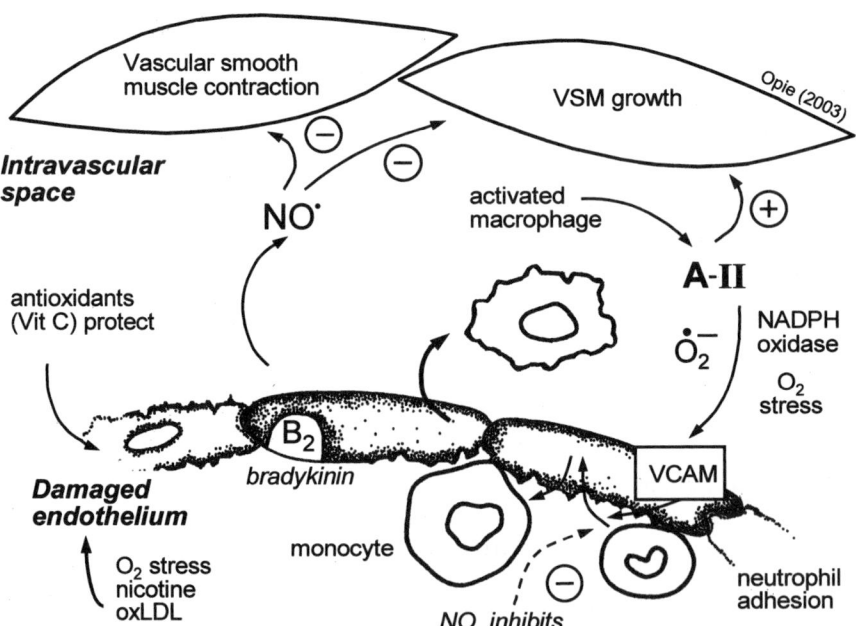

FIG. 9-11. Vascular disease. Role of angiotensin II (*A-II*) and nitric oxide (*NO*). Note the adverse effects of oxidative stress induced by local formation of A-II in promoting leukocyte adhesion to the damaged endothelium and monocyte penetration with macrophage activation. In contrast, the healthy endothelium produces protective NO. *oxLDL*, oxidized low-density lipoprotein; *VSM*, vascular smooth muscle; *VCAM*, vascular cell adhesion molecule.

Nuclear Factor-κB

Normally NF-κB lies in the cytoplasm and is inactivated by the inhibitory chaperone I-κB (Fig. 9-10). When the latter is phosphorylated, for example, as part of a growth pathway stimulus, NF-κB becomes activated and travels from the cytoplasm to the nucleus where it combines with its response element to enhance nuclear transcription of a wide variety of genes. Activated NF-κB is "extremely promiscuous, interacting with a large number of transcription factors" (39). At least some of these genes are involved in cardiac hypertrophy. NF-κB is also activated by another path involving an ROS-activated kinase, apoptosis signal-regulating kinase. This alternate path operates in response to A-II and other agonists linked to the G protein G_q (40). Apoptosis signal-regulating kinase is bifunctional and, as the name implies, also promotes apoptosis, for example, in response to TNF-α.

REACTIVE OXYGEN SPECIES AND NITRIC OXIDE

As defined in Chapter 19, *free radicals* are highly reactive chemical groups that differ from standard compounds in having unpaired electrons in their outer orbitals, therefore being potentially very unstable. ROS is the collective term applied to those radicals that are derived from oxygen, such as superoxide and the hydroxyl radical (Table 19-2). An important physiologic source of ROS is complex III in the electron transport chain in the mitochondria (Fig. 19-4). Normally, enzymes such as superoxide dismutase break down ROS, but when rates of production are enhanced, ROS accumulates. Initially, ROS was thought to have only adverse effects, causing *oxidative stress*, and was proven to be a major pathogen in vascular disease. Atherogenesis progresses when ROS production rates are enhanced under the influence of A-II, which stimulates nicotinamide adenine dinucleotide phosphate (reduced form) oxidase, a process producing superoxide (Fig. 9-11). ROS also mediates reperfusion injury and apoptosis (Fig. 9-8).

Gradually, however, a new role for ROS has emerged, that of an important physiologic signal. The concept that free radicals can transmit physiologic signals is already firmly established for *reactive nitrogen species* that include NO. ROS may promote cell growth by activating a kinase that in turn activates NF-κB (Fig. 9-10) (39). ROS also helps to mediate protective preconditioning signaling (Fig. 19-11), possibly by directly activating the protective mitochondrial potassium–adenosine 5′-triphosphate channel (41). High rates of mitochondrial metabolism may be self-regulating, producing more superoxide that is converted to hydrogen peroxide. The latter is freely diffusible and, hypothetically, decreases the rate of pyruvate entry into mitochondria (4).

Probably small degrees of stimulation by the ROS are physiologic, whereas excessive or prolonged stimulation can have abnormal and pathologic consequences. Thus, depending on the circumstances, such signals may be variably good or bad in their effects. For example, ROS may deliver both apoptotic and growth-promoting signals via the same kinase (19).

Nitric Oxide Signaling

In 1998, the Nobel prize for medicine/physiology went to Furchgott, Ignarro, and Murad for describing the fundamental role of the *NO messenger system* in the cardiovascular system. NO is formed in different sites by different isoforms of NO synthase (NOS). For example, that formed in the endothelium travels swiftly to the surrounding smooth muscle cells to stimulate the soluble cytosolic enzyme guanylate cyclase to produce vasodilatory cyclic guanosine 3′,5′-monophosphate (Fig. 9-12). NO is a free radical with a very short half-life, measured in seconds or even less, so that there is almost no "downstream" activity. NO acts locally, just at the site or close to where it is formed. During exercise, enhanced blood flow promotes shear stress on the endothelium to increase formation of NO and to give exercise-induced vasodilation (42). Conversely, when blood flow is low, as in coronary disease, release of NO is decreased, and vasoconstrictive forces dominate. NO also directly protects the vascular endothelium

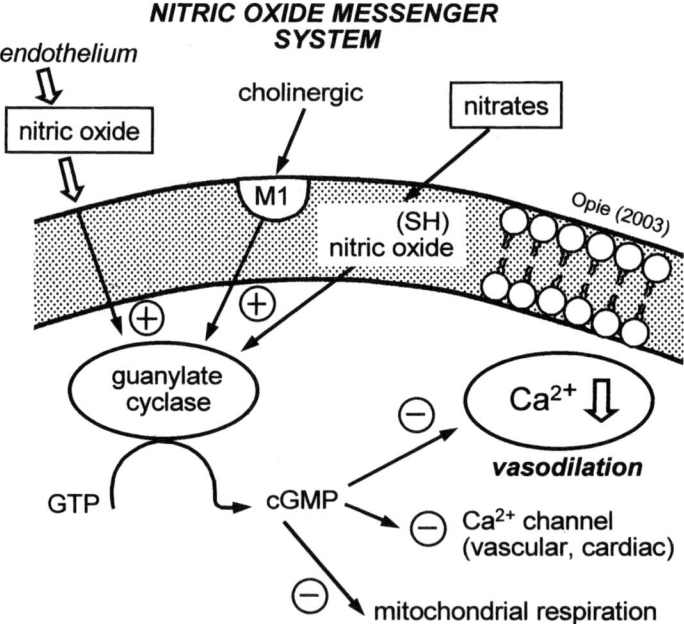

FIG. 9-12. Nitric oxide messenger system. Proposed role in stimulating soluble guanylate cyclase and cyclic guanosine 3′,5′-monophosphate to cause vasodilation and possibly a negative inotropic effect. Antianginal nitrates also cause coronary vasodilation by this mechanism. M_1, muscarinic receptor, subtype 1.

by decreasing the release of endothelin, a vasoconstrictive and potentially damaging peptide. Additionally, NO has major nonvascular cardiac effects. These include participation in the heart-rate slowing effects of cholinergic stimulation and in the downward regulation of cardiac oxygen metabolism.

Physiologic Synthesis of Nitric Oxide by Endothelial or Neuronal Nitric Oxide Synthase

NO is synthesized in endothelial cells from L-arginine and oxygen in response to a complex messenger system involving receptors, IP_3, and calcium. The enzyme concerned is *endothelial NOS*, which is calcium sensitive (43) and requires several complex cofactors. Because NO is so labile and difficult to measure, one common way to assess its contribution to vasodilator activity to inhibit its formation by L-arginine analogues (L-NG-monomethyl arginine and nitro-L-arginine methyl ester). Many studies with these compounds have shown, for example, that the rate of formation of NO in hypertension states is diminished. In addition, NO can, with difficulty, be measured directly. "Puffs" of NO are formed the heart in diastole (44). Abruptly increasing the ventricular load increases this pulsatile NO production, which probably comes from the endothelium, thereby theoretically facilitating diastolic ventricular filling and preventing platelet aggregation (44). However, NO plays little direct role in the regulation of myocardial contractility, whether in health or disease (45). An indirect effect by autonomic modulation of heart rate remains more likely (46).

The *neuronal NOS isoform* synthesizes NO in *nitrergic (nitroxidergic)* neurons (47). In the sinoatrial node, locally made NO enhances vagal slowing of the heart rate and limits sympathetic tachycardia (Fig. 7-18). Such autonomic effects of NO occur presynaptically with release of acetylcholine, cholinergic activation, and adrenergic withdrawal (48). The bradycardia induced by exercise training may be explained, in part, by increased synthesis of iNOS (48).

Inducible Nitric Oxide

This enzyme is normally not expressed but must be induced (hence the name) at the transcriptional level. In disease states, inflammatory cytokines and endotoxins stimulate the mRNA for iNOS, which is found in biopsy specimens from humans with septic shock. Inhibition of cardiac contraction may be mediated by peroxynitrite ($ONOO^-$), formed when the excess NO interacts with superoxide. In human dilated cardiomyopathy, increased iNOS may contribute to depressed contraction (45).

Excess Nitric Oxide and Peroxynitrite

Excess NO inhibits cytochrome c, critical in the mitochondrial respiratory chain (Chapter 11). In ischemia, the low tissue oxygen tension facilitates this inhibition (49); thus, the rate of oxidative metabolism decreases. Hypothetically, free radical formation is increased, the mitochondrial membrane is damaged, and cytochrome c is released with the risk of apoptosis (50). Although some of these effects may be directly attributed to NO, formation of the toxic free radical peroxynitrite contributes to cardiac damage in a mouse model of cardiomyopathy (51). These indirect adverse effects of NO are reflected in the "two faces of NO" (52). However, peroxynitrite is not only a "bad guy." It is normally formed from NO and in small amounts mediates cardioprotection by nitration of the protective PKC-ε isoform (11).

Nitric Oxide: Conclusions

One major physiologic function of NO is vasodilation via cyclic guanosine $3',5'$-monophosphate generated by guanylate cyclase. Second, NO modifies sympathovagal activity at the terminal sympathetic neurons where the action of acetylcholine is facilitated and the release of norepinephrine is inhibited. Exercise training may act in part by promoting sympathetic inhibition by NO. Third, NO, itself cardioprotective, may be converted to another free radical, the potentially toxic peroxynitrite, which is harmful to the vascular endothelium.

METABOLIC CONTROL OF GENES

Peroxisome Proliferator-Activated Receptors

PPARs received their name due to the ability of fibrates (cholesterol-lowering agents) to promote peroxisome proliferation in rat livers. In reality, PPARs are nuclear transcription factors that are activated by ligands (in addition to being activated by signaling kinases) such as by fibrates (53). The receptor component in the name is confusing because the ligand binds to PPAR in the nucleus as opposed to classical cell surface receptor–ligand interactions (e.g., insulin–insulin receptor, TNF-α and its receptors). Interestingly, in the heart, the α-isoform of PPAR is the most prevalent (54), and the major role of PPAR-α activation is to produce genes that regulate fatty acid oxidation. The concept of metacrine regulation is that the metabolic substrate long chain fatty acid acts as a ligand to activate PPAR-α. PPAR-α interacts (dimerizes) with another nuclear hormone receptor, the retinoid receptor (RXR) (Fig. 9-13) to activate transcription of target genes.

Physiologically, the results of gene activation by PPAR-α include induction of the gene's encoding fatty acid thereby regulating almost every step of fatty acid utilization including β oxidation (55). Pathologically, overload hypertrophy down-regulates PPAR-α expression to decrease fatty acid metabolism and hence to increase glucose metabolism so that oxygen is conserved (Chapter 13). Conversely, PPAR-α overexpression increases fatty acid oxidation and decreases glucose uptake and oxidation, thereby closely resembling the diabetic state (56).

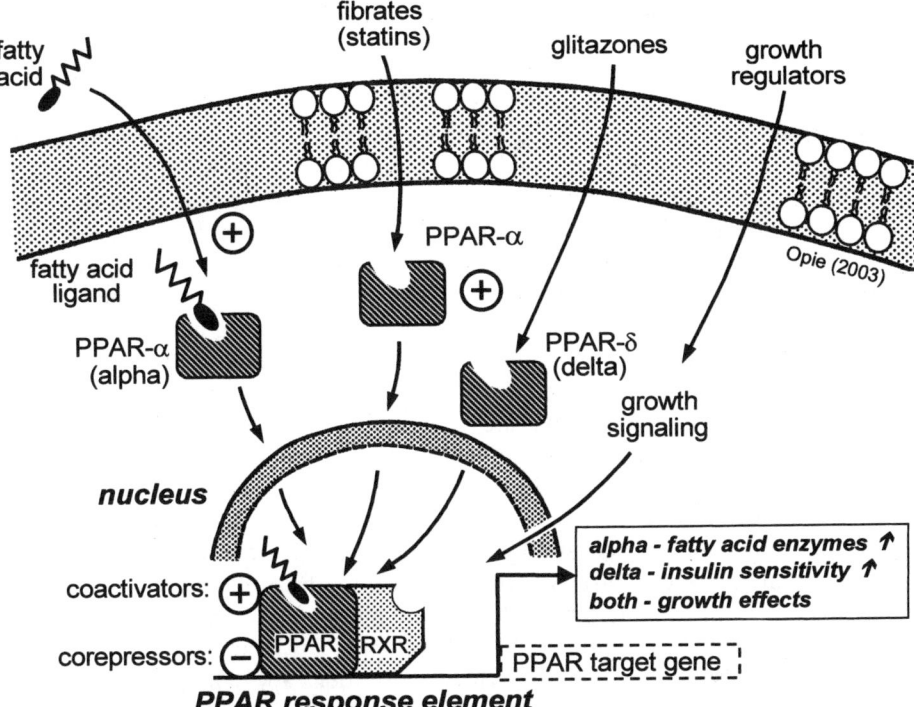

FIG. 9-13. Role of peroxisome proliferator-activated receptors (*PPARs*) in regulation of fatty acid and carbohydrate metabolism. PPARs are compounds that stimulate the PPAR receptors. They are activated in response to ligands such as fatty acids in the case of PPAR-α. PPARs act as transcription factors (Fig. 9-5) at the nuclear peroxisome response elements (*PPRE*), in the presence of the essential cofactor retinoid X receptor (*RXR*). Transcription proceeds to promote the formation of PPAR-responsive genes that, respectively, help to govern fatty acid oxidation in the case of PPAR-α and insulin sensitivity in the case of PPAR-γ. Thus, PPAR-α transactivates multiple genes encoding enzymes required for mitochondrial β oxidation.

In contrast, PPAR-γ is enriched in adipose tissue and controls the programs of fat storage by regulating lipolysis, hence influencing insulin resistance and glucose metabolism. In addition, PPAR-γ may transduce antihypertrophic signaling in the heart (54). The mechanism may either be overlap activation of the PPAR-α receptor or inhibition of the growth factor NF-κB.

Control by Fatty Acids and Glucose

Not only do enzyme activities regulate metabolic paths, but also metabolic flow regulates enzymes actively at the level of gene expression (Fig. 9-13). Thus, when the plasma free fatty acid level is high, increasing cardiac tissue free fatty acids activate PPAR-α, promoting the synthesis of the enzymes of fatty acid oxidation and of pyruvate dehydrogenase kinase. The latter inhibits pyruvate dehydrogenase and hence decreases glycolysis (Fig. 11-10), thereby increasing the contribution of fatty acids to metabolism (57).

In cardiac hypertrophy and heart failure, fatty acid oxidation enzyme gene expression is down-regulated, specifically that of the enzyme medium chain acyl–coenzyme A dehydrogenase (58). This is part of the induction of the fetal gene program, meaning reversion to the fetal pattern of metabolism with its greater reliance on glucose and glycolysis than on fatty acid metabolism. Additionally, the genes for atrial natriuretic peptide, glucose transporter 1 (GLUT-1), and other fetal genes are expressed. In the failing human heart, this process is accomplished simply by repression of the adult metabolic genes, thereby exposing the fetal genes and allowing them to be dominant (59). A key mechanism explaining the substrate switch from adult preference for fatty acids to the fetal reliance on glycolysis is down-regulation of PPAR-α. This induces a range of changes including the down-regulation of medium chain acyl–coenzyme A dehydrogenase (60). If PPAR-α is reactivated in the hypertrophic heart by an appropriate agonist, then the substrate switch is blocked and the isolated heart rapidly fails (60). Therefore, the proposal is that the substrate switch from fatty acid to carbohydrate metabolism is essential to maintain the mechanical function of the hypertrophic rat heart (60). The current challenge is to assess the extent to which these ideas apply to human left ventricular hypertrophy and heart failure.

SUMMARY

1. *The balance of life versus death.* The myocardium is in a constant state of flux, with factors promoting cell growth and survival being balanced by those promoting cell death. Cell growth occurs in response to stimulation of surface membrane receptors that respond to agonists, whether circulating or synthesized locally in the heart. Cell death occurs by several modes, with most attention currently devoted to programmed cell death or apoptosis. Transcription factors that act on the promoter regions of DNA are activated by kinase signaling sequences such as the MAP kinases.
2. *A-II is a crucial component of the renin–angiotensin–aldosterone regulatory system.* A-II stimulation activates diverse paths that lead to vasoconstriction, myocardial growth, and apoptosis. Common to these divergent effects are the A-II receptor with its subtypes, the G_q protein, the enzyme phospholipase C, and activation of PKC. Thereafter follows activation of the kinases that lead to the MAP kinase complex. Different responses to A-II, still not well understood, may be explained by the existence of receptor subtypes (AT-1 and AT-2), several PKC isoforms, different components of the MAP kinase complex, and two isoforms of p38 MAP kinase. Mobilization of calcium also plays a prominent role in the vasoconstriction.

3. *MAP kinases.* Many of the growth and prosurvival signals converge on the MAP kinase family that transit the signals from the cytosol to the nuclei where they promote the formation of mRNAs that lead to peptide generation, which, in turn, orchestrate prosurvival or proapoptotic consequences. The MAP kinase cascade carries the signals from the cell surface receptors by a series of kinases that sequentially phosphorylate and activate the next kinase, until reaching the MAP kinase complex. In general, but not always, stimulation of ERK is prosurvival, JNK is proapoptotic, and p38 MAP kinase can be either.
4. *Insulin promotes both growth and inhibits apoptosis.* Crucial signals are PI-3 kinase and Akt. Insulin stimulates the formation of insulin-like growth factor in myocardial cells, to further increase growth.
5. *Transcription factors.* Growth signals including A-II and insulin ultimately stimulate transcription factors via MAP kinases in the case of A-II and via Akt in the case of insulin. Transcription factors act on the promoter region of DNA to up-regulate the transcription of mRNA, which in turn conveys the signal to the ribosomes where polypeptide chains are made.
6. *Apoptosis, or programmed cell death,* is promoted by death receptor pathways and by mitochondrial release of cytochrome c. Both may converge on caspase-3, which churns up the cell nuclei to turn them into apoptotic bodies with cell death.
7. *Cytokines such as TNF-α may have cell protective or cell destructive effects,* mediated by different pathways and dependent on the strength and duration of the cytokine stimulation of the TNF-receptor. Corticotrophin-1 stimulates another receptor, gp-130, to mediate a protective path by activating JAK-STAT3.
8. *NF-κB* is a cytosolic factor that when activated travels to the nucleus where it is extremely promiscuous and potentially promotes the formation of a large number of genes. Several of the paths that it stimulates are growth promoting.
9. *ROS have definite adverse effects* and, for example, play a major role in the genesis of atheroma, apoptosis, and reperfusion injury. Nonetheless, they too have a physiologic function, being produced by the mitochondrial electron transfer chain and mediating protective signaling during the process of preconditioning.
10. *NO is a ubiquitous but short-lived messenger,* for example, conveying vasodilator signals from the vascular endothelium to vascular smooth muscle. This is a principle also used pharmacologically when the nitrate drugs are used to bring more blood to the oxygen-deprived heart. NO is also synthesized in the autonomic nervous system where it enhances the activity of the parasympathetic nervous system. When produced in excess, as when its production is up-regulated in septic shock, inhibitory effects on contraction and mitochondrial metabolism become evident.
11. *PPARs activate gene transcription to exert overall control over major metabolic pathways.* For example, PPAR-α is concerned with regulation of fatty

acid metabolism, and PPAR-γ with insulin resistance and glucose metabolism. Whereas PPAR-α promotes cardiac hypertrophy, PPAR-γ is antihypertrophic. These effects are still in the early stage of characterization, and the mechanisms not well understood.

12. *Metabolic gene expression.* In the failing heart, gene expression reverts to the fetal gene expression pattern with metabolism more dependent on glucose than on fatty acids.

REFERENCES

1. Gulick T, et al. The peroxisome proliferator-activated receptor regulates mitochondrial fatty acid oxidative enzyme gene expression. *Proc Natl Acad Sci U S A* 1994;91:11012–11016.
2. Sack MN, et al. Tumor necrosis factor in myocardial hypertrophy and ischaemia—an anti-apoptotic perspective. *Cardiovasc Res* 2000;45:688–95.
3. Sack MN. Tumour necrosis factor-a in cardiovascular biology and the potential role for anti-tumour necrosis factor-a therapy in heart disease. *Pharmacol Ther* 2002;94:1–13.
4. Nemoto S, et al. Role of mitochondrial oxidants as regulators of cellular metabolism. *Mol Cell Biol* 2000;20:7311–7318.
4a. Flesch M, et al. Differential regulation of mitogen-activated protein kinases in the failing human heart in response to mechanical unloading. *Circulation* 2001;104:2273–2276.
4b. Beltrami AP, et al. Evidence that human cardiac myocytes divide after myocardial infarction. *N Engl J Med* 2001;344;1750–1757.
4c. Gonzalez A, et al. Stimulation of cardiac apoptosis in essential hypertension. Potential role of angiotensin II. *Hypertension* 2002:39:75–80.
5. Sabri A, et al. Dual actions of the Ga_q agonist *Pasteurella multocida* toxin to promote cardiomyocyte hypertrophy and enhance apoptosis susceptibility. *Circ Res* 2002;90:850–857.
6. Crackower MA, et al. Angiotensin-converting enzyme 2 is an essential regulator of heart function. *Nature* 2002;417:822–828.
7. Yamada T, et al. Angiotensin II type 2 receptor mediates programmed cell death. *Proc Natl Acad Sci U S A* 1996;93:156–160.
8. Opie LH, et al. Enhanced angiotensin II activity in heart failure: reevaluation of the counterregulatory hypothesis of receptor subtypes. *Circ Res* 2001;88:654–658.
9. Minamino T, et al. MEKK1 is essential for cardiac hypertrophy and dysfunction induced by Gq. *Proc Natl Acad Sci U S A* 2002;99:3866–3871.
10. Abe J-C, et al. Kinase signaling in the cardiovascular system. In: Sperelakis N, ed. *Heart physiology and pathophysiology*, 4th ed. San Diego: Academic Press, 2001:657–677.
11. Balafanova Z, et al. Nitric oxide (NO) induces nitration of protein kinase Ce (PKCe), facilitating PKCe translocation via enhanced PCKe-RACK2 interactions. A novel mechanism of NO-triggered activation of PKCe. *J Biol Chem* 2002;277:15021–15027.
12. Tian R, et al. Long-term expression of protein kinase C in adult mouse hearts improves postischemic recovery. *Proc Natl Acad Sci U S A* 1999;96:13536–13541.
13. Baines CP, et al. Mitochondrial PKCi and MAPK form signaling modules in the murine heart. *Circ Res* 2002;90:390–397.
14. Takeishi Y, et al. Responses of cardiac protein kinase C isoforms to distinct pathological stimuli are differentially regulated. *Circ Res* 1999;85:264–271.
15. Pass JM, et al. Enhanced PKCbII translocation and PKCbII-RACK1 interactions in PKCe-induced heart failure: a role for RACK. *Am J Physiol* 2001;281:H2500–H2510.
16. Kalra D, et al. Angiotensin II induces tumour necrosis factor biosynthesis in the adult mammalian heart through a protein kinase C-dependent pathway. *Circulation* 2002;105:2198–2205.
17. Kholodenko BN. MAP kinase cascade signaling and endocytic trafficking: a marriage of convenience? *Trends Cell Biol* 2002;12:173–177.
18. Chien KR. Molecular basis of cardiovascular disease. In: Chien KR, ed. *A companion to Braunwald's heart disease*. Philadelphia: WB Saunders, 1999:221–221.
19. Sugden PH, et al."Stress-responsive" mitogen-activated protein kinases (c-Jun N-terminal kinases and p38 mitogen-activated protein kinases) in the myocardium. *Circ Res* 1998;83:345–352.

20. Abe J, et al. Role of mitogen-activated protein kinases in ischemia and reperfusion injury. The good and the bad. *Circ Res* 2000;86:607–609.
21. Bueno OF, et al. The MEK1-ERK 1/2 signaling pathway promotes compensated cardiac hypertrophy in transgenic mice. *EMBO J* 2000;2000:6341–6350.
22. Wang Y, et al. Cardiac muscle cell hypertrophy and apoptosis induced by distinct members of the P38 mitogen-activated protein kinase family. *J Biol Chem* 1998;273:2161–2168.
23. Thielmann M, et al. Myocardial dysfunction with coronary microembolization. Signal transduction through a sequence of nitric oxide, tumour necrosis factor-a, and sphingosine. *Circ Res* 2002;90:807–813.
24. Tamura S, et al. Regulation of stress-activated protein kinase signaling pathways by protein phosphatases. *Eur J Biochem* 2002;269:1060–1066.
25. Brand NJ, et al. Myocardial molecular biology: an introduction. *Heart* 2002;87:284–293.
26. White MF, et al. The insulin signalling system. *J Biol Chem* 1994;269:1–4.
27. Jonassen AK, et al. Myocardial protection by insulin at reperfusion requires early administration and is mediated via Akt and a p70s6 kinase cell-survival signaling. *Circ Res* 2001;89:1191–1198.
28. Matsui T, et al. Akt activation preserves cardiac function and prevents injury after transient cardiac ischemia in vivo. *Circulation* 2001;104:330–335.
29. Sugden PH, et al. Akt like a woman. Gender differences in susceptibility to cardiovascular disease. *Circ Res* 2001;88:975.
29a. Linzbach AJ. Heart failure from the point of view of quantitative anatomy. *Am J Cardiol* 1960;5:370–382.
30. Anversa P, et al. Myocyte growth and cardiac repair. *J Mol Cell Cardiol* 2002;14:91–105.
31. Haunstetter A, et al. Toward antiapoptosis as a new treatment modality. *Circulation* 2000;86:371–376.
32. Finkel E. The mitochondrion: is it central to apoptosis? *Science* 2001;292:624–626.
33. Eskes R, et al. Bid induces the oligomerization and insertion of bax into the outer mitochondrial membrane. *Mol Cell Biol* 2000;20:929–935.
34. Sawyer DB, Loscalzo J. Myocardial hibernation. Restorative or preterminal sleep? *Circulation* 2002;105:1517–1519.
35. Bradham WS, et al. Tumor necrosis factor-alpha and myocardial remodeling in progression of heart failure: a current perspective. *Cardiovasc Res* 2002;53:822–830.
36. Yamauchi-Takihara K, et al. A novel role for STAT3 in cardiac remodeling. *Trends Cardiovasc Med* 2000;10:298–303.
37. Palmieri EA, et al. Differential expression of TNFα, IL-6 and IGF-1 by graded mechanical stress in normal rat myocardium. *Am J Physiol* 2001;282:H926–H934.
38. Schultz JEJ, et al. TGF-β1 mediates the hypertrophic cardiomyocyte growth induced by angiotensin II. *J Clin Invest* 2002;109:787–796.
39. Force T, et al. Apoptosis signal-regulating kinase/nuclear factor-κB. A novel signaling pathway regulates cardiomyocyte hypertrophy. *Circulation* 2002;105:402–404.
40. Hirotani S, et al. Involvement of nuclear factor-κb and apoptosis signal-regulating kinase 1 in G-protein-coupled receptor agonist-induced cardiomyocyte hypertrophy. *Circulation* 2002;105:509–515.
41. Zhang DX, et al. Characteristics and superoxide-induced activation of reconstituted myocardial ATP-sensitive potassium channels. *Circ Res* 2001;89:1177–1183.
42. Smiesko V, et al. The arterial lumen is controlled by flow-related shear stress. *News Physiol Sci* 1993;8:34–38.
43. de Belder AJ, et al. Nitric oxide in the clinical arena [Editorial]. *J Hypertens* 1994;12:617–624.
44. Pinsky DJ, et al. Mechanical transduction of nitric oxide synthesis in the beating heart. *Circ Res* 1997;81:372–379.
45. Paulus WJ, et al. Nitric oxide and cardiac contractility in human heart failure. Time for reappraisal. *Circulation* 2001;104:2260–2262.
46. Chowdhary S, et al. L-arginine augments cardiac vagal control in healthy human subjects. *Hypertension* 2002;39:51–56.
47. Esplugues JV. NO as a signalling molecule in the nervous system. *Br J Pharmacol* 2002;135:1079–1095.
48. Paterson DJ. Nitric oxide and the autonomic regulation of cardiac excitability. *Exp Physiol* 2001;86:1–12.
49. Trochu J-N, et al. Role of endothelium-derived nitric oxide in the regulation of cardiac oxygen metabolism. Implications in health and disease. *Circ Res* 2000;87:1108–1117.

50. Moncada S, et al. Does nitric oxide modulate mitochondrial energy generation and apoptosis? *Nat Rev* 2002;3:214–220.
51. Mungrue IN, et al. Cardiomyocyte overexpression of iNOS in mice results in peroxynitrite generation, heart block and sudden death. *J Clin Invest* 2002;109:735–743.
52. Hoit BD. Two faces of nitric oxide. Lessons learned from the NOS2 knockout [Editorial]. *Circ Res* 2001;89:289–291.
53. Kelly DP. The pleiotropic nature of the vascular PPAR gene regulatory pathway. *Circ Res* 2001;89:935–937.
54. Frey N, et al. Modulating cardiac hypertrophy by manipulating myocardial lipid metabolism. *Circulation* 2002;105:1152–1154.
55. Kelly DP. Peroxisome proliferator-activated receptor a as a genetic determinant of cardiac hypertrophic growth. Culprit or innocent bystander? [Editorial]. *Circulation* 2002;105:1025–1027.
56. Finck BN, et al. The cardiac phenotype induced by PPARa overexpression mimics that caused by diabetes mellitus. *J Clin Invest* 2002;109:121–130.
57. Taegtmeyer H, et al. Adaptation and maladaptation of the heart in diabetes: part I. General concepts. *Circulation* 2002;105:1727–1733.
58. Sack MN, et al. Fatty acid oxidation enzyme gene expression is downregulated in the failing heart. *Circulation* 1996;94:2837–2842.
59. Razeghi P, et al. Metabolic gene expression in fetal and failing human heart. *Circulation* 2001;104:2923–2931.
60. Young ME, et al. Reactivation of peroxisome proliferator-activated receptor a is associated with contractile dysfunction in hypertrophied rat heart. *J Biol Chem* 2001;276:44390–44395.

PART IV

The Heart

10

Oxygen Supply: Coronary Flow

Lionel H. Opie and Gerd Heusch

No single mechanism predominates in control of coronary vascular tone: neural, humoral, and local metabolic control mechanisms all participate.

Muller et al. (1)

Because the work production and energy requirement of the heart vary so much from rest to exercise, there must be some system of variable oxygen delivery to the myocardium. Blood reaches the cardiac myocytes from the coronary circulation (Fig. 10-1). Changes in the coronary flow rate control the delivery of oxygen (Fig. 10-2). Blood leaving the heart in the coronary sinus is markedly deoxygenated and dark in color, and in response to myocardial hypoxia, little further extraction of oxygen is possible. When the heart needs more oxygen (as during exercise), the coronary blood flow must increase. Simultaneously, Gerlach in Germany and Berne (2) proposed that the myocardium communicates its oxygen requirements to the coronary arteries by the rate of production of adenosine. According to Berne's hypothesis, when the heart lacks oxygen (as during ischemia), the breakdown of only a small quantity of high-energy phosphate compounds, such as adenosine 5'-triphosphate (ATP), produces enough adenosine for powerful coronary vasodilation. This theory fails to explain events during exercise, so that there must be other vasodilator mechanisms, such as nitric oxide (NO) and activation of the ATP-sensitive potassium channel K_{ATP}. The activity of the autonomic nervous system plays an important ancillary role, in that neurogenic stimuli may restrain the extent of coronary vasodilation. The rate of release of norepinephrine from the terminal sympathetic neurons is subject to *neuromodulation*. Thus, vagal muscarinic activity decreases the rate of norepinephrine release, whereas angiotensin II increases the release (Fig. 10-3). The major vasodilator influence is the release of NO from the healthy endothelium. When the endothelium is damaged, it releases vasoconstrictive endothelin.

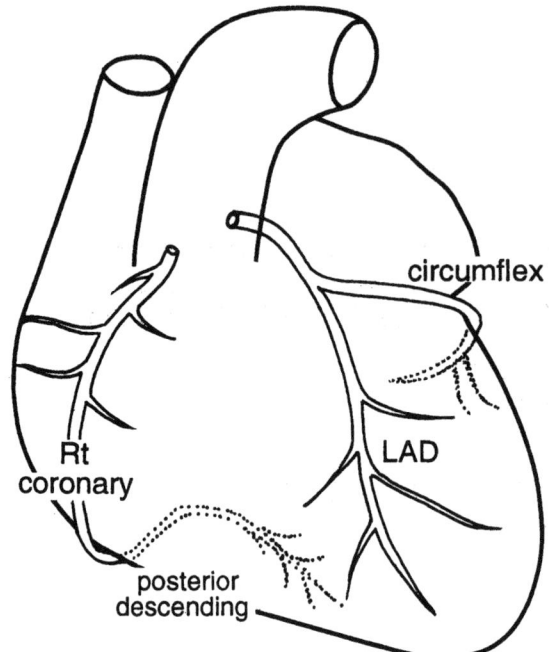

FIG. 10-1. Anatomy of major coronary arteries. LAD, left anterior descending.

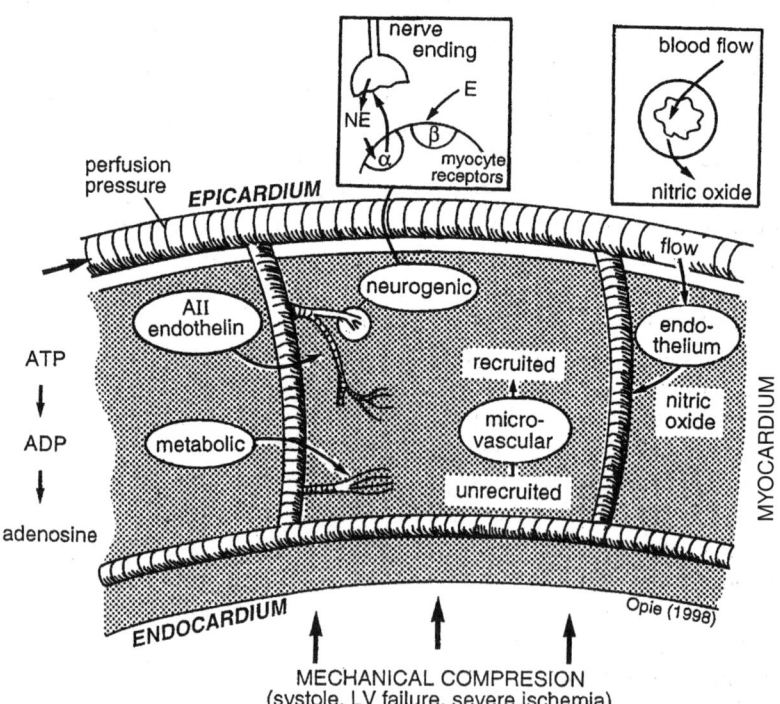

FIG. 10-2. Metabolic versus neurogenic control of the coronary circulation. Metabolic control is the basic mechanism, whereas neurogenic control is ancillary. *A-II*, angiotensin II; NE, norepinephrine; E, epinephrine.

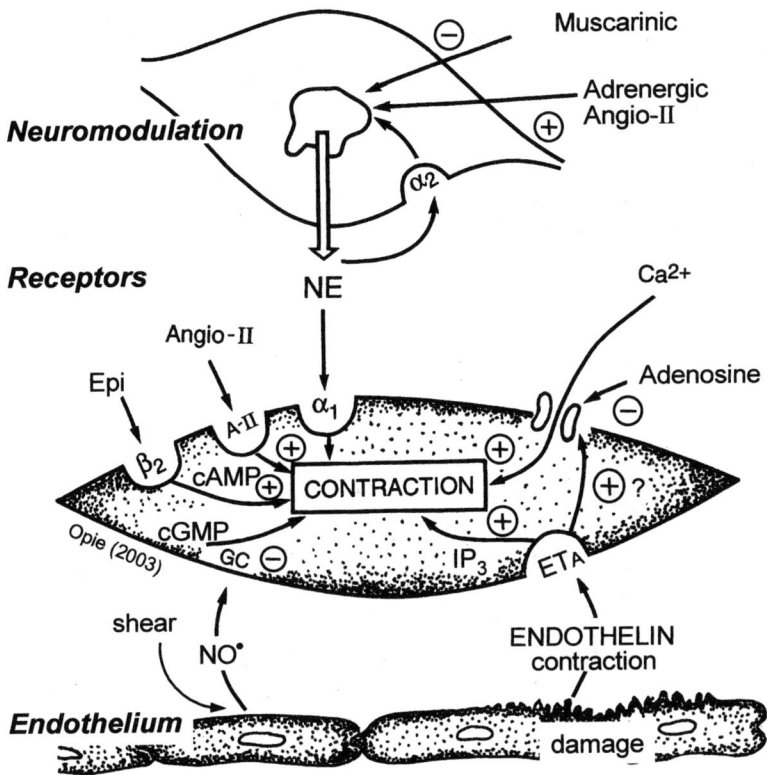

FIG. 10-3. Triple control of vascular contraction by neuromodulation, vascular receptors, and endothelium. Neuromodulation governs the rate of release of vasoconstrictive norepinephrine (*NE*), which is increased by adrenergic activation and angiotensin II (*AII*). The second site of control is at vascular receptors. Vasoconstrictive agonists include α_1- and α_2-adrenergic activity, angiotensin II, and endothelin. Vasodilatory stimuli include β_2-adrenergic agonist activity with formation of cyclic adenosine 3′,5′-monophosphate and the formation of nitric oxide with the formation of cyclic guanosine 3′,5′-monophosphate via guanylate cyclase (*Gc*). The endothelium may promote either relaxation via nitric oxide or, when damaged, vascular contraction by release of endothelin. Other endothelial factors not shown but involved include vasodilatory prostacyclin and vasoconstrictive thromboxane A_2. *Epi*, epinephrine; IP_3, inositol 1,4,5-triphosphate; ET_A, endothelin receptor subtype A. For guanylate cyclase, see Figure 9-12.

CORONARY CIRCULATION

The two major coronary arteries run from the base of the aorta to the left and right ventricles, respectively, before giving off branches that run down the surface of the heart toward the apex. The left coronary artery usually supplies the left ventricular wall. Its major branch is the left anterior descending coronary artery (anterior interventricular artery), which supplies part of the septum. This pattern varies from species to species and from individual to individual. In humans, the coronary arteries have attracted popular attention because when partially or completely occluded by coronary atherosclerosis (coronary artery disease), the myocardial oxygen supply becomes inadequate and the myocardium starts to suffer from the effects of lack of oxygen.

Resistance Versus Conductance Arterial Vessels

Just as the peripheral vascular resistance can be calculated from the aortic pressure divided by the cardiac output (Fig. 14-1), the coronary vascular resistance (CVR) is approximated by the formula

$$CVR = (aortic\ pressure/coronary\ flow)$$

From the point of view of regulation of coronary flow, there are two major types of arterial vessels: the small *resistance arterioles* because they are narrow and the resistance increases by a power of four as the radius decreases (Poiseuille law, Fig. 2-14), constituting the major resistance to flow and the large *conductance arteries* that govern the quantity of blood arriving at the resistance vessels. The coronary blood flow is proportional to the driving pressure across the coronary bed (coronary arterial pressure or blood pressure) divided by the resistance. Anatomically, the major coronary vascular resistance lies in the small coronary arterioles less than 150 µm in diameter (3), also called the autoregulatory vessels (see section on autoregulation).

Capillary Microcirculation

The control of the myocardial oxygen supply lies in the *coronary arterioles*, which keep on branching until the very small, thin-walled capillaries are formed. The microcirculation is that part of the coronary circulation concerned with the regulation of the terminal arterioles and capillaries, directly responsible for the transfer of oxygen from the oxygenated arterial blood to the myocardial tissues. These aspects of the coronary circulation are remarkably similar to the peripheral circulation. Capillary flow is governed not by the properties of the capillary itself but by tone of the feeder arteriole (Fig. 2-15).

In the normal heart, there are more than 2,000 capillaries per square millimeter, of which normally only between 60% and 80% are open and functioning. There is approximately one capillary per myofiber (Table 10-1). The number of function-

TABLE 10-1. *Microanatomy of oxygen supply of a myocardial cell*[a]

Capillaries per square millimeter; left ventricle	~2,500
Muscle fibers (myocytes) per square millimeter	~2,500
Muscle fiber diameter (µm)	17–18
Fiber-capillary ratio	1.0
Mean capillary diameter	3–4 µm
Intercapillary distance	17 µm
Diffusion distance (half of intercapillary)	8.5 µm

[a]Data from references 3a–3e.

TABLE 10-2. Recruitment of capillaries[a]

	Intercapillary distance (μm)	Diffusion distance (μm)
Normal	17	8.5
Exercise, estimated	14	7.0
Hypoxia	14.5	7.3
Prolonged anoxia	11	5.5
Maximal recruitment	6.5	3.3

[a]Data from references 3a–3e.

ing capillaries increases by recruitment if the arterial oxygen tension decreases (Tables 10-1 and 10-2). Each capillary is extremely narrow so that the myocardium accommodates this astonishing abundance of open capillaries. With a mean capillary diameter of approximately 3 to 4 μm, less than 5% of tissue volume is occupied. The normal intercapillary distance is approximately 17 μm (Table 10-1). During *arterial hypoxia*, the precapillary sphincters relax, more capillaries are recruited, and the intercapillary distance shrinks to 14.5 μm (Table 10-1). Prolonged anoxia reduces this distance further to 11 μm. These findings support Krogh's early idea of the regulation of capillary density by the metabolic demands of the tissue. In exercise, the coronary blood flow might double, but unless there is recruitment of capillaries with a reduction in intercapillary distance, the oxygen demands of the tissue cannot be met. Even reducing the intercapillary distance from 17 to 14 μm allows the oxygen to diffuse only to an additional 1.5 μm, which is an important adjustment to avoid tissue anoxia. Only after such microvascular changes have occurred and if oxygen deprivation is still severe are the reserves of oxygen dissolved in the tissue and in myoglobin used up.

Tissue Myoglobin

Myoglobin is an oxygen-binding hemoglobin-like compound found in low concentrations in the heart, approximately 0.25 mmol/L or 0.4 g/100 g. Even the small amounts of oxygen associated with myoglobin (as oxymyoglobin) may be important in intracellular oxygen transport because the partial pressure of oxygen required for half-maximal saturation of myoglobin is very low (2.4 mmHg) (4). In the normal heart, oxygen bound to myoglobin or tissue hemoglobin or dissolved in tissue water can maintain the heart for approximately 8 seconds or eight contractions in the absence of any coronary blood flow. Myoglobin is not only a reservoir for small amounts of oxygen but also facilitates the transport of oxygen (5).

Tissue Oxygen Tension

The cytochrome oxidase system in which oxygen acts in the mitochondria requires a remarkably low oxygen tension of less than 0.05 mmHg (O_2 concentration, 10^{-7} mol/L). This is the minimal effective tissue oxygen tension for oxidative phosphorylation (6). The oxygen tension required for mitochondrial function is approximately 2,000 times less than that in arterial blood (i.e., 100 mmHg). The average myocardial tissue P_{O_2} (oxygen tension) should lie between these values. To measure tissue oxygen tension with a needle microelectrode requires intracellular penetration and trauma, which can be circumvented by measuring P_{O_2} on the surface of the beating heart or calculating the P_{O_2} from the hemoglobin oxygen saturation in frozen myocardium. The same message emerges irrespective of the technique: there is a marked variation both in the oxygen content of the capillary hemoglobin and in the oxygen tension of myocardial tissue, with some values apparently approaching zero. Because of the wide variety of tissue P_{O_2} values, any given state of oxygenation is best described by a scatter diagram. As the P_{O_2} decreases, so does the scatter diagram change until most of tissue oxygen tensions are less than 5 mmHg. In addition, measurements of the state of oxygenation of various intracellular respiratory pigments show the probable existence of an intracellular gradient of oxygen tension from the cytosol to the mitochondria. The phasic patency of precapillary sphincters suggests that at any given overall level of capillary recruitment, some of the capillaries are opening and others closing all the time.

REGULATION OF CORONARY VASCULAR TONE

The metabolic needs of the myocardium are met by the control of the coronary blood flow, which is tightly coupled to the energy status of the cell. During increased heart work or ischemia, myocardial metabolism, sensitive to the workload and the prevailing oxygen tension of the medium, self-regulates energy metabolism mainly by release of adenosine and other vasodilator mediators. The latter act largely on the small coronary resistance arterioles and not on the large conductance arteries. Such metabolic vasodilation is restricted by approximately 30% by adrenergic vasoconstriction, mediated by α-adrenergic receptors (Table 10-3).

TABLE 10-3. *Coronary neurogenic control*

Innervation	Messenger	Receptor	Site and function
Adrenergic sympathetic	NE	α	Vasoconstrictive
		α_1	Larger conductance vessels
		α_2	Resistance vessels
	NE, E	β	Vasodilatory
		β_1	Larger vessels
		β_2	Resistance vessels
Cholinergic parasympathetic	ACh	Muscarinic	Vasodilation via nitric oxide (vasoconstriction when endothelium damaged)
Nonadrenergic noncholinergic nerves	CGRP[a]	CGRP receptors	Modest vasodilation by opening K_{ATP} channel[b]

NE, norepinephrine; E, epinephrine; ACh, acetylcholine; CGRP, calcitonin gene related peptide.
[a]Reference 6a.
[b]Reference 6b.

Vasoconstrictors Versus Vasodilators

Several neurogenic vasoconstrictor influences oppose metabolic vasodilation (Figs. 10-3 and 10-4). Adrenergic activation of α-receptors involves two types of postsynaptic receptors: the α_1 and α_2 subtypes. Both of these promote vasoconstriction, acting at least in part through the inositol 1,4,5-trisphosphate messenger system (Fig. 7-14). The net result of these vasoconstrictive stimuli is an increase in free cytosolic calcium in the vascular smooth cells with activation of myosin light chain kinase that leads to actin–myosin interaction. Vasoconstrictive adrenergic influences are opposed by vasodilatory influences such as the β-adrenergic vascular receptors and metabolic mechanisms such as NO, adenosine, and activation of the vascular ATP-dependent potassium channels (K_{ATP}). In addition, there are several platelet-derived substances, such as serotonin, that are vasodilatory only when the vascular endothelium is intact but become vasoconstrictive when the endothelium is damaged. Cholinergic stimulation, normally vasodilatory because it releases NO, also becomes vasoconstrictive when the endothelium is damaged. Thus, there are at least three essential regulators of

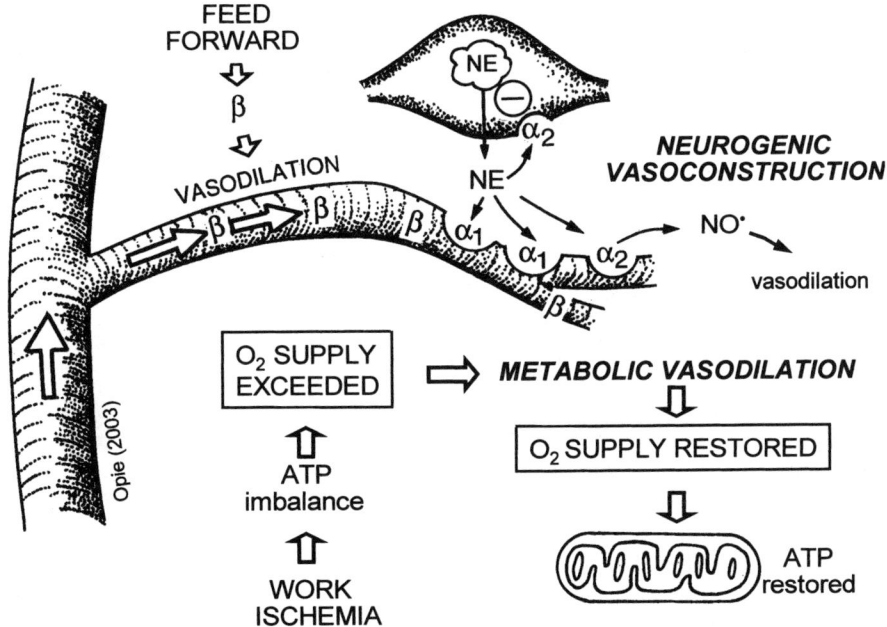

FIG. 10-4. Metabolic vasodilators. The role of vasodilators, including adenosine and nitric oxide (NO), in local metabolic control of the coronary circulation and the contrasting role of neurogenic vasoconstriction. As a result of heart work or ischemia, the rate at which the oxygen supply to the mitochondria can synthesize adenosine 3',5'-triphosphate (ATP) is temporarily exceeded so that ATP breaks down to form adenosine. NO is released from the healthy endothelium. Neurogenic factors are both vasodilatory (β-adrenergic) and vasoconstrictive (α-adrenergic). NE, norepinephrine.

coronary tone: (a) the metabolic vasodilatory system, (b) the neurogenic control system (more vasoconstrictive than vasodilatory), and (c) the vascular endothelium, which can be either vasodilatory by releasing NO or vasoconstrictive by releasing the peptide endothelin-1.

Endothelin-1 is one of the most powerful vasoconstrictors, especially in the diseased atherosclerotic arteries where endothelial damage is extensive (7). In addition, endothelin contributes to normal *coronary tone*, the latter being another term for the physiologic coronary vascular resistance. Another potential vasoconstrictor is angiotensin II, which couples to the same inositol 1,4,5-trisphosphate vasoconstrictive signal system as does endothelin and α-adrenergic receptor activation. Such angiotensin II–mediated vasoconstriction is probably of major significance only in diseased states. Of these complex control mechanisms, there is a major role for metabolic vasodilation in response to situations requiring an increased coronary blood flow, such as augmented heart work or ischemia.

Metabolic Vasodilation of Coronary Circulation

Local metabolic control appears to be the most important mechanism that matches increases in the oxygen consumption and metabolic demand of the heart to the required increase in coronary blood flow. Adenosine plays a critical but not solitary role in the local metabolic regulation of changes in the coronary circulation (Fig. 10-2). It does not help to maintain coronary vascular tone in basal or in normal physiologic conditions. *Adenosine* is formed within the myocardial cells when, as a result of hypoxia, ischemia, or vigorous heart work, high-energy phosphate compounds are broken down. Because the molar ratio of ATP to adenosine is very high, perhaps approximately 1,000:1, only a small decrease in ATP can activate the pathways producing adenosine, acting particularly at the level of the 5′-nucleotidase (Fig. 10-5). This enzyme converts adenosine 5′-monophosphate to adenosine at the inner border of the sarcolemma. Most of the adenosine leaves the cell to reach the extracellular space, where it acts on the arteriolar vessel wall as a vasodilator. Adenosine does not have to penetrate the vascular cell to vasodilate. It can dilate even when firmly attached to molecules that prevent penetration. It is supposed, however, that adenosine usually penetrates the vascular muscle cell, where it acts to vasodilate and then leaves into the extracellular space. Such adenosine reaches the circulation, where it is broken down by *adenosine deaminase* (Fig. 10-6), present both in red cells and in the vessel wall. Agents such as dipyridamole inhibit adenosine deaminase to allow large amounts of adenosine to accumulate. Thus, vasodilation is induced in both the ischemic and nonischemic zones, from which coronary collateral arteries bring blood into the ischemic zone. With vasodilation in the nonischemic zone, the driving pressure for the blood flow into the ischemic zone decreases. Less blood flows to the ischemic zone along the collaterals. This "collateral steal" means that these vasodilator agents have limited antianginal potential. The methylxanthines, including the bronchodilator theophylline, compete with adenosine for the vascular sites, thereby inhibiting the vasodilation caused by adenosine.

10. OXYGEN SUPPLY: CORONARY FLOW

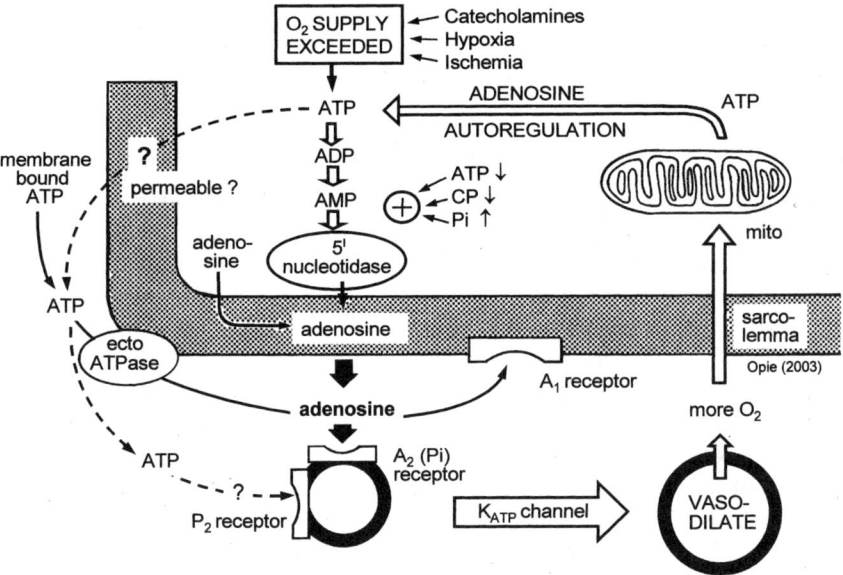

FIG. 10-5. Adenosine as a vasodilator. Adenosine formed from adenosine 3′,5′-triphosphate (*ATP*) in conditions of increased myocardial work or hypoxia interacts with a vascular A_2 receptor (Table 7-1) to cause vasodilation. ATP may be an additional dilator acting on the purinergic receptor (P_2, subtype 2). *CP*, creatine phosphate; *Pi*, inorganic phosphate; *ADP*, adenosine 5′-disphosphate; *AMP*, adenosine 5′-monophosphate; *MITO*, mitochondria.

Purinergic Receptors

Adenosine is a purine compound and acts on purinergic receptors. These are further subdivided into the P_1-receptors sensitive to adenosine and the P_2-receptors sensitive to ATP (Fig. 10-5). The P_1-receptors can be further subdivided into the *A_1-myocardial receptors* and *A_2-vascular receptors* (Table 7-1). The myocardial receptors inhibit the formation of cyclic AMP and hyperpolarize nodal cells (Fig. 5-8), so that adenosine in high doses can arrest the heart. The vascular A_2-receptors situated on the vascular smooth muscle cells stimulate the formation

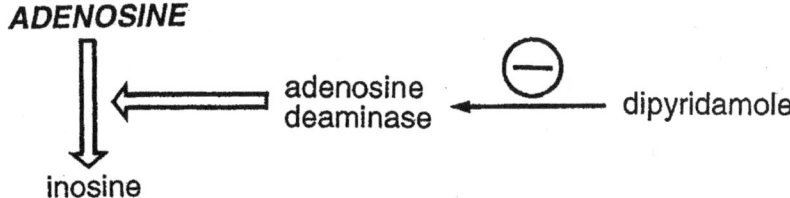

FIG. 10-6. Coronary vascular reserve is measured by the principle of maximal vasodilation achieved, for example, by the inhibition of adenosine deaminase activity by the drug dipyridamole.

of vasodilatory cyclic adenosine 3′,5′-monophosphate (Fig. 10-3). There are additional mechanisms for vasodilation by adenosine, involving production of NO by the endothelium (8) and vasodilation via the K_{ATP} channel.

Nitric Oxide and Endothelium-Dependent Dilation

An intact vascular endothelium is crucial in determining vascular smooth muscle tone (Fig. 10-3). In response to well-defined stimuli, healthy endothelial cells liberate a very short-lived vasodilatory factor, NO. NO vasodilates because it stimulates guanylate cyclase in the vascular smooth muscle to form vasodilatory cyclic guanosine 3′,5′-monophosphate (Fig. 9-12) and inhibits platelet aggregation by increasing the platelet level of cyclic guanosine 3′,5′-monophosphate to decrease platelet cytosolic calcium. Therefore, the risk of occlusion of small arterioles in response to physiologically induced platelet aggregation is decreased. NO is released by vascular shear forces associated with increased coronary flow (9) (Fig. 10-3). When the coronary perfusion pressure increases, as in exercise, the flow also tends to follow suit. The increased blood flow releases more NO from the endothelium. Adenosine, acting on the endothelial K_{ATP} channels, also elicits the production of NO (8).

When the endothelium is damaged, as in coronary artery disease, the release of NO is diminished and the release of vasoconstrictive endothelin is increased. In the presence of coronary artery disease and endothelial damage, platelet aggregation occurs and is likely to release vasoconstrictive factors from the endothelium, which may precipitate myocardial ischemia. In such conditions, the vasoconstrictive stimuli overcome metabolic vasodilation.

Interactive Roles of Adenosine, Nitric Oxide, and K_{ATP} Channel

The adenosine hypothesis is widely accepted as explaining part of the coronary vasodilation resulting from hypoxia or ischemia. During physiologic exercise, the evidence that adenosine plays a dominant role is conflicting, and factors such as endothelium-dependent formation of NO and activation of the K_{ATP} channel are probably at work. When the vascular K_{ATP} channel opens, it hyperpolarizes the vascular smooth muscle cells to cause coronary vasodilation (Fig. 17-6). These channels are normally inhibited by ATP, even in low concentrations, which explains why they contribute to the basal coronary tone (10). Adenosine is one of the factors that relieve the ATP inhibition. Thus, when adenosine formation is increased, as in severe heart work or ischemia (Fig. 11-20), this mechanism may operate. The interaction between these three metabolic vasodilators (i.e., adenosine, NO, and the K_{ATP} channel) is not fully determined. In dogs, opening of the K_{ATP} channels is the main mechanism, with adenosine and NO coming into play when these K channels are blocked by the antidiabetic drug glibenclamide (11). In contrast, in pigs, sequential blocking of each of these three vasodilators show that they operate in parallel (12). Some evidence suggests that humans are more like pigs than dogs (12).

Other Metabolic Vasodilators

A decreasing tissue oxygen and increasing carbon dioxide tension (PCO_2) may account for approximately 40% of the changes in coronary flow during pacing. Hypoxia may act as a vasodilator by opening the ATP-sensitive potassium channels. An increasing PCO_2 may act similarly to intracellular acidosis.

Protons produced by anaerobic metabolism have a direct effect in causing coronary vasodilation and sensitize the coronary arteries to the effects of added adenosine.

ATP is normally found within the cell and does not cross the sarcolemma, and there is an unexpected and controversial proposal that small amounts of superficial ATP (Fig. 10-4) liberated by hypoxic or working heart muscle into the circulation can have a vasodilatory effect. Measurements of ATP and adenosine in the effluent from the hypoxic heart argue against a direct vasodilatory role of ATP.

Potassium in a modestly increased concentration is also vasodilatory, whereas very high values vasoconstrict. The mechanisms involved are complex and include effects on neurotransmitters and adrenergic receptors as well as release of NO by potassium. When extracellular potassium is sufficiently high, it will depolarize the cell membrane to increase the opening probability of the calcium channel, leading to vasoconstriction.

Atrial natriuretic peptide is released from the atria in response to stretch and promotes diuresis and renal loss of sodium. In addition, atrial natriuretic peptide is an arterial vasodilator, acting on guanylate cyclase.

Prostaglandins can be released into coronary venous blood when angina is provoked by rapid pacing of the heart. It is not surprising, therefore, that prostaglandins have been regarded as physiologic vasodilators. These early observations have been supported by the isolation of *prostacyclin*, which is produced by the endothelium and powerfully relaxes coronary arteries and inhibits platelet aggregation. The real role, if any, for other prostaglandins in the control of the coronary circulation is still controversial.

AUTONOMIC CONTROL

Sympathetic stimulation activates vasoconstrictive α-adrenergic receptors in the coronary arteries (Fig. 10-7). Whether such α-mediated vasoconstriction serves any physiologic function, as opposed to a clear role in disease (13), is still not clear. One view is as follows: Suppose that during exercise, as part of sympathetic stimulation, there is increased α-adrenergic receptor activation with constriction of arterioles greater than 100 μm in diameter, then the lowered pressure in the downstream arterioles could induce myogenic vasodilation.

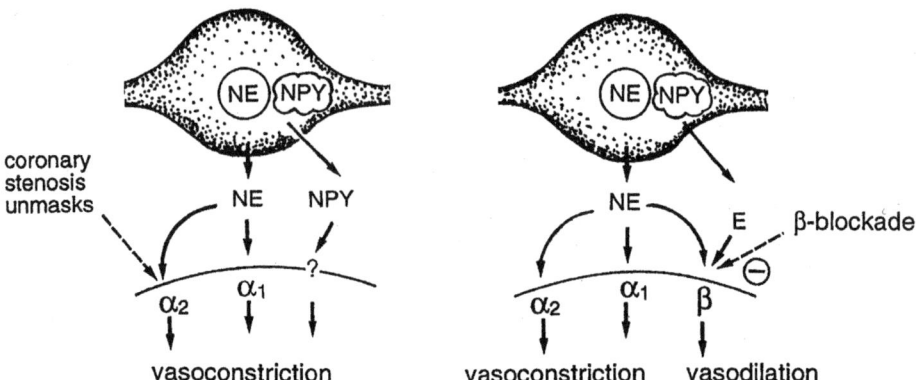

FIG. 10-7. Neurogenic vasodilation. Physiologically, the catecholamines norepinephrine (*NE*) and epinephrine (*E*) both mediate coronary vasodilation by β-adrenergic effects. Their positive inotropic effect will also indirectly promote vasodilation. In coronary disease, norepinephrine released from the terminal neurons (shown above) may cause vasoconstriction. Increasing coronary stenosis may unmask α_2-mediated vasoconstriction. β-Adrenergic blockade by propranolol may promote unopposed vasoconstriction. *NPY*, neuropeptide Y, a vasoconstrictor coreleased with norepinephrine (35) and hypothetically playing a role in coronary spasm.

Adrenergic Receptor Subtypes

α_1-Receptor–mediated coronary vasoconstriction acts mainly on the larger coronary arteries, whereas both α_1- and α_2-receptor activity are involved in regulating the degree of vasoconstriction of the smaller resistance vessels (13). Enhanced sympathetic tone may increase flow through small arterioles when the circulation is healthy. When there is a decrease in coronary perfusion pressure, then vasoconstriction mediated by both receptor subtypes occurs throughout the coronary microcirculation (1). Thus, in the presence of coronary disease, adrenergic stimuli such as emotional stress, cold exposure, or smoking could lead to a relative preponderance of α-adrenergic vasoconstrictive mechanisms, with increased risk of myocardial ischemia (13). α_2-Postjunctional adrenergic receptors could have greater functional significance when adrenergic activity is enhanced, as in heart failure. Experimentally, coronary stenosis unmasks α_2-adrenergic activity, perhaps because endothelial damage removes the vasodilatory effects of NO. Studies on patients show a distribution of α_1- and α_2-adrenergic receptors similar to that found in animals (14).

Neuropeptide Y is costored and coreleased with norepinephrine from adrenergic terminal neurons, and the ratio of its release to that of norepinephrine increases with sympathetic stimulation (Fig. 10-7). Neuropeptide Y is concentrated around the coronary arteries and is a potent and long-lasting vasoconstrictor. It contributes to myocardial ischemia in patients with coronary artery disease (15).

Vasodilatory Coronary Vascular β-Adrenergic Receptors

In addition to vasoconstrictive α-adrenergic receptors, there are coronary β-adrenergic receptors that should, when stimulated, lead to vasodilation. It might be expected that coronary β-receptors should be of the noncardiac $β_2$ subtype, yet the contrary may be true (16). Different β-receptor subtypes may regulate coronary resistance in the small vessels ($β_2$-receptors) than in the larger vessels (mainly $β_1$). In large human coronary arteries, $β_1$-receptors dominate and are localized to the muscular medial layer (16). According to the *feedforward* hypothesis, β stimulation by norepinephrine causes vasodilation of healthy coronary arteries, independently of any increase in heart rate or contractility (17). In the presence of a diseased endothelium, however, norepinephrine is likely to have predominantly coronary vasoconstrictive effects.

Cholinergic Coronary Vasodilation

Acetylcholine, the cholinergic messenger, is a powerful coronary vasodilator when given in supraphysiologic doses by the intracoronary route in the presence of an intact endothelium, acting by release of NO. Yet with vagal stimulation, the dilator response is transient and weak.

To summarize these extremely complex control mechanisms, the major effect of sympathetic α-adrenergic stimulation is vasoconstriction to increase the tone of both large and small coronary arteries, and this is overridden by metabolic vasodilation. The net effect is coronary vasodilation during exercise when the coronary arteries are healthy, but when they are diseased and the endothelium does not secrete NO, then overall vasoconstriction is more likely (13).

CORONARY FLOW VARIATIONS

Reactive hyperemia is a phenomenon somewhat better explained by the metabolic than by the neurogenic theories of coronary control. When the coronary arteries are transiently occluded and then reperfused, there is a period of apparent overperfusion as the blood flow increases substantially for a short period. Such reactive hyperemia can be found in patients in whom the coronary artery is briefly occluded by a balloon during percutaneous transluminal angioplasty, a procedure used increasingly to relieve some types of coronary artery disease. Adenosine appears to be involved because when adenosine receptors are blocked by theophylline, reactive hyperemia is reduced by 40% to 100% (18). Also, in response to intracoronary adenosine, there is marked coronary hyperemia similar to that caused by papaverine (18). Additionally, flow-induced vasodilation may be operative (1). The complex mechanisms, mainly metabolic, whereby coronary blood flow can increase severalfold to meet the increased demands placed on the circulation during exercise emphasize the capacity for coronary vasodilation.

Phasic Coronary Flow

The changing intraventricular pressures during the cardiac cycle will alter coronary flow (Fig. 10-8). During systole, subendocardial but not subepicardial arteries are compressed (19). An important hypothesis is that systolic blood flow in the subendocardium decreases and even stops as the left ventricular pressure increases to compress the arteriolar lumen, whereas conversely, subendocardial blood flow increases in diastole. Of the total coronary flow, most occurs in diastole. The remaining component occurs in systole but mainly in the epicardial zone. Early diastolic flow, which is the peak flow rate, can be impaired when the rate of myocardial relaxation in early diastole decreases, as in ischemia and reperfusion (20). When the coronary perfusion pressure is increased experimentally, for example, by an increased pulse pressure (Fig. 10-9), then both systolic and diastolic components of epicardial flow increase, with diastolic flow dominating (21).

When the normal phasic coronary flow is impaired, there is greater risk of periodic platelet aggregation, especially in the presence of endothelial damage, which can worsen the reduction in the cyclical flow.

Coronary Autoregulation

The process whereby coronary flow is regulated independently of the arterial perfusion pressure is called *coronary autoregulation*, which basically means that coronary blood flow stays relatively constant within wide limits of blood pres-

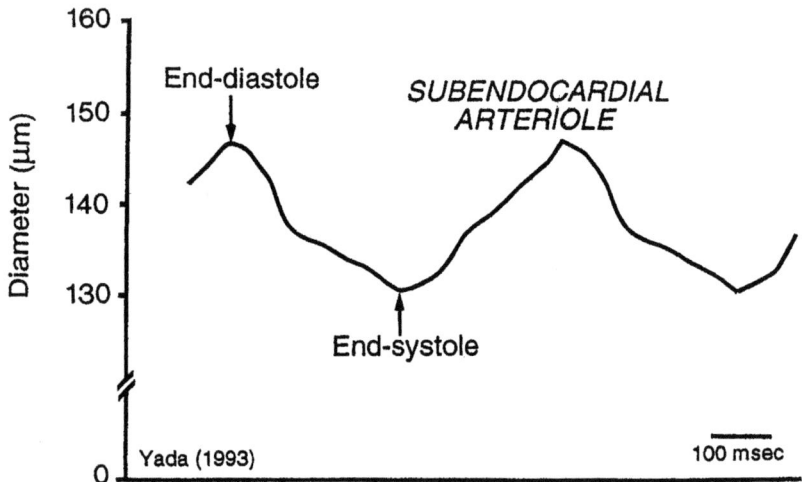

FIG. 10-8. Subendocardial arteriolar diameter in systole and diastole. (Adapted from Yada T, et al. In vivo observation of subendocardial microvessels of the beating porcine heart using a needle-probe videomicroscope with a CCD camera. *Circ Res* 1993;72:939–946.)

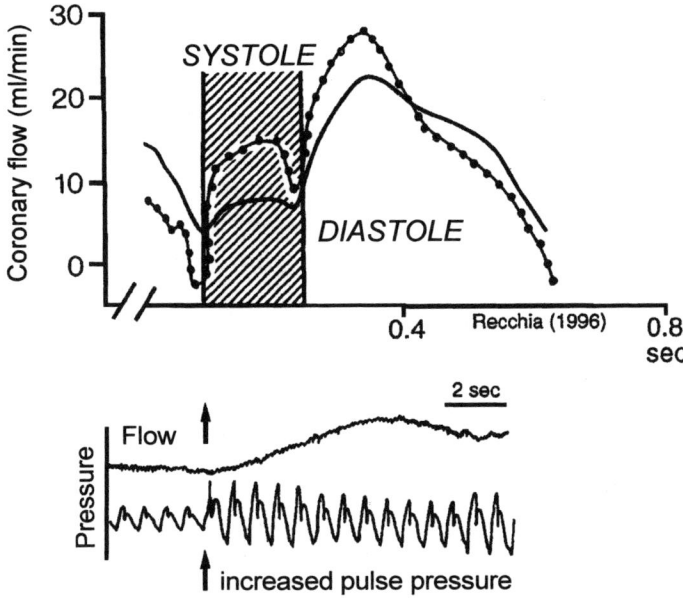

FIG. 10-9. Phasic coronary flow: effects of systole and diastole on phasic coronary flow in dogs. The *dotted lines* indicate increased pulse pressure (bottom panel) as may occur during exercise. (Adapted from Recchia FA, et al. Pulse pressure-related changes in coronary flow in vivo are modulated by nitric oxide and adenosine. *Circ Res* 1996;79:849–856.)

sure changes (Fig. 10-10). This mechanism helps to protect the myocardium against sudden changes in blood pressure. Most of the autoregulation takes place in coronary arterioles larger than 150 μm in diameter, but smaller arterioles can be recruited as the perfusion pressure progressively decreases (22). There are definite limits to autoregulation above which an increased perfusion will augment coronary flow and below which myocardial ischemia will result. In the presence of severe coronary stenosis, when the coronary perfusion pressure drops to less than 50 mmHg, coronary autoregulation is progressively lost. The signal systems involved in autoregulation are not fully understood. At the lower end of the range, formation of adenosine and NO and opening of the vascular K_{ATP} channel may all play a role.

Myogenic Control

Such control originates in the intrinsic properties of the vascular smooth muscle (hence the name myogenic). Vascular smooth muscle responds to increased force by contracting, so that an alternate name is stretch-induced contraction. That is, as the distending pressure across the vessel wall increases, so does the inherent vascular tone and vice versa. The inherent tendency of an increased

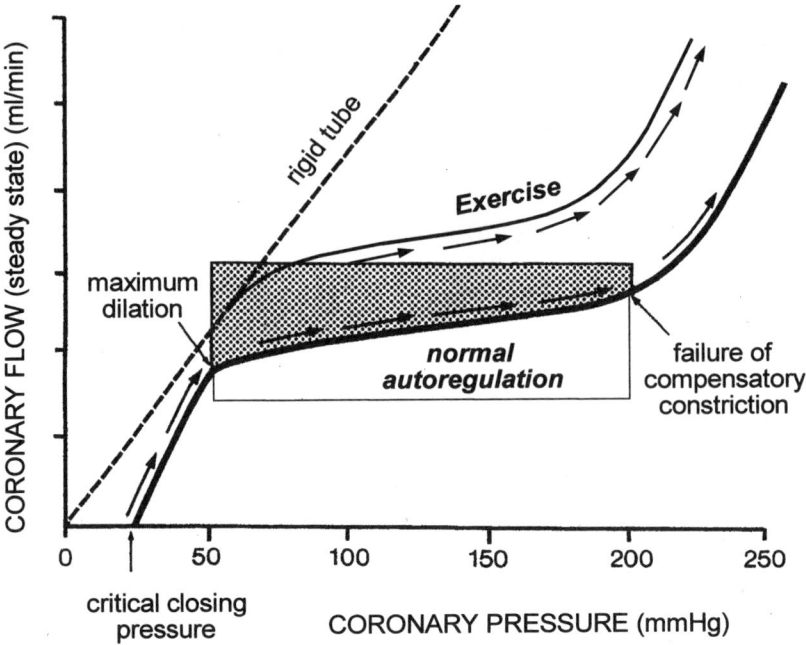

FIG. 10-10. Coronary autoregulation maintains coronary flow within a rather narrow range despite large variations in coronary perfusion pressure. When maximal metabolism-induced dilation at low pressures becomes inadequate, then the relationship between coronary pressure and flow becomes like that of a rigid tube. At the other extreme, with very high pressures, compensatory neuroconstriction fails with much increased coronary flow. Note that exercise-induced vasodilation provides a greater coronary flow throughout the range of autoregulation.

intravascular pressure to distend the vessel is opposed, so that myogenic control could contribute to coronary autoregulation, particularly in coronary arterioles less than 100 μm in diameter (1). The mechanism of myogenic tone is not understood, but stretch-activated channels could be important.

Exercise

Coronary blood flow can more than double during acute exercise in conscious dogs (9), and in humans, the flow may increase threefold during heavy exercise. The explanation includes the greater pulse pressure of exercise (Figs. 10-9 and 15-8). Factors improving coronary flow may include β-adrenergic–induced vasodilation and flow-induced formation of NO. When NO synthesis is inhibited, then the coronary vasodilation of exercise is much lower. Such formation of NO is probably induced by the effect of mechanical shear stress on the endothelium, with perhaps the release of adenosine playing a role (8). NO may have an additional metabolic effect by decreasing the myocardial oxygen uptake for a given workload (23), i.e., rendering the heart more efficient and decreasing the oxygen requirement.

The "Garden Hose" and "Erectile" Effects

To review, the accepted view is that the coronary arteries dilate in response to an increased myocardial oxygen demand. There is also some evidence of an opposite sequence of events, as originally found by Gregg (24). The proposed explanation may be that the greater coronary flow may stiffen the ventricle, thereby increasing the oxygen demand (25). Colorful names such as the "garden hose" or "erectile" effect have perhaps given this phenomenon more prominence than it deserves. Nonetheless, it is logical that as coronary flow decreases during coronary occlusion, there will be a reversed erectile effect as the arteries empty, so that the ischemic segments will have less work to do (26).

MYOCARDIAL ISCHEMIA AND CORONARY FLOW

Before considering the complex and highly variable effects of coronary disease on coronary flow, we need to evaluate the consequences of ischemia (an inadequate coronary blood flow). Experimental ischemia vasodilates by at least two mechanisms. First, there will be a breakdown of ATP to adenosine (Fig. 10-5). Second, a decreasing local level of ATP (and accumulation of adenosine 5'-diphosphate and adenosine) will activate the ATP-sensitive potassium channel K_{ATP}. Opening of this channel may contribute to early potassium loss from the ischemic myocardium and to the associated electrocardiographic changes (Fig. 17-6). Even during exercise, such ischemia-induced vasodilation is not maximal, possibly owing to the influence of neurogenic vasoconstriction induced by α-adrenergic receptor stimulation (13) or the commonly associated endothelial dysfunction. Hypothetically, drugs closing this channel, such as the oral antidiabetic agent glibenclamide, may prevent ischemia-mediated vasodilation. Therefore, in diabetic patients with acute myocardial infarction, it is preferable to avoid such oral agents and to change antidiabetic therapy to insulin.

Coronary Artery Disease

The effects of coronary artery disease on the coronary arteries are highly variable, from diffuse damage to a localized narrowing or stenosis. The direct hemodynamic effect of coronary stenosis is to decrease the coronary perfusion pressure in the distal segment of the diseased artery. Second, the indirect effect of tissue ischemia causes contractile failure, thereby increasing the left ventricular end-diastolic pressure, which in turn compresses subendocardial tissue and reduces coronary perfusion further to increase ischemia (Fig. 10-8). Third, as discussed in the preceding section, ischemia has direct vasodilatory effects on the coronary circulation, acting by the formation of adenosine and NO, and opening of the vascular K_{ATP} channels. Fourth, because the vascular endothelium is damaged in coronary artery disease, such vasodilatory stimuli are usually overcome by a variety of vasoconstrictive forces including neurohumoral mechanisms (27) and endothelin.

To reduce coronary flow by stenosis requires a very large decrease in arterial lumen. The most important factor is the severity of the stenosis and the consequent increase in resistance to blood flow across the stenosis. The resistance increases by a power of 4 as the radius decreases (Poiseuille law), and reducing the internal diameter from 80% to 90% dramatically elevates the resistance (Fig. 10-11). Resting flow is not affected until the stenosis is very severe, and one estimate is that a 70% reduction in internal diameter with a 90% to 95% decrease in luminal area is required for basal coronary flow to decrease. When the internal diameter is reduced beyond 30%, the response to those stimuli normally increasing coronary flow starts to be impaired.

For a given severity of stenosis, the longer the stenotic segment, the more marked the effects of any given degree of occlusion. For any given degree of *fixed coronary stenosis*, there are complex additional factors, such as the degree of turbulence across the stenosis and added vascular spasm, which may further decrease the flow (*dynamic stenosis*). The mechanism is probably by enhanced release of endothelin-1 from the damaged endothelium (7).

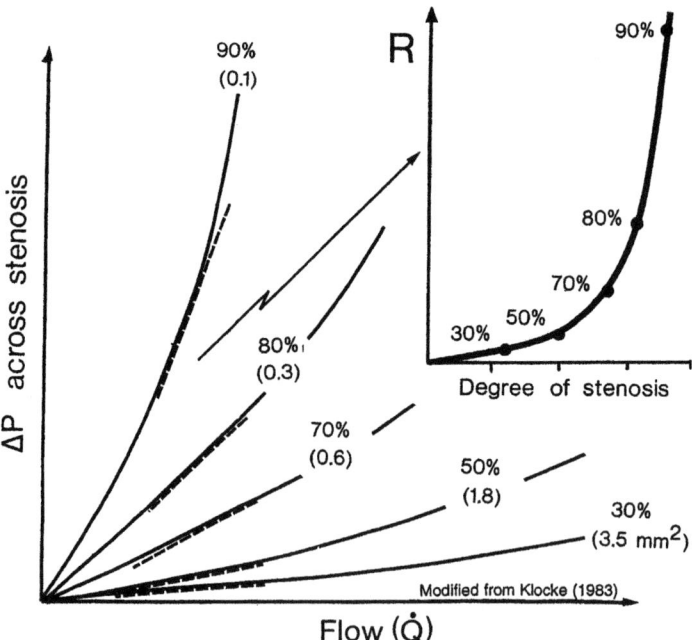

FIG. 10-11. Coronary stenosis and vascular resistance. The effect of the severity of coronary stenosis (internal diameter) on vascular resistance (*R*) (36), %, percentage of reduction in internal diameter.

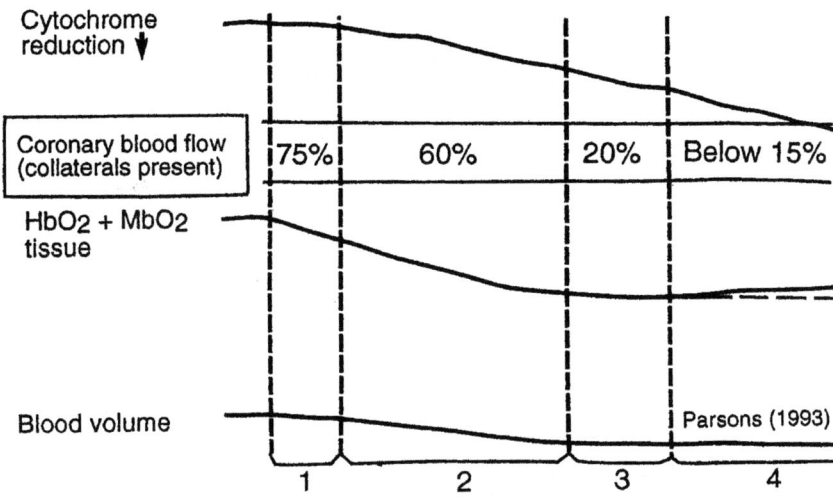

FIG. 10-12. Progressive flow reduction in left anterior descending coronary artery in the dog. Note the initial protective role of tissue oxygen stores during progressive chemical reduction of respiratory chain cytochrome enzymes. HbO_2 and MbO_2, oxygenated forms of hemoglobin and myoglobin. (Modified from Parsons WJ, et al. Myocardial oxygenation in dogs during partial and complete coronary artery occlusion. *Circ Res* 1993;73:458–464.)

As the coronary blood flow decreases to less than the limits of autoregulation (Fig. 10-10), the extraction of oxygen from the arterial blood increases. Nonetheless, because extraction is normally nearly complete (28), this mechanism cannot fully compensate so that tissue oxygen stores of hemoglobin and myoglobin decrease, and the respiratory chain cytochromes become less oxidized. When the myocardial blood flow decreases to less than 50% of control, tissue oxygen stores decrease to a minimum (Fig. 10-12), and any further flow reduction means that the respiratory chain becomes even less oxidized (Fig. 10-12). The result is the development of anaerobic metabolism (Fig. 11-2).

Anatomic Site of the Occluded Artery: Collateral Flow

The severity of ischemia is greater when a main left coronary artery rather than a branch is restricted, probably because collateral flow is better maintained with smaller ischemic lesions resulting from branch occlusions. Once severe subendocardial ischemia has occurred, left ventricular failure compresses the coronary arteries further, and an advancing wavefront phenomenon occurs and the epicardial zones are eventually involved (Fig. 10-13). At the other end of the spectrum, mild ischemia, detected only during exercise, can cause a small reversible decrease of regional function (29).

The *collateral flow* is the coronary blood flow reaching the ischemic zone by means of alternate arteries that have developed and supply the zone that was for-

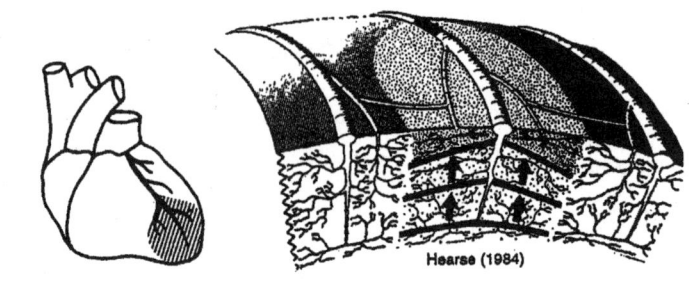
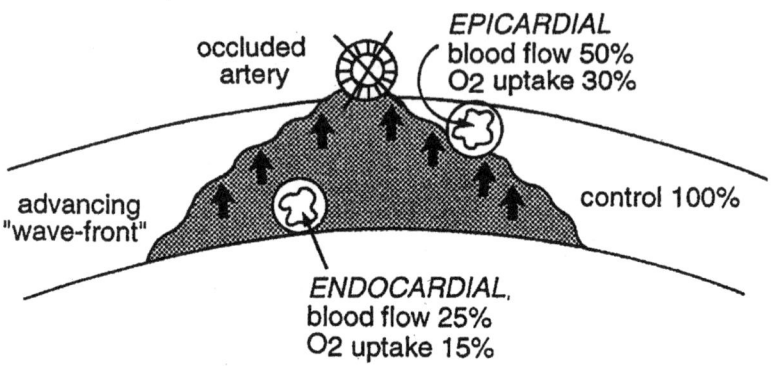

FIG. 10-13. Complete coronary occlusion damages subendocardial tissue first. A wavefront phenomenon then involves the epicardial zones, according to the model of Reimer et al. (*Circulation* 1977;56:786–794). The mechanism is probably by a progressive increase in subendocardial pressure as the left ventricle fails. %, percentage of control. (Upper right panel courtesy of Prof. David Hearse, St. Thomas' Hospital, London, UK.)

merly reached by the occluded artery (*collateral*, coming in from the side). In some species, such as the guinea pig, collateral flow is so extensive that even complete coronary artery occlusion by ligation results in no detectable ischemia. In other species, such as the rat, the flow is so low that very severe ischemia results, as Schaper (30) so eloquently stated, "guinea pigs win the rat race." In humans, it is thought that gradual coronary occlusion provokes a variable growth of collateral arteries, and the results of complete arterial occlusion vary significantly from patient to patient. Never is the collateral flow high enough in humans to align them to guinea pigs.

Subendocardial Ischemia

A traditional point of view has been that the subendocardial zone of the heart has a lower oxygen tension and a more anaerobic type of metabolism. The lower oxygen tension should cause a lower oxygen uptake. In reality, subendocardial

TABLE 10-4. Metabolic vasodilation

Agent	Site of action	Signal system
Adenosine	Resistance arterioles	A_2 receptor, promotes formation of vasodilatory cAMP
Nitric oxide	Resistance arterioles	Guanylate cyclase, cGMP
ATP	ATP-sensitive K^+ channel	Decreased ATP and increased adenosine remove inhibition by ATP on channel opening

cAMP, cyclic adenosine 3′, 5′-monophosphate; cGMP, cyclic guanosine 3′, 5′-monophosphate; ATP, adenosine 5′-triphosphate.

layers, being subject to greater mechanical stress, require an increased oxygen uptake, which accounts for the lower tissue oxygen tension and higher rates of oxidative metabolism (Table 10-4). A higher rather than lower capillary density in the endocardial zones also supports the idea of a higher rate of oxidative metabolism in the subendocardium. These metabolic factors may, in addition to blood flow factors, account for the increased vulnerability of the subendocardium to ischemic damage with increased risk of necrosis (Fig. 10-13).

CORONARY ARTERY VASOCONSTRICTION AND SPASM

Besides anatomic stenosis resulting from coronary artery disease, a second mechanism of coronary artery narrowing is by vasoconstriction (Fig. 10-14). Sometimes, especially in the large epicardial arteries, intense vasoconstriction is focal and called *coronary spasm*. When the narrowing caused by such spasm is added to organic coronary artery disease, the term is *dynamic stenosis*, which can be relieved by drugs inducing coronary vasodilation, such as the nitrates or calcium antagonists. Clinically, the degree of vasoconstriction or coronary spasm is thought to be variable, with the critical finding being the induction of myocardial ischemia at rest and not by effort as in the case of classic angina. The result can vary from a minor degree of vasoconstriction shown only by particular changes on the electrocardiogram (asymptomatic ST-segment deviations, thought to result from different degrees of ischemic loss of potassium) to transmural ischemia with severe chest pain at rest and the typical ST-segment elevation of what is called *Prinzmetal's angina*.

There are two explanations for the association of spasm and organic stenosis. First, platelet thrombi may form at the stenotic site to liberate agents, such as serotonin and thromboxane A_2, which are vasoconstrictive in the presence of endothelial damage. Leukocytes may liberate other vasoconstrictive substances called *leukotrienes*. Second, coronary atheroma damages the vascular endothelium with decreased production of several vasodilating substances, including NO and the vasodilatory prostaglandin (PGI_2), and enhanced production of vasoconstrictive mediators, including endothelin and angiotensin II (27). Endothelin is actively produced at sites of organic stenosis by macrophages and can medi-

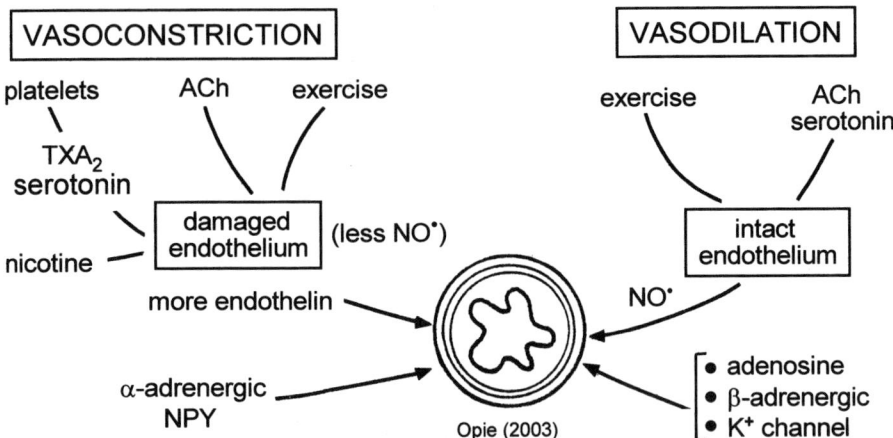

FIG. 10-14. Endothelium and coronary diameter. The endothelium plays an important role in determining the degree of coronary vasoconstriction or coronary vasodilation in response to some stimuli such as acetylcholine (*ACh*), exercise, and serotonin released from damaged platelets. When the endothelium is intact, exercise, acetylcholine, and serotonin are all vasodilatory, acting by release of nitric oxide (*NO*). Exercise may act by the release of adenosine, by β-adrenergic stimulation, by stimulation of the K_{ATP} channel (K^+ channel), and by flow-mediated release of NO. With endothelial damage, these factors promote vasoconstriction, possibly by the release of endothelin. In addition, β-adrenergic stimuli become vasoconstrictive instead of vasodilatory. Besides releasing serotonin, platelets also release thromboxane A_2 (*TXA₂*). Vasoconstrictive stimuli enhance the risk of coronary vasoconstrictive spasm. *NPY*, neuropeptide Y. See Figure 10-7.

ate the increased tone (7). Cigarette smoking promotes coronary spasm (31) hypothetically by causing endothelial damage. Nonetheless, the exact vasoconstrictive mechanism in coronary artery spasm in humans still has not been identified despite intensive studies.

Abnormal Coronary Vasomotion

The normal coronary response to exercise is vasodilation, whereas in coronary disease, there is vasoconstriction, also called abnormal vasomotion (13). Likewise in hypertensives, there is impaired coronary vasodilation on exercise, even when there is no visible angiographic evidence of coronary artery disease (32). The most probable explanation is that both coronary disease and hypertension cause endothelial dysfunction.

MYOCARDIAL BLOOD FLOW MEASUREMENTS

Whereas coronary blood flow can be measured experimentally by several techniques, including flow probes, the actual rate of delivery of blood to the myocardium requires different techniques. In animals, *microspheres* provide a very accurate index of regional myocardial blood flow. Such microspheres are injected into the circulation and are then caught in the capillaries throughout the heart. The dissected tissue is analyzed, and the flow in that segment of tissue is proportional to the counts. Using this method, coronary blood flow can be measured even in minute areas of the myocardium. If different radionuclide traces are used, coronary blood flow before or after an intervention can be quantified precisely. Microsphere data in dogs show a normal resting myocardial blood flow of approximately 100 mL/100 g per minute with approximately 70 mL/100 g per minute in pigs. *Positron emission tomography* (PET) in humans uses ^{13}N-ammonia as an indicator of myocardial blood flow (33). The principle is that dynamic imaging monitors the uptake and retention of the tracer ^{13}N-NH$_3$. Technical refinements allow the separation of the first arrival phase, dependent on blood flow, with distinction from the later myocardial retention phase, which depends on conversion of the ammonia into the amino acid glutamine. It is assumed that the rate of conversion of ammonia to glutamine remains constant and can be compensated for mathematically. Even if uncorrected, however, this factor is only approximately 10%. The rate constant (K_1) for delivery of ^{13}N-NH$_3$ into the tissue incorporates a mass factor (i.e., positrons emitted per unit mass), so that the myocardial blood flow is ultimately given as, for example, 90 to 100 mL/100 g per minute (33). Similar values are found if H$_2$^{15}O is used as the tracer; this technique allows more frequent repetition of flow measurements because of the shorter half-life of ^{15}O than of ^{13}N, but the image quality is better with ^{13}N (34). Values for myocardial blood flow obtained by PET in humans correspond well with those of other techniques and with microsphere data in large animals such as dogs and pigs. PET can also image glucose extraction. It is possible, therefore, to compare the uptake of ^{18}F-deoxyglucose relative to that of ^{13}N-ammonia, the ratio being increased in reversible ischemia. The major problems with PET are its great expense and limited spatial and transmural resolution.

Thallium-201 (^{201}Tl) is an analogue of potassium, and its uptake by the myocardium is impaired in ischemia. The myocardial distribution of ^{201}Tl is the result of two processes. The initial distribution reflects the distribution of the coronary blood flow to the various zones of the myocardium. The second phase of redistribution reflects actual uptake by the myocardial cells. The uptake of thallium by the myocardium depends on the same sodium–potassium pump (Na$^+$/K$^+$/ATPase) that transports potassium, but thallium binds 10 times more avidly at two sites instead of one site for potassium. In the underperfused but potentially viable myocardium, both the uptake and washout of ^{201}Tl are slow, so that in time, the levels of radioactivity in the normal and ischemic zones tend to equalize. In infarcted, scarred myocardium, the tissue cannot take up ^{201}Tl, and no equalization can occur. These differences can be useful in distinguishing the potential viability of poorly contracting myocardial segments. Nonetheless, thallium studies do not give absolute blood flow measurements.

Quantitative coronary angiography with blood flow measurements can be achieved by combining angiography to give the coronary diameter and Doppler ultrasonography to give the flow velocity. Such a combination yields continuous measurement of coronary blood flow but does not give myocardial perfusion (13).

CORONARY FLOW RESERVE

The *coronary vascular reserve* (or coronary vasodilatory reserve or coronary flow reserve) is measured by the ratios of the coronary flow found during the period of reactive hyperemia and the basal coronary flow. Methods of achieving maximal flow include (a) intracoronary administration of the drug dipyridamole, which inhibits the breakdown of adenosine (Fig. 10-6) and (b) the evocation of maximal hyperemic flow after the transient ischemia caused by injection of the radioopaque contrast material used for coronary angiography or after percutaneous transluminal angioplasty. Coronary vascular reserve is reduced in ischemic heart disease, by chronic smoking, and in the hypertrophied myocardium of chronic hypertension or aortic stenosis. Mechanisms by which coronary vascular reserve is reduced in the hypertrophied myocardium, even in the absence of any apparent coronary artery disease, may relate either to small vessel damage (microvascular disease) or to endothelial damage evoked by the shear forces associated with a sustained blood pressure increase.

SUMMARY

1. *Capillaries.* The myocardium has a very rich supply of capillaries, with approximately one capillary for each myofiber. Normally, not all the capillaries are open. Recruitment, or opening up of capillaries, occurs when the myocardial oxygen demand increases during exercise or ischemia, so that the available oxygen has a shorter distance to diffuse to the mitochondria where it is required.
2. *Regulation of the caliber of the coronary arterial tree.* There are five major systems. First, there is the resting coronary vascular tone. Second, metabolic mechanisms increase coronary flow in response to exercise or ischemia. A small fraction of the ATP broken down is converted ultimately to the vasodilator adenosine, which, however, is less important than previously expected. Third, the healthy vascular endothelium produces the important vasodilator NO. Fourth, neural stimulation also regulates the extent of vasodilation. Adrenergic stimulation causes both vasodilatory β-adrenergic stimuli and vasoconstrictive α-adrenergic stimuli. Fifth, myogenic control at the level of the muscles of the arterioles is still poorly understood but important.

3. *During exercise,* coronary flow increases substantially. Flow-mediated release of NO from the endothelium is important, but all the exact signals are not yet known.
4. *Ischemia promotes vasodilation,* acting both by formation of adenosine and by opening of the ATP-sensitive potassium channels.
5. *In coronary artery disease,* the vascular endothelium is damaged, with decreased release of NO and increased activity of vasoconstrictive mediators. The normal vasodilatory effect of ischemia per se is often overcome by the effects of associated endothelial dysfunction, which results in endothelium-mediated coronary vasoconstriction or even spasm.
6. *PET measures coronary blood flow* in humans by monitoring the uptake of ^{13}N-NH_3. It is a powerful tool when combined with the uptake of glucose to estimate the viability of tissue in coronary artery disease.

STUDENT QUESTIONS

1. Describe the autonomic control of the coronary arteries.
2. What is NO and where and how is it formed? What are its physiologic effects in the coronary system?
3. What is the coronary vascular resistance? Why is it important?
4. What is coronary autoregulation? Propose a mechanism for this effect.
5. How does metabolic vasodilation take place?

CARDIOLOGIST-IN-TRAINING QUESTIONS

1. Why does the coronary blood flow increase during exercise?
2. What role does the vascular endothelium play in the physiologic regulation of coronary blood flow?
3. What is endothelial dysfunction and what role may it play in altering the response to ischemia?
4. How may coronary disease alter normal physiologic coronary vascular responses?
5. Describe the principles of measurement of myocardial blood flow in humans.

REFERENCES

1. Muller JM, et al. Integrated regulation of pressure and flow in the coronary microcirculation. *Cardiovasc Res* 1996;32:668–678.
2. Berne RM. Regulation of coronary blood flow. *Physiol Rev* 1964;44:1–29.
3. Balaban RS, et al. Function, metabolic and flow heterogeneity of the heart. The view is getting better. *Circ Res* 2001;88:265–267.
3a. Bourdeau-Martini J, et al. Dual effect of oxygen on magnitude and uniformity of coronary intercapillary distance. *Am J Physiol* 1974;226:800–810.
3b. Honig CR, Bourdeau-Martini J. Extravascular component of oxygen transport in normal and hypertrophied hearts with special reference to oxygen therapy *Circ Res* 1974;34/35[Suppl 2]:97–103.

3c. Kreuzer, Turek. In: Tenhoor et al., ed. *Oxygen supply of heart and brain*. The Hague: Dutch Heart Foundation, 1979:48–62.
3d. Tomanek et al. Quantitative changes in the capillary bed during developing, peak, and stabilized cardiac hypertrophy in the spontaneously hypertensive rat. *Circ Res* 1982;51:295–304.
3e. Wittenburg JB. Myoglobin facilitated oxygen transport diffusion: role of myoglobin in oxygen entry into muscle. *Physiol Rev* 1970;50:559–636.
4. Tamura M, et al. Optical measurements of intracellular oxygen concentration of rat heart in vitro. *Arch Biochem Biophysiol* 1978;191:8–22.
5. Merx MW, et al. Myoglobin facilitates oxygen diffusion. *FASEB J* 2001;15:1077–1079.
6. Chance B. Pyridine nucleotide as an indicator of the oxygen requirements for energy-linked functions of mitochondria. *Circ Res* 1976;38[Suppl I]:I-31–I-38.
6a. Yaoita H, et al. Nonadrenergic noncholinergic nerves regulated basal coronary flow via release of capsaicin-sensitive neuropeptides in the rat heart. *Circ Res* 1994;75:780–788.
6b. Nelson MT, Braydin JE. Regulation of arterial tone by calcium-dependent K^+ channels and ATP-sensitive K^+ channels. *Cardiovasc Drugs Therap* 1993;7:605–610.
7. Kinlay S, et al. Role of endothelin-1 in the active constriction of human atherosclerotic coronary arteries. *Circulation* 2001;104:1114–1118.
8. Hein TW, et al. cAMP-independent dilation of coronary arterioles to adenosine. Role of nitric oxide, G proteins and K_{ATP} channels. *Circ Res* 1999;85:634–642.
9. Wang J, et al. Chronic exercise enhances endothelium-mediated dilation of epicardial coronary artery in conscious dogs. *Circ Res* 1993;73:829–838.
10. Farouque HMO, et al. Effect of ATP-sensitive potassium channel inhibition on resting coronary vascular responses in humans. *Circ Res* 2002;90:231–236.
11. Ishibashi Y, et al. ATP-sensitive K^+ channels, adenosine and nitric oxide-mediated mechanisms account for coronary vasodilation during exercise. *Circ Res* 1998;82:346–359.
12. Merkus D, et al. Coronary blood flow regulation in exercising swine involving parallel rather than redundant vasodilator pathways. *Am J Physiol Heart Circ Physiol* 2003 (*in press*).
13. Heusch G, et al. α-Adrenergic coronary vasoconstriction and myocardial ischemia in humans. *Circulation* 2000;101:689–694.
14. Gregorini L, et al. Effects of selective α_1- and α_2-adrenergic blockade on coronary flow reserve after coronary stenting. *Circulation* 2002;106:2901–2907.
15. Gullestad L, et al. Postexercise ischemia is associated with increased neuropeptide Y in patients with coronary artery disease. *Circulation* 2000;102:987–993.
16. Amenta F, et al. Autoradiographic localization of β-adrenergic receptors in human large coronary arteries. *Circ Res* 1991;68:1591–1599.
17. Miyashiro JK, et al. Feedforward control of coronary blood flow via coronary β-receptor stimulation. *Circ Res* 1993;73:252–263.
18. Wilson RF, et al. Effects of adenosine on human coronary arterial circulation. *Circulation* 1990;82: 1595–1606.
19. Yada T, et al. In vivo observation of subendocardial microvessels of the beating porcine heart using a needle-probe videomicroscope with a CCD camera. *Circ Res* 1993;72:939–946.
20. Domalik-Wawrzynski LJ, et al. Effect of changes in ventricular relaxation on early diastolic coronary blood flow in canine hearts. *Circ Res* 1987;61:747–756.
21. Recchia FA, et al. Pulse pressure-related changes in coronary flow in vivo are modulated by nitric oxide and adenosine. *Circ Res* 1996;79:849–856.
22. Chilian WM, et al. Coronary microvascular responses to reductions in perfusion pressure. Evidence for persistent arteriolar vasomotor tone during coronary hypoperfusion. *Circ Res* 1990;66: 1227–1238.
23. Heusch G, et al. Endogenous nitric oxide and myocardial adaptation to ischemia. *Circ Res* 2000;146: 146–152.
24. Gregg DE. Effect of coronary perfusion pressure or coronary flow on oxygen usage of the myocardium. *Circ Res* 1963;13:497–500.
25. Iwamoto T, et al. Coronary perfusion related changes in myocardial contractile force and systolic ventricular stiffness. *Cardiovasc Res* 1994;28:1331–1336.
26. Schulz R, et al. No effect of coronary perfusion on regional myocardial function within the autoregulatory range in pigs. Evidence against the Gregg phenomenon. *Circulation* 1991;83:1390–1403.
27. Zhang C, et al. Divergent roles of angiotensin II AT_1 and AT_2 receptors in modulating coronary microvascular function. *Circ Res* 2003;92:322–329.

28. Parsons WJ, et al. Myocardial oxygenation in dogs during partial and complete coronary artery occlusion. *Circ Res* 1993;73:458–464.
29. Lee J-D, et al. Exercise-induced regional dysfunction with subcritical recovery stenosis. *Circulation* 1986;73:596–605.
30. Schaper W. Experimental infarcts and the microcirculation. In: Hearse DJ, et al., eds. *Therapeutic approaches to myocardial infarct size limitation*. New York: Raven Press, 1984:79–90.
31. Sugiishi M, et al. Cigarette smoking is a major risk factor for coronary spasm. *Circulation* 1993;87:76–79.
32. Frielingsdorf J, et al. Normalization of abnormal coronary vasomotion by calcium antagonists in patients with hypertension. *Circulation* 1996;93:1380–1387.
33. Camici PG, et al. The impact of myocardial blood flow quantitation with PET on the understanding of cardiac diseases. *Eur Heart J* 1996;17:25–34.
34. De Silva R, et al. Role of positron emission tomography in the investigation of human coronary circulatory function. *Cardiovasc Res* 1994;28:1595–1612.
35. Warner MR, et al. Sinus and atrioventricular nodal distribution of sympathetic fibers that contain neuropeptide gamma. *Circ Res* 1990;67:713–721.
36. Klocke FJ. Measurements of coronary blood flow and degree of stenosis: current clinical implications and continuing uncertainties. *J Am Coll Cardiol* 1983;1:31–41.

11

Fuels: Aerobic and Anaerobic Metabolism

Lionel H. Opie and Gary D. Lopaschuk

"Metabolism—the lost child of cardiology."
Taegtmeyer (1)

Every day the human heart uses between 3.5 and 5 kg of adenosine 5'-triphosphate (ATP) to keep pumping. For this process, it needs a continuous supply of oxygen, delivered by a coronary circulation that is sufficiently flexible to meet increases in energy needs (e.g., during exercise). The heart also requires a constant supply of fuels, mainly glucose or fatty acids, which are delivered by the coronary circulation. When taken up into the heart cells, these fuels are broken down by the pathways of intermediary metabolism to the two-carbon fragment acetyl-CoA, which can enter the citrate cycle in the mitochondria (Fig. 11-1).

The uptake of fuels by the heart depends partly on their arterial concentrations and partly on the energy demand. When the blood supply is normal, the supply of oxygen and fuels is also normal, and the heart derives energy from the breakdown and oxidation of either fatty acids or glucose. When there is lack of oxygen, as in coronary artery disease or during exercise, oxidative metabolism decreases and glycolysis (the breakdown of glucose) is stimulated (Fig. 11-2). Glycolysis can provide limited amounts of energy in the form of ATP even in the absence of oxygen (anaerobic ATP). Note that although anaerobic means without air (from the Greek), this term is often more loosely used to indicate partial rather than total lack of oxygen. When the blood flow is substantially reduced, as in severe ischemia, the delivery of both oxygen and glucose decreases, and glycolysis may decrease. Thus, severe ischemia causes metabolic changes that limit the capacity of the tissue to survive.

WHY METABOLISM MATTERS

These patterns of substrate metabolism are not just of theoretical interest. Physiologic facts are now being translated into clinical understanding and therapy. As

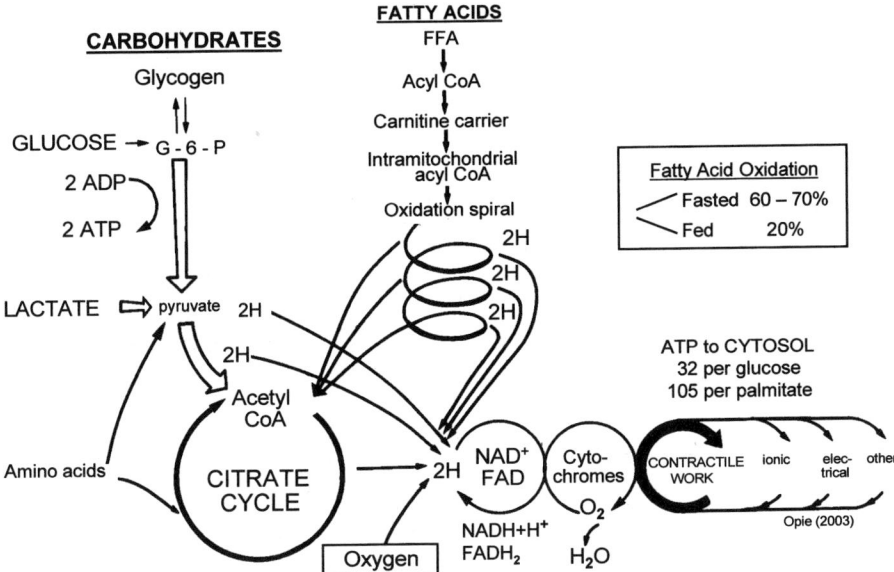

FIG. 11-1. How carbohydrates and fatty acids yield energy for contractile work. The crucial processes are those by which the fuels (glucose and fatty acids) are simplified for entry into the Krebs cycle that lies within the mitochondria. There production of protons (*H*) within the yields energy in the form of adenosine 5′-triphosphate that is mostly used for contractile work.

is argued, glucose metabolism and glycolysis protect the threatened heart, whereas fatty acid metabolism is harmful to the ischemic heart. Myocardial ischemia, as occurs in angina pectoris (Chapter 17), is a metabolic condition resulting from the oxygen lack, so that metabolic therapy becomes appropriate. In acute heart attacks (myocardial infarction), severe oxygen lack is not the only factor that kills cells. The accompanying stress reaction leads to excess β-adrenergic stimulation with high blood levels of free fatty acids (FFAs) that in turn are taken by the heart to turn off glucose metabolism. In severe myocardial hypertrophy and heart failure (Chapter 16), the heart undergoes gene reprogramming, so that the normal adult pattern of metabolism, described previously, is replaced by a fetal program so that "regulated pathways become misregulated pathways," with major therapeutic implications that we are now just beginning to understand (2).

FUELS OF THE HUMAN HEART

For its major sources of energy, the heart alternates between carbohydrates in the fed state and fatty acids in the fasted state, as suggested by Bing (2b) in the early 1950s. In the fasted state, blood FFAs are high. The high rates of uptake of fatty acids are preferentially used for oxidative metabolism (Table 11-1, Fig. 11-3), so that fatty acids become the major source of energy (3,4). When fatty acids

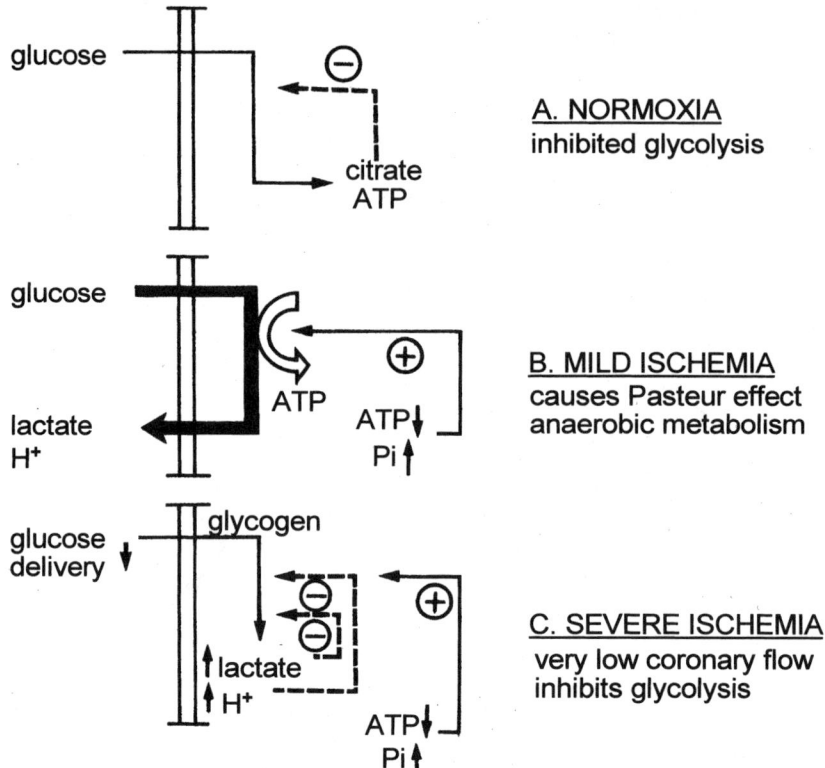

FIG. 11-2. Glycolysis. A: In the normally oxygenated heart, free fatty acids are the preferred fuel, and tissue citrate and adenosine 5′-triphosphate (*ATP*) are high, to inhibit glycolysis. **B:** When coronary flow is mildly decreased (mild ischemia), glycolysis is stimulated. **C:** In severe ischemia (severe deprivation of both oxygen and coronary flow), the decreased delivery of glucose and glycogen depletion as well as the accumulation of lactate and protons all inhibit glycolysis despite any tendency to acceleration by a low cardiac content of ATP. *Pi*, inorganic phosphate.

TABLE 11-1. *Fuels for oxidative metabolism of the human heart: ratio of oxygen uptake accounted for by extraction of various substrates if fully oxidized*

Conditions	Glucose (OER %)	Pyruvate (OER %)	Lactate (OER %)	Total CHO (OER %)	FFA + (TG) (OER %)
Insulin, low glucose[a]	6	44	51	101	3
Feeding	–	–	–	92	5
CHO meal[b]	68	4	28	100	–
Lipid meal	10	–	10	20	30 + (50)
Fasting, few hours[c]	31	2	28	61	34
Exercise	16	0	61	77	21
Exercise, recovery	21	2	36	59	36
Fasting overnight	27	1	11	38	62 + (14)

[a]Reference 2a.
[b]Subjects studied 2 to 3 hours after a light, low-fat breakfast.
[c]Subjects studied in the early afternoon after a light breakfast.
OER, oxygen extraction ratio; CHO, carbohydrate; FFA, free fatty acids; TG, triglyceride; –, absence of data.

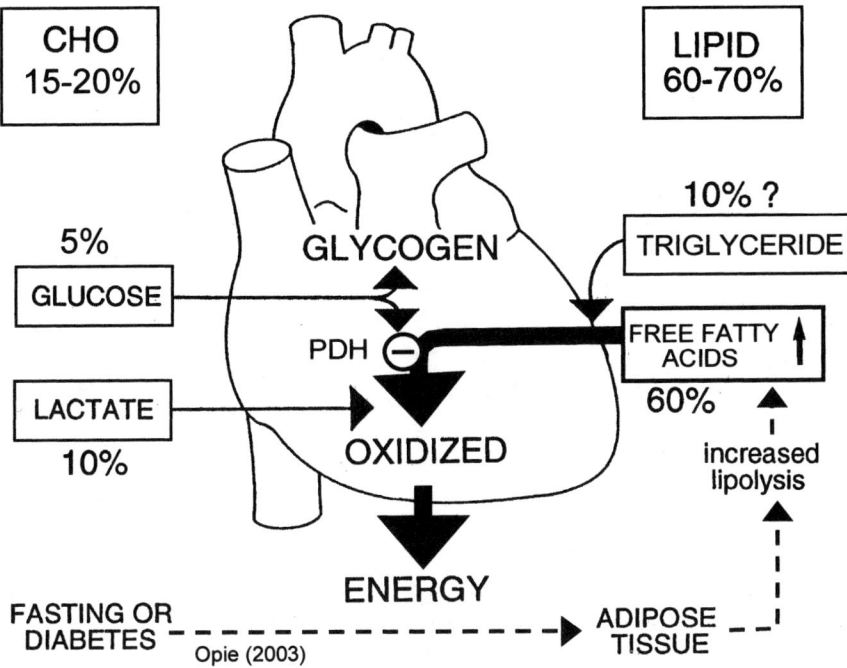

FIG. 11-3. Substrate metabolism: fasted state. Patterns of substrate metabolism when blood levels of free fatty acids are high, as in the fasted state or poorly controlled diabetes mellitus. High levels of blood free fatty acids are oxidized by the heart in preference to glucose and lactate. Use of lipid accounts for 60% to 70% of the oxygen uptake of the heart, whereas use of carbohydrate accounts for less than 20%. Potential errors in the indirect methods used mean that the sum of the oxidation extraction ratios (Tables 11-1 and 11-2) will not exactly equal 100%. *CHO*, carbohydrate.

are oxidized, glucose oxidation is inhibited and the glucose taken up is increasingly converted to glycogen, the glucose-sparing effect of fatty acid oxidation (5). Conversely, in the carbohydrate-fed state (Fig. 11-4), when circulating glucose and insulin are high, the circulating fatty acid levels are suppressed. The uptake of fatty acids by the heart decreases, the inhibition of glycolysis by fatty acids is removed, and glucose oxidation increases. Nonetheless, even in the carbohydrate-fed state, the rates of glucose oxidation when measured directly are only approximately one-fourth to one-half of the chemical glucose uptake (contrast values in Table 11-1 with those in Table 11-2). The missing part of the glucose uptake may yet undergo delayed oxidation after initial conversion to storage carbohydrate (glycogen).

The marked variation in the relative roles of glucose and fatty acid as major fuel between the fed and fasted states is impressive (Figs. 11-3 and 11-4) and forms the basis of the *glucose–fatty acid cycle*, first described by Randle et al. (5). An updated form of this cycle allows additional control of blood fatty acid levels by the newly described hormone leptin and gene regulation of the

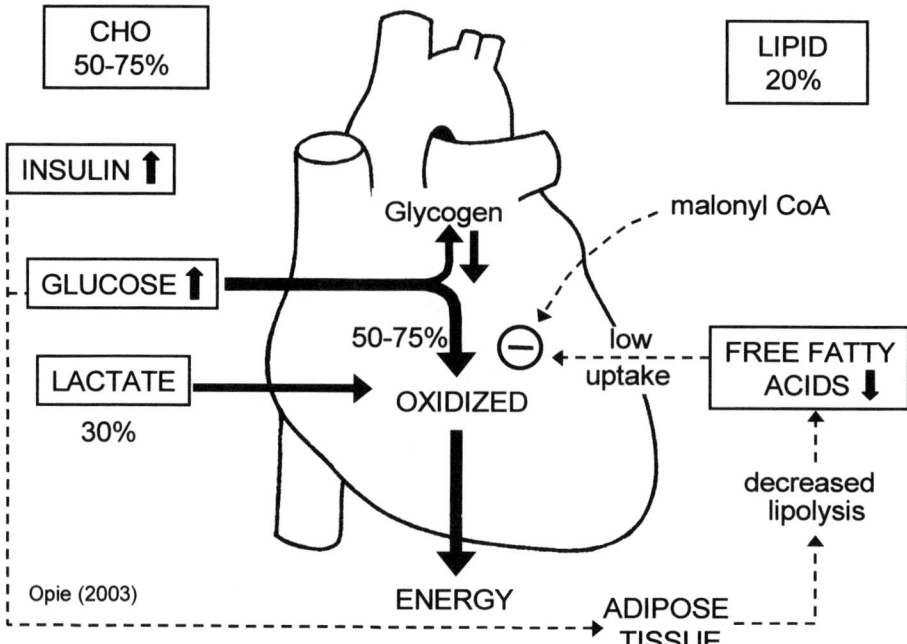

FIG. 11-4. Substrate metabolism: fed state. After a high carbohydrate meal or glucose feeding, blood glucose and insulin are high, and blood free fatty acids are low. Glucose becomes the major fuel of the heart, and carbohydrates can account for 50% to 75% of the oxygen uptake. *CHO*, carbohydrate.

TABLE 11-2. *Fuels for oxidative metabolism of the human heart: radioisotope data*

Conditions	Glucose-glycogen (OER %)	Lactate (OER %)	Total CHO (OER %)	FFA (OER %)
Glucose infusion[a]	25–50	27	50–75	20[c]
Exercise, moderate[b]	14	28	42	64[c]
Fasting overnight	3	13	16	62[d]

[a]See reference 5a. Mean glucose level, 10.8 µmol/mL; insulin level, 30 µmol/mL; FFA level, approximately 0.150 mmol/L. Measured glucose oxidation, 24%, as much as 50% via glycogen oxidation.
[b]Young, healthy, highly trained volunteers (5b).
[c]Free fatty acids, calculated oxygen extraction ratio not in paper but assuming 84% rapid oxidation (5c).
[d]Arteriovenous difference data, see Table 11-1.
OER, oxygen extraction ratio; CHO, carbohydrate; FFA, free fatty acids.

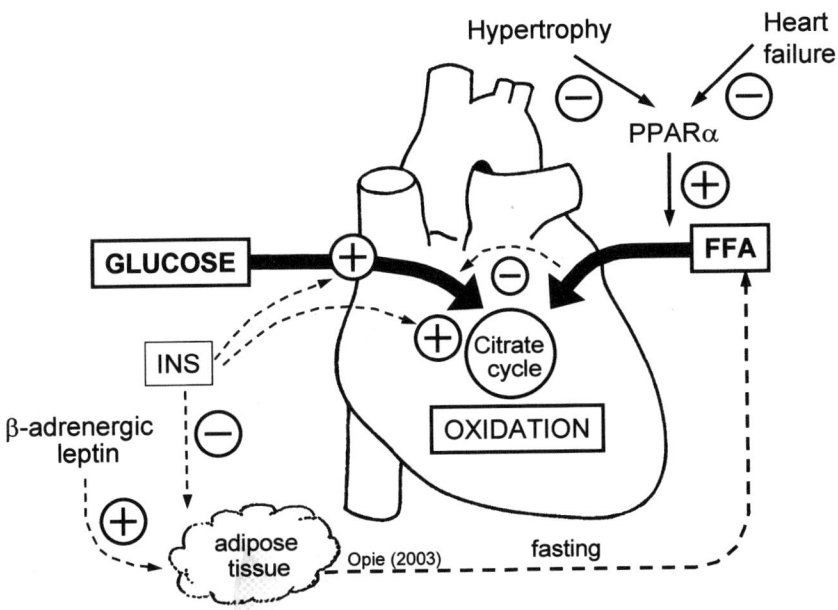

FIG. 11-5. Substrate metabolism: regulation of glucose–free fatty acid (*FFA*) interaction. Insulin (*INS*) promotes glucose uptake and its entry into the citrate cycle while inhibiting the release of FFAs from adipose tissue. β-Adrenergic stimulation and the hormone leptin both release FFAs from adipose tissue. The metabolism of FFAs is promoted by the nuclear transcription factor peroxisome proliferator–activated receptor α (Fig. 9-13), which in turn is inhibited in myocardial hypertrophy or failure. FFAs are preferentially used by the normal myocardium so that glucose oxidation is inhibited.

enzymes of fatty acid oxidation (Fig. 11-5). When the blood and oxygen supply is limited, as in patients with coronary artery disease, there is competition between glucose and fatty acids for the residual albeit diminished oxygen supply (Fig. 11-6). How does this residual oxygen supply reach the ischemic zone? Some blood flow reaches the ischemic zone from arteries running in from healthy nonischemic parts of the heart. This is called the *collateral circulation*. Although glucose uptake and glycolysis are stimulated, the enzyme pyruvate dehydrogenase is inhibited (see later, Fig. 11-9) so that little of the glucose uptake and glycolytic flux enters the citrate cycle. FFAs are better able to capture the residual oxygen uptake, which is reduced but not stopped by the ischemia. Thus, fatty acids win the fight for the residual oxygen; they steal oxygen from glucose only to waste much of it (see later in this chapter).

INSULIN AND GLUCOSE TRANSPORT

The uptake of glucose from the bloodstream across the sarcolemma and into the cells of the heart is controlled by the glucose transporters GLUT-1 and especially GLUT-4 (Fig. 11-7). These are stereospecific and prefer to transport glu-

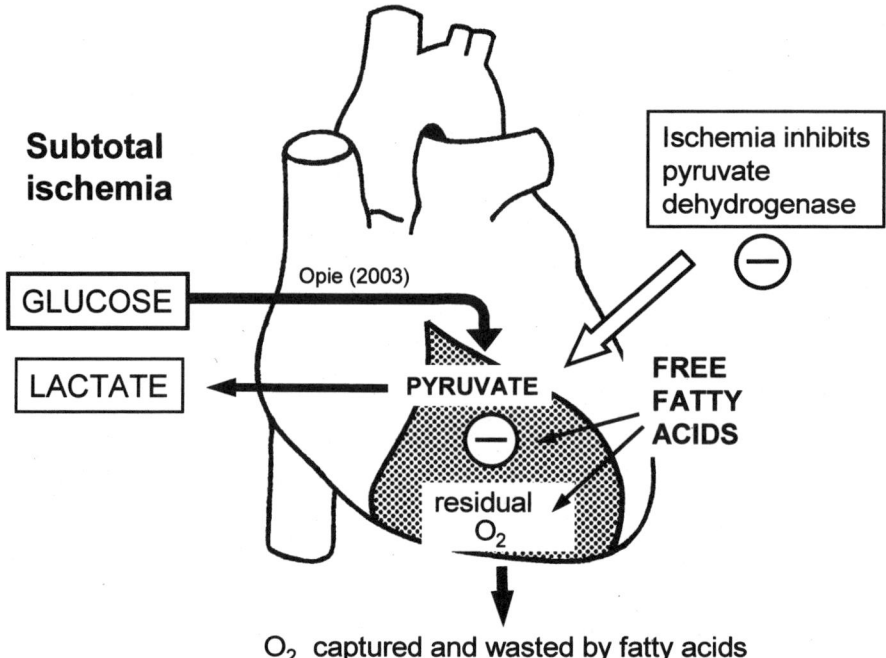

FIG. 11-6. Fatty acids steal oxygen from glucose in subtotal ischemia. Glucose uptake and glycolysis are stimulated, but pyruvate dehydrogenase is inhibited (Fig. 11-9) so that little of the glucose uptake and glycolytic flux enter the citrate cycle. Free fatty acids (FFAs) are better able to capture the residual oxygen uptake, which is reduced but not stopped by the ischemia. FFAs, however, waste much of the oxygen.

cose rather than any other circulating sugars (6,7). No energy is required for such glucose transport because the glucose concentration in the extracellular space is so much higher than in the cytosol. The uptake of glucose increases whenever the glucose transporter is stimulated, as in the fed state and during increased heart work, hypoxia, and ischemia. All these conditions also enhance glycolysis. Conversely, the uptake of glucose is inhibited when blood fatty acid levels are high, as in the fasted state or severe diabetes mellitus.

Insulin is a circulating hormone. Its level increases in the fed state to enhance glucose uptake by two major mechanisms. First, insulin decreases the release of FFAs from adipose tissue, thereby removing the inhibitory effects of FFAs on glucose uptake and glycolysis. Second, insulin increases the number of active glucose carriers (Fig. 11-7). Insulin translocates the glucose carrier GLUT-4 and, to a much lesser extent, GLUT-1 from internal unavailable sites to external sarcolemmal sites (8,9). Thus, insulin stimulates the rates at which the carriers are recycled between internal and external sites. Promotion of glucose uptake increases glycolysis and the glucose contribution to myocardial respiration. Complex signaling paths convey the "message" of insulin from the cell surface receptor to multiple internal sites of action. Insulin binds to specific insulin receptors, consisting of an external α subunit and an internal β subunit. When insulin occupies the external subunit, there is a rapid self-phosphorylation (*autophosphorylation*) of the β-subunit. This greatly amplifies the effect of insulin and in turn activates peptide kinases to phosphorylate tyrosine. Tyrosine phosphorylation increases the activity of the insulin receptor substrate 1. Thereafter, the downstream events are becoming clearer. Increasing emphasis is placed on the central role of a pathway leading, via the enzymes phosphatidylinositol-3 kinase and Akt (also called protein kinase B), to various critical end points such as increased glucose transport or glycogen synthesis or growth.

Other Hormones

β-Adrenergic stimulation to some extent directly stimulates glycolysis as shown in isolated heart preparations, but in the whole animal or in humans, it largely acts by mobilizing FFAs from adipose tissue, thereby promoting a metabolic condition similar to fasting with predominant fatty acid metabolism by the heart (Fig. 11-5). *Leptin*, a complex hormone that regulates food intake,

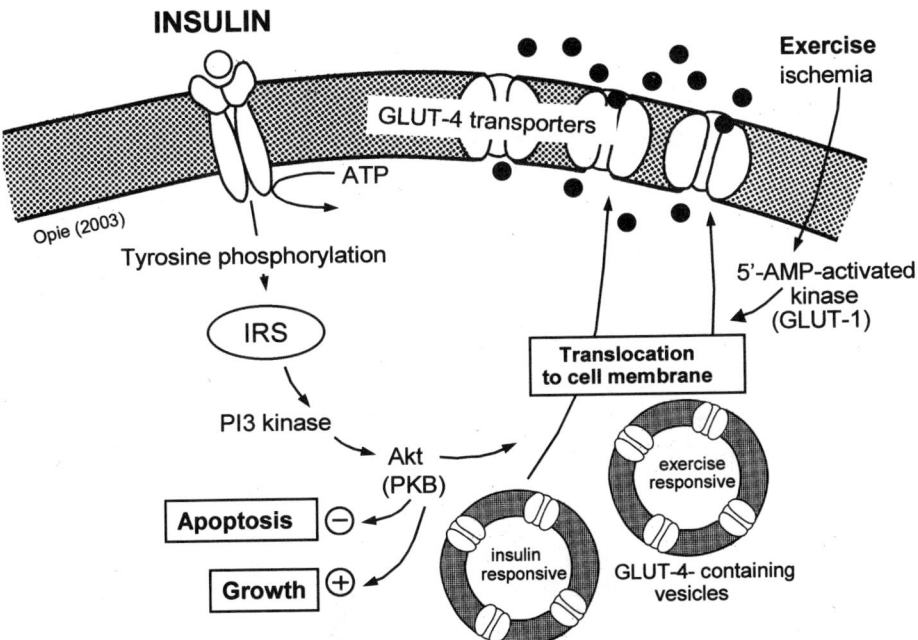

FIG. 11-7. Multiple roles of insulin. In the heart, besides translocation of glucose transporters (GLUT-4) to increase inward transport of glucose, insulin promotes prosurvival pathways, shown in Figure 9-1, by inhibiting apoptosis and stimulating growth. Protein kinase B (*PKB*) plays a key role. *Glut-4*, glucose transporter 4; *IRS*, insulin receptor substrate; *PI*, phosphatidylinositol.

increases blood fatty acids by two mechanisms. First, it decreases food intake, and, second, it promotes sympathetic activity via the hypothalamus, thereby increasing the release of FFAs from adipose tissue (Fig. 11-5). Furthermore, leptin directly stimulates fatty acid metabolism in the isolated heart (10).

PATHWAYS OF GLYCOLYSIS

Glycolysis is the metabolic pathway that responds to oxygen lack by converting glucose to pyruvate. During normal oxidative metabolism, glycolytically produced pyruvate is then oxidized in the citrate cycle. Under anaerobic conditions, pyruvate is converted to lactate (Fig. 11-8). Thus, ATP is produced from glycolysis not only during anaerobic (oxygen-lacking) conditions, but also under aerobic conditions; although it is mainly during anaerobiosis that the relatively small amounts of glycolytic ATP are of importance in preserving membrane function.

Very little free glucose is found in the cytosol, so that any glucose taken up in cardiac myocytes is trapped and rapidly converted by the unidirectional enzyme *hexokinase* to glucose 6-phosphate. The latter compound is then directed either

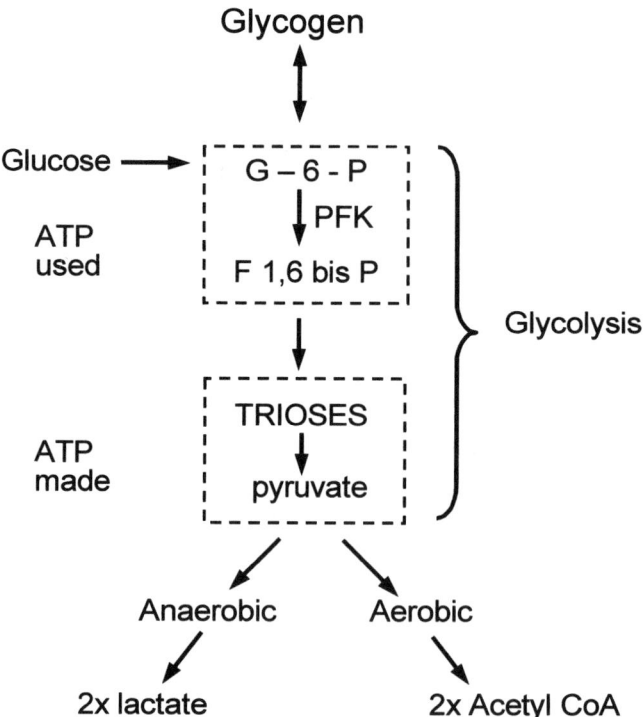

FIG. 11-8. Glycolysis simplified. *G-6-P*, glucose 6-phosphate; *PFK*, phosphofructokinase; *F 1,6 bisP*, fructose 1,6-bisphosphate.

to glycogen synthesis or to glycolysis (Fig. 11-8). Glycolysis converts glucose 6-phosphate into a compound containing two phosphate groups, fructose 1,6-diphosphate (fructose 1,6-bisphosphate) under the influence of the enzyme phosphofructokinase (PFK). Of the many enzymes participating in the reactions of the glycolytic pathway, PFK is one of the few that actually regulate flux. When its activity increases, as in hypoxia, glucose 6-phosphate is converted at an increased rate via fructose 6-phosphate to fructose 1,6-bisphosphate:

$$\text{Glucose} + \text{ATP} \rightarrow \text{glucose 6-phosphate} + \text{ADP}$$
$$\text{Glucose 6-phosphate} \rightarrow \text{fructose 6-phosphate}$$
$$\text{F-6-P} + \text{ATP (enzyme: PFK)} \rightarrow \text{fructose 1,6 bisphosphate} + \text{ADP}$$

Thereafter, glycolysis converts each six-carbon hexose biphosphate into two three-carbon triose phosphates. During the next stages of glycolysis that form two molecules of pyruvate, four molecules of ATP are made independently of oxygen: fructose 1,6-bisphosphate + 4 ADP → 2 × pyruvate + 4 ATP.

There is a coordinated intracellular control of glycolysis in that glucose uptake, glucose phosphorylation, and the activity of PFK and pyruvate dehydrogenase can all speed up or slow down simultaneously in response to increased heart work and other stimuli (Table 11-3).

Fructose 2,6-bisphosphate is an additional product of glycolysis, not an intermediate, with the capacity for potent stimulation of PFK that overrides the inhibitory effects of ATP and citrate on PFK. It is produced from fructose 6-phosphate by an enzyme (PFK-2) whose activity increases when glycolytic flow is increased in response to insulin or increased heart work (11).

In addition to the production of anaerobic ATP, does glycolysis have a role in normal aerobic conditions? Such aerobic glycolysis provides energy for the maintenance of normal ATP-requiring membrane functions such as the sodium pump and the ATP-sensitive potassium channels (12). Key glycolytic enzymes are situated near the sarcolemma and may be involved in membrane-related glycolysis. More controversial functions of glycolysis are to sustain maximal heart work and to promote diastolic relaxation especially during ischemia (13).

TABLE 11-3. *Major factors controlling glycolysis and sites of action*

Conditions	Glucose uptake	Glycogen content	Activity of phosphofructokinase	Activity of pyruvate dehydrogenase
Increased heart work	+	↓	+	+
Inotropic agents	+	↓	+	+
Fed state, insulin	+	↑	+	+
Starvation, high blood fatty acids or ketones	−	↑	−	−
Hypoxia, mild ischemia	+	↓	+	−
Severe ischemia	−	↓	−	−

+, stimulation; −, inhibition; ↓, decreased content; ↑, increased content.

Pyruvate and Lactate

Pyruvate is a three-carbon compound formed from either lactate taken up by the heart or glycolysis. In the anaerobic heart, pyruvate forms lactate (Fig. 11-9). In the aerobic heart, pyruvate is fully oxidized in the Krebs citrate cycle but must first be shortened to a two-carbon compound (technical term: oxidative decarboxylation) through the action of the enzyme complex pyruvate dehydrogenase, which is found in the inner mitochondrial membrane. The products of the multi-stage reaction include acetyl-CoA, which is ready to enter the citrate cycle, and nicotinamide adenine dinucleotide (reduced form) ($NADH_2$), which will eventually form ATP by oxidative phosphorylation. Pyruvate dehydrogenase can exist in

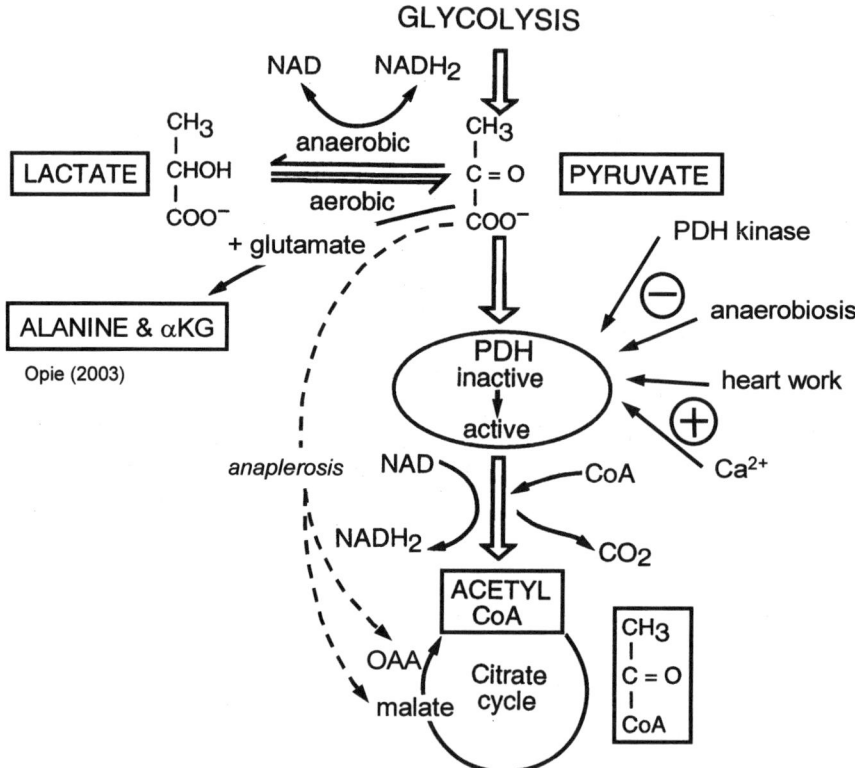

FIG. 11-9. Major fates of pyruvate. In the normal aerobic heart, lactate is taken up and converted to pyruvate, the major part of which enters the citrate cycle. Transamination is a pathway of minor significance. In the anaerobic heart, lactate is produced from pyruvate derived from glycolysis. There is also formation of alanine and the possibility of adenosine 5′-triphosphate production via guanosine 5′-triphosphate as succinate is ultimately formed. During postischemic reperfusion, pyruvate can be converted to malate and oxaloacetate (*OAA*) to help to replenish the citrate cycle intermediates by anaplerosis. PDH, pyruvate dehydrogenase; αKG, α-ketoglutarate.

either active or inactive forms. Normally, this enzyme is largely inactive but is activated by increased heart work, catecholamines, or the high glycolytic rates of the fed state (Table 11-3). Conversely, the enzyme is inhibited by $NADH_2$ formed by ischemia or hypoxia or by fatty acid oxidation. Inhibition of pyruvate dehydrogenase is the key factor that slows down glycolysis during oxidation of fatty acids (14).

Lactate is taken up by the aerobic heart and is produced during anaerobiosis, so that its release into coronary sinus blood was used as a sign of myocardial ischemia. Now, however, it is appreciated that the heart may produce lactate from glucose during some aerobic conditions, such as after a high carbohydrate meal. The contribution of lactate to the energy needs of the well-oxygenated myocardium increases as much as 60% when the circulating lactate levels are high (e.g., during and soon after some types of vigorous exercise) and as much as 90% during a lactate infusion. Lactate is a much less important fuel when its level is low or the FFA level is high. The uptake of lactate by the heart depends on a specific transport system because the sarcolemma is not freely permeable to lactate. When taken up, intracellular lactate is converted into pyruvate by lactate dehydrogenase and thus joins the pool of pyruvate in the cytosol. The reaction catalyzed by lactate dehydrogenase is freely reversible: lactate + NAD^+ ↔ NADH + H^+.

The myocardial activity of lactate dehydrogenase (with five isoenzymes) is high enough to make is unlikely that it could be a controlling step for lactate metabolism by the heart.

Malate–Aspartate Cycle

For glycolysis to proceed requires disposal of the $NADH_2$ (NADH + H^+) that is continuously generated. During normal oxygenation, cytoplasmic $NADH_2$ is removed by the malate–aspartate cycle, which depends on continued mitochondrial respiration and therefore slows or stops in ischemia (Figs. 11-10 and 11-11). In hypoxia or ischemia, $NADH_2$ is converted back to NAD as pyruvate forms lactate, so that the expected accumulation of $NADH_2$ is less than expected. Nonetheless, the cytoplasmic $NADH_2$/NAD ratio will be forced toward $NADH_2$ as the tissue lactate increases in relation to the pyruvate level because of the equilibrium relationship. $NADH_2$ accumulation in the cytosol means more protons so that intracellular acidosis is promoted. During hypoxia or ischemia, the regulatory enzyme pyruvate dehydrogenase is inhibited by $NADH_2$ so that less pyruvate enters the citrate cycle, more lactate forms, and the ratio $NADH_2$ to NAD increases further. Because of a lack of oxygen, $NADH_2$ also accumulates in the mitochondria with adverse effects: (a) there is inhibition of dehydrogenase enzymes at several sites so that any residual activity of the citrate cycle is decreased and (b) intramitochondrial calcium increases, probably because increased intramitochondrial H^+ influences exchange systems across the mitochondrial membrane in such a way that the internal calcium rises.

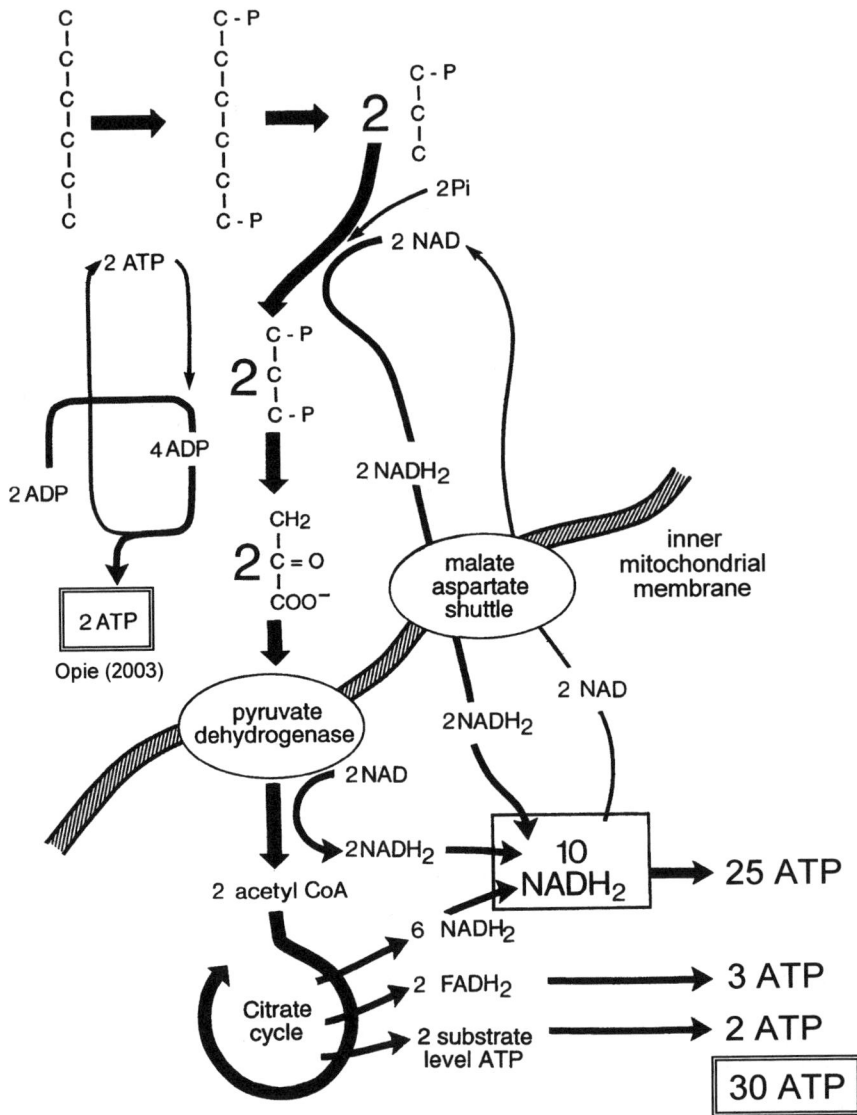

FIG. 11-10. Energy balance during oxidative metabolism of glucose. Top: The basic structure of six-carbon hexose units where adenosine 5'-triphosphate (ATP) is used, then broken down to two trioses where ATP is produced in low amounts before entry into citrate cycle via pyruvate dehydrogenase with much more production of ATP. Note that the values for ATP production per glucose molecule are lower than standard, based on the "modern" phosphorylation to oxidation ratios, as in Table 11-5.

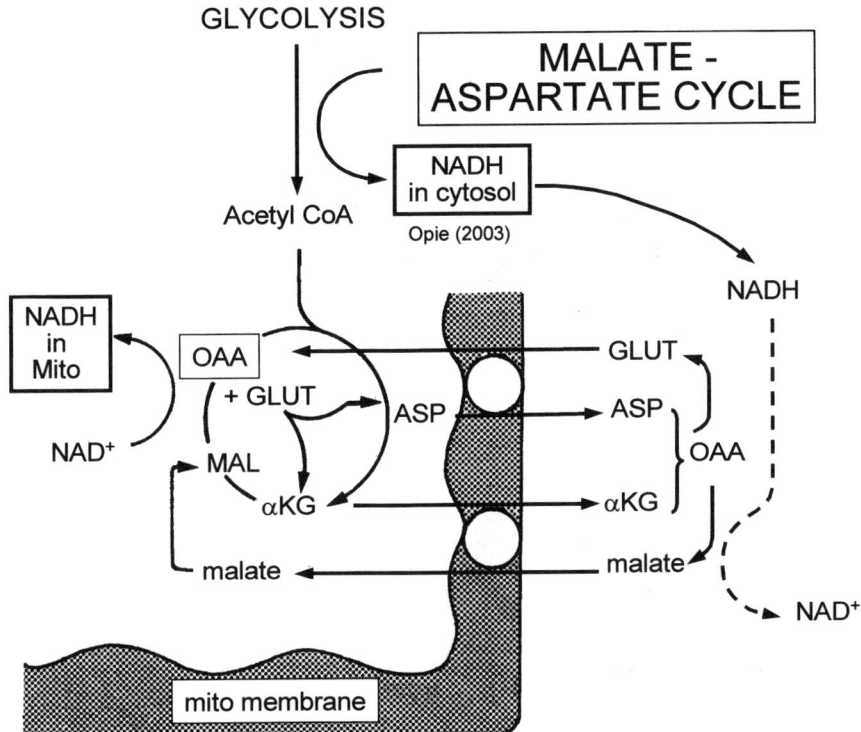

FIG. 11-11. Malate–aspartate cycle. By means of this cycle, $NADH_2$ ($NADH + H^+$) produced by glycolysis in the cytosol enters the mitochondrial space to provide protons for adenosine 5′-triphosphate production (Fig. 11-17). During ischemia or hypoxia, $NADH_2$ is converted back to NAD as pyruvate dehydrogenase forms lactate (Fig. 11-9).

GLYCOGEN

Glycogen is a polysaccharide (i.e., a combination of many molecules of glucose) that forms large granules in the cytoplasm of the heart. Although frequently thought of as a storage carbohydrate, glycogen molecules are in a constant state of turnover as a result of variable rates of synthesis and degradation. The pathways of *glycogen synthesis* function separately from those of glycogen breakdown because two different enzyme systems are involved. Nonetheless, they all seem to be held in close physical apposition by the molecular scaffolding proteins. *Glycogen synthesis* (Fig. 11-12) proceeds at a high rate in the fed state under the influence of insulin, which both increases glucose uptake and stimulates the synthase (through a complex and controversial mechanism). Glycogen synthesis also takes place after intense heart work or after ischemia has depleted glycogen. Low glycogen levels promote glycogen synthesis. In the fasted state, despite the lack of insulin, glycogen synthesis can still proceed,

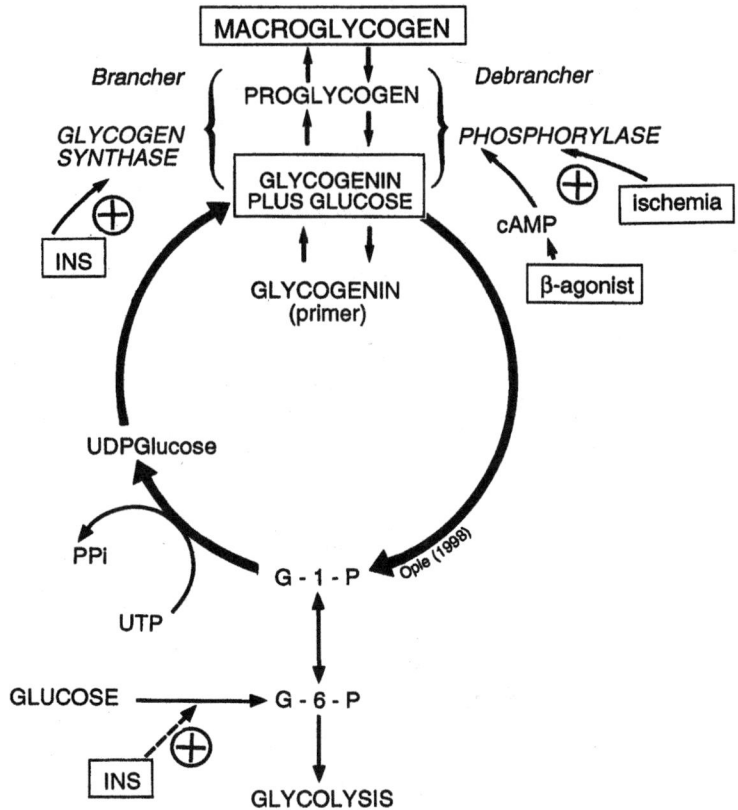

FIG. 11-12. Glycogen synthesis and breakdown. Note different pathways for synthesis, which is controlled by glycogen synthase (= synthetase), when compared with glycogen breakdown, which is controlled by glycogen phosphorylase. *INS*, insulin; *cAMP*, cyclic adenosine 3',5'-monophosphate; *PPi*, inorganic pyrophosphate; *UTP*, uridine triphosphate; *G-1-P*, glucose 1-phosphate; *G-6-P*, glucose 6-phosphate.

albeit at a lower rate. Now glycogen synthase is stimulated by the high myocardial levels of glucose 6-phosphate resulting from the FFA-induced block of glycolysis. The energy required for glycogen synthesis is derived from a special high-energy phosphate, uridine triphosphate, which is formed from ATP.

The two major mechanisms underlying glycogen breakdown are activation of phosphorylase by cyclic adenosine 3',5'-monophosphate (cAMP), as during β-adrenergic stimulation and, in ischemia, by a decrease in high-energy phosphate levels (Fig. 11-12). An increase in cAMP promotes the cascade of events that eventually converts the inactive enzyme phosphorylase *b* to the highly active phosphorylase *a*: catecholamine stimulus → β-receptor → adenylate cyclase → cAMP activation of protein kinase A → activation of phosphorylase *b* kinase → change of phosphorylase *b* to *a* → breakdown of glycogen.

An unexpected finding is that calmodulin, an intracellular calcium–binding protein, is one of the subunits of phosphorylase b kinase, which explains why calcium ions are required for the formation of phosphorylase a. Phosphorylase is the enzyme controlling the initial burst of glycogenolysis during hypoxia or ischemia, and thereafter the activity of the *debranching enzyme* becomes significant. Another unexpected and difficult-to-understand finding is that the kinase switching on glycogen synthase (glycogen synthase kinase 3) inhibits myocardial hypertrophy by complex mechanisms involving the growth factor calcineurin (15).

Function of Cardiac Glycogen

Cardiac glycogen is a potential source of myocardial energy, producing three ATP units during glycolysis and the standard amount of ATP through the citrate cycle in aerobic conditions. It has an established role as an energy source during short-lived conditions such as a work jump, soon after the onset of enhanced β-adrenergic stimulation, and in response to myocardial hypoxia or ischemia. In addition, a generous proportion of exogenous glucose, after uptake and conversion to glucose 6-phosphate, "passes through" glycogen on the way to glycolytic breakdown. Then, glucose derived from glycogen is preferentially used rather than exogenous glucose to enter glycolysis and then to be oxidized (16). These proposals provide a physiologic role for glycogen.

Glycogenin and Proglycogen

Glycogenin is a primer or backbone for glycogen synthesis, which is well described in the liver and presumably is present in the heart. It is autocatalytic in that it glycosylates itself before incorporation into glycogen (17). Proglycogen is an abundant stable glycogen precursor molecule found in the heart. Hypothetically, glycogen may oscillate between proglycogen and the higher molecular weight storage glycogen called *macroglycogen* depending on energy supply and demand (17).

Glycogen Storage Disease of the Heart

In the lysosomes of the heart, the breakdown of some of the glycogen is mediated by a different pathway dependent on α-1,4-glucosidase (acid maltase). The congenital absence of this enzyme has drastic consequences because the heart cells become filled with glycogen, and the fatal condition of cardiomegalic glycogenolysis or Pompe disease results. There is emerging evidence that mutations of the enzyme activated by the breakdown to ATP to adenosine 5′-monophosphate (AMP), AMP protein kinase, can cause another type of glycogen storage disease associated with cardiomyopathy (18).

FREE FATTY ACIDS DURING AEROBIC METABOLISM

Although long-chain FFAs are the major myocardial fuel during fasting, their oxidation in the mitochondria can only take place after complex but essential transformational steps. In ischemia, when mitochondrial metabolism is inhibited, accumulation of long-chain metabolites exert adverse influences on the myocardial cell membranes. Myocardial metabolism of FFA starts with the blood level because the higher the FFA level and the greater the FFA/albumin molar ratio are, the greater the uptake of FFA by the myocardium. FFA molecules traversing the sarcolemma bind to intracellular *fatty acid binding protein* before further metabolism (19). Eventually, if sufficient FFAs are taken up, accumulated intracellular intermediates will limit the fatty acid activation (Fig. 11-13).

After uptake into the myocardial cell, a series of intricate steps changes the long-chain fatty acid into acetyl-CoA that can enter the citrate cycle, which in turn will yield ATP. This complex sequence has been reviewed in detail (20). The first step is the activation of the intracellular fatty acid by CoA to form fatty acyl-CoA derivatives. The mitochondrial membrane is not permeable to these acyl-CoA molecules, which need transformation and transfer from the cytosol to within the mitochondria by a staged transfer system that requires carnitine and formation of acylcarnitine, transport into the mitochondrial space, and conversion of acylcarnitine back to acyl-CoA. Thereafter, the long-chain acyl-CoA molecules are progressively broken into two-carbon units of acetyl-CoA by β-oxidation, and finally acetyl-CoA is oxidized in the citrate cycle. Any activated

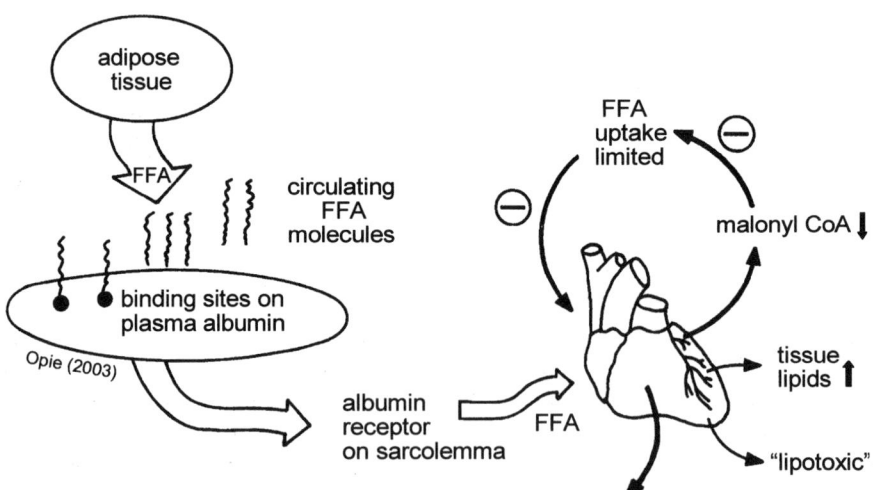

FIG. 11-13. Uptake of free fatty acids (FFA) at high circulating levels, exceeding the tight binding sites on plasma albumin (*two black circles*) is uncontrolled and may give rise to toxic effects. For details of tissue CoA and acyl-CoA, see Figure 11-14.

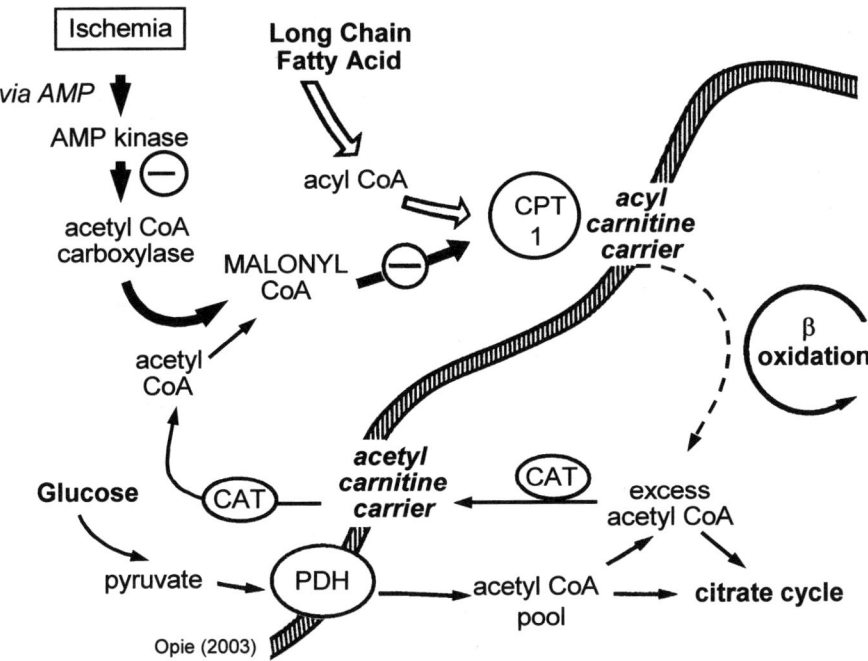

FIG. 11-14. **Long-chain fatty acid transfer into mitochondria for oxidation.** The acylcarnitine carrier transfers activated fatty acid (acyl-CoA) into the mitochondrial space for oxidation in the fatty acid oxidation cycle. For details, see text. *Acyl CoA*, long-chain acyl-CoA compounds; *CPT*, carnitine palmityl transferase; *acylcarnitine*, long-chain acylcarnitine compounds; *CAT*, carnitine acetyltransferase; *PDH*, pyruvate dehydrogenase.

intracellular fatty acid not oxidized can be stored as triglycerides or be transformed to structural lipids by lengthening and alterations in the degree of saturation to myocardial membrane lipids. Tissue triglyceride (also called triacylglycerol) may be a reserve source of fatty acids when the circulating levels are low. Complex intracellular controls exist to prevent any undue accumulation of lipid intermediates that may have toxic effects.

The overall steps can be summarized as follows (20). Palmitate is the standard example, although the main fatty acid taken up in humans is oleic acid (Table 11-4). Therefore, in the schema that follows, palmityl (or palmitoyl) is more correctly given as acyl (Fig. 11-14).

1. Extramitochondrial palmityl-CoA forms from palmitate: palmitate + CoA + ATP → palmityl-CoA + AMP + inorganic pyrophosphate.
2. Extramitochondrial palmityl carnitine forms from extramitochondrial palmityl-CoA, catalyzed by the enzyme carnitine palmitoyltransferase 1.
3. The enzyme carnitine acylcarnitine translocase transfers extramitochondrial palmityl carnitine to within the space between outer and inner mitochondrial membranes.

TABLE 11-4. Myocardial uptake of plasma free fatty acids in fasting humans

Fatty acid	Structure	Site of unsaturated bonds	Percentage of total plasma FFA[a,b]	Percentage of uptake of FFA by human heart
Palmitic	C16:0	–	~25	16
Palmitoleic	C16:1	9	2	2
Stearic	C18:0	–	14	7
Oleic	C18:1	9	30–45	53
Linoleic	C18:2	9, 12	10–14	7
Linolenic	C18:3	6, 12, 15	8 in guinea pig	No data
Arachidonic	C20:4	5, 8, 11, 14	5	No data on humans, no uptake in dog heart[c]
Erucic	C22:1	13	Normally low	No data but may increase with rapeseed seed ingestion

[a]Reference 20a.
[b]Calculated from data of Rothlin and Bing (20b).
[c]Reference 20c.
FFA, free fatty acid.

4. Mitochondrial carnitine palmityltransferase 2, located on the inner membrane, allows intramitochondrial palmityl carnitine to react with CoA to liberate intramitochondrial palmityl-CoA and carnitine; the carnitine is exported to the mitochondrial intermembrane space.
5. Intramitochondrial palmityl-CoA enters the fatty acid β-oxidation spiral to form acetyl-CoA, which enters the citrate cycle.
6. During high rates of FFA uptake and subsequent metabolism by the above steps, more acetyl-CoA may form than can enter the citrate cycle. Such acetyl-CoA can also react with intramitochondrial carnitine via the enzyme carnitine acetyltransferase to form acetylcarnitine. The latter is transported outward from the mitochondria by the enzyme carnitine acetyltranslocase, and in the process cytoplasmic acetyl-CoA is formed. This can then undergo transformation into malonyl-CoA, which provides feedback inhibition.

Oxidation of Excess Free Fatty Acids Limited by Malonyl-CoA

To summarize and simplify the complexities of FFA metabolism, FFAs must be converted to acyl-CoA to enter the mitochondria where β-oxidation converts the long chain into two-carbon acetyl-CoA units that enter the citrate cycle, thereby providing energy in the form of ATP. When excess FFAs reach the mitochondria, there is risk of uncoupling of oxidation from phosphorylation with oxygen wastage. To prevent this sequence, the entry of acyl-CoA into mitochondria should be limited. This task is performed by *malonyl-CoA*. This forms whenever high cytosolic levels of acetyl-CoA are produced (21) (e.g., from excess β-oxidation). Malonyl-CoA potently inhibits step 2 (Fig. 11-14) to switch off FFA metabolism. The enzyme that synthesizes malonyl-CoA, acetyl-CoA carboxylase, is inhibited by another enzyme, *AMP-activated protein kinase* (AMP protein kinase). The latter is stimulated into activity whenever ATP breaks down to AMP (e.g., by a work jump, ischemia) (see later, Fig. 11-20). During severe ischemia, AMP protein kinase becomes active and malonyl-CoA formation is inhibited, so that more long-chain fatty acids enter the mitochondria as acyl-CoA, there to "steal" the residual oxygen at the expense of energy-friendly glycolysis (Fig. 11-6). Thus, the protective effects of malonyl-CoA in limiting oxidation of FFAs is lost.

β-Oxidation

β-Oxidation converts intramitochondrial long-chain acyl-CoA to the two-carbon unit acetyl-CoA. The fatty acid oxidation spiral continuously removes acetyl-CoA from the carboxyl (–COOH) end of the chain. The enzymes of β-oxidation are loosely organized into a multienzyme complex in which the intermediates never leave the complex except for entering and departing. The products of each reaction are simply displaced by the arrival of fresh substrates for that reaction to move on in the spiral. The net ATP production per palmitate molecule is only 105 according to current thought, although it is often still regarded as 130 (Table 11-5). During anaerobiosis, there is impaired β-oxidation owing to decreased electron transport. Intermediates of fatty acid metabolism accumulate, including β-hydroxy fatty acids, acylcarnitine, and acyl-CoA. These intermediates damage heart cell membranes.

Structural Lipids of the Heart

Phospholipids, the major structural lipids of the heart, form an important part of the various cell membranes, including the sarcolemma. In phospholipid mol-

TABLE 11-5. *Comparative energy yields of various fuels per molecule fully oxidized*

Molecule	ATP yield per molecule		ATP yield per carbon atom		ATP yield per oxygen atom taken up to (P/O ratio)	
	Old[a]	New	Old	New[a]	Old	New
Glucose	38[b]	32[c]	6.3	5.2	3.17	2.58
Lactate	18	14.75	6.0	4.9	3.00	2.46
Pyruvate	15	12.25	5.0	4.1	3.00	2.50
Palmitate[d]	130	105	8.1	6.7	2.83	2.33

[a]Old, conventional; new, revised (see reference 21a).
[b]Thirty-six via mitochondria, two via glycolysis.
[c]Thirty via mitochondria, two via glycolysis.
[d]For palmitate details, see reference 21b.
ATP, adenosine 5'-triphosphate; P/O, phosphorylation/oxidation.

ecules, both the free base group (choline, ethanolamine, serine, and inositol) and the phosphate are charged in such a manner that the polar head contrasts with the nonpolar tail. This polarity of the molecule allows the formation of the lipid bilayer of the cell membranes. The polar heads point outward, and the nonpolar tails inward. Various complex proteins are inserted into the lipid bilayer, including enzyme systems that may require specific phospholipids for optimal activity. Such lipid–enzyme complexes include adenylate cyclase and the sarcolemmal sodium–potassium pump. In prolonged ischemia, all membranes are damaged, and products of phospholipid breakdown are formed. One view is that ischemic injury becomes irreversible when the molecular structure of the cell membranes is damaged beyond repair.

ADENOSINE 5'-TRIPHOSPHATE SYNTHESIS AND EXPORT

The breakdown of ATP is the only immediate source of energy for contraction, the maintenance of ion gradients, and other vital functions. The complex metabolic pathways already described transform the major fuels (glucose, FFAs, and lactate) to acetyl-CoA, which enters the citrate cycle to produce $NADH_2$ ($NADH + H^+$). $NADH_2$ is the reduced form of the cofactor nicotinamide adenine dinucleotide. The 2H units, in turn, yield the protons that are pumped across the mitochondrial membrane, and the electrons that flow along the cytochrome chain, with the conversion of ADP into ATP by oxidative phosphorylation as the result. After being produced in the mitochondria, ATP must be transported outward to the cytosol by the ATP/ADP transport system for use in the cytoplasm, mainly in contraction. As cytosolic ATP is used, it is replenished by synthesis from ADP in the mitochondria. The rates of synthesis and breakdown of ATP are therefore closely linked.

The rate at which the Krebs citrate cycle (Fig. 11-15) operates is a major factor controlling the rate of production of ATP by the heart. The standard dogma is that each turn of the cycle produces 12 molecules of ATP, but actually (allowing for technical factors often ignored) it is closer to 10 (Table 11-6). The citrate cycle accelerates with increased heart work. Conversely, decreased rates of operation of the cycle occur during states of oxygen deprivation, such as hypoxia, ischemia, and cardioplegic arrest.

Increased Heart Work and Citrate Cycle

How can the activity of the citrate cycle be matched to the varying energy requirements of the heart (Fig. 11-16)? Hypothetically, as the heart works harder, more ATP is broken down to ADP to drive oxidative phosphorylation, which in turn uses H^+ from $NADH_2$, so that the $NAD/NADH_2$ ratio within the mitochondria increases, thereby stimulating the activity of some key enzymes of the citrate cycle (e.g., isocitrate dehydrogenase, α-ketoglutarate dehydrogenase, malate dehydrogenase). The change in the mitochondrial $NAD/NADH_2$ ratio toward

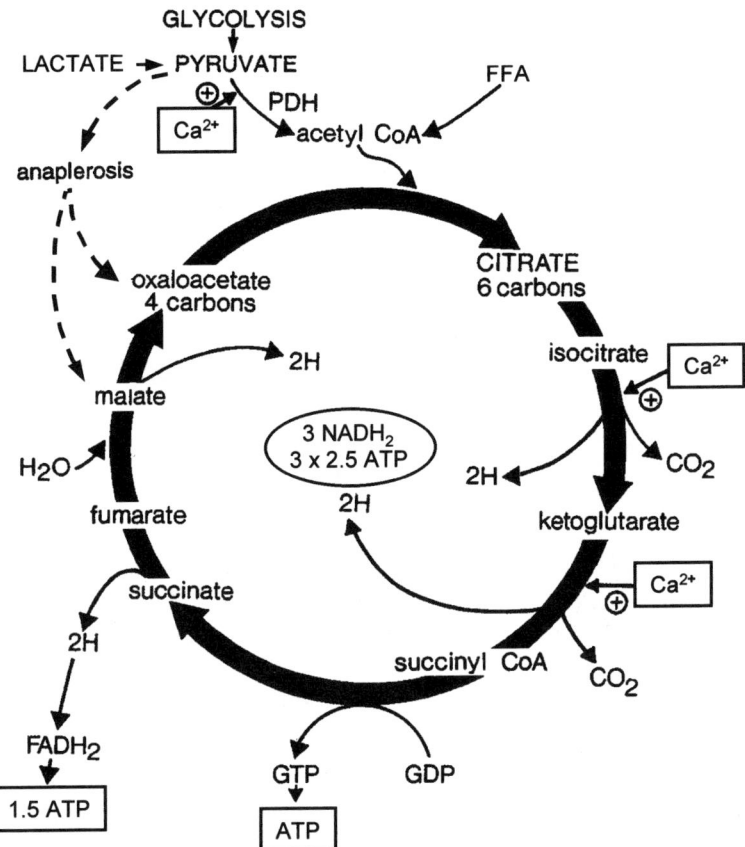

FIG. 11-15. **The citrate cycle of Krebs.** In reality, the following reactions are readily reversible: citrate → isocitrate; succinate → oxaloacetate via the intervening reactions. The most important potential sites of control are citrate synthase, isocitrate dehydrogenase, α-ketoglutarate dehydrogenase, and malate dehydrogenase (by regulating the supply of oxaloacetate). Of these, isocitrate dehydrogenase and α-ketoglutarate dehydrogenase are calcium sensitive as is pyruvate dehydrogenase (*PDH*). These dehydrogenases respond to increased cytosolic calcium (as in inotropic stimulation) by increased activity. *NADH₂*, nicotinamide adenine dinucleotide (reduced form); *FADH₂*, flavin adenine dinucleotide (reduced form); *GTP*, guanosine 5'-triphosphate; *GDP*, guanosine 5'-diphosphate.

NAD also helps the formation of oxaloacetate from malate. Oxaloacetate is one of the substrates for the key enzyme citrate synthase that regulates the formation of citrate. The other substrate for citrate synthase is acetyl-CoA, the formation of which also is stimulated during increased heart work by increases in the rates of glycolysis and the fatty acid oxidation spiral. The above sequence is supported by direct measurement of the mitochondrial ratio of NAD to NADH₂, which decreases at the start of increased work in the isolated heart (22).

TABLE 11-6. Sites of production of $2H^+$, CO_2, and high-energy phosphates in the citrate cycle

Product	Sites of production	Fate
4 × 2H⁺ in total	Isocitrate dehydrogenase	Formation of NADH plus H⁺ (NADH₂) and electron transport to produce 2.5 ATP
	α-Ketoglutarate dehydrogenase	As above
	Succinate dehydrogenase	FADH₂ formation and electron transport via CoQ to produce 1.5 ATP
	Malate dehydrogenase	2.5 ATP as above
GTP	Succinate dehydrogenase by substrate level phosphorylation	1 ATP ultimately
One turn of citrate cycle	Various dehydrogenase reactions as above	10 ATP[a]

[a]For conventional data with a phosphorylation/oxidation ratio of 3.0, see Table 11-5; likewise, there would be 12 ATP per turn of cycle.

NADH, nicotinamide adeninine dinucleotide (reduced form); ATP, adenosine 5'-triphosphate; FADH₂, flavin adenine dinucleotide (reduced form); CoQ, coenzyme Q; GTP, guanosine 5'-triphosphate.

When the heart must suddenly increase ATP production as during a work jump, it is controversial which one of several potential factors limits oxidative phosphorylation: the rate of formation of ADP from ATP, the supply of oxygen from the coronary circulation, or the rate of the malate–aspartate cycle to transport cytosolic NADH₂ to the mitochondria to help to drive the citrate cycle.

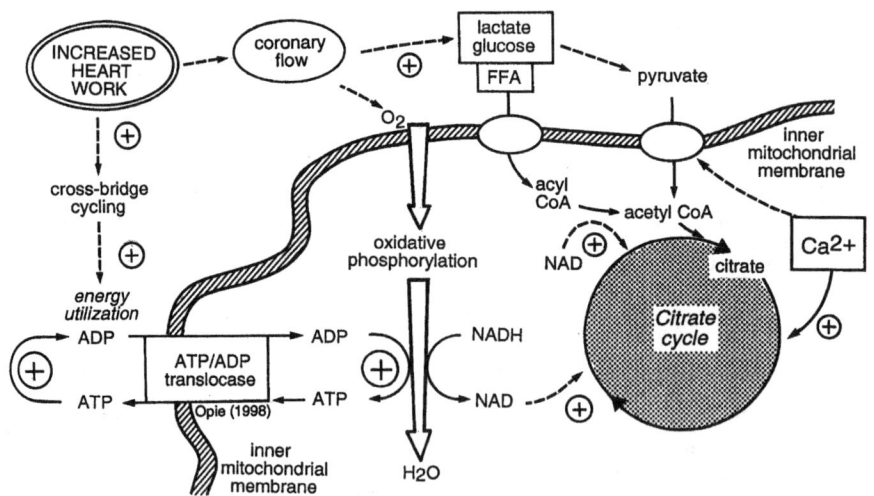

FIG. 11-16. Mechanical work and citrate cycle. The proposed effects of increased heart work in providing an increased supply of circulating substrates and in stimulating oxidative phosphorylation and citrate cycle activity. *FFA*, free fatty acids; *NAD*, nicotinamide adenine dinucleotide; *ADP*, adenosine 5'-diphosphate; *ATP*, adenosine 5'-triphosphate; *NADH*, nicotinamide adenine dinucleotide (reduced form).

Inotropic Stimulation and Regulation of Citrate Cycle by Calcium

For practical purposes, it may be accepted that the citrate cycle responds to the decrease in the ATP/ADP and NAD/NADH$_2$ ratios when a volume or a pressure load increases the oxygen uptake of the heart. When the primary stimulus to heart work is increased contractility, as during enhanced β-adrenergic stimulation, the cytosolic concentration of calcium ions increases. The intramitochondrial calcium concentration also increases as the cytosolic level increases and stimulates the activity of two dehydrogenases of the citrate cycle: isocitrate dehydrogenase and α-ketoglutarate dehydrogenase (22). Calcium also converts the inactive to the active form of pyruvate dehydrogenase (Fig. 11-9). In addition, because the positive inotropic effect of calcium by definition increases heart work, increased provision of ADP to the mitochondria will promote the rate of oxidative phosphorylation (22).

Respiratory Control

By mitochondrial respiration is meant all those processes concerned with the uptake of oxygen and the associated production of ATP, including the activity of the citrate cycle and the respiratory chain. In addition to the evident need for oxygen, there are three important regulators of the respiratory rate: (a) the supply of ADP that regulates respiration by its rate of transfer into the mitochondria, (b) the ratio of NAD/NADH$_2$ in the mitochondria, which regulates the activity of citrate cycle dehydrogenases (Fig. 11-16), and (c) the mitochondrial calcium concentration, which also regulates these dehydrogenases (23). With the exception of the regulatory role of calcium, these key factors can be deduced from the overall equation for phosphorylation of ADP to ATP: NADH + H$^+$ + 2.5 ADP + 3 inorganic phosphate (P$_i$) + ½ O$_2$ → NAD$^+$ + H$_2$O + 2.5 ATP.

The traditional view would make it 3 ADP and 3 ATP in this equation (Table 11-5). The response of mitochondria to oxygen is dramatic, needing only minute amounts of oxygen for full operation. Therefore, in conditions of oxygen lack, the mitochondria are probably fully functioning until suddenly switched off as the mitochondrial oxygen tension decreases. If there is sufficient oxygen, the processes of respiration are regulated such that ATP is resynthesized as rapidly as it is used, so that the level tends to stay constant.

Calcium Uptake and Release by Mitochondria

Calcium is an important controller of mitochondrial respiration. Calcium uptake by the mitochondria occurs by a uniporter system that is not linked to the transport of any other ion. Inward transport of calcium is increased when cytosolic calcium increases. This uptake of calcium ions by mitochondrial matrix effectively requires energy to pump the protons out to balance the charges brought in with calcium ions. The fact that mitochondria contain much less calcium than previously thought suggests that the main function of calcium transfer in and out of the mitochondria is to regulate internal matrix calcium and thereby Krebs cycle activity.

Calcium release from mitochondria occurs by an antiporter system, whereby two sodium ions are taken up for each calcium ion released. This carrier system is electrically neutral, and two sodium ions are taken up for each calcium ion released. There are separate pathways and separate control mechanisms for calcium uptake and release. The flux of calcium ions can be varied in either direction so that the mitochondrial pool of calcium can act as a calcium buffer for the cytosol.

The uptake of *excess calcium* in conditions of cytosolic calcium overload is serious. It impairs the proton gradient across the mitochondrial membranes, thereby reducing the ability of mitochondria to synthesize ATP. Irreversible reperfusion damage may be mediated by calcium (Chapter 19). Approximately two calcium ions and one phosphate ion accumulate for each pair of electrons passing through each energy-conserving site of the respiratory chain. Calcium forms insoluble calcium phosphate in the mitochondrial matrix, seen as irreversible granular densities on electron microscopy.

COUPLED OXIDATIVE PHOSPHORYLATION

Oxidation is an increase in positive charges or loss of negative charges; reduction is the reverse. When an electron donor donates e^-, it undergoes oxidation. When an electron acceptor accepts e^-, it undergoes reduction. Transfer of hydrogen is regarded as an equivalent process (because the hydrogen atoms equal $H^+ + e^-$).

The exact mechanisms linking the oxidation of $NADH_2$ (formed from the activity of the citrate cycle or pathways of substrate breakdown) to the formation of ATP are still poorly understood, despite the obvious importance of this critical process (Fig. 11-17). The basic oxidative reaction in coupled oxidative phosphorylation is the oxidation of $NADH_2$ (which is more correctly given in the ionized form as NADH and H^+): $NADH + H^+ + \frac{1}{2} O_2 \rightarrow NAD^+ + H_2O$.

This is coupled to phosphorylation of ADP: $2.5\ ADP + 2.5\ P_i \rightarrow 2.5\ ATP$.

Classically, it has been taught that three molecules of ATP are formed for each atom or half-molecule of oxygen taken up [phosphorylation/oxygen reuptake (P/O) ratio of 3]; however, current evidence favors a lower value of approximately 2.5 (Table 11-5). Production of ATP is coupled to proton production, and four protons produce enough proton motive force for one ATP. Thus, according to these current views and depending on the substrate oxidized, the P/O ratio may vary from 2.30 to 2.58, in contrast to the "old" values of 2.80 to 3.17. That means that the oxygen uptake required for a given rate of ATP production can be changed by approximately 12% from total glucose to total fatty acid utilization. Furthermore, fatty acids in high concentrations uncouple the mitochondria to further waste oxygen.

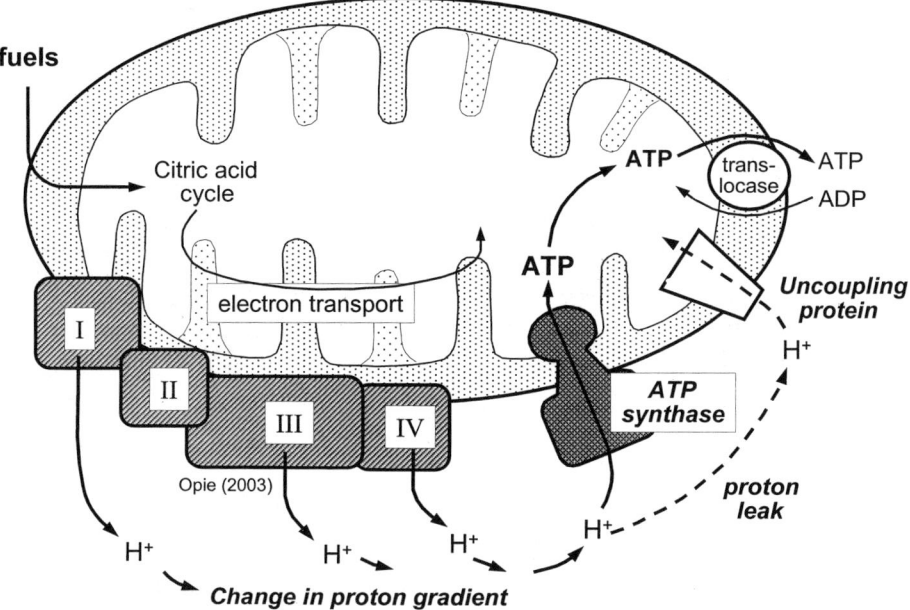

FIG. 11-17. Proton pumping and adenosine 5′-triphosphate (*ATP*) synthesis. According to Mitchell's chemiosmotic hypothesis, the electron transfer components of the respiratory chain (I to IV) are arranged spatially and in sequence so that alternate electron and proton transfers occur. The consequence is that protons are transferred from the mitochondrial matrix space out across the inner membrane and a membrane potential is generated. The result is the establishment of an electrochemical proton gradient across the mitochondrial inner membrane (the proton motive force) made up of a proton concentration gradient and a charge separation or membrane potential. Coupling of the proton motive force to the synthesis of ATP from adenosine 5′-diphosphate and inorganic phosphate occurs via the ATP synthase as protons reenter the mitochondrial matrix. Note role of uncoupling proteins that lead to proton leaks.

Electron Transport through the Respiratory Chain

Electrons derived from $NADH_2$ ($NADH + H^+$) flow along the respiratory transport (electron transmitter) chain as follows: $NADH + H^+ +$ flavoprotein (FP) $\rightarrow$ FP + $2e^- + NAD^+ + 2H^+$, FP + $2e^-$ + coenzyme Q (CoQ) $\rightarrow$ reduced CoQ (ubiquinone) + FP, reduced CoQ + cytochromes $\rightarrow$ reduced cytochromes + CoQ, reduced cytochromes + $2H^+ + \frac{1}{2} O_2 \rightarrow$ cytochromes + H_2O.

Electrons are transferred through the cytochromes, which are electron-transferring proteins containing iron porphyrin (heme) groups. The iron atoms undergo reversible changes in valency from the ferrous to the ferric form and vice versa. Heart mitochondria, with their high rate of respiration and extensive surface area of inner membranes, each contain 60,000 to 70,000 molecules of cytochrome in all, compared with 17,000 in each liver mitochondrion (24).

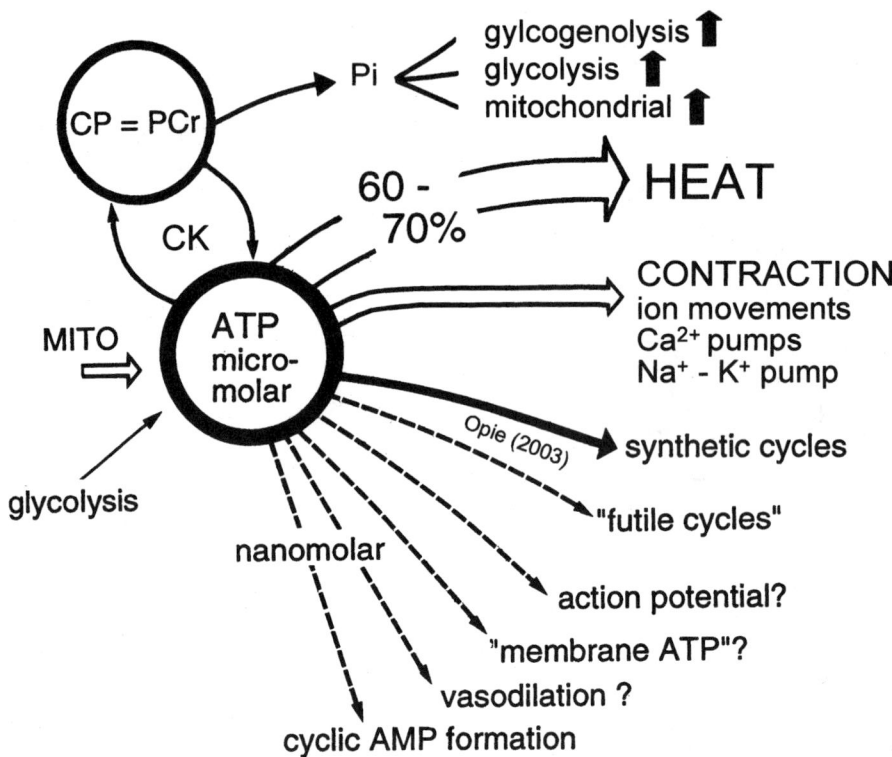

FIG. 11-18. Functions of adenosine 5′-triphosphate (*ATP*) and creatine phosphate (*CP*). Note major use in heat production, then contraction and related activities, such as ion transfer across membranes. *PCr*, phosphocreatine; *cyclic AMP*, adenosine 3′,5′-monophosphate; *MITO*, mitochondria.

The respiratory chain may be divided into three spans, each associated with the pumping of protons and with the production of ATP (Fig. 11-17). Site 1 is the span between NADH and CoQ_{10}, site 2 is the span between cytochrome b and cytochrome c, and site 3 is the span between cytochrome c and oxygen. Together, these sites transfer 10 protons outward across the mitochondrial membrane, and each four protons produce one ATP according to the current view. The mitochondrial oxidation of three molecules of $NADH_2$ produced by the citrate cycle, therefore, yields 2½ molecules of ATP per atom of oxygen reduced (with a P/O ratio of 2.5). Other reactions (e.g., pyruvate dehydrogenase) forming $NADH_2$ will also have a P/O ratio of 2.5, but reactions feeding into the chain at the level of CoQ will have a lower P/O ratio (succinate dehydrogenase produces $FADH_2$, which reacts with CoQ so that only eight protons are transferred with the potential for the synthesis of 2 ATP).

Proton Pumping and Adenosine 5'-Triphosphate Synthesis

The actual mechanism for ATP manufacture is closely linked with the fate of protons rather than electrons; thus, hydrogen atom = proton + electron and $H = H^+ + e^-$.

It is simple to suppose that the two H^+ link up with the two electrons and with oxygen eventually to form water. According to Mitchell's theory of oxidative phosphorylation, protons are pumped outward across the inner mitochondrial membrane to yield a gradient of H^+ across the membrane (Fig. 11-17). This H^+ gradient is the driving force for phosphorylation of ADP because protons reenter the mitochondrial matrix through a complex of membrane proteins called the *ATP synthetase*, which is a protein ionophore. Formation of ATP from ADP is driven by proton movements caused by the transmembrane proton gradient.

To review, for oxidative phosphorylation to proceed requires a continuous supply of (a) oxygen delivered by the coronary circulation, (b) protons and electrons delivered by the citrate cycle, and (c) ADP. Both ADP and ATP are large, highly charged molecules that must be transported rapidly and continuously across the impermeable inner mitochondrial membrane. Such counterexchange of ADP inward and ATP outward across the inner membrane occurs by the activity of a very active transport system, the ADP-ATP carrier, or antiporter, also called the *translocase*. It is the most abundant protein in cardiac mitochondria. The carrier system is highly selective, transporting only ADP and ATP. The entry process of the translocase greatly prefers ADP to ATP, possibly by more than 50 times. As the cytosolic ATP is converted to ADP during increased heart work, ADP transport to within the mitochondrial matrix is encouraged. Thus, there is an inverse relationship between the external ATP/ADP ratio and the oxygen uptake.

Oxygen Wastage and Uncoupling

When the heart is exposed to high circulating levels of circulating catecholamines and/or FFAs, the oxygen uptake may increase much more than expected from the change in respiratory quotient in switching from carbohydrate to fatty acids as fuel (10). This phenomenon, also found in humans (25), is not fully understood. Probably a major cause is the uncoupling effect of fatty acids on the respiratory chain so that much more oxygen is required for the same rate of production of ATP (26). An attractive but thus far unproven hypothesis is that fatty acids act on cardiac mitochondria to promote the activity of *uncoupling proteins*, which promote proton leaks (Fig. 11-18), to bypass the ATP synthase (27). Thus, the efficiency of converting oxygen to ATP (the P/O ratio) decreases. There may also be an increased turnover of intracellular *futile cycles*, repetitively synthesizing and breaking down triglycerides, thereby also wasting ATP. Last, pathways of respiration producing not ATP but free oxygen radicals may be enhanced.

TABLE 11-7. *Compensatory metabolic pathways sensitive to falls of adenosine 5′-triphosphate and creatine phosphate and increase of adenosine 5′ diphosphate, adenosine 5′-monophosphate, and inorganic phosphate*

Pathway	Site of regulation	Mode of regulation
Glycogenolysis	Phosphorylase	CP inhibits; AMP and Pi stimulate phosphorylase *b*
Glycolysis	Phosphofructokinase (and glucose uptake)[a]	ATP and CP inhibit; increase of AMP and Pi stimulates
Adenosine formation	5′-nucleotidase	Fall in energy status activates
ATP synthesis	Oxidative phosphorylation	ADP and Pi stimulate mitochondrial oxidative phosphorylation

[a]Regulated by coronary flow rate and glucose transporters, GLUT 4 and GLUT 1.
CP, creatinine phosphate; AMP, adenosine 5′-monophosphate; Pi, inorganic phosphate; ATP, adenosine 5′-triphosphate.

HOW IS THE ENERGY USED?

How is the vast amount of ATP that is made every day by the heart actually used? Quite simply, most is for heat production, then contraction (Fig. 11-18), and all the associated essential phenomena, such as calcium uptake by the sarcoplasmic reticulum. Approximately 11% to 15% of ATP may be used for active transport by the sodium–potassium pump (Table 11-7). Very little (less than 5%) is used for the actual generation of the action potential or the conduction of the cardiac impulse. Very small amounts of ATP are needed to phosphorylate the proteins in response to the formation of protein kinase or to form cAMP. An ill-defined small percentage is used for the futile cycles of glycogen and triglyceride turnover and of mitochondrial calcium uptake and release, and a further small percentage is used for protein synthesis. In pathologic states, ATP wastage occurs if futile cycles speed up or if abnormal, nonphosphorylating pathways of oxygen uptake are stimulated by excess FFAs (oxygen wastage). In all these calculations, it must be appreciated that the actual energy liberated by ATP hydrolysis is largely converted to heat. Thus, only approximately 20% to 25% of the ATP used is actually converted into mechanical work. The source of this heat is the flux of protons through the uncoupling proteins (Fig. 11-17). When allowance is made for this inevitable loss of heat, the heart is in fact very efficient in its ability to convert free energy into mechanical work plus heat.

Creatine Phosphate as Reserve Energy

At first sight, it would appear that creatine phosphate [(CP) also called phosphocreatine] rather than ATP is the immediate source of energy for contraction. In several types of pathologies such as heart failure and mild ischemia, loss of CP exceeds that of ATP. Yet, the overall evidence is that ATP and not CP is used directly in muscular contraction because ATP causes isolated actomyosin threads to shorten. It is logical (and in agreement with the classic concepts of skeletal muscle physiology) that the ATP concentration in the myocardial cell should be maintained at the expense of CP, with the pool of CP having a more marked depletion than the pool of ATP.

Energy Transfer between Adenosine 5′-Triphosphate and Creatine Phosphate

The transfer of energy from CP to ATP occurs under the influence of creatine kinase [(CK), creatine phosphokinase], which catalyses the following reaction: CP + ADP → ATP + creatine, and the equilibrium favors formation of ATP by approximately 50 times. The function of CP as a reserve of energy can be seen during the abrupt onset of intense exercise as modeled by an acute work jump in the isolated heart. Why does the content of ADP increase rather than decrease, as would be expected from the above equation? This is partly because the initial event is ATP hydrolysis. ATP (enzyme: myosin ATPase) → ADP + P_i + free energy. However, ATP is reformed from CP and ADP. Therefore, combining these two equations, ATP should not decrease at all: creatine phosphokinase → creatine + P_i + free energy.

In reality, ATP decreases and ADP increases, showing that the rate of ATP hydrolysis during the work jump can exceed the rate at which ATP is formed from CP.

Creatine Kinase (Creatine Phosphokinase)

The heart has a high content of CK, and the loss of this enzyme in large amounts into the circulation is taken as proof of cell necrosis in acute myocardial infarction. The larger proportion of the cardiac CK exists in the cytosol as the *MB isoenzyme* [having one subunit of muscle (M) type and one of brain (B) type]. The MM isoenzyme is present in small amounts in the myofibrils and possibly the microsomes. Different localization of isoenzymes within the extramitochondrial space could be one way in which local aliquots of energy are transferred from CP to ATP, so that ATP can be used at various localized sites in the cytoplasm (Fig. 11-19). This process is the *CP shuttle*, which transfers energy from one site in the cytosol to another (28). The very low cytosolic concentration of free ADP (most is protein bound) means that ADP produced by heart work could not rapidly diffuse to the mitochondria.

A *mitochondrial CK isoenzyme* is situated on the outside of the inner mitochondrial membrane where it is thought to be in close juxtaposition to the adenine nucleotide translocase. The kinetic properties of the enzyme support its role in dealing with ATP newly synthesized and newly exported from mitochondria. ATP produced in the mitochondria by oxidative phosphorylation is transferred by the mitochondrial CK isoenzyme to cytoplasmic CP. Thus, the real end product of oxidative phosphorylation in the heart is CP (29). The latter compound then transfers high-energy phosphate bonds back to ATP at the site of ATP use,

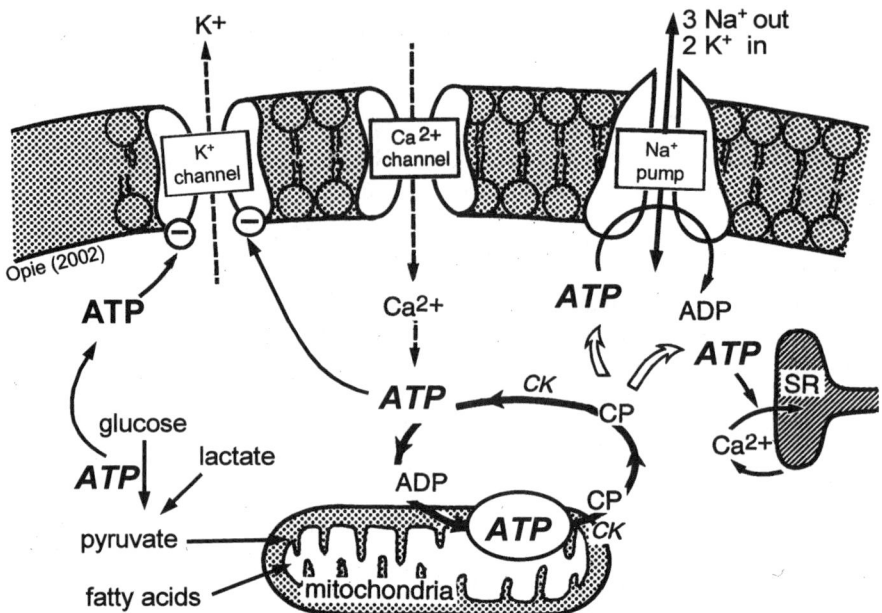

FIG. 11-19. Adenosine 5′-triphosphate (*ATP*) pools and compartments. The major ATP compartments are mitochondrial and cytosolic. Minor localized pools are associated with (a) the potassium channel, where ATP acts as a regulatory ligand and (b) external surface ATP, which may function as a vasodilator. ATP is used in many noncontractile processes, such as sodium pumping and uptake of calcium by the sarcoplasmic reticulum (*SR*). Creatine kinase (*CK*) has an important role in the functional compartmentalization of ATP. The mitochondrial CK isoenzyme is situated between the inner and outer mitochondrial membranes to form creatine phosphate (*CP*) from creatine. The outer mitochondrial membrane is freely permeable to CP, which can then reform ATP from adenosine 5′-diphosphate (*ADP*) generated by cellular activity, such as contraction. This is the function of the cytoplasmic CK isoenzyme.

under the influence of a cytosolic isoenzyme of CK (Fig. 11-19). When creatine transport is inhibited by a specific inhibitor, heart failure ensues, which again supports the concept of the importance of the CP shuttle for cardiac contractile function (28,29). A corollary of this proposal is that ADP produced by the mitochondrial CK should have preferential access to the translocase. Thus, CK plays a vital role in the maintenance of cytosolic ATP at the expense of cytosolic CP. By transferring energy-rich bonds from ATP as it emerges from the mitochondria to cytosolic CP, and then back again to ATP, CK also controls the transport of energy in the cytosol.

During irreversible ischemia, the sarcolemma becomes permeable and various enzymes leak into the circulation, including CK. When the blood level of CK increases above a particular arbitrary level, the diagnosis of cardiac cell necrosis (myocardial infarction) is made.

ADENOSINE 5'-TRIPHOSPHATE COMPARTMENTS

At the onset of ischemia, there is a surprising discrepancy between the rapid cessation of contraction and the small decrease in the level of myocardial ATP. Cellular compartmentation of ATP is one of several possible explanations. Compartmentation means that some compounds are not distributed uniformly throughout the cell. Rather, different concentrations are found in different compartments within the cell. Compartmentation of ATP between its site of production in mitochondria and its site of use in the cytoplasm is well accepted. At least 90% of the ATP is found in the cytosol. During acute heart work, the ATP in the cytosol is broken down so that the very small amount of cytosolic ADP doubles. Cytosolic ADP will, therefore, increase with increased work to drive mitochondrial respiration, according to the classic concept that the rate of mitochondrial respiration is set by ADP.

The possibility of *cytosolic subcompartments of ATP* has in the past provoked much controversy (Fig. 11-19). Evidence favoring cytoplasmic subcompartmentation is as follows. First, unequal distribution of CK isoenzymes throughout the cytoplasm could form more ATP from CP in specific cytosolic sites. Second, the existence of a small subcompartment of rapid-turnover ATP would explain those situations in which small changes in total ATP occur but appear to have large effects, such as the abrupt loss of contractile activity in ischemic hearts while the ATP is still relatively high. Depletion of only a small pool of ATP could cause contractile failure, but it is equally possible that other factors, such as an increase in tissue P_{CO_2} or P_i, could cause contractile failure (Table 17-1). Third, ATP produced by glycolysis appears to have a special function in protecting the cell membrane, particularly the activity of the ATP-sensitive potassium channel (12) and the sodium pump (30). When ischemic contracture develops in underperfused hearts, it is the source of ATP and not the total ATP that is important in preventing contracture. Thus, ATP made by glycolysis is effective, whereas ATP from residual mitochondrial metabolism is not (31).

Despite such evidence favoring ATP compartments, the high activity of the CK shuttle means that there is constant production of ATP at local sites where it is needed. It is only when the CK shuttle decreases in activity as in ischemia (28) that added production of ATP from glycolysis improves myocardial function (32).

PHYSIOLOGIC BREAKDOWN OF ADENOSINE 5'-TRIPHOSPHATE

To release energy from ATP requires its breakdown to ADP and P_i (Fig. 11-20), which form during each cardiac contraction cycle. It is usually forgotten that there is a proton produced and that ATP is chelated to magnesium.

Thus, the standard equation ATP $\rightarrow$ ADP + P_i + free energy becomes $MgATP^{2-} \rightarrow MgADP^{1-} + P_i^{2-} + H^+$ + free energy. The exact charges depend on the intracellular pH. ADP can (a) reform ATP via the CK reaction, (b) be further split to form ATP and AMP by the adenylate kinase reaction, or (c) enter the mitochondria under the influence of the adenine nucleotide translocase to stimulate respiration. The proton produced is important during anaerobic glycolysis, when it is the major source of the intracellular acidosis (33).

The total content of ADP in the normal heart is approximately 0.5 to 1.0 µmol/g wet weight. However, the real concentration dissolved in cell water (as opposed to the overall level) is difficult to assess because most ADP is bound to actin, some to myosin, and only a smaller portion is freely dissolved in the cytosol. The breakdown of even small amounts of cytosolic ATP to ADP can markedly increase the concentration of free ADP in the cytosol (estimated at only 0.02 µmol/g wet weight), thereby stimulating mitochondrial metabolism. AMP can also be formed from ATP (e.g., during ischemia or a work jump).

Under the influence of myosin ATPase, 2 ATP → 2 ADP + 2 P_i + 2(free energy) is followed by the action of the enzyme *adenylate kinase* (myokinase) 2 ADP → ATP + AMP. This reaction is reversible and will proceed toward formation of AMP only when ADP is elevated. Because myosin ATPase again catalyzes, ATP → ADP + P_i + free energy, the overall reaction is 2 ATP → ADP + AMP + 3 P_i + (free energy).

This pattern of ATP breakdown liberates 1.5 times as much high-energy phosphate as does simple ATP hydrolysis to ADP (compare previous equations). The extra energy provided by the added breakdown of ATP beyond ADP to AMP is followed by further metabolism of AMP to inosine 5'-monophosphate and adenosine. Because the ratio of ATP to adenosine is so high, perhaps approximately 1,000:1, the breakdown of only a small amount of ATP to adenosine can markedly increase the levels of the latter.

Adenosine 5'-Monophosphate–Activated Protein Kinase: Masterminding Energy Metabolism

During acute work stress (imagine primitive man suddenly running away from the lion), the heart needs all the energy that it can get. There should be a mechanism to make "all systems go." However, as already described, fatty acids can inhibit glucose metabolism. Conversely, glycolysis can inhibit fatty acid metabolism via the formation of malonyl-CoA. Although increased work drives the citrate cycle by increased NAD and increased calcium (Fig. 11-16), what is also needed is stimulation of the pathways of both glycolysis and fatty acid metabolism so that more acetyl-CoA units can enter the citrate cycle. The crucial switch is the breakdown of ATP not just to ADP but further to AMP, as occurs during a work jump in the rat heart (Fig. 11-20). The AMP in turns stimulates a kinase, AMP-activated protein kinase, which is the "fuel gauge of the heart" (21). AMP kinase inhibits the formation of malonyl-CoA, a metabolite that limits the entry of acyl-CoA into the mitochondria (Fig. 11-15). Therefore, AMP kinase indirectly enhances the entry of acyl-CoA into the mitochondria and promotes fatty acid oxidation. More specifically, AMP kinase inactivates acetyl-CoA carboxy-

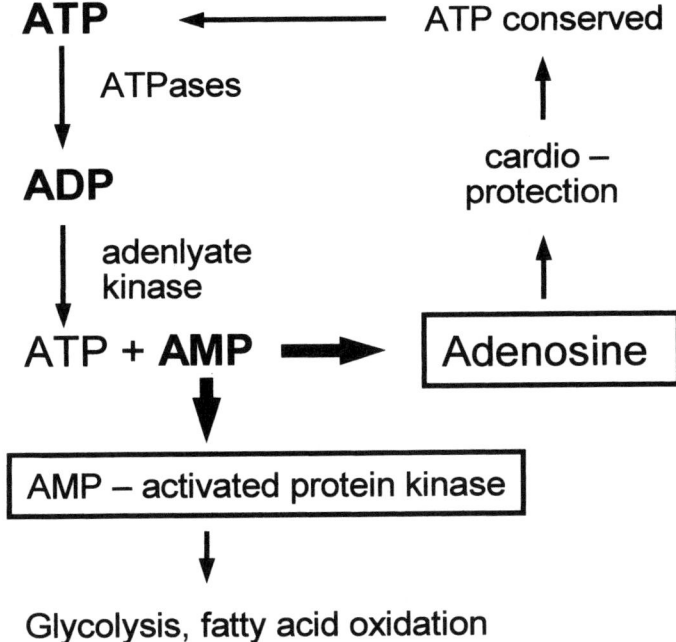

FIG. 11-20. Adenosine 5'-triphosphate (*ATP*) breakdown. The influence of oxygen supply on the extent of ATP breakdown. In normoxia, ATP is broken down by heart work (myosin ATPase) to adenosine 5'-diphosphate (*ADP*) and inorganic phosphate (*Pi*), which are resynthesized to ATP in the mitochondria. In hypoxia, further breakdown yields more energy and stimulates glycolysis to provide anaerobic energy and causes a compensatory vasodilation (probably via adenosine). *MITO*, mitochondria.

lase needed for the synthesis of malonyl-CoA (21). AMP kinase also increases glucose uptake by translocating glucose transporters to the sarcolemma and stimulating glycolysis (11). During subtotal ischemia, when there is much more breakdown of ATP to AMP than during acute heart work, there is considerable activation of AMP kinase that drives the fatty acid metabolism to "steal" the residual oxygen from glucose and glycolysis. A genetic mutation in AMP kinase causes one type of cardiomyopathy (Fig. 16-3) (18).

Adenosine

Adenosine is a naturally generated cardioprotective agent linked to multiple signal systems (Fig. 11-21). First, it interacts with three receptors: the A_1 and A_3 myocardial receptors and the A_2 vascular receptors. The key physiologic function of adenosine is to act on the vascular A_2 receptors, thereby keeping energy metabolism in balance by providing compensatory coronary vasodilation whenever the myocardial ATP runs down, as in ischemia. When adenosine acts on the

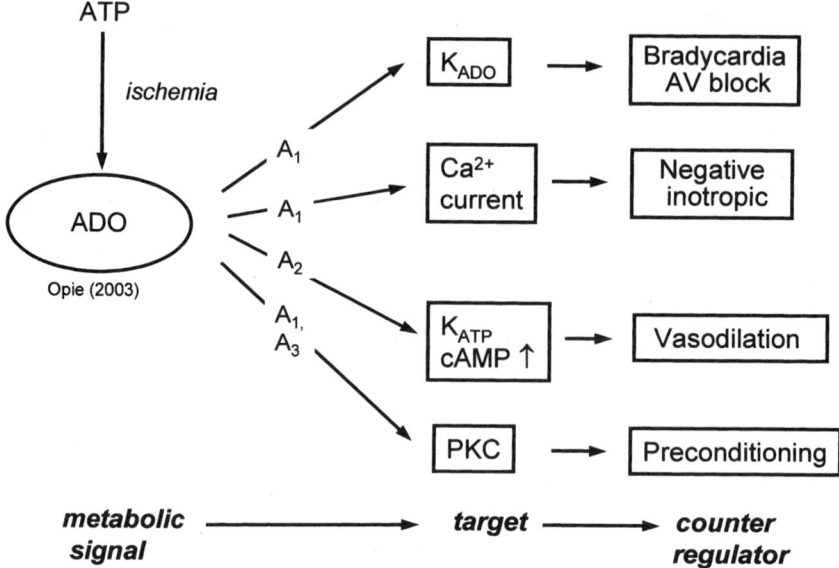

FIG. 11-21. Adenosine (ADO) signaling. A_1-receptor stimulation activates the potassium channel (K_{ADO}), inhibiting the sinoatrial node with bradycardia and the atrioventricular (AV) node with therapeutic AV block (Fig. 20-5), and inhibits ventricular contraction by increasing calcium channel closing times. A_2-receptor stimulation opens vascular adenosine 5′-triphosphate (ATP)–sensitive potassium channel (K_{ATP}) with vasodilation. A_1- or A_3-receptor stimulation activates protein kinase (PKC) with preconditioning (Fig. 19-12). For function of adenosine in coronary flow regulation, see Figure 10-5.

A_1 receptors, there are several cardioprotective effects, including potassium channel opening, catecholamine antagonism, therapeutic inhibition of the atrioventricular node in supraventricular tachycardias, and an important role in a type of cardioprotection called preconditioning (Fig. 19-12). This is where the A_3 receptor also becomes relevant (34).

Adenosine 5′-Triphosphate Products and Energy Status

A decrease in ATP stimulates both the primitive energy supply systems of glycogenolysis and glycolysis and the more evolved mitochondrial oxidative systems. Stimulation of the latter is assisted by an increased coronary blood flow via adenosine formation and provides more oxygen to increase oxidative phosphorylation in the mitochondria. The detailed mechanisms whereby the decline in ATP acts on the different pathways vary (Table 11-7), but the principle is constant. It is not the level of ATP itself that regulates the compensatory pathways but the ATP breakdown products (AMP, P_i, adenosine) that act as regulators. Breakdown of only a small amount of ATP potentially can markedly increase the cellular levels of the real regulators, such as AMP and adenosine. The *phospho-*

rylation potential relates change in high-energy phosphates to mitochondrial metabolism (23).

$$\text{phosphorylation potential} = \frac{(ATP)}{(ADP)(P_i)}$$

AMP is omitted because it does not play a direct role in the regulation of mitochondrial respiration. The value of this ratio is that it is reciprocally related to the rate of mitochondrial oxidative metabolism. The problem is that the cytosolic ADP concentration is required and cannot readily be measured but only calculated.

In humans, the ratio of CP/P_i can be measured by ^{31}P nuclear magnetic resonance techniques and, therefore, assessed *in vivo*. This ratio is a simple approach to measuring the energy status because it is closely related to the breakdown of ATP to ADP and P_i. Another nuclear magnetic resonance ratio that has been used on the human heart is CP/ATP, the principle being that in conditions of myocardial metabolic stress, ATP is maintained at the expense of CP.

METABOLISM OF ISCHEMIA

Ischemia means inadequate coronary flow (Chapter 17) such that the tissue oxygen tension decreases (hypoxia). When ischemia is very severe, with no coronary flow at all, there is no oxygen (anoxia). In clinical conditions such as angina pectoris and acute myocardial infarction, there still is some collateral flow to the ischemic zone, so that there is subtotal ischemia. In this situation, various therapeutic agents can still reach the ischemic cells. In cardiac surgery, when the heart is arrested, there is no coronary flow at all, and the ischemia is total. When extrapolating from animal data to human disease, it is therefore important to distinguish between subtotal and total ischemia. Only subtotal ischemia has a continued albeit much diminished oxygen supply to the ischemic zone, as in ischemic heart disease in patients (Fig. 17-1). Therefore, most of the following discussion concentrates on subtotal ischemia.

Anaerobic Glycolysis in Ischemia

Strictly, anaerobic means "no oxygen" but that does not mean "no life." Anaerobic metabolism refers to any state of suboptimal oxygenation that accelerates glycolysis and increases the production of lactate (Fig. 11-22). Anaerobic glycolysis is part of the defense mechanism that allows sufficient production of oxygen-independent energy to sustain the noncontractile ischemic myocardium (Table 11-7). To explain how glycolysis is accelerated during hypoxia and ischemia requires an analysis of the properties of two crucial enzymes, PFK and glyceraldehyde 3-phosphate dehydrogenase. The PFK reaction is ideally suited for metabolic control of glycolysis during hypoxia because it is so sensitive to the energy status of the myocardial cells. Low molecular weight metabolites, such

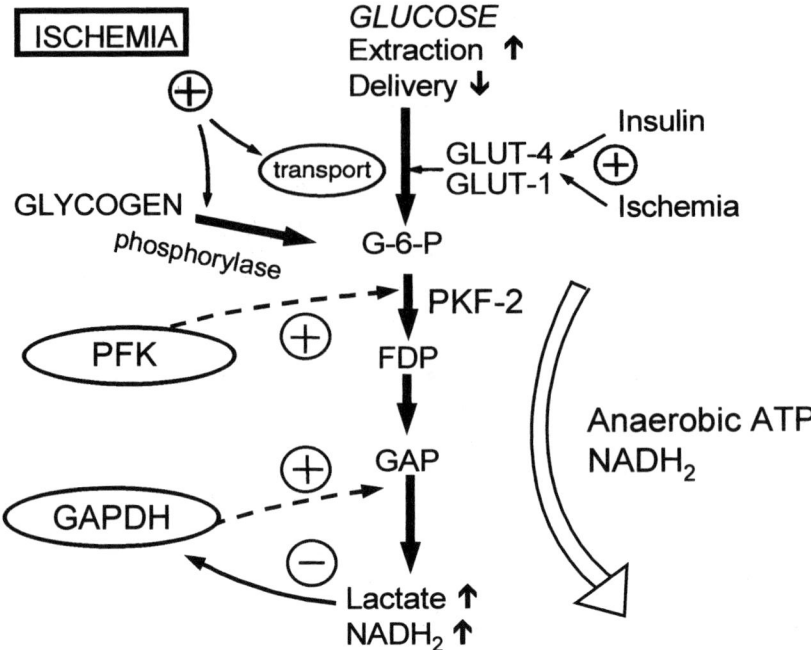

FIG. 11-22. Regulation of glycolysis in ischemia. In mild ischemia, glycolysis is stimulated (Fig. 11-2). Two major hypotheses are rate-limiting steps as shown in ovals and "top-down" control, regulated by rates of decreased rates of glucose delivery or glycogenolysis. *G-6-P*, glucose 6-phosphate; *FDP*, fructose 1,6-bisphosphate; *GAP*, glyceraldehyde 3-phosphate; GAPDH, glyceraldehyde 3-phosphate dehydrogenase; GLUT, glucose transporter; *PFK*, phosphofructokinase.

as ATP, AMP, ADP, and P_i, interact with the enzyme at *allosteric sites* (allo, alongside; steric, configuration) that are distant from the site of interaction between substrates and enzyme. During hypoxia and mild ischemia, ATP levels decrease and those of ADP, AMP, and P_i increase. These changes enhance the activity of the enzyme (increased anaerobic glycolysis). Furthermore, the activity of the closely related enzyme PFK-2 also increases in ischemia, albeit through a different mechanism involving AMP kinase (11). During severe ischemia, glycolysis is inhibited by low rates of delivery of glucose, glycogen depletion, and intracellular acidosis, which all inhibit the enzyme PFK. In addition, just before the onset of irreversible damage in severe ischemia, PFK is translocated from cytosol to myocardial membranes and thereby inactivated (35).

A second and equally important control step is that regulating the flow through glycolysis at the level of the enzyme glyceraldehyde 3-phosphate dehydrogenase (36), which is inhibited in severely ischemic tissue by the end products of anaerobic glycolysis, such as lactate, protons, and $NADH_2$. However, such inhibition is not as severe as previously supposed because the major limitation to glycolytic flux in ischemia lies in decreased glucose delivery, the direct result of decreased coronary flow (37).

Thus, to review, mild ischemia stimulates glycolysis and has potentially beneficial effects by provision of oxygen-independent ATP, whereas severe ischemia inhibits glycolysis mainly by decreasing the delivery of glucose to the ischemic cells but also by glycogen depletion and enzyme inhibition.

Inadequate Energy Production by Anaerobic Glycolysis

Strictly speaking, anaerobic glycolysis means that glycolysis is occurring in the total absence of air and hence anoxia. The term is commonly applied to the acceleration of glycolysis with production of lactate that occurs in response to lesser degrees of oxygen lack. To produce as much ATP by glycolysis during true anaerobiosis would require an acceleration of glycolysis by nearly 20 times, in contrast to the more modest acceleration that even total anoxia produces when coronary flow is maintained artificially. The anaerobic heart, therefore, develops a severe deficit of energy unless arrested by high potassium (Fig. 11-23) or

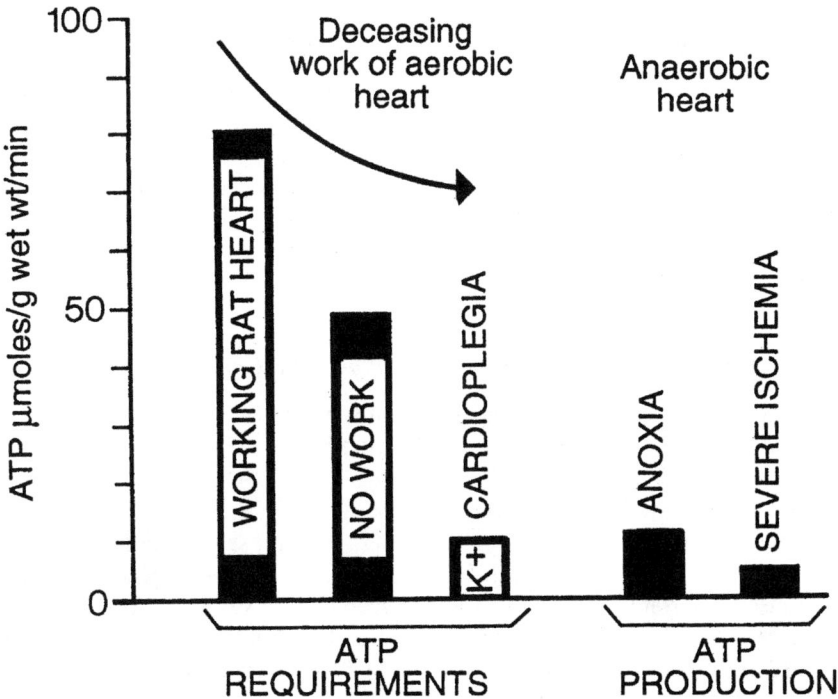

FIG. 11-23. Adenosine 5'-triphosphate (*ATP*) requirements versus ATP production during oxygen lack. Anaerobic ATP production cannot meet energy needs of the heart unless it is arrested by cardioplegia, even when ATP is produced at maximal rates (anoxia with sustained coronary flow). During total ischemia, the rate of anaerobic glycolysis decreases so that the best way to preserve the ischemic myocardium is to reduce the ATP demand (cardioplegia + hypothermia). For details of calculations, see Opie LH. Substrate utilization and glycolysis in the heart. *Cardiology* 1971; 56: 2–21.

hypothermia, which is the basis of cardioplegia. When glucose is the source of glycolysis, the whole glycolytic path uses two ATP and produces four ATP, i.e., the net production is two. When glycogen is the source, ATP production is three per six-carbon molecule passing through glycolysis. An important point is that glycolytic ATP will be made whenever glucose 6-phosphate is converted to pyruvate even during oxidative metabolism.

Anaerobic glycolysis changes the normal uptake of lactate by the aerobic myocardium to discharge, and the level in the coronary sinus may exceed that in arterial blood during myocardial ischemia. This is not a very sensitive procedure because apparent net uptake of lactate can mask local lactate production by the ischemic zone (38). The formation of protons during anaerobic glycolysis is, strictly speaking, not from glycolysis itself but from the associated breakdown of ATP. The *malate–aspartate shuttle* is crucial in transferring protons in the form of $NADH_2$ from the cytosol to the mitochondria (Fig. 11-11). During anaerobic glycolysis, such protons accumulate in the cytosol and may contribute to the loss of contractile function that occurs (Table 17-1).

Adenosine 5'-Triphosphate Breakdown in Ischemia

When ATP is broken down acutely, as in hypoxia or ischemia, it is protected by CP. Then, release from the heart of breakdown products of ATP can be expected. During regional ischemia, the concentration of P_i in the coronary sinus increases. This phosphate is derived only in part from ATP, with a larger component coming from the breakdown of CP. Adenosine, inosine, and hypoxanthine can all cross the cell membrane, and, therefore, it is not surprising that the ischemic myocardium releases these compounds.

Does Decreased Adenosine 5'-Triphosphate Cause Cell Death?

A simplistic view of cell death in ischemia would be that ATP decreases to a critical level, vital functions cease, and all is over. Considering the pains to which the cell goes to maintain and replenish its ATP, it would not be surprising if there were a critical level of ATP required to keep the cell alive. Nonetheless, this concept is oversimplified. ATP levels less than those regarded as critical are still compatible with cell survival. In the *nonischemic zone* after coronary occlusion, muscle contracted normally and survived at ATP values as low as 1.5 to 2.0 μmol/g wet weight (39). In *reperfusion* after ischemic arrest (40), ATP might decrease to as low as 1 μmol/g wet weight and the heart could still survive. Such evidence shows that it is very unlikely that there is a single critical level of ATP, although chronic depletion of ATP is marker of metabolic deterioration and poor prognosis for human heart failure (41). Furthermore, cell death occurs not only by necrosis but also by apoptosis (Fig. 9-9). Here ATP depletion is not required. Instead, a crucial process is the release of cytochrome c from mitochondria damaged by several different stimuli including ischemia (Figs. 9-18 and 18-6).

CLINICAL APPLICATIONS OF ENERGY METABOLISM

Cardioplegia

This is the most successful and widely used application of metabolic principles to myocardial preservation (Fig. 11-23). A low temperature diminishes the ATP requirements by decreasing the rate of enzyme reactions and the force of contraction, whereas a high external potassium mechanically arrests the heart by depolarization.

Insulin Resistance

This diagnosis is of increasing clinical importance and is applied to a variety of common clinical conditions that share the inability of skeletal muscle to respond to insulin by adequately increasing the glucose uptake. These conditions include obesity, diabetes mellitus, some cases of hypertension, and patients with postinfarction heart failure. Circulating FFAs are elevated in conditions associated with insulin resistance, such as obesity and maturity-onset diabetes. Thus, glucose uptake by muscle is inhibited, with less response to insulin. The excess circulating glucose level induces phosphorylation of the serine/threonine components of the insulin receptor, which diminishes the capacity of this receptor to undergo the required phosphorylation in response to insulin (42), thereby further decreasing the response to insulin.

For the patient, the major problem with insulin resistance is that it is potentially a self-perpetuating vicious circle because as it progresses, the blood levels of glucose and FFAs are both likely to increase. As a result, the diabetic state could worsen or the patient without diabetes could come closer to developing frank diabetes. In heart failure or hypertension, these adverse trends could be exaggerated by concurrent diuretic or β-blocker therapy, which may promote the diabetic state. A new principle is that the glitazone drug group lessens insulin resistance by stimulating the formation of peroxisome proliferator–activated receptor (PPAR)-γ in adipocytes (Fig. 9-15), resulting in decreased release of FFAs. Development of overt diabetes can also be prevented by increased exercise, weight loss, and diet. Exercise training increases glucose transport into both skeletal and heart muscle.

Lipid Metabolites in Myocardial Injury

During ischemia, the concentrations of long-chain fatty acid intermediates in both cytosol and mitochondria increase substantially with adverse effects on cardiac cell membranes (Fig. 11-24). Some of these inhibit the activity of the sodium–potassium pump at concentrations likely to be present in the ischemic tissue. The ensuing loss of potassium is also arrhythmogenic. *Lysophosphoglycerides* are membrane-active fatty acids that are released from the phospholipids of the sarcolemma and other membranes during ischemia. These also have

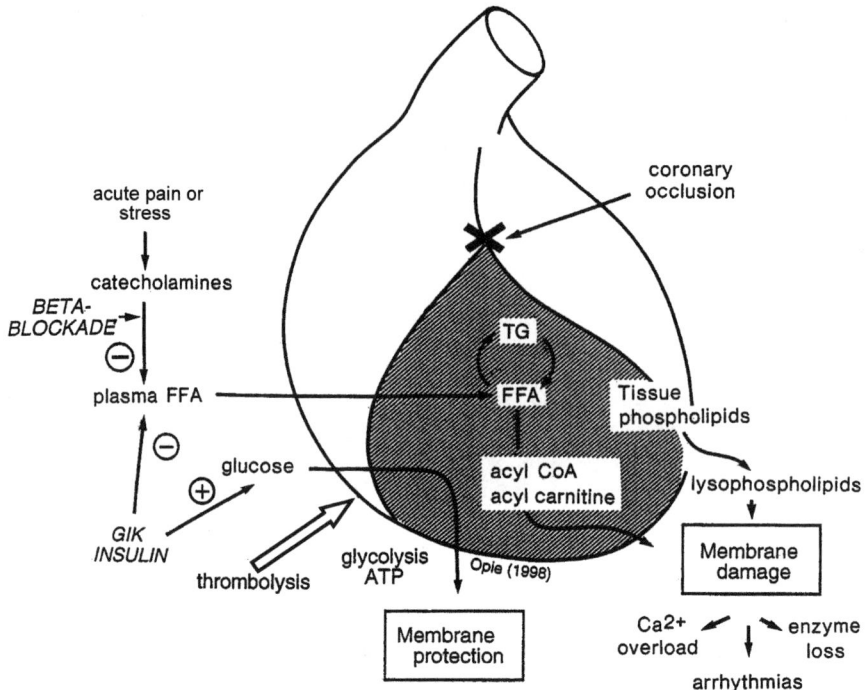

FIG. 11-24. Ischemic myocardium. Mechanisms of fatty acid toxicity and metabolic protection by glycolysis. *FFA*, free fatty acids; *TG*, triglyceride; CoA, coenzyme; *GIK*, glucose/insulin/potassium; ATP, adenosine 5'-triphosphate; –, negative effect; +, positive effect.

arrhythmogenic properties. No therapy is available to limit such lipid accumulation; several trials with carnitine or propionylcarnitine have not been promising. However, these compounds do decrease fatty acid oxidation rates and do help in ischemia by increasing the activity of pyruvate dehydrogenase and thereby indirectly increasing the rates of glucose oxidation. *Lipotoxicity* is an extreme experimental condition of cardiac lipid overload, experimentally found, for example, when excess accumulation of myocardial triglyceride occurs as in severe diabetic cardiomyopathy.

Metabolic Imaging: Positron Emission Tomography

Pathways of intracellular metabolism, previously studied only in animal tissues, can now be traced in humans by the technique of positron emission tomography (PET) scanning. Radiolabeled 2-deoxyglucose (^{18}F-fluorodeoxyglucose) can be visualized by PET (Fig. 11-25) when it is given in tracer amounts that accumulate within myocardial cells as the phosphorylated compound, without glycolysis being inhibited. In addition, the compound $^{13}NH_3$ can be used to measure coronary blood flow (Chapter 10). As expected, mild ischemia increases the

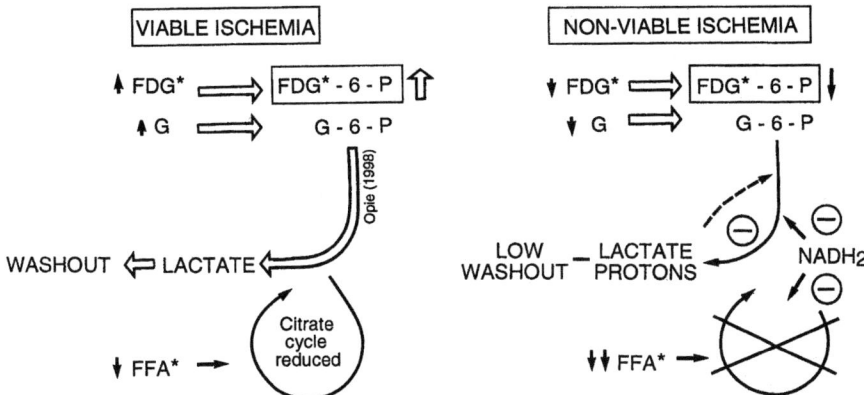

FIG. 11-25. **Glucose imaging and viability.** Proposed use of ^{18}F-fluorodeoxyglucose (*FDG**) acting as a marker for glucose uptake. FDG-6-phosphate is not metabolized. Hence, the intensity of extraction of fluorodeoxyglucose by the myocardium as detected by positron emission tomography is an index of viability. In "mismatch," glucose extraction is increased in relation to coronary blood flow measured by NH_3. In very severe ischemia or infarction, glucose delivery is decreased, glycolysis is inhibited, and extraction of FDG decreases.

glucose extraction, so that the metabolic severity of ischemia can be measured and used clinically to distinguish between those myocardial segments that are ischemic but viable (increased glucose extraction in relation to decreased coronary flow, "mismatch" pattern). In contrast, those segments that are nonviable have both decreased glucose extraction and low coronary flow. This test has practical potential in diagnosing hibernation (Fig. 19-8) and hence in selecting patients with a hibernating heart who will benefit from coronary artery surgery. ^{11}C-acetate is used to measure oxidative metabolism. The benefits of β-blockade in the failing heart can in part be explained by decreased uptake and metabolism of fatty acids, as shown with ^{18}F-labeled long-chain fatty acids (43). What is still missing is a PET imaging agent to trace glucose oxidation.

Heart Failure and High-Energy Phosphates

Nuclear magnetic resonance techniques (^{31}P-NMR) allow repetitive measurements of ATP and CP in the animal heart *in situ*. In heart failure, there are defects in energy production. Mitochondrial CK activity decreases, and adenylate kinase becomes more active in energy transfer (44). In human heart failure, the ratio of CP to ATP decreases in relation to the severity of failure (41).

METABOLIC THERAPIES FOR ISCHEMIA

The principles of metabolic therapy (Fig. 11-24) are fourfold. First, promotion of maximal rates of glycolysis, thereby providing more protective glycolytic

ATP, as by glucose-insulin-potassium (32). Second, glycolysis should be coupled to glucose oxidation, thereby passing along the $NADH_2$ made by glycolysis to the mitochondria for oxidation and decreasing the rate of production of adverse protons. The best way to achieve this aim is by increasing the activity of pyruvate dehydrogenase. Third, oxygen-wasting fatty acid metabolism should be diminished. Fourth, reperfusion damage can be minimized by insulin. These therapies act independently of hemodynamic therapy, such as reduction of the heart rate by β-adrenergic blockers to decrease myocardial oxygen demand.

Promotion of Protective Glycolysis by Glucose/Insulin/Potassium

Experimentally, provision of glycolytic ATP is crucial to the survival of ischemic cells (Fig. 11-23). Thus, promotion of glycolysis by a high circulating glucose concentration and insulin is logical. In isolated hearts in which coronary flow is reduced to only 10% of normal, high glucose and insulin concentrations not only increased glycolysis but produced higher ATP and CP concentrations with lower P_i and greater free-energy yield from ATP hydrolysis (32). In patients, strong data favor glucose-insulin-potassium infusions for acute myocardial infarction in patients with diabetes (45,46). There is a large trial currently underway of those without diabetes. Such an infusion may work, in part, by suppression of blood FFA levels, which tend to be high in patients with diabetes. In all patients with acute myocardial infarction, severe ischemia limits glycolysis by the low rate of delivery of glucose, so that reperfusion by thrombolysis or primary angioplasty is an important procedure to accelerate glycolysis.

Linking (Coupling) of Glycolysis to Glucose Oxidation

This is an important concept of Lopaschuk (47). In low-flow ischemia, glycolysis is stimulated but its end products, such as pyruvate, $NADH_2$, and protons, cannot readily enter the citrate cycle so that glycolysis is uncoupled from glucose oxidation. Lopaschuk proposed that the protons produced when glucose oxidation is low (i.e., uncoupled glycolysis from glucose oxidation) are primarily responsible for the marked decrease in cardiac efficiency in the presence of high levels of fatty acids. Each proton produced is derived from ATP breakdown and eventually requires one ATP for its clearance (directly or indirectly). There is the potential for a very large increase in efficiency if glucose oxidation is indirectly stimulated by inhibiting fatty acid oxidation. The fundamental step in enhancing glucose entry into the citrate cycle is increased activity of pyruvate dehydrogenase, whether achieved by inhibition of fatty acid oxidation or pharmacologic agents such as dichloroacetate.

Inhibition of Fatty Acid Metabolism

During ischemia, the activity of AMP kinase (Fig. 11-20) increases severalfold with the result that more fatty acid in the form of acyl-CoA enters mitochondria to be oxidized and to produce $NADH_2$ (14). The latter inhibits pyruvate dehydrogenase. Thus, fatty acids are preferentially oxidized and "steal" the residual oxygen from glucose, thereby uncoupling respiration, especially in the presence of a high adrenergic drive as occurs when patients feel threatened by the chest pain that accompanies cardiac ischemia. Various conditions decrease fatty acid oxidation, including a decrease in circulating fatty acid levels (one of the effects of the insulin in glucose-insulin-potassium) as well as the pharmacologic agents ranolazine and trimetazidine that are becoming available for clinical use in angina.

Postreperfusion Abnormalities

These are multiple. Experimentally, increased fatty acid oxidation and reduced glucose oxidation are adverse. There is also a postischemic run down of citrate cycle intermediates that can be remedied by conversion of pyruvate to malate (Fig. 11-9). This "topping-up" process is called *anaplerosis* (48). Excessive cytosolic calcium in the reperfused myocardium can be normalized by promotion of glycolysis (49), which provides the cytosolic ATP required for the uptake of calcium by the sarcoplasmic reticulum and for extrusion of sodium by the sodium pump. Promotion of glycolysis is not enough to prevent low rates of glucose oxidation and poor cardiac performance (50). Levels of malonyl-CoA can be very low, the proposed result of an accumulation of AMP, which in turn activates AMP kinase to inhibit the synthesis of malonyl-CoA and thereby promote adverse fatty acid oxidation (50). Increased glucose oxidation and cardiac function may be achieved by activation of pyruvate dehydrogenase (e.g., by dichloroacetate, by provision of pyruvate, and by inhibition of fatty acid oxidation). Another protective intervention is insulin, in this case acting independently of glucose to decrease reperfusion-induced apoptosis (51). None of these measures has been subject to clinical trials, although there is indirect evidence favoring the use of insulin as part of glucose-insulin-potassium in reperfused patients with acute myocardial infarction (45).

Gene Therapy

The transcription factor PPAR-α is very likely to be a key regulator of the gene changes that cause substrate switching from protective glucose use to adverse fatty acid use in the hypertrophic and failing heart (Fig. 16-11), at least in animals (2). A promising experimental therapy is enhancing the genes that promote the synthesis of glucose transporters, thereby preventing the hypertrophied heart from dilating and failing (52).

Dietary Protection by Long-Chain ω-3 Polyunsaturated Fatty Acids

Increased dietary ω-3 fatty acids, such as in fish and canola oils, protect against as sudden death (53). This fits with substantial experimental data showing that animals fed on such diets are protected from fatal ventricular fibrillation as provoked by regional myocardial ischemia (Chapter 20).

SUMMARY

1. *Myocardial fuels.* The heart is omnivorous in its requirements for fuels that it can convert to energy required mainly for contractile purposes. Glucose is the major myocardial fuel only after a high carbohydrate meal. Glucose is transported into heart cells by the insulin-sensitive transporter GLUT-4 to undergo phosphorylation to glucose 6-phosphate. Glycogen is a reserve fuel that can be broken down to glucose 6-phosphate in emergency situations, such as the sudden onset of heart work or ischemia. Glycolysis is the process common to glucose uptake and glycogen breakdown, which converts glucose 6-phosphate to two molecules of pyruvate. In anaerobic conditions (lack of oxygen), pyruvate is converted to lactate, whereas aerobically it forms the two-carbon compound acetyl-CoA, which enters the citrate cycle.
2. *Energy yield.* During glycolysis (glucose 6-phosphate to pyruvate), there is a net yield of two ATP and two H^+ (the latter from the dehydrogenation step). The two H^+ cannot immediately form water but must first interact with an important carrier molecule, NAD, to form $NADH_2$, which enters the mitochondrial space by a shuttle mechanism to yield aerobic energy. The additional energy yield of the oxidative metabolism of glucose is approximately 30 ATP molecules per glucose molecule, with a total yield of 32 ATP (these are lower than values previously given).
3. *Role of FFAs.* Long-chain FFAs, usually the major myocardial fuel, readily pass through the sarcolemmal membrane before irreversible activation to acyl-CoA, which cannot penetrate the mitochondrial barrier without a carnitine carrier system. Acyl-CoA is carried into the mitochondria as acylcarnitine, there to enter the pathways of β-oxidation that sequentially "chop off" two carbon fractions to form acetyl-CoA, which in turn enters the citrate cycle. Acyl-CoA that is not taken up into the mitochondria cannot be oxidized and forms triglyceride and myocardial structural lipids, the latter by changes in the degree of saturation and chain length.
4. *Citrate cycle.* The citrate cycle functions within the mitochondrial matrix to produce both carbon dioxide and hydrogen atoms and, ultimately, ATP by oxidative phosphorylation. The last process takes place as hydrogen atoms are transferred outward across the mitochondrial membrane by the process of proton pumping, which is coupled with the generation of high-energy phosphate compounds. Normally one ATP molecule is made for every four protons transferred, with a P/O ratio of 2.5, not 3, as previously held. An important mechanism regulating the activity of the citrate cycle is the mitochondrial ratio of $NAD/NADH_2$ (the redox state), which decreases during increased heart work when more cytosolic ATP is also broken down to ADP per unit time. The increased supply of cytosolic ADP is transferred to within

the mitochondria by the ADP-ATP translocase, and this stimulates mitochondrial oxidative phosphorylation, using up both reducing equivalents and oxygen to form ATP and H_2O.

5. *Ischemia.* In ischemia, when oxidative metabolism is impaired, the use of ATP decreases dramatically. The ATP content of the myocardium also falls, but less rapidly, because ischemic arrest of contractility decreases the use of ATP and because of replenishment from CP. As ATP decreases, the level of breakdown products such as ADP, AMP, adenosine, inosine, and hypoxanthine all increase to stimulate various pathways and restorative processes. In the phase of recovery from ischemic arrest (reperfusion), ATP can be reformed either by salvage pathways or by *de novo* synthesis. It seems unlikely that there is a fixed critical ATP level below which the cell dies, although ATP is always low in dying cells.

6. *Adenosine.* Adenosine is probably the most important breakdown product of ATP. It has multiple protective functions including compensatory coronary vasodilation. It also slows the heart rate (by the current K_{ADO}), inhibits the calcium current, and probably plays an important role in preconditioning by activation of protein kinase C.

7. *Anaerobic glycolysis.* During anaerobiosis, metabolism shifts from predominant dependence on oxygen-requiring fatty acids to glycolysis. Lactate is produced instead of being taken up by the myocardium. Pyruvate is converted to lactate because $NADH_2$ formed cannot enter the anaerobic mitochondria. Formation of ATP by glycolysis may be important for the survival of ischemic cells. Hypothetically, glycolytic ATP can protect the membrane by providing energy for the membrane-related pumps, such as the sodium pump and the calcium uptake pump of the sarcoplasmic reticulum.

8. *Unlinking of glycolysis from oxidation.* When circulating FFAs are high, fatty acid oxidation by the ischemic myocardium is enhanced relative to that of glucose. This process occurs as result of stimulation of the AMP-activated protein kinase by ischemia, which indirectly enhances the rate of entry of activated fatty acid into the mitochondria. There the fatty acids inhibit the oxidation of glucose and "steal" the residual oxygen from glucose. The result is that glycolysis is accelerated, but pyruvate cannot enter the citrate cycle, so that glycolysis is uncoupled from oxidation and forms more harmful protons. Further harm comes from the accumulation of the membrane-active intermediates of lipid metabolism, such as intracellular FFA, acyl-CoA, and acylcarnitine.

9. *Insulin resistance.* This is a clinically common condition, occurring in diverse situations such as obesity, type 2 diabetes, hypertension, and as recently found in severe heart failure. The mechanism is not well understood, but may be related to excess blood FFA levels. The resulting impairment of glucose transport into muscle can precipitate or exaggerate the diabetic state.

10. *PET.* This technique of allows noninvasive monitoring of myocardial metabolic pathways. For example, ^{18}F-fluorodeoxyglucose is extracted more by

the viable but poorly contracting "hibernating myocardium" than by normal myocardium. This increase relative to the coronary blood flow is called "mismatch." In severely injured tissue, the extraction is decreased. Thus, myocardial viability may be defined by mismatch, which helps to select patients for coronary artery surgery.

STUDENT QUESTIONS

1. Which are the major fuels of the heart in the fasting and the fed states? Explain why these differences exist.
2. Outline the pathways of glycolysis and the major rate-controlling steps. In which conditions are these pathways increased and decreased?
3. In which conditions is fatty acid oxidation increased and decreased?
4. How is ATP produced in mitochondria? Discuss P/O ratios.
5. What is the effect of oxygen deprivation (anaerobiosis) on myocardial use of fuels? How well are the energy needs of the myocardium covered during anaerobiosis?

CARDIOLOGIST-IN-TRAINING QUESTIONS

1. During increased heart work in a patient with coronary artery disease, the blood supply is limited and ischemia develops. What changes in the patterns of myocardial energy utilization can be expected?
2. Glycolytic flux is important during ischemia. Critically consider procedures to increase this flux.
3. Insulin resistance is found in a number of clinically diverse conditions. List these conditions. Does insulin resistance matter to the patient? If so, what are the therapeutic implications?
4. "Adenosine can be harnessed for endogenous cardioprotection." Do you agree? Give reasons.
5. What is the scientific basis for the concept of "mismatch" whereby particular changes in myocardial metabolism, detectable by PET, can indicate myocardial viability or otherwise?

REFERENCES

1. Taegtmeyer H. Metabolism—the lost child of cardiology [Editorial]. *J Am Coll Cardiol* 2000;36: 1386–1388.
2. Taegtmeyer H. Switching metabolic genes to build a better heart. *Circulation* 2002;106:2043–2045.
2a. Ferrannini E, Santoro D, Bonadonna R, et al. Metabolic and hemodynamic effects of insulin on function. *Am J Physiol* 1993;264:E308–E315.
2b. Bing RJ, et al. Metabolic studies on the human heart *in vivo*. *Am J Med* 1953;15:284–296.
3. Opie LH. Metabolism of the heart in health and disease. Part 1. *Am Heart J* 1968;76:685–698.
4. Neely JR, et al. Relationship between carbohydrate and lipid metabolism and the energy balance of heart muscle. *Annu Rev Physiol* 1974;36:413–459.
5. Randle PJ, et al. The glucose fatty acid cycle: its role in insulin sensitivity and the metabolic disturbances of diabetes mellitus. *Lancet* 1963;April 13:785–789.

5a. Wisneski JA, Stanley WC, Neese RA, et al. Effects of acute hyperglycemia on myocardial glycolytic activity in humans. *J Clin Invest* 1990;85;1648–1656.
5b. Gertz EW, Wisneski JA, Stanley WC, et al. Myocardial substrate utilization during exercise in humans. *J Clin Invest* 1988;82:2017–2025.
5c. Wisneski JA, Gertz EW, Neese RA, et al. Myocardial metabolism of free fatty acids. Studies with 14C-labeled substrates in humans. *J Clin Invest* 1987;79:359–366.
6. Pessin JE, et al. Mammalian facilitative glucose transporter family: structure and molecular regulation. *Rev Physiol* 1992;54:911–930.
7. Lopaschuk GD, et al. Glucose metabolism in the ischemic heart. *Circulation* 1997;95:313–315.
8. Young LH, et al. Low-flow ischemia leads to translocation of canine heart GLUT-4 and GLUT-1 glucose transporters to the sarcolemma in vivo. *Circulation* 1997;95:415–422.
9. Russell RR, et al. Insulin stimulates translocation of both GLUT4 and GLUT 1 in the heart. *Circulation* 1996;94(suppl 1):1–308(abst).
10. Atkinson LL, et al. Leptin activates cardiac fatty oxidation independent of changes in the AMP-activated protein kinase-acetyl-CoA carboxylase-malonyl-CoA axis. *J Biol Chem* 2002;277: 29424–29430.
11. Hue L, et al. Insulin and ischemia stimulate glycolysis by acting on the same targets through different opposing signaling pathways. *J Mol Cell Cardiol* 2002;34:1091–1097.
12. Weiss JN, et al. Glycolysis preferentially inhibits ATP-sensitive K+ channels in isolated guinea pig cardiac myocytes. *Science* 1987;238:67–70.
13. Apstein CS, et al. Determinants of a protective effect of glucose and insulin on the ischemic myocardium. Effects of contractile function, diastolic compliance, metabolism, and ultrastructure during ischaemia and reperfusion. *Circ Res* 1983;52:515–526.
14. Lopaschuk GD, et al. Metabolic modulation. A means to mend a broken heart. *Circulation* 2002; 105:140–142.
15. Antos CL, et al. Activated glycogen synthase-3^b suppresses cardiac hypertrophy *in vivo*. *Proc Natl Acad Sci U S A* 2002;99:907–912.
16. Henning SL, et al. Contribution of glycogen to aerobic myocardial glucose utilization. *Circulation* 1996;93:1549–1555.
17. Alonso MD, et al. A new look at the biogenesis of glycogen. *FASEB J* 1995;9:1126–1137.
18. Arad M, et al. Constitutively active AMP kinase mutations cause glycogen storage disease mimicking hypertrophic cardiomyopathy. *J Clin Invest* 2002;109:357–362.
19. van der Vusse GJ, et al. Cardiac fatty acid uptake and transport in health and disease. *Cardiovasc Res* 2000;45:279–293.
20. Kantor PF, et al. Myocardial energy metabolism. In: Sperelakis N, et al., eds. *Heart physiology and pathophysiology*, 4th ed. San Diego: Academic Press, 2001.
20a. Spector AA, Soboroff JM. Utilization of fatty acids complexed to human plasma lipoproteins by mammalian cell suspensions. *J Lipid Res* 1971;12:545–555.
20b. Rothlin ME, Bing RJ. Extraction and release of individual free fatty acids by the heart and fat deposits. *J Clin Invest* 1961;40:1380.
20c. Van der Vusse GJ, Roemen TH, Prinzen FW, et al. Uptake and tissue content of fatty acids in dog myocardium under normoxic and ischemic conditions. *Circ Res* 1982;50:538–546.
21. Dyck JRB, et al. Malonyl CoA control of fatty acid oxidation in the ischemic heart. *J Mol Cell Cardiol* 2002;34:1099–1109.
21a. Hinkle PC, Kumar MA, Resetar A, et al. Mechanistic stoichiometry of mitochondrial oxidative phosphorylation. *Biochemistry* 1991;30:3576–3582.
21b. Brand MD, et al. The causes and functions of mitochondrial proton leak. *Biochem Biophys Acta* 1994;1187:132–139.
22. Brandes R, et al. Intracellular Ca^{2+} increases the mitochondrial NADH concentration during elevated work in intact cardiac muscle. *Circ Res* 1997;80:82–87.
23. Brown GC. Control of respiration and ATP synthesis in mammalian mitochondria and cells. *Biochem J* 1992;284:1–13.
24. Lehninger AL. *Biochemistry*, 2nd ed. New York: Worth Publishers, 1975.
25. Simonsen S, et al. The effect of free fatty acids on myocardial oxygen consumption during arterial pacing and catecholamine infusion in man. *Circulation* 1978;58:484–491.
26. Challoner DR, et al. Metabolic effect of epinephrine on the QO_2 of the arrested isolated perfused rat heart. *Nature* 1965;205:602–603.
27. Boss O, et al. Uncoupling proteins 2 and 3: potential regulators of mitochondrial energy metabolism. *Diabetes* 2000;49:143–156.

28. Ingwall JS. *ATP and the heart.* Boston: Kluwer Academic Publishers, 2002.
29. Ye Y, et al. High-energy phosphate metabolism and creatine kinase in failing hearts. A new porcine model. *Circulation* 2001;103:1570–1576.
30. Cross HR, et al. Is a high glycogen content beneficial or detrimental to the ischemic rat heart? *Circ Res* 1996;78:482–491.
31. Owen P, et al. Glucose flux rate regulates onset of ischemic contracture in globally underperfused rat hearts. *Circ Res* 1990;66:344–354.
32. Cave AC, et al. ATP synthesis during low-flow ischemia. Influence of increased glycolytic substrate. *Circulation* 2000;101:2090–2096.
33. Gevers W. Generation of protons by metabolic processes in heart cells. *J Mol Cell Cardiol* 1977;9:867–874.
34. Maddock HL, et al. Adenosine A_3 receptor activation protects the myocardium from reperfusion/reoxygenation injury. *Am J Physiol* 2002;283:H1307–H1313.
35. Hazen SL, et al. The rapid and reversible association of phosphofructokinase with myocardial membranes during myocardial ischemia. *FEBS Lett* 1994;339:213–216.
36. Mochizuki S, et al. Control of glyceraldehyde-3-phosphate dehydrogenase in cardiac muscle. *J Mol Cell Cardiol* 1979;11:221–236.
37. King LM, et al. Glucose delivery is a major determinant of glucose utilization in the ischemic myocardium with a residual coronary flow. *Cardiovasc Res* 1998;39:381–392.
38. Gertz EW, et al. Myocardial substrate utilization during exercise in humans: dual carbon-labeled carbohydrate isotope experiments. *J Clin Invest* 1988;82:1409–1416.
39. Gudbjarnason S, et al. Functional compartmentation of ATP and creatine phosphate in heart muscle. *J Mol Cell Cardiol* 1970;1:325–330.
40. Schaper J, et al. Ultrastructural, functional, and biochemical criteria for estimation of reversibility of ischaemic injury: a study on the effects of global ischaemia on the isolated dog heart. *J Mol Cell Cardiol* 1979;11:521–541.
41. Neubauer S, et al. Myocardial phosphocreatine-to-ATP ratio is a predictor of mortality in patients with dilated cardiomyopathy. *Circulation* 1997;96:2190–2196.
42. Pillay TS, et al. Glucose-induced phosphorylation of the insulin receptor. *J Clin Invest* 1996;97:613–620.
43. Wallhaus TR, et al. Myocardial free fatty acid and glucose use after carvedilol treatment in patients with congestive heart failure. *Circulation* 2001;103:2441–2446.
44. Dzeja PD, et al. Adenylate kinase-catalyzed phosphotransfer in the myocardium. Increased contribution in heart failure. *Circ Res* 1999;84:1137–1143.
45. Opie LH. Proof that glucose-insulin-potassium provides metabolic protection of ischaemic myocardium? [Editorial]. *Lancet* 1999;353:768–769.
46. Malmberg K, et al. Randomized trial of insulin-glucose infusion followed by subcutaneous insulin treatment in diabetic patients with acute myocardial infarction (DIGAMI Study): effects on mortality at one year. *J Am Coll Cardiol* 1995;26:57–65.
47. Lopaschuk GD, et al. An imbalance between glycolysis and glucose oxidation is a possible explanation for the detrimental effects of high levels of fatty acids during aerobic perfusion of ischemic hearts. *J Pharmacol Exp Ther* 1993;264:135–144.
48. Taegtmeyer H. Metabolic support for the postischaemic heart. *Lancet* 1995;345:1552–1555.
49. Jeremy RW, et al. The functional recovery of post-ischaemic myocardium requires glycolysis during early reperfusion. *J Mol Cell Cardiol* 1993;25:261–276.
50. Kudo N, et al. High rates of fatty acid oxidation during reperfusion of ischemic hearts are associated with a decrease in malonyl-CoA levels due to an increase in 5′-AMP-activated protein kinase inhibition of acetyl-CoA carboxylase. *J Biol Chem* 1995;270:17513–17520.
51. Jonassen AK, et al. Myocardial protection by insulin at reperfusion requires early administration and is mediated via Akt and a p70s6 kinase cell-survival signaling. *Circ Res* 2001;89:1191–1198.
52. Liao R, et al. Cardiac-specific overexpression of GLUT1 prevents the development of heart failure attributable to pressure overload in mice. *Circulation* 2002;106:2125–2131.
53. Albert CM, et al. Blood levels of long-chain n-3 fatty acids and the risk of sudden death. *N Engl J Med* 2002;346:1113–1118.

12

Ventricular Function

Lionel H. Opie and Mark G. Perlroth

"The rate of relaxation of the heart in diastole is quite as important a feature as is the systolic contraction."

Henderson (1)

THE CARDIAC CYCLE

The Wiggers diagram (2) is one of the most frequently reproduced and modified figures in cardiology (Color Plate 8-1). Although conceived by Wiggers, the earliest complete diagram showing the phases of the cardiac cycle and the pressures in aorta, ventricles, atria, and veins as well as the relationship to the electrocardiogram and heart sounds was by Sir Thomas Lewis in 1920. The message of this cycle is so important that every student of cardiology must commit it to memory. A simplified version is shown in Figure 12-1. The basic events are (a) left ventricular (LV) contraction, (b) LV relaxation, and (c) LV filling (Table 12-1). These events generate the pressure to propel blood received from the lungs to the body via the aorta. Similarly, right ventricular contraction, undergoing a similar sequence of events, propels blood to the lungs and from there to the left heart. For simplicity, we focus on events in the left side of the heart where the pressure changes are greater and the ventricle is correspondingly thicker. This increased wall thickness of the left ventricle is a natural adaptation to the higher pressures in the aorta and left ventricle than in the pulmonary artery and right ventricle.

The Ventricle Contracts: Systole

LV pressure increases when the arrival of calcium ions at the contractile protein starts to trigger actin–myosin interaction. On the electrocardiogram, the arrival of the wave of depolarization that opens the L-calcium channels is indicated by the peak of the R wave (Color Plate 8-12). Soon the LV pressure builds up to exceed that in the left atrium (normally 5 to 12 mmHg), followed approximately 30 milliseconds later by the mitral component of the first sound, M_1. The exact relationship of M_1 to mitral valve closure is still open to debate (3,4).

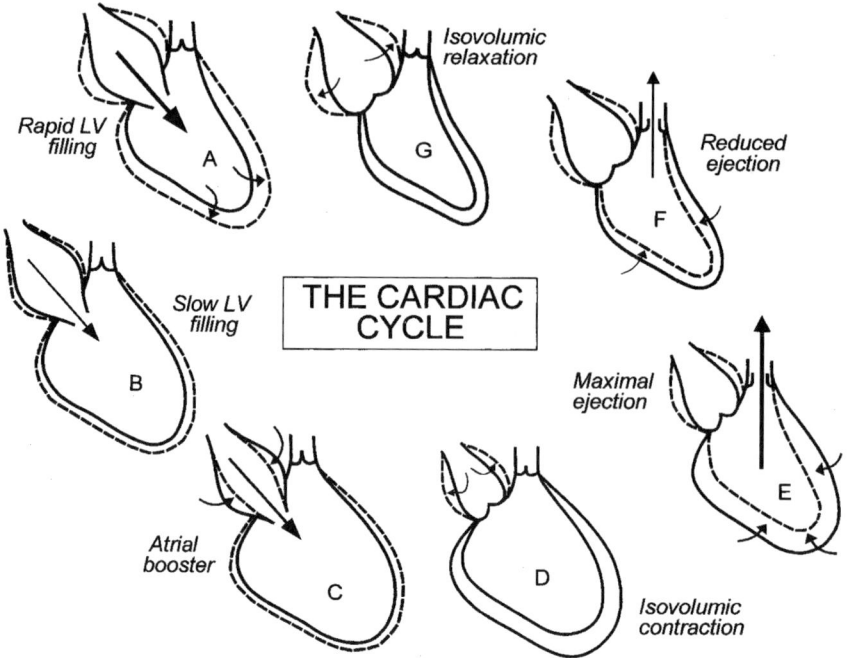

FIG. 12-1. The cardiac cycle. Visual phases of the ventricular cycle are modified from Shepherd, Vanhoutte. *The human cardiovascular system.* New York: Raven Press, 1979:68. For explanation of phases A through G, see Table 12-1.

Mitral valve closure, often thought to coincide with the crossover point at which the LV pressure initially exceeds the left atrial pressure, is in reality delayed because the valve is kept open by the inertia of the blood flow (5). The second component of the first heart sound, T_1, occurs shortly thereafter, as pressure increases in the right ventricle, similarly to that in the left ventricle, although lesser in magnitude. The result is that the tricuspid valve closes, creating the sec-

TABLE 12-1. *The cardiac cycle*

LV contraction
   Isovolumic contraction (D)
   Maximal ejection (E)
LV relaxation
   Start of relaxation and reduced ejection (F)
   Isovolumic relaxation (G)
   Rapid LV filling and LV "suction" (A)
   Slow LV filling (diastasis) (B)
   Atrial booster (C)

The letters A through G refer to the phases of the cardiac cycle shown in Figure 12-1. For overall hemodynamic changes, see the Wiggers diagram, Color Plate 8-12.
LV, left ventricular.

ond component of the first heart sound. These two components cannot be distinguished clinically under normal circumstances.

Isovolumic contraction occurs between the times of mitral closure and aortic valve mitral closure and opening. The LV volume is fixed because both these valves are shut, and causes pressure development to proceed as the interaction of actin and myosin increases. Thereafter, the aortic valve opens when the pressure in the left ventricle exceeds that in the aorta. Opening of the aortic valve is followed by *rapid ejection*. The speed of ejection of blood is determined both by the pressure gradient across the aortic valve and the elastic properties of the aorta and arterial tree. The aorta, in particular, undergoes systolic expansion (Fig. 1-8). The pattern of contraction of the whole heart is a complex wringing motion, with the apex swinging up to the chest wall and the base rotating in the opposite direction, around a relatively fixed equatorial mid zone (6).

Ventricular Relaxation

After the LV pressure increases to a peak, it then starts to decrease. As the cytosolic calcium is taken up into the sarcoplasmic reticulum under the influence of phosphorylated phospholamban, more and more myofibers enter the state of relaxation. As a result, the rate of ejection of blood into the aorta decreases (*phase of reduced ejection*). While LV pressure is decreasing faster than aortic pressure [with aortic pressure marginally exceeding LV pressure (7)], forward blood flow decelerates but is maintained by momentum. Next, as ejection halts and the aortic valve closes, forward aortic flow is assisted by the recoil of the aorta. The first component of the second sound, A_2, results from aortic valve closure, and the second component, P_2, results from closure of the pulmonary valve as pressure in the right ventricle decreases to less than that in the pulmonary artery. In contrast to S_1, the two components of S_2 are clinically distinguishable. Thereafter, the ventricle relaxes without changing its volume (*isovolumic relaxation*) because it is sealed off as both aortic and mitral valves are closed. Next, the mitral valve opens as the LV pressure decreases to less than that in the left atrium. The filling phase of the cardiac cycle starts (Color Plate 8-12). Mitral valve opening, normally silent, may be audible as an opening snap in mitral stenosis.

Ventricular Filling

Just after mitral valve opening, as the LV pressure decreases to less than that in the left atrium, the *phase of rapid or early filling* accounts for most of ventricular filling. Active diastolic relaxation of the ventricle (*ventricular suction*) may also contribute to early filling, particularly during exercise. A physiologic third heart sound (S_3) may result from rapid filling during exercise or with sinus tachycardia. LV filling temporarily stops as pressures in the atrium and ventricle equalize, called the *phase of diastasis*, which means separation. *Atrial systole* or

TABLE 12-2. Origins of the heart sounds

Sound	Origin
First	
Mitral component (M_1)	Mitral valve closure
Tricuspid component (T_1)	Tricuspid valve closure
Second	
Aortic component (A_2)	Aortic valve closure
Pulmonary component (P_2)	Pulmonary valve closure
Third	
Physiologic	Rapid left ventricular filling
Pathologic	Ventricular wall vibrations
Fourth	
Pathologic	Enhanced atrial systole

the *left atrial booster* increases the pressure gradient from the atrium to the ventricle to renew filling. When the LV fails to relax normally, as in LV hypertrophy, the increased left atrial contraction can enhance late filling (8), producing a fourth heart sound that is not normally audible (Table 12-2).

Definitions of Systole and Diastole

Systole is the contraction phase and *diastole* is the relaxation phase. Systole means contraction in Greek, and diastole is derived from two Greek words for send and apart. For the physiologist, systole starts with isovolumic contraction when LV pressure crosses the atrial pressure (Color Plate 8-12). Physiologic diastole commences as the LV pressure starts to decrease (Table 12-3). For the cardiologist at the bedside, systole is demarcated by the heart sounds, lasting from the first heart sound (M_1) to the closure of the aortic valve (A_2). The remainder of the cardiac cycle is cardiologic diastole. Mitral valve closure (M_1) actually occurs approximately 30 milliseconds after the onset of physiologic systole at the crossover point of pressures. Thus, cardiologic systole starts and ends later than physiologic systole. The term *protodiastolic* (early diastole) for the

TABLE 12-3. *Physiologic versus cardiologic definitions of systole and diastole*

Physiologic systole	Cardiologic systole
Isovolumic contraction	From M_1 to A_2
Maximal ejection	Only part of isovolumic contraction[a] includes maximal and reduced ejection phases.
Physiologic diastole	Cardiologic diastole
Reduced ejection	A_2–M_1 interval (filling phases included)
Isovolumic relaxation	
Filling phases	

[a]Note that M_1 occurs with a definite delay after the start of left ventricular contraction.

physiologist is the early part of the relaxation phase from the time when aortic flow begins to decline until the mitral valve opens. For the cardiologist, protodiastole is the early phase of rapid filling, when the third heart sound (S_3) may be heard. This sound probably reflects ventricular wall vibrations during rapid filling and is accentuated during youth, exercise, and pregnancy. A pathologic S_3 (protodiastolic gallop) results from increased wall stiffness secondary to an increase in LV diastolic pressure as in heart failure, hypertrophy, and infiltrative disease of the ventricle.

PRELOAD AND AFTERLOAD

To understand how increased venous return, as during exercise, enhances ventricular function, a simple circuit diagram can be proposed (Fig. 12-2). *Preload* is the load present before contraction has started and is provided by venous return that fills the atrium and empties into the left ventricle during diastole. During systole, the left ventricle contracts against the *afterload* (load after the ventricle starts to contract). When the preload increases (Fig. 12-2), the left ventricle distends and the stroke volume increases. This mechanism explains at least in part the increased cardiac output of exercise or of volume expansion (infusion of intravenous fluids). Increased heart rate increases cardiac output not only by multiplying the number of beats per minute but also by enhancing contractility (see later, Fig. 12-8).

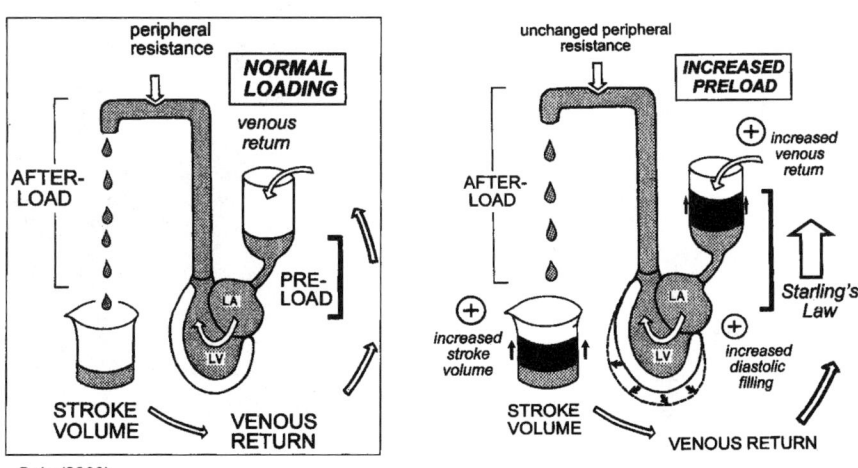

FIG. 12-2. Simplified model of circulation, normal loading, and increased preload. Left: Venous return provides preload, and afterload is regulated by the peripheral (systemic) vascular resistance. *LA*, left atrium; *LV*, left ventricle. **Right:** Effects of increasing preload on stroke volume and cardiac output. Note the effect on LV volume. For Starling's actual observations, see Figure 12-3.

The Starling Law of the Heart

The Starling law may be stated in many forms, one of which is that the energy of contraction is a function of the initial length of the muscle fiber: "Within physiological limits, the larger the volume of the heart, the greater the energy of its contraction and the amount of chemical change at each contraction" (9).

Put differently, increased venous pressure stretches the fibers more at the end of diastole and systolic contraction is more vigorous with an increased stroke volume. To obtain the end-diastolic fiber length and the stroke volume, Starling measured the heart volume, stroke volume, and cardiac output (Fig. 12-3). Because heart volume is difficult to determine even with modern echocardiographic techniques, the LV end-diastolic *filling pressure* or mean left atrial pressure is often taken as a surrogate for heart volume. As the filling pressure increases, so does the preload on the myocardium with attendant changes in ventricular performance (Fig. 12-4). However, LV pressure and volume are not linearly related because the myocardium cannot continue to stretch indefinitely (see later, Fig. 12-22). Rather, as the LV end-diastolic pressure increases, stroke volume reaches a plateau.

An invasive procedure, the transvenous insertion of a Swan–Ganz catheter through the right heart into the distal pulmonary arterial tree, measures both the LV filling pressure (as reflected by the pulmonary capillary pressure) and cardiac output by the indicator dilution method using a temperature-sensitive device at the tip of the catheter (Fig. 16-13).

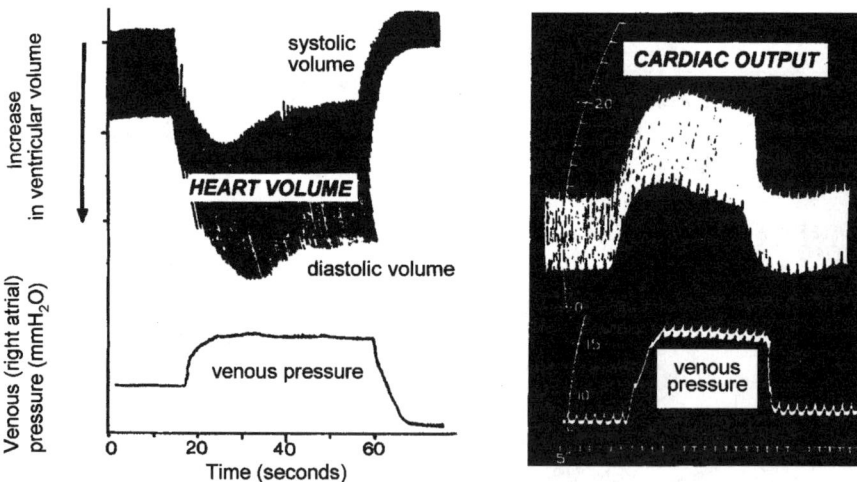

FIG. 12-3. The Starling law of the heart as applied to preload (venous filling pressure). As preload increases (bottom in both parts), the heart volume increases (on left at top), as does cardiac output (on right at top). Both stroke volume and heart rate would have increased. Starling's explanation was "the output of the heart is a function of its filling; the energy of contraction depends on the state of dilatation of the heart's cavities." (Left panel adapted from Patterson et al. *J Physiol* 1914;48:465; right panel adapted from Halliburton, McDowall. *Handbook of physiology and biochemistry*. London: John Murray, 1942.)

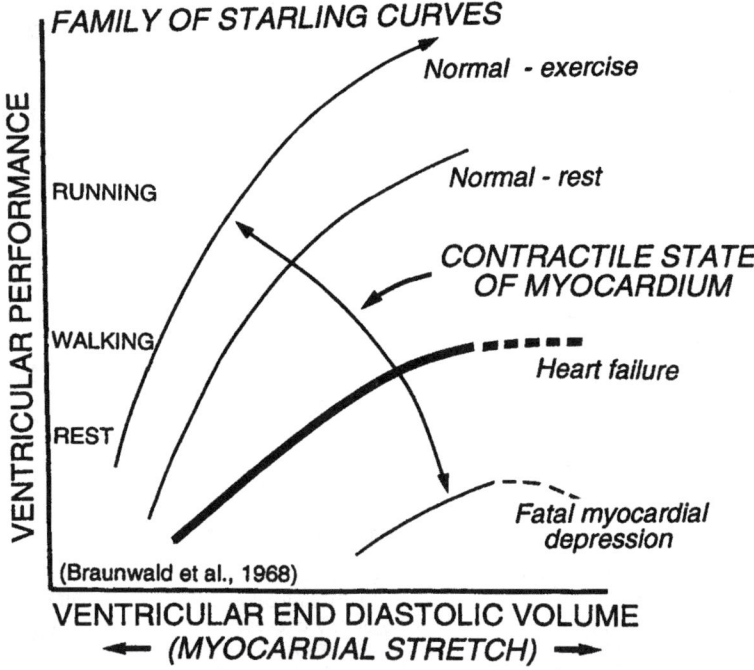

FIG. 12-4. Family of Starling curves. According to the Starling law, increased stretch of myocardial fibers, which increases the ventricular end-diastolic volume, results in greater ventricular performance. However, as illustrated, cardiac performance can be modified without changing the end-diastolic volume by moving to a different curve at a higher or lower inotropic state. The line for heart failure is based on that shown in Figures 1 and 2 of Holubarsch et al. (13). (Modified from Braunwald et al. *Mechanisms of contraction the failing heart.* Boston: Little Brown, 1968.)

Force–Length Relationship and the Starling Law

In the past, optimal sarcomere length was linked to the Starling law. Supposedly, ventricular stretch gives rise to such optimal overlap of actin and myosin with an increased force of contraction. Although the overlap theory holds for skeletal muscle, in the heart, the situation is different (Fig. 12-5). In the case of skeletal muscle, Fuchs (10) pointed out that each actin filament projects approximately 1 μm from each side of the Z disk, so that the active force would decline when the sarcomere length was less than the sum of the lengths of the individual actin filaments, i.e., less than 2.0 to 2.2 μm. In cardiac muscle, however, only 10% or less of the maximal force is developed, even at 80% of the optimal length (Fig. 12-5). Thus, cardiac sarcomeres must function near the upper limit of their maximal length (L_{max}), which is 2.2 μm (11).

The favored explanation for this steep length–tension relationship of cardiac muscle is *length-dependent activation*, an enhanced sensitization of the actin–myosin filaments to available calcium transients (Color Plate 8-7). Direct

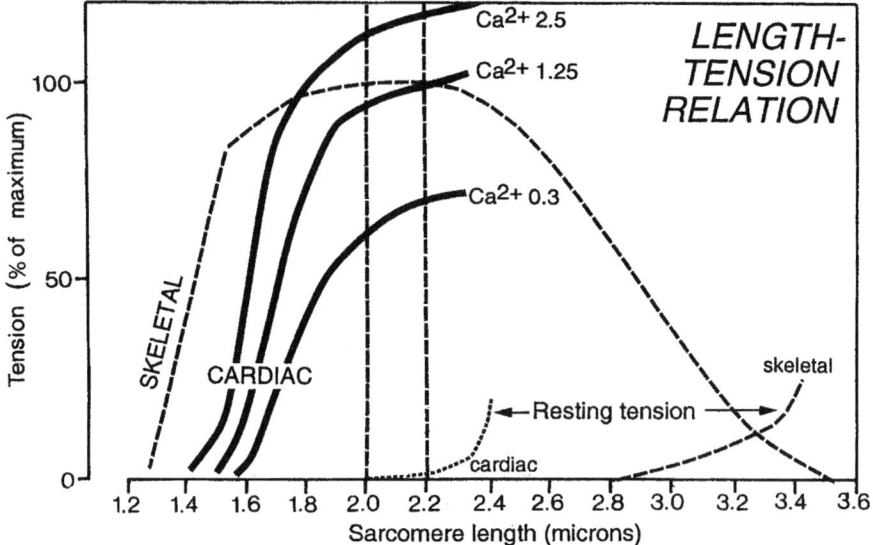

FIG. 12-5. Effect of sarcomere length on tension. The relationship between sarcomere length and tension for cardiac muscle compared with skeletal muscle. Note the effect of increasing calcium ion concentration and the absence of any decrease in tension at maximal sarcomere lengths, so that there is no basis for the descending limb of the Starling curve. Recent sophisticated laser-diffraction techniques invalidate previous curves based on apparent sarcomere length–tension relationships of imperfect papillary muscle preparations. For data on failing human heart, see Holubarsch et al. (13).

evidence of this point of view is that the calcium transient does not increase as the sarcomere length is extended (12). In contrast, when forces increase by a true inotropic intervention such as β-adrenergic stimulation, there is also an increase in the calcium transient.

Frank and Isovolumic Contraction

Whereas Starling emphasized the role of increasing the initial length of the muscle fiber by increasing the heart volume, it was his German predecessor, Frank, who, in 1895, established another important principle. When an isolated heart was filled to several increasing volumes, each of which was fixed throughout the cardiac cycle through an ingenious perfusion system, the isovolumically (Greek, *iso*, equal) contracting heart could generate an increasing and decreasing pressure trace (Fig. 12-6). The greater the initial volume was, the more rapid the rate of increase, the greater the peak pressure reached, and the faster the rate of relaxation. Frank was, therefore, able to show that an increasing diastolic heart volume stimulated the ventricle to contract more rapidly and more forcefully, which is a positive *inotropic effect* (Greek, *ino*, fiber; *tropus*, move). Thus, the observation of Frank explained the mechanical performance of the heart dur-

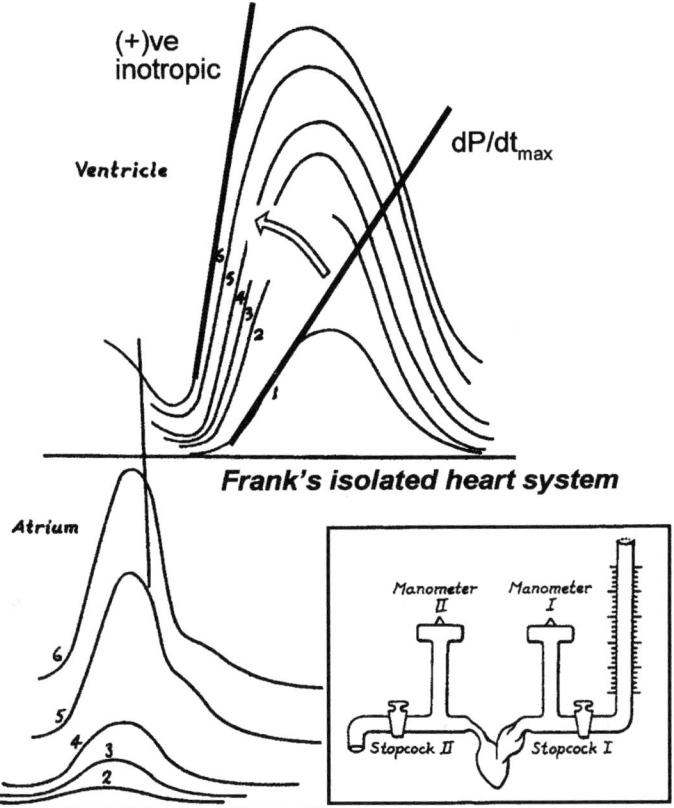

FIG. 12-6. Frank family of isometric (isovolumic) curves. Top: Intraventricular pressure. **Bottom:** Left atrial filling pressure progressively increased to give greater initial filling of the left ventricle (44). Then inlet and outlet valves were closed to produce isovolumic conditions. Curves 2 through 6 have a progressively greater velocity of pressure generation reflecting greater contractility. Hence, the initial fiber length (volume of ventricle) can influence contractility. This effect of initial fiber length on contractility has recently been rediscovered. One index of contractility is the maximal rate of change of the intraventricular pressure (max dP/dt) that could be obtained, indicated by the two tangential lines added to the curves of the original figure of Frank. The line on curve 6 has the much steeper slope and therefore indicates a greater rate of contraction or greater contractility, in contrast to the line drawn on curve 1, which ascends more slowly and indicates a lower contractile state.

ing the operation of the Starling law. These findings of Frank and Starling are so complementary that they often referred to as the Frank–Starling law.

Measurement of Afterload

Starling and colleagues gave a simple picture of the how afterload could influence an isolated muscle: "The extent to which it will contract depends on . . . the amount of the weight which it has to overcome" and "the tension aroused in it."

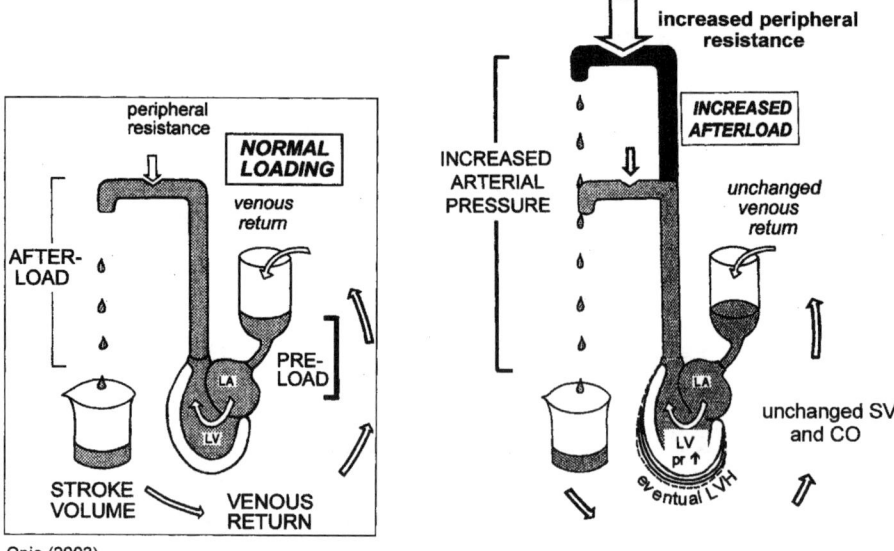

FIG. 12-7. Effect of increasing afterload by increasing peripheral vascular resistance and hence arterial blood pressure. Left ventricular (LV) pressure development is enhanced because of increased performance as result of increased LV end-diastolic volume after increased peripheral vascular resistance. Normal loading conditions are shown for comparison. For constancy of stroke volume during abrupt increase in blood pressure, see Markwalder, Starling. *J Physiol* 1914;48:348. Eventually chronically increased LV pressure causes LV hypertrophy (*LVH*).

Hypothetically, increased afterload stimulates sarcolemma stretch receptors to allow cytosolic calcium levels to increase. Generally, in clinical practice, the arterial blood pressure can be taken as one important measure of afterload if there is no significant aortic stenosis. Increased afterload by itself will increase the intraventricular pressure that has to be generated to open the aortic valve and the pressure against which the myocardium contracts during the ejection phase (Fig. 12-7). These increases will translate themselves to an increased wall stress, which can be measured either as an average value throughout systole or at a given phase of systole. A second important component of afterload lies in *aortic compliance*, the extent to which the aorta can "yield" during systole. *Aortic impedance* is an index of afterload and is the aortic pressure divided by the aortic flow at that instant, so that afterload varies continuously during ejection. Factors reducing aortic flow, such as high arterial blood pressure or aortic valve narrowing (stenosis), will increase impedance and hence afterload.

Preload and Afterload Are Interlinked

The preceding approach presumes that preload and afterload are two separate unconnected entities. Nonetheless, supposing that the LV end-diastolic pressure increases, as during exercise, preload increases by definition. When the left ventricle starts to contract, the tension (or wall stress) in the LV wall will be higher because of greater distention of the left ventricle by the greater pressure. The load during systole also will increase, and afterload will increase. Another example is heart failure when there is a depressed contractile state. One of the compensations is an increase in the peripheral (systemic) vascular resistance, initiated chiefly by an increased sympathetic drive. In that situation, the poorly functioning myocardium cannot cope as effectively with afterload, and the relative amount of blood ejected with each contraction (ejection fraction) becomes less, more blood is retained in the left ventricle, and the heart equilibrates at a higher preload. Therapy aimed at reducing afterload (arterial vasodilator therapy) will improve myocardial performance, allow the left ventricle to empty better, and reduce the end-diastolic volume and preload. Once again, in the intact circulation, it is difficult to separate preload from afterload. Nonetheless, it is useful to emphasize that, in general, preload is related to the degree to which the myocardial fibers are stretched at the end of diastole, and afterload is related to the wall stress generated by those fibers during systole.

HEART RATE AND THE FORCE–FREQUENCY RELATIONSHIP

The heart rate is one of the three basic mechanisms that acutely regulate the contractile state; the other two are the Frank–Starling law and autonomic control by the sympathetic and parasympathetic systems (13). The heart rate is also one of the three major determinants of the myocardial oxygen demand; the others are myocardial wall stress and velocity of contraction. As expected, increased heart rate increases the myocardial oxygen demand when the stroke volume is fixed by increasing the external work of the heart. Unexpectedly, increased heart rate also increases the oxygen demand by progressively enhancing the force of ventricular contraction (Figs. 12-8 and 12-9). This phenomenon is called the Bowditch staircase effect or the *treppe* (German for steps) effect or the positive inotropic effect of activation or the force–frequency relationship. Conversely, decreased heart rate has a negative staircase effect. To explain the treppe effect during rapid stimulation, the proposal is that more sodium and calcium ions enter the myocardial cells than can be handled by the sodium pump. Sodium overload leads to an increase in cytosolic calcium by the sodium–calcium exchanger, with an increased force of contraction.

Force–Frequency Relationship in Humans

In the failing human heart, there is a very different response to an increased frequency of stimulation (Fig. 12-9). At a fixed muscle length (*isometric contraction*), peak contractile force occurs at approximately 150 to 180 stimuli per minute (14), which is the human equivalent of the treppe phenomenon. In patients with atrial fibrillation, the variable filling interval influences contrac-

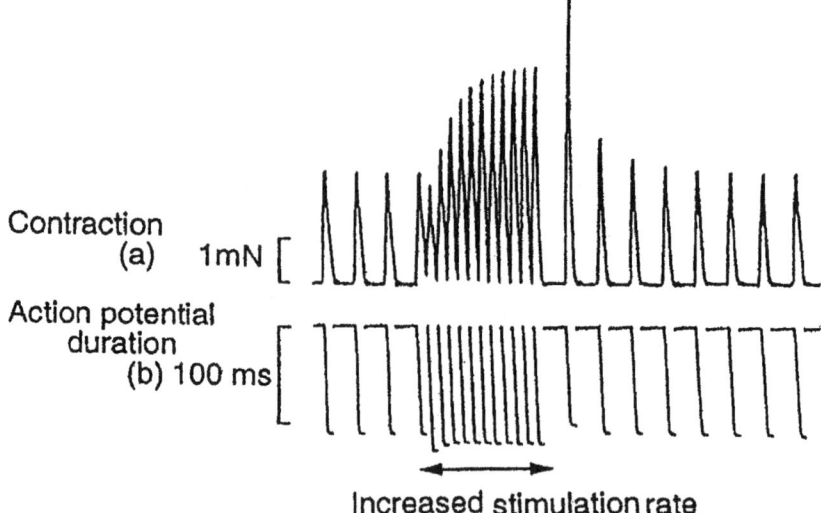

FIG. 12-8. The Bowditch or treppe phenomenon, whereby a faster stimulation rate **(bottom)** increases the force of contraction **(top).** The stimulus rate is shown as the action potential duration of an analog analyzer. The tension developed by papillary muscle contraction is shown in millinewtons. On cessation of rapid stimulation, the contraction force gradually decreases. Hypothetically, the explanation for the increased contraction during more rapid stimulation is repetitive Ca^{2+} entry with each depolarization and, hence, an accumulation of cytosolic calcium. (From Noble MIM. Excitation-contraction coupling. In: Drake-Holland AJ, Noble MIM, eds. *Cardiac metabolism.* Chichester: John Wiley, 1983:49–71, with permission.)

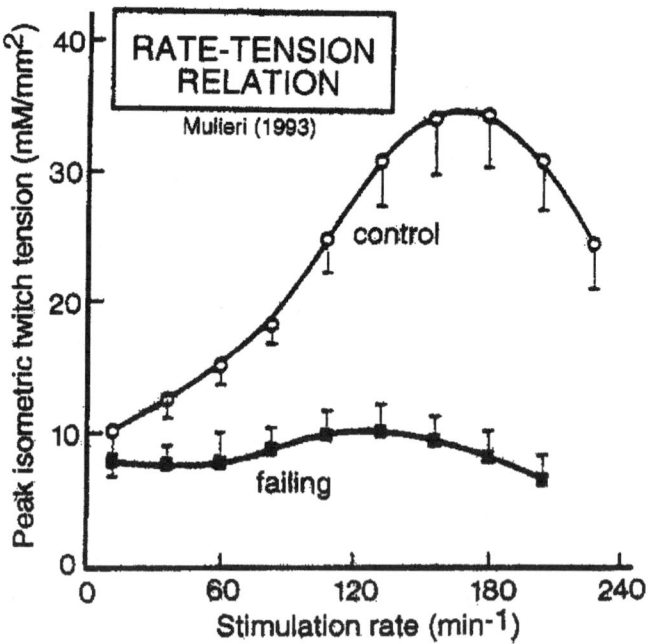

FIG. 12-9. Heart rate–tension relationship. Plot of average steady-state isometric twitch tension versus stimulation frequency. Each point represents the mean ± standard error of the mean of eight nonfailing, control preparations and eight failing, mitral regurgitation preparations. Temperature 37°C. Data from Mulieri et al. (14).

tion, with longer filling intervals and greater diastolic stretch causing stronger contractions (15).

In the human heart *in situ*, electrically stimulated pacing rates of as high as 150 beats per minute can be tolerated with 1:1 conduction, whereas higher rates cause atrioventricular block. However, during exercise, a maximal heart rate of 170 beats per minute or more can be tolerated, presumably because of the enhanced rate of conduction through the atrioventricular node associated with β-adrenergic stimulation. A current concept is that incessant or chronic tachycardias can cause or contribute to LV failure.

CONTRACTILITY OR THE INOTROPIC STATE

Although difficult to define with exactness, increased contractility results in a greater velocity of contraction, which reaches a greater peak tension or force when other factors determining the myocardial oxygen uptake, such as the heart rate, preload, and afterload, are kept constant. An alternate name for contractility is the *inotropic state*. Because changes in contractility in the intact circulation alter tension development and ejection by the heart, preload and afterload will change simultaneously, making it difficult in practice clearly to separate myocardial performance, the inotropic state, and contractility. Contractility is an important regulator of the myocardial oxygen uptake. Factors that increase contractility include adrenergic stimulation, digitalis, and other inotropic agents. At a molecular level, an increased inotropic state is an enhanced load-independent interaction between calcium ions and the contractile proteins. Such an interaction could result from either increased calcium transients or sensitization of the contractile proteins to a given level of cytosolic calcium, as during the action of particular drugs acting through this mechanism. With conventional inotropes, as internal calcium increases within physiologic limits (Fig. 8-6), so does the myosin ATPase activity and maximal tension development.

Force–Velocity Relationship and Idealized Contractility

If the concept of contractility is truly independent of load and heart rate, then unloaded heart muscle stimulated at a fixed rate should have a maximal value of contractility for any given magnitude of the cytosolic calcium transient. This value, the V_{max} of muscle contraction, is defined as the *maximal velocity of contraction* when the isolated muscle is not loaded at all (Fig. 12-10). β-Adrenergic stimulation increases V_{max} and converse changes are found in the failing myocardium. V_{max} is also termed V_0 (the maximal velocity at zero load). The problem with this relatively simple concept is that V_{max} cannot be measured directly but is generated from the curves defining the velocity of contraction at progressively smaller afterloads with fixed preloads (Fig. 12-10). The rate of force development in unloaded muscle is obtained from the extrapolated intercept on the velocity axis. This is usually termed the force–velocity relationship.

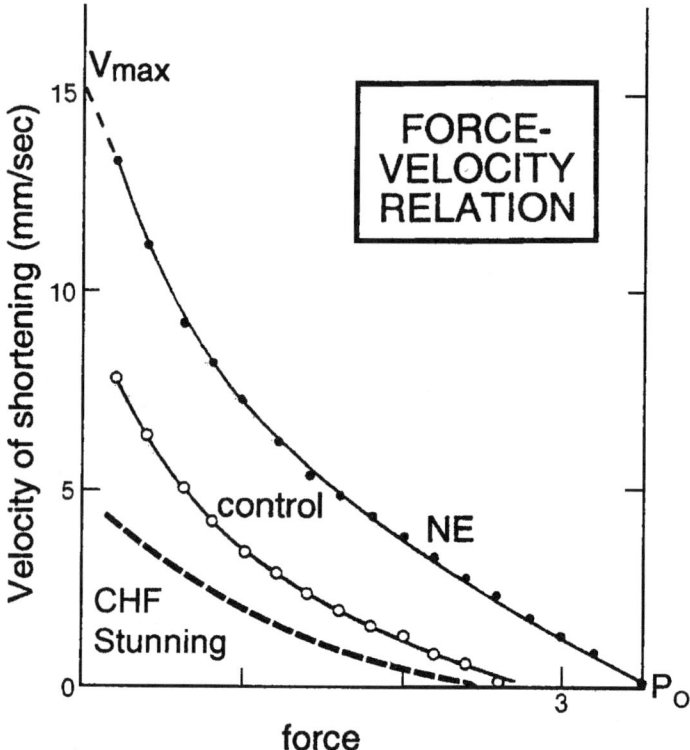

FIG. 12-10. Force–velocity relationship. Norepinephrine (*NE*) induces an increase in the velocity of shortening, maximal force, isometric contraction (P_O), and maximal velocity of zero-load shortening (V_{max}). Cat papillary muscle preparation. The *dashed line* adds hypothetical data from congestive heart failure (*CHF*). For stunning, see McDonald et al. (45). (Modified from Braunwald E, et al. Normal and abnormal circulatory function. In: Braunwald E, ed. *Heart disease: a textbook of cardiovascular medicine*, 4th ed. Philadelphia: WB Saunders, 1992:351–392.)

The peak velocity (V_{max}) is defined at zero load when there is no external force development. In another extreme condition, there is no muscle shortening at all (zero shortening), and all the energy goes into development of pressure (P_0) or force (F_0). This situation is an example of *isometric shortening* (Greek, *iso*, the same; *metrikos*, length). Although isometric conditions can be found in the whole heart as an approximation during isovolumic contraction, complete unloading is impossible. Therefore, the applications of force–velocity or force–length relationships to the heart *in vivo* are limited.

Isotonic Contraction

When muscle is experimentally allowed to shorten against a steady load, the conditions are *isotonic* (Greek, *iso*, same; *tonic*, contractile force). Isotonic conditions cannot prevail physiologically because the load is constantly changing during the ejection period. Therefore, data from isolated heart muscle contracting isotonically cannot directly be applied to humans.

β-Adrenergic Effects

Norepinephrine can increase V_{max} (Fig. 12-10). The data are best explained by an effect of β-adrenergic stimulation on enhancing calcium ion entry (Fig. 7-9), although there is an added effect on contractile proteins. Either isoproterenol (β stimulant) or protein kinase A (intracellular messenger) can increase V_{max} by approximately 40%, concurrently with phosphorylation of troponin I and C protein in an isolated ventricular myocyte preparation (16). Hypothetically, such phosphorylations increase the rate of cross-bridge cycling (17) and the rate of relaxation.

Problems with the Contractility Concept

The concept of contractility has at least two serious defects: (a) the absence of any potential index that can be measured *in situ* and is free of significant criticism and, in particular, the absence of any acceptable noninvasive index and (b) the impossibility of separating the cellular mechanisms of contractility changes from those of an altered load. The first objection is increasingly being overcome by new tissue Doppler imaging techniques, such as the rate of myocardial acceleration during isovolumic contraction (see page 384). But the second objection remains. Increased preload involves increased fiber stretch, which in turn causes length activation, explicable by sensitization of the contractile proteins to the prevailing cytosolic calcium concentration. Increased preload or afterload may increase cytosolic calcium through stretch-sensitive channels. Hence, the traditional separation of inotropic state from load/heart rate effects as two independent regulators of cardiac muscle performance is no longer simple now that the underlying cellular mechanisms have been uncovered. In clinical terms, it nonetheless remains important to separate the effects of a primary increase in load or heart rate from a primary increase in contractility.

In congestive heart failure, this distinction between load and contractility is especially relevant when attempting to dissect the multiple hemodyamic abnormalities found. The basic abnormality of a decreased contractility could result in increased afterload, preload, and heart rate, all of which then predispose to a further decrease in myocardial performance. Thus, decreased contractility is eventually self-augmenting. Because muscle length can influence load-independent measurements of contractile behavior, and the end-diastolic length may be maximal in dilated failing hearts, the traditional separation of length and inotropic state into two independent regulators of cardiac muscle performance becomes difficult to sustain in pathophysiological situations. In practical clinical terms, it still remains useful to separate the effects of a primary increase of load from a primary change in contractility in the assessment and management of severe heart failure. In this situation, the preload is abnormally high due to back pressure from the poorly contracting left ventricle (Figs. 16-13 and 16-15), leading to two different therapies. Diuretic therapy can lessen blood volume and reduce the preload, whereas an increased positive inotropic effect can be achieved by drugs such as the β-adrenergic stimulants that have a calcium-dependent positive inotropic effect independent of loading conditions (Fig. 12-10). Drugs that increase cyclic AMP levels and have a similar signaling chain to that shown in the frontispiece include the β-adrenergic stimulant dobutamine and the phosphodiesterase inhibitor milrinone. But these agents bring the risk of calcium-induced arrhythmias (Fig. 20-15), so that the current approach is increasingly to develop agents that do not change cystolic calcium but act by sensitizing the contractile apparatus to the prevailing calcium levels (the calcium-sensitizing drugs).

WALL STRESS

Myocardial wall stress or *wall tension* increases when the myofilaments slide over each other during cardiac contraction as they are squeezing blood out of the ventricles into the circulation. *Tension* exists when the two forces are applied to an object so that the forces tend to pull the object apart. When a spring is pulled by a force, tension is exerted; when more force is applied, the spring stretches, and the tension increases.

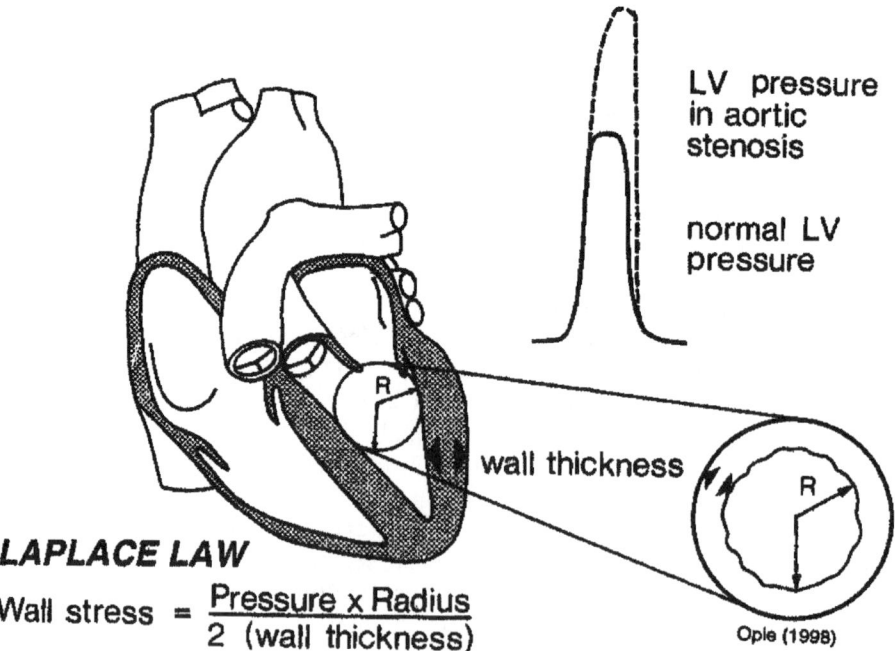

LAPLACE LAW

Wall stress = $\dfrac{\text{Pressure} \times \text{Radius}}{2 \text{ (wall thickness)}}$

FIG. 12-11. Laplace law. Wall stress and afterload. As afterload increases, so does the wall stress. The formula is derived from the Laplace law. The increased left ventricular (*LV*) pressure in aortic stenosis is compensated for by LV wall hypertrophy, which decreases the denominator on the right side of the equation, thereby maintaining wall stress at control levels.

12. VENTRICULAR FUNCTION

Stress develops when tension is applied to a cross-sectional area, and the units are force per unit area. According to the *Laplace law* (Fig. 12-11), the formula for wall stress (σ) in a thin-walled sphere is wall stress (σ) = (pressure × radius)/(2 × wall thickness).

The concept that wall tension in a confined fluid-containing space will vary as a function of the radius can be examined in a simple model. If a sausage-shaped party balloon is partially inflated and then tied off, the portion of the balloon that is expanded can be compared with the unexpanded tip (Fig. 12-12). Note that there are equal internal pressures throughout the balloon. The difference in wall tension at the two sites, which is a function of radius and not of pressure, can be readily palpated.

Thus, increased wall thickness owing to compensatory ventricular hypertrophy balances increased pressure and/or volume loads, and wall stress remains unchanged. In congestive heart failure or with chronic volume loads (as with aortic or mitral regurgitation), the heart dilates, the radius increases, and so does wall stress. Furthermore, in congestive heart failure, because ejection of blood is inadequate, the radius stays too large throughout the contractile cycle, and both end-diastolic and end-systolic tensions are higher. However, there are limitations

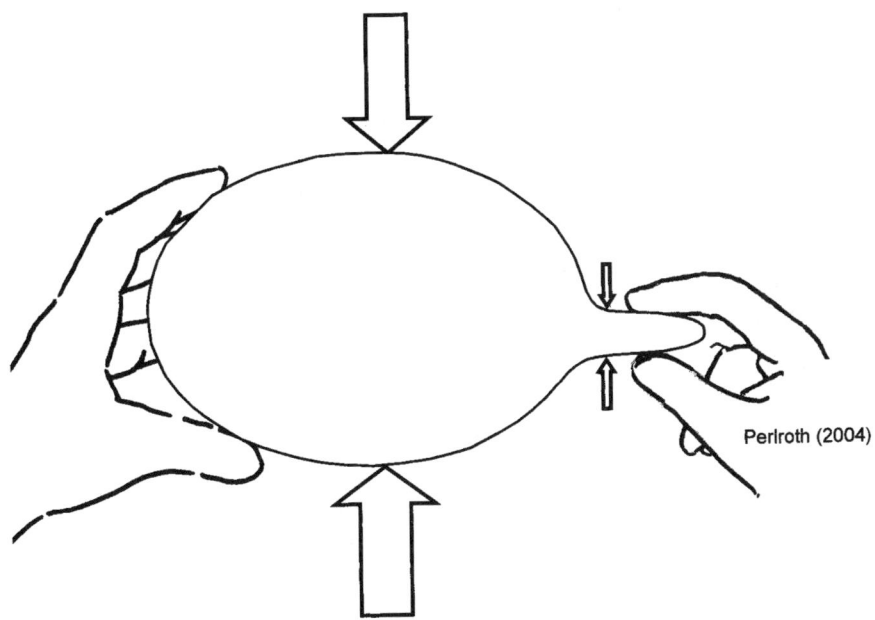

FIG. 12-12. Model of wall tension as a function of radius in a partially inflated balloon. The internal pressure is equal in all directions, but the resistance of the wall of the balloon to deformation is much greater in the portion that is more expanded to the larger diameter than it is in the unexpanded nipple. The higher wall tension in the larger part (*larger arrows*) will cause it to burst sooner as the pressure within increases, whereas the smaller nipple with the much lower wall tension is much more resistant to a pressure increase.

on the interpretation of hypertrophy and failure in relation to the Laplace law. First, because the shape of the ventricle is not a true sphere and wall thickness is not uniform, the Laplace calculation should only be considered a useful approximation. Second, hypertrophy is much more complex than stress normalization, as is discussed in Chapter 13.

Wall Stress, Preload, and Afterload

Wall stress is a useful concept in the understanding of preload and afterload in the human heart. Preload can be defined as the wall stress at the end of diastole and therefore at the maximal resting length of the sarcomere (Fig. 12-5). Measurement of wall stress *in vivo* is difficult because the radius of the left ventricle (see preceding sections) neglects the confounding influence of the complex anatomy of the left ventricle. Surrogate measurements of the indices of preload include LV end-diastolic pressure (more accurately the transmural LV-intrathoracic pressure difference at the end of diastole) or dimensions (the latter being the major and minor axes of the heart in a two-dimensional echocardiographic view). Afterload, the load on the contracting myocardium, is the wall stress during LV ejection. Increased afterload means that increased intraventricular pressure has to be generated first to open the aortic valve and then during the ejection phase. These increases translate into increased myocardial wall stress, which can be measured as either an average value or a given phase of systole, such as end systole. Systolic wall stress reflects the two major components of afterload: arterial blood pressure and arterial compliance. Decreased arterial compliance (increased stiffness) and increased afterload can be anticipated when there is aortic dilation as in severe systemic hypertension or as a consequence of atherosclerosis and aortic calcification in the elderly. Generally, in clinical practice, it is a sufficient approximation to take arterial blood pressure as a measure of afterload if there is no significant aortic stenosis.

Wall Stress and Myocardial Oxygen Demand

It is not only external work that determines the requirement for adenosine 5′-triphosphate (ATP). Instead, tension development (increased wall stress) is oxygen requiring even without external work being done. The difference between tension development and external work can be epitomized by a person standing and attempting unsuccessfully to lift a heavy suitcase, doing no external work but developing tension and becoming very fatigued, compared with the act of lifting the suitcase and doing external work. As predicted by the Laplace equation, the greater the LV chamber size is, the greater the radius is, and for a given wall thickness, the greater the wall stress (Fig. 12-

11). Hence, ejection of the same stroke volume from a large left ventricle against the same blood pressure will produce as much external work (external work = pressure × stroke volume) as ejection of an equal stroke volume by a normal-size left ventricle, but with much greater wall stress in the case of the larger ventricle. Therefore, more oxygen will be required. In clinical terms, heart size is an important determinant of myocardial oxygen uptake, and in a patient with angina and a large left ventricle, the appropriate therapy to reduce LV size will also reduce the myocardial oxygen demand with relief of symptoms.

Wall stress allows for energy required for generation of muscular contraction that does not result in external work. Furthermore, in states of enhanced contractility, wall stress is increased. Thus, thinking in terms of wall stress provides a more comprehensive approach to the problem of myocardial oxygen uptake. Apart from a metabolic component (usually small but occasionally prominent in special circumstances, such as when circulating free fatty acids are abnormally high), changes in heart rate, contractility, and wall stress account for most of the clinically relevant changes in myocardial oxygen uptake.

OXYGEN COST OF HEART WORK

To what extent is external work a determinant of the myocardial oxygen uptake? External work is done, for example, when a mass is lifted a specific distance, as in the ejection of blood against pressure (Fig. 12-2). In terms of the heart, cardiac output is the mass moved, and the resistance against which it is moved is afterload, mainly blood pressure. The following definitions may be helpful:

force = pressure × area (cm^3)
work = force (gm) × distance (cm) = pressure (F/cm^2) × volume (cm^3)
cardiac output (CO) = heart rate × stroke volume (liters/minute)
power = work/time = (F × cm)/time = pressure (F/cm^2) × CO_3 (cm^3/time)
stroke volume (SV) = end-diastolic volume (EDV) − end-systolic volume
ejection fraction = SV/EDV (%)
stroke work (clinical approximation) = mean BP × SV
stroke work index = stroke work/body surface area (m^2)
minute work (clinical approximation) = mean BP × CO

Force

Although force is a much-used word in relation to muscle mechanics, it is difficult to define. A practical definition is given above (force = pressure × area). Force is usually measured in grams, i.e., the force exerted by the earth (gravity) on a mass of 1 g. In many cases, it is not possible to define force exactly, but, in general, force has the following properties. First, force is always applied by one object (such as muscle) on another object (such as a load). Second, force is characterized by both the direction in which it acts and its magnitude. Hence, it is a vector, and the effect of a combination of forces can be established by the principle of vectors. Third, each object exerts a force on the other, so that in a state of rest or constant velocity, force and counterforce are equal and opposite (third law of motion of Newton).

An analogy to the force of the heart is the human effort required to squeeze a ball in the palm of the hand (Fig. 12-13). A small rubber ball can be compressed easily. A larger rubber ball (size of a tennis ball) is compressed less readily, and two large rubber balls or one really large ball could be compressed only with the greatest difficulty. As the size of the object in the hand increases, so does the total force (force = pressure × area) required to compress it. One solution is a

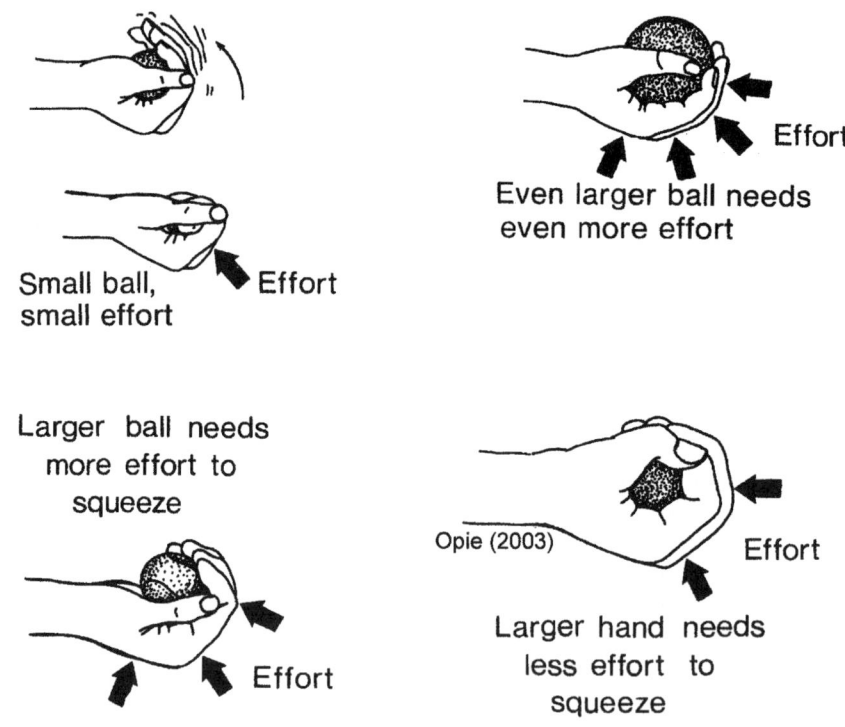

FIG. 12-13. Model of force. The effort required to squeeze a ball in the hand has some analogies to force development in the heart. When the volume of the ventricle is increased, more force is required to expel the blood. When the heart hypertrophies, the greater force developed by the thicker ventricle allows a larger volume of blood in the ventricle to be ejected more easily. The analogy is that more force (effort) is required to compress a larger ball and that a larger hand needs less effort to squeeze the large ball than does a smaller hand.

larger hand to deal with the larger ball, similar to the situation in ventricular hypertrophy in which the thicker wall (with more myofilaments) can generate more force to propel the blood against the increased afterload imposed on the ventricle.

Kinetic Versus Pressure Work

In strict terms, the work performed (*power production*) needs to take into account not only pressure but kinetic components. Thus far, it is pressure work that has been discussed. It is the larger component, and an approximate clinical index of pressure work is the product of cardiac output and peak systolic pressure. The *kinetic work* is that component required to accelerate the blood against the pressure of the arterial system. Kinetic work depends on cardiac output, the density of the blood, the cross-sectional area of the major resistance site (e.g., the aortic valve), and the ejection time. Normally, kinetic work is only a small fraction of the total work (18), but it increases substantially in aortic stenosis.

The formulae for work production are

$$\text{pressure power} = K_1 \times P_s \times \text{cardiac output}$$

$$\text{Kinetic power} = K_2 \times \frac{(CO)^3}{A^2} \times \left(\frac{T}{T_e}\right)^2$$

where P_s is peak systolic pressure in millimeters of mercury, CO is cardiac output in milliliters per minute, A is area of aortic valve in square centimeters, T is total cycle time, T_e is ejection time, and the units for power are milliwatts (i.e., millijoules per second). Instead of the peak systolic pressure, another formula uses the mean systolic pressure. Even these formulae are simplifications because in reality the pressure power is the product of the integrated sum of the instantaneous arterial pressure and the instantaneous aortic flow, which changes continuously throughout ejection.

Work Diagram of the Left Ventricle

Bearing in mind that the major factor in cardiac work is the product of pressure and volume, it follows that external work can be quantified by the integrated pressure–volume area that represents the product of the systolic pressure and stroke volume. This sequence can be depicted as a loop with counterclockwise rotation (a → b → c → d in Figure 12-14). As contractile force develops in the LV wall in systole, the pressure builds up in the cavity (a → b in Figure 12-14) until the moment when the aortic valve opens to eject the blood (b), and the isovolumic phase of LV contraction is over. When the aortic valves opens, the flow of blood commences and the ventricular pressure still increases because the pressure in the aorta must be overcome, whereas the LV volume decreases (b → c). The intraventricular pressure is highest at the peak of ejection before point c.

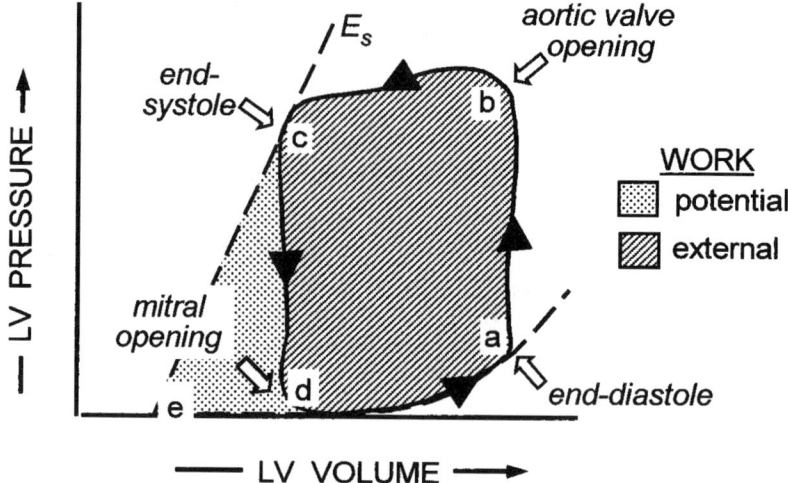

FIG. 12-14. Pressure–volume loop. Normal left ventricular pressure–volume relationship. The aortic valve opens at b and closes at c. The mitral valve opens at d and closes at a. External work is defined by a, b, c, d and potential energy by e, d, c. The pressure–volume area is the sum of external and internal (potential) work.

As the heart relaxes in early diastole, the pressure decreases to nearly zero (c → d), and the volume is at its nadir. Then, as the mitral valve opens and the left ventricle fills, the volume increases as the pressure stays low (d → a). When systole starts, the cycle is repeated. This sequence should be studied in conjunction with the Wiggers diagram (Color Plate 8-12).

Components of Work and Oxygen Consumption

To relate work to the oxygen consumption, both the external work (the area a, b, c, d) and the volume–pressure triangle joining the end-systolic volume–pressure point to the origin (the area c, d, e) must be taken into account. Although this area has been called internal work, more strictly it should be called *potential energy* that is generated within each contraction cycle but not converted to external work. The concept of internal work dates back many years, being well described in muscle preparation contracting but doing no external work (19). Intuitively, internal work is done whenever the heart works externally. The potential energy of the elastic component of the heart at the end of systole (point c) may be likened to the potential energy of a compressed spring. The total oxygen requirement is the combined areas for external work and for potential energy (20) that is the sum of the areas for external work (a, b, c, d in Figure 12-14) and potential energy (c, d, e in Figure 12-14). An additional small portion of the work of moving the blood can be accounted for by factors external to the left ventricle, such as atrial contraction and venous return.

Pressure Versus Volume Work

In analyzing the difference between oxygen cost of pressure work and volume work, Suga et al. (20) made the following proposals. To keep the stroke work the same, the area within the loop a → b → c → d has to be the same, so that the stroke volume during a pressure load is initially less (to compensate for the higher pressure). However, the remaining area between the pressure–volume loop and the end-systolic pressure–volume relationship line (c → d → e in Figures 12-14 and 12-15) is greater for the same amount of external work done under the increased pressure.

With a *volume load*, the increased work that the heart must perform is met by an increased end-diastolic volume (Fig. 12-15, left). An example is mitral regurgitation (Fig. 16-6) in which the mitral valve "leaks" and part of the stroke volume is ejected into the left atrium, thereafter returning to the left ventricle during the subsequent diastole. The diastolic stretch of the myofibers evokes the phenomenon of length-dependent activation (Color Plate 8-7). The primary adaptation to increased heart volume is an increased fiber length and not

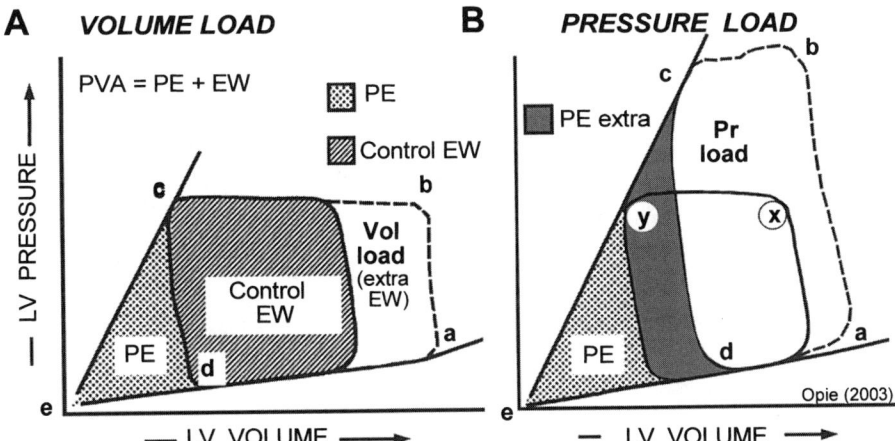

FIG. 12-15. Pressure versus volume work. In artificial circumstances, and using an isovolumic preparation, it is possible to compare equal amounts of stroke work performed by volume loading **(left)** and pressure loading **(right)**, which have different consequences for the oxygen uptake (20). Both external work (*EW*; a, b, c, d) and potential energy (*PE*; c, d, e) are oxygen requiring. The *hatched area* **(left)** enclosed by the solid loop indicates the control condition for external work (control EW). The *stippled triangles* (c, d, e) to the left of the pressure–volume loops in each part represent the requirement for potential energy. The total pressure–volume area (*PVA*) predicts the myocardial oxygen consumption at a steady heart rate (46). The areas added in each partly reflecting extra stroke work (and bounded by *dashed lines*) are the same for the volume-loaded as for the pressure-loaded heart. The *shaded area* during the pressure load indicates the extra internal work or potential energy and hence the extra oxygen requirement of the pressure-loaded heart when compared with the volume-loaded heart. Therefore, the pressure-loaded heart needs greater oxygen uptake than a volume-loaded heart for the same increment in external work. **Right:** x and y indicate upper limits of the pressure–volume loop corresponding to control external work **(left)**.

increased pressure development, so that the amount of external work done is more, but that against the internal resistance is unchanged so that the efficiency increases. A secondary and later adaptation to a sustained volume load is fiber slippage (during which adjacent layers of myocardium are displaced relative to each other, as in the extension of a telescope) so that the ventricular wall thins and becomes more compliant.

With a pressure load as during severe hypertension or narrowing of the aortic valve by aortic stenosis, cardiac work is increased to overcome the greater afterload (Fig. 12-15, right). The peak systolic pressure in the left ventricle must increase (Fig. 12-11), and pressure power increases. However, the area defining potential energy, c → d → e, greatly increases so that for a given amount of external work, more oxygen is taken up for the same amount of external work. The result is that the efficiency of external work (next section) decreases. An extreme example of the loss of efficiency during pressure work would be if the aorta were completely occluded, so that none of the work would be external and all would be internal.

β-Adrenergic stimulation shifts point c of the pressure–volume loop to the left, increasing the slope of E_s in the pressure–volume diagram (Fig. 12-16), which is an index of the positive inotropic effect. Concurrently, the lusitropic effect of this intervention pushes down the diastolic filling curve d → a. External work increases substantially, with little increase in internal work. Thus, the ratio of external to internal work increases so that the heart becomes more efficient. Conversely, during β-adrenergic blockade, external work decreases more than internal work (Fig. 12-16, right), so that efficiency is less.

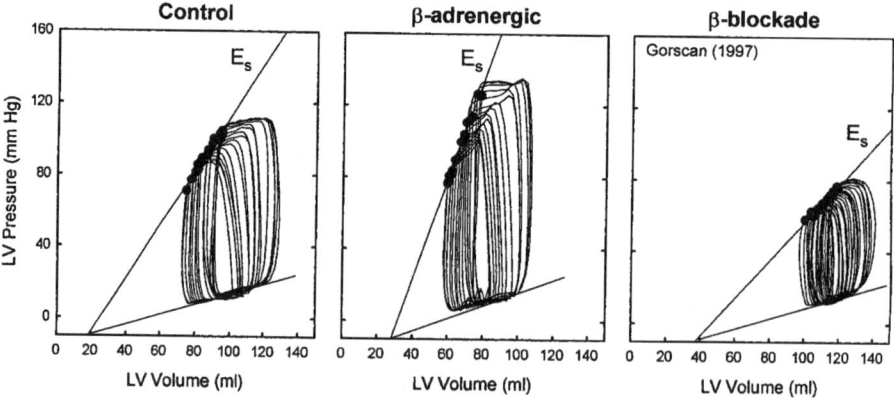

FIG. 12-16. **Contractility changes: effects on pressure–volume loops.** Control **(left)** versus β-adrenergic stimulation by dobutamine **(middle)** versus β-blockade **(right)**. Note much steeper E_s (end-systolic pressure–volume relationship) slope during β-adrenergic stimulation than during β-adrenergic blockade by esmolol. These data provide further evidence of the use of E_s as an inotropic index. Data from Gorcsan et al. (28).

Efficiency of Work

The efficiency of work relates the amount of external work performed to the myocardial oxygen uptake. An ideal definition of efficiency of work would be efficiency = work performed/maximal work possible. The denominator of this equation cannot be measured. There are many definitions of efficiency. One simple measure of efficiency is to relate the external measured work to the oxygen uptake: efficiency = work performed/oxygen uptake.

To improve the efficiency of work requires an analysis of whether it requires more oxygen to increase pressure or volume work. To conserve the myocardial oxygen balance, it would be desirable to achieve more work for the same oxygen uptake (improved efficiency). In practice, this means less pressure and more volume work, an aim that can be achieved therapeutically by arterial vasodilation. Conversely, increasing internal work (e.g., by allowing aortic stenosis to progress) promotes inefficient pressure work, which is one reason why aortic stenosis is so deleterious to patients with coronary artery disease.

Heat Production and the Efficiency of Work

The assessment of heat production is most useful when trying to marry the analyses of skeletal muscle mechanics by A.V. Hill to the much more complex mechanics of cardiac muscle (21). From the metabolic view, however, all heat production is nothing other than the use of ATP, partly for contraction and relaxation but also for ionic movements. However, the production of heat is the major product of ATP hydrolysis. A major requirement of all tissue, including the heart, is to be at the optimal temperature (37°C) for enzyme activity so that the generation of heat by ATP hydrolysis is teleologically desirable. Furthermore, the percentage of ATP converted to heat cannot be substantially changed except by breaking ATP down further than adenosine 5′-diphosphate. Taking these facts into account may explain why the efficiency of external work of the heart is only 15% to 25%, although in some experimental conditions, the range may become 20% to 40% (21).

Efficiency of Work in Heart Failure

The failing myocardium is unable to generate enough pressure to keep arterial blood pressure high enough without compensatory support mechanisms such as increased peripheral arteriolar vasoconstriction (Fig. 16-14). In the pressure–volume loop, external work is much decreased, whereas much more potential energy is generated (Fig. 12-17). Thus, the failing myocardium produces less external work at the cost of a much greater oxygen consumption and the efficiency of work declines. This harmful situation can be countered by reducing afterload with vasodilators (22).

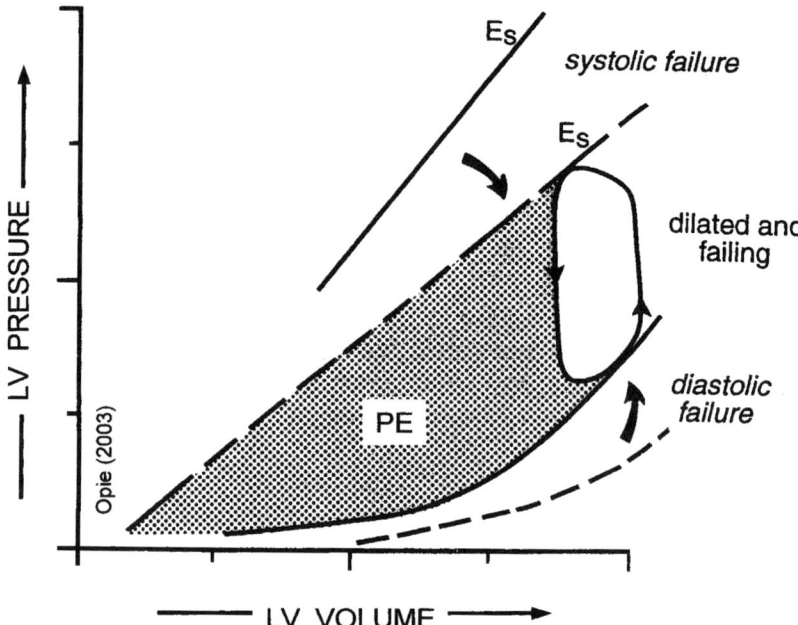

FIG. 12-17. Severe heart failure: pressure–volume loop. There is severe left ventricular failure with both systolic and diastolic failure. The dilated failing ventricle gives a larger end-diastolic volume (compare with normal in Figure 12-14). Decreased compliance with diastolic failure moves the end-diastolic pressure–volume curve upward and to the left. Decreased contractility (systolic failure) moves the pressure–volume slope E_s to the right. Decreased stroke volume is indicated by the smaller volume changes. Compare with Figure 12-15 and note the greatly increased potential energy (*PE*) related to internal work, with much less external work (area within the open loop).

TABLE 12-4. *Mechanisms for parameters of mechanical cardiac function*

Parameter of function	Definition	Proposed explanation
End-diastolic fiber length	Acts by the Starling law	Increased fiber sensitivity to Ca^{2+}
Peak force (peak tension increment); developed pressure	Difference between maximal systolic tension and minimal diastolic tension	Total number of cross-bridges attached since beginning of systole; a function of (a) initial fiber length, (b) systolic Ca^{2+} increase; (c) calcium responsiveness of filaments; (d) myosin light chain phosphorylation; (e) loading
V_{max} of isolated papillary muscle	Maximal rate of shortening at zero load (see Figure 12-4)	Proportional to (a) myosin ATPase activity, (b) rate-limiting steps in cross-bridge cycle, (c) rate of increase and peak level of cytosolic Ca^{2+}
P_0	Maximal tension at zero shortening rate	Related to number of attached cross-bridges and to peak Ca^{2+}
Indices of contractility	See Table 12-5	As for V_{max} but variously influenced by preload and afterload

CLINICAL INDICES OF CONTRACTILITY

Although it is relatively easy for the clinician to approximate preload or afterload of the heart by measuring the LV filling pressure or blood pressure and to relate these to the stroke volume, it is very difficult to assess the inotropic state (or the contractile state) of the myocardium. By definition, the types of studies undertaken on papillary muscle to obtain V_{max} are virtually impossible in humans, and various indices are used (Tables 12-4 and 12-5).

Left Ventricular Function Curves

Ventricular function curves can be obtained by varying the end-diastolic volume with repetitive measurements during a volume load (intravenous infusion). These curves are based on the Starling relationship (Fig. 12-4) indirectly assessed by Swan–Ganz catheterization using neither the heart volume nor the end-diastolic fiber length but the pulmonary capillary pressure (approximating LV end-diastolic pressure) as a surrogate (Fig. 16-13). The extrapolation from the one to the other usually is reasonable barring acute changes in LV compliance (see section on compliance). Furthermore, to produce an LV function curve by altering the preload over a wide range in humans is not easy. Yet another problem is the wide overlap among the different patterns of LV function curves, so that it is not a simple matter to decide whether a given function curve decreases into the normal category, into impaired LV function without clinical heart failure, or into clinical heart failure. Nonetheless, by comparing the LV end-diastolic pressure with the stroke volume and relating this point to the normal range (Fig. 16-13), an approximation of cardiac function can be obtained in real time and the immediate effect of therapeutic interventions such as volume loading or inotropic drugs can be observed.

Maximal Rate of Left Ventricular Pressure Generation

In relation to the cardiac contraction–relaxation cycle, it is easiest to consider LV function during the early period of isovolumic contraction (Fig. 12-18). During this period of isovolumic contraction, preload and afterload are constant, and the maximal rate of pressure generation should be an index of the inotropic state: inotropic index = maximal dP/dt, where P is LV pressure, t is time, and d indicates rate of change. This index has stood the test of years and gives some absolute values. Unfortunately, this index is not fully independent of the preload, which when increased will enhance the contractile state by length activation.

The measurements required for dP/dt can be obtained with sufficient precision only by LV catheterization with transducer-tipped catheters, except in mitral regurgitation when Doppler echocardiography can measure changes in the LV-atrial pressure gradient (23). Bearing in mind that LV pressure is changing during the period of isovolumic contraction, some workers prefer to make a correc-

TABLE 12-5. *Some applicable clinical indices of myocardial contractile (inotropic) state*

Index	Advantage	Comment
Isovolumic indices		
dP/dt_{max}	Classical invasive index	Requires LV catheterization; preload sensitive
Noninvasive $+dP/dt$	Can be determined by echocardiogram and phonocardiogram or MRI	dt measured from M_1 (phono) to AO (echo); dP from aortic diastolic pr and assuming LVEDP
Load-sensitive indices		
Ejection fraction	Noninvasive radionuclide scan or from echocardiographic volumes	Volume ejected during systole compared with initial ventricular volume; index of LV systolic function; load dependent; normal >55% (EDD-ESD)/(EDD), like ejection fraction, is load dependent
Percentage of fractional shortening	Simple, noninvasive echocardiographic technique	Compares well with fractional shortening
Long to minor axis shortening	Echocardiographic index claimed to be sensitive	Calculated from end-systolic and end-diastolic diameters and ejection time; consider end-systolic wall stress
V_{cf}	Noninvasive echocardiographic technique	
End-systolic indices		
End-systolic volume	Echocardiographic or MRI	Normal mean 34 mL in males, 29 in females; limit 55 mL (26,42)
End-systolic pressure–volume relationship	Echocardiographic or radionuclide determination; end-systolic pressure can be measured noninvasively	A small end-systolic volume reflects high contractility but is also afterload dependent
End-systolic wall stress/V_{cf}	Corresponds approximately to force-velocity relationship of isolated papillary muscle	Needs complex echocardiographic analyses
End-systolic stress/end-systolic volume	Corresponds approximately to one end point of pressure–volume loop	Wall stress difficult to measure (42)
Pressure–volume loop	Part of loop can be monitored noninvasively as end-systolic pressure–volume relationship	Increased slope (of end-systolic pressure–volume relationship) indicates increased contractility
Tissue Doppler imaging: systolic acceleration (isovolumic contraction)	Noninvasive; not influenced by preload or afterload (29)	Increased rate of acceleration shows increased contractility

For dP/dt_{max}, see Figure 12-6.
LV, left ventricular; phono, phonocardiography; AO, aortic valve opening; EDD, end-diastolic dimension; ESD, end-systolic dimension; V_{cf}, velocity of circumferential fiber shortening; MRI, magnetic resonance imaging.

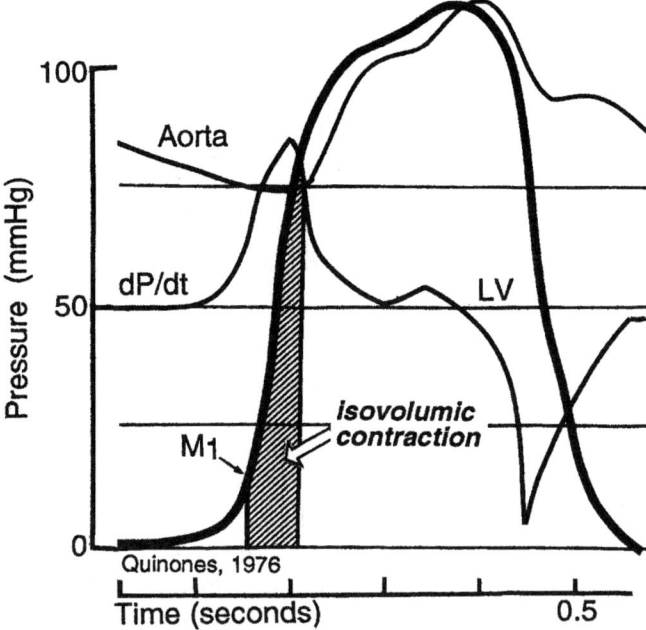

FIG. 12-18. Isovolumic contraction phase and maximal dP/dt, which measures the peak rate of contraction during the isovolumic period when theoretically there should be no effect of afterload. Based on original data of Quinones et al. (7). For dP/dt_{max}, see Table 12-5.

tion for the change in pressure by dividing dP/dt by P at the maximal rate of pressure development, (dP/dt)/P. Another correction is to divide dP/dt by the end-diastolic volume (24).

Ejection Phase Indices of Contractile State

During the ejection phase, the left ventricle contracts against the afterload. Hence, all indices of function in this period are afterload dependent (Table 12-5), a problem that is especially serious in the case of the failing myocardium, which is adversely affected by afterload increases.

The *ejection fraction* of the left ventricle, measured by radionuclide, angiographic, or echocardiographic techniques, or by magnetic resonance imaging, is one of the most frequently used indices and one of the least sensitive. The ejection fraction relates stroke volume to end-diastolic volume and is therefore an index of the extent of LV fiber shortening. Nonetheless, this index is easy to obtain and particularly useful in evaluating the course of systolic heart failure. The ejection fraction is by definition afterload sensitive. A second defect is that the ejection fraction relates the systolic emptying to the diastolic volume without measuring that volume. A third and major defect is that it gives no information on diastolic heart function or failure. Even in patients developing serious diastolic heart failure with high LV end-diastolic pressures and pulmonary edema, the systolic ejection fraction may be normal (25). Thus, the correlation between the degree of clinical heart failure and the ejection fraction is sometimes imperfect.

Echocardiographic Indices of Contractile State

The major advantages of echocardiographic indices is that the techniques are available at the bedside, are noninvasive, and relatively rapid. The *fractional shortening* uses the percentage of change of the minor axis (defined in the next paragraph) of the LV chamber during systole (Fig. 12-1). An approximation often used by clinicians is to estimate the ejection fraction from fractional shortening. Despite the obvious defects mentioned, this easily defined index is pragmatically useful in the management of heart failure. More accurately, ejection fraction can be determined from volume measurements. The end-systolic volume reflects the contractile state because the normal left ventricle ejects most of the blood present at the end of diastole (ejection fraction exceeds 55%). Impaired contractility, shown by an abnormally increased end-systolic volume, is a powerful predictor of adverse prognosis after myocardial infarction (26). The end-diastolic volume is a less powerful predictor but essential for the accurate measurement of the ejection fraction.

Much more sophisticated measurements of the pumping function of the heart can also be obtained by echocardiography. In particular, the velocity at which the circumference of the heart in its minor axis changes during systole is a useful index of myocardial contractility (Table 12-5). The minor axis of the heart is the distance from the left side of the septum to the opposite endocardial wall. The major axis lies parallel to the direction of the septum, which introduces an additional factor, septal contraction, so that major axis changes cannot be used to assess contractile activity. The mean velocity of circumferential fiber shortening (mean V_{cf}) can be determined from echocardiographic measurements of the end-diastolic and end-systolic sizes and the rate of change. The difference between the calculated circumferences is divided by the duration of shortening, which is the ejection time. The mean V_{cf} compares favorably with more sophisticated invasive measurements of the contractile state.

Tissue Doppler imaging is relatively new, very sensitive, and state of the art. It records high-amplitude, low-frequency Doppler shifts, thereby capturing systolic and diastolic myocardial velocities. For example, in LV hypertrophy, tissue Doppler imaging picks up subtle systolic abnormalities in patients who would otherwise be classified as having diastolic heart failure with "normal" systolic function as measured by the ejection fraction (27). There are several tissue Doppler imaging indices to measure LV contractile function, including endocardial velocity (28) and myocardial acceleration during isovolumic contraction (29).

Contractility Indices Based on Pressure–Volume Loops

There are two fundamental aspects of the Frank–Starling relationship that can be seen readily in a pressure–volume loop (Fig. 12-14). First, as the preload increases, the LV volume increases. Conversely, for any given preload (initial volume of contraction), a positive inotropic agent increases the amount of blood ejected, and for the same final end-systolic pressure, there is a smaller end-systolic volume. Thus, the slope of the end-systolic pressure–volume relationship (E_s) is increased (Figs. 12-16 and 12-17). It follows that relating pressure to volume is one way to assess both the Starling effect and the contractility of the left ventricle.

Accordingly, measurements of pressure–volume loops are among the best of the current approaches to the assessment of the contractile behavior of the intact heart, and hence the key to one of the major determinants of the myocardial oxygen demand. The end-systolic pressure–volume relationship can be estimated noninvasively from the (mean) arterial systolic pressure (which approximates arterial pressure at the moment of end-systolic ejection, i.e., point c on the pressure–volume loop in Fig. 12-14) and the end-systolic echocardiographic dimension. Invasive measurements of the LV pressure are required for definition of the full loop, which is an indirect measure of the Starling relationship between the force developed (as measured by the LV pressure) and the muscle length (measured indirectly by the volume). A higher contractile activity (increased inotropic state) will have higher end-systolic pressures for any given end-systolic volume and a steeper slope E_s (Figs. 12-16 and 12-17). This means correspondingly higher oxygen uptakes. Because the slope of the end-systolic pressure–volume relationship is constant over a range of arterial and LV end-diastolic pressures, it is relatively preload and afterload independent compared with other indices.

DIASTOLE AND DIASTOLIC FUNCTION: "DIASTOLOGY"

Phases of Diastole

Hemodynamically, diastole can be divided into four phases (Fig. 12-19), using the clinical definitions of diastole according to which diastole extends from aortic valve closure to the start of the first heart sound. The first phase of diastole (see preceding section) is the isovolumic phase, which, by definition, does not contribute to ventricular filling. The second phase of rapid or early filling provides most (approximately 80%) of ventricular filling. The third phase of slow filling or diastasis accounts for only 5% of the total filling. The final atrial booster phase normally accounts for the remaining 15%.

Cellular Factors That Influence Relaxation

Among the many complex cellular factors influencing ventricular relaxation, four are mainly of interest. First, the cytosolic calcium level must decrease to

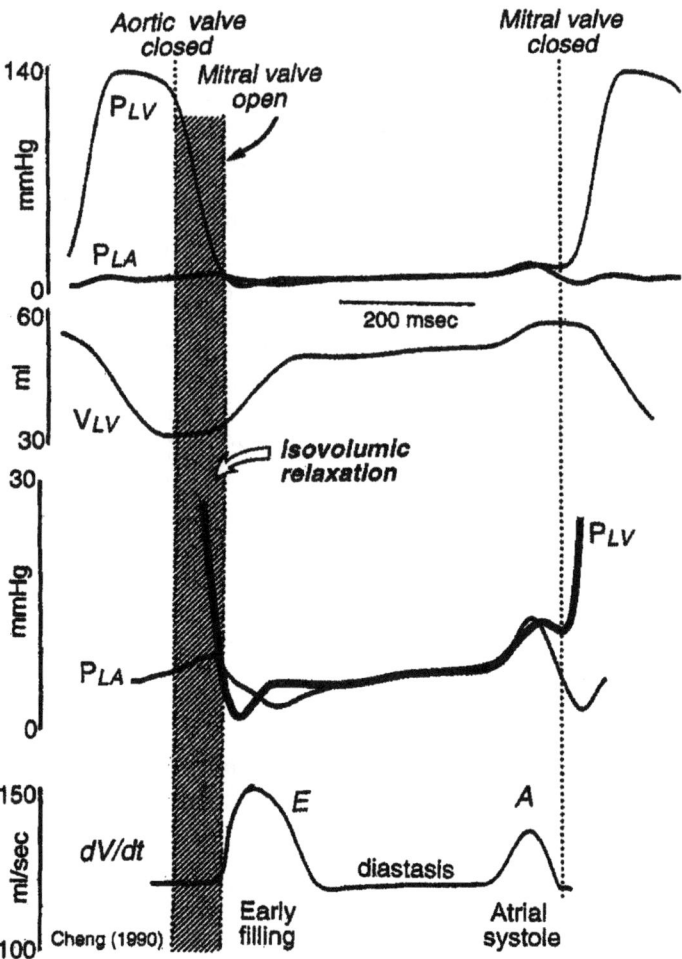

FIG. 12-19. Diastolic filling phases. Left ventricular filling occurs early in diastole and during atrial systole in response to pressure gradient from the left atrium to the left ventricle. The early diastolic pressure gradient is generated as left ventricular pressure decreases below left atrial pressure and the late diastolic gradient is generated as the atrial contraction increases the left atrial pressure to more than the left ventricular pressure. Recording of left ventricular pressure (P_{LV}), left atrial pressure (P_{LA}), left ventricular volume integrated over time (dV/dt), which indicates the rate of left ventricular filling. Data from Cheng et al. Circ Res 1990;66:814.

cause the relaxation phase, a process requiring ATP and phosphorylation of phospholamban for uptake of calcium into the sarcoplasmic reticulum (Fig. 12-20). Second, increased phosphorylation of troponin I enhances the rate of relaxation (30). Third, the inherent viscoelastic properties of the myocardium are important. In the hypertrophied heart, relaxation occurs more slowly. Fourth, relaxation is influenced by the systolic load. The history of contraction affects

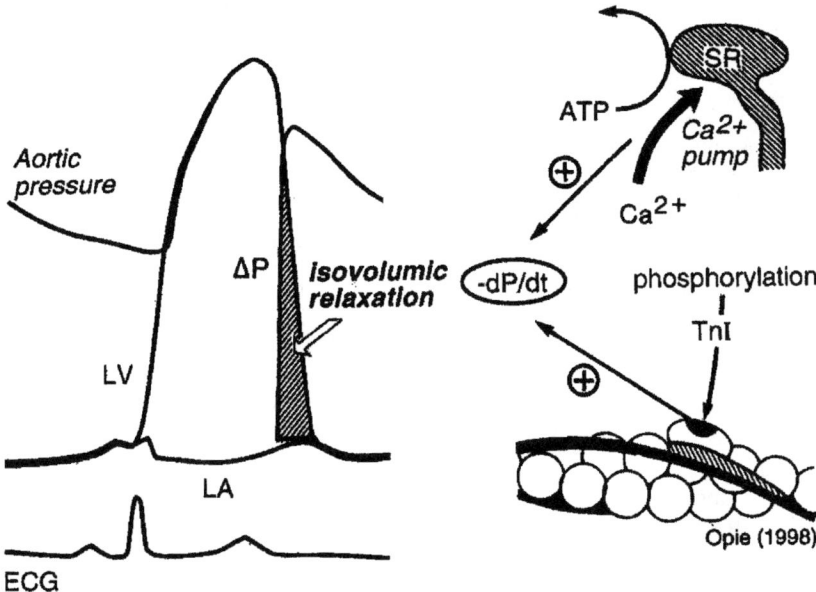

FIG. 12-20. Regulation of isovolumic relaxation. This phase of the cardiac cycle is shown in the *shaded area*. It extends from the aortic second sound (A_2) to the crossover point between the left ventricular and left atrial pressures (Color Plate 8-12). The rate of relaxation is given by –dP/dt. This is influenced by the rate of uptake of calcium ions into the sarcoplasmic reticulum (*SR*) and the degree of phosphorylation of troponin I (*TnI*), as shown in Figure 8-3. *LA*, left atrial pressure.

cross-bridge relaxation (31). Within limits, the greater the systolic load is, the faster the rate of relaxation is. This complex relationship has been explored in detail by Zile and Brutsaert (32) but could perhaps be simplified as follows. When the workload is high, peak cytosolic calcium is also thought to be high. High end-systolic cytosolic calcium means that the rate of decrease in calcium also can be greater if the uptake mechanisms are functioning effectively. In this way, a systolic pressure load and the rate of diastolic relaxation can be related. Yet, when the systolic load exceeds a particular limit, the rate of relaxation is delayed (31), perhaps because of too great a mechanical stress on the individual cross-bridges. Thus, in congestive heart failure caused by an excess systolic load, the delay in relaxation is increasingly afterload dependent, so that reduction of the systolic load should improve LV relaxation.

Isovolumic Relaxation Phase

The isovolumic relaxation phase of the cardiac cycle is energy dependent, requiring ATP for the uptake of calcium ions by the sarcoplasmic reticulum (Fig. 12-20), which is an active process. Impaired relaxation is an early event in

TABLE 12-6. *Some indices of diastolic function*

Isovolumic relaxation
  $(-)dP/dt_{max}$
  Aortic closing, mitral opening interval
  Peak rate of left ventricular wall thinning
  Time constant of relaxation, τ^a
Early diastolic filling
  Relaxation kinetics on ERNA (rate of volume increase)
  Early filling phase (E phase) on Doppler transmitral velocity trace
  Early filling phase (E phase) on Doppler of velocity of mitral valve annulus motion
Diastasis
  Pressure–volume relationship indicates compliance
Atrial contraction
  Invasive measurement of atrial and ventricular pressures
  Doppler transmitral pattern (late or A phase)
E/A ratios
  Normally E > A unless A increased by age or disease, further decreased left ventricular compliance again increases E to A (43)

[a]For noninvasive measurements by continuous wave Doppler velocity profile in mitral regurgitation, see Chen et al. (33).
ERNA, equilibrated radionuclide angiography.

angina pectoris. A proposed metabolic explanation is that there is impaired generation of energy that diminishes the supply of ATP required for the early diastolic uptake of calcium by the sarcoplasmic reticulum. In congestive heart failure, diastolic relaxation also is delayed and irregular, as is the rate of decay of the cytosolic calcium elevation. Most patients with coronary artery disease have a variety of abnormalities of diastolic filling, probably related to those also found in angina pectoris. Theoretically, such abnormalities of relaxation are potentially reversible because they depend on changes in patterns of calcium ion movement. Indices of the isovolumic phase and other indices of diastolic function are shown in Table 12-6.

The rate of such relaxation can be measured by negative dP/dt_{max} with invasive catheterization (Fig. 12-19). Tau, the time constant of relaxation, describes the rate of decrease in LV pressure during isovolumic relaxation and also requires invasive techniques for precise determination (33). In practice, tau is often measured echocardiographically (33). Tau is increased as the systolic LV pressure increases. Another echocardiographic index of relaxation is the peak rate of wall thinning. The isovolumic relaxation time, because it lies between aortic valve closure and mitral valve opening, can be measured by signals of valve movements on Doppler echocardiography. In each case, precise measurement is difficult, and the range of normality is large.

Early Diastolic Velocity

E/A ratios (early phase of atrial filling phases, see later, Fig. 12-24) may reflect the compensatory increase in the late (atrial) filling phase found when the hypertrophic LV fails to relax normally during diastole. The result is that the E/A ratio on the mitral Doppler pattern decreases or reverses. In time, with both increased LV hypertrophy and the development of fibrosis, LV chamber compliance decreases and the E wave again becomes more prominent. Thus, it becomes difficult to separate E/A ratios that are truly normal from pseudonormal patterns of mitral inflow. This is where Doppler tissue imaging gives a more accurate answer (34,35). This technique can measure the actual velocity of tissue relaxation of the mitral valve annulus or the posterior wall (34).

Does the Left Ventricle "Suck" During Early Filling?

Whether the LV suction by active relaxation could increase the pressure gradient from left atrium to left ventricle during the early filling phase remains controversial although well supported by data. An LV suction effect can be found by carefully comparing LV and left atrial pressures; it occurs especially in the early diastolic phase of rapid filling (Fig. 12-21). The sucking effect may be most important in mitral stenosis, when the mitral valve does not open as it otherwise should in response to diastolic suction. During catecholamine stimulation, and

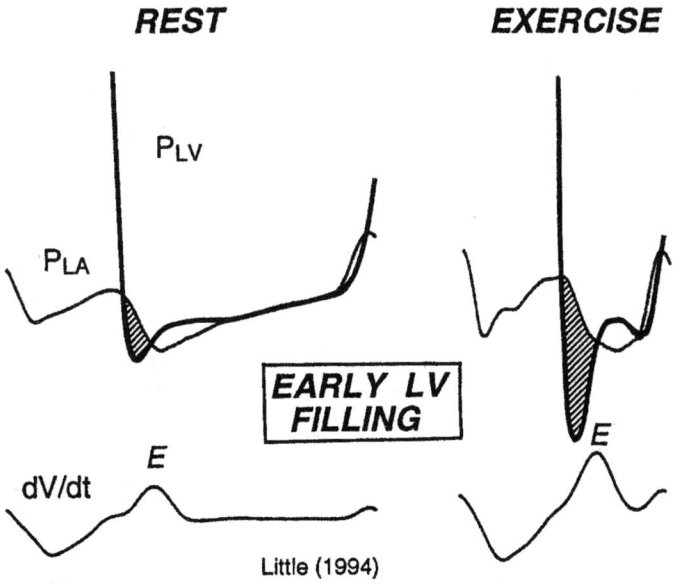

FIG. 12-21. Apparent left ventricular (LV) sucking effect. During exercise, the lowest LV pressure decreases without any increase in left atrial pressure. This leads to an increase in the peak mitral valve gradient and produces a larger peak filling rate (E). Recording of LV pressure (P_{LV}) and left atrial pressure (P_{LA}) and the rate of change of LV volume (dV/dt) at rest and during exercise. (From Little, Cheng. Modulation of diastolic dysfunction in the intact heart. In: Lorell, Grossman, eds. *Diastolic relaxation of the heart.* Boston: Kluwer Academic Publishers, 1994:167, with permission.)

hence during exercise, the rate of relaxation may increase to enhance the sucking effect and to prolong the period of filling. Such active relaxation may reside in the properties of the giant molecule titin (Color Plate 8-3). The proposal is that at very short sarcomere lengths, as may be found in the contracting ventricle during early diastole, myosin is pulled into the space between the two anchoring segments of titin to lower the intraventricular pressure to below that in the atrium (36).

Diastolic Left Ventricular Dysfunction

"Diastolic dysfunction is the primary mechanism for dyspnea in patients with heart failure, irrespective of the presence or severity of systolic dysfunction" (34). This statement is now open to challenge as the new tissue Doppler technique with measurement of mid-wall velocity reveals that systolic dysfunction often accompanies clinical diastolic heart failure (35). The concept of diastolic dysfunction with virtually normal systolic function does, however, remain as a cause of cardiac disability (35).

In hypertrophic hearts, as in chronic hypertension or severe aortic stenosis, echocardiographic abnormalities of diastolic function are common and may precede clinical diastolic heart failure (35). Conceptually, impaired relaxation must be distinguished from prolonged systolic contraction with delayed onset of normal relaxation (32). Experimentally, there are several defects in early hypertensive hypertrophy including decreased rates of contraction and relaxation and decreased peak force development (37). Loss of the load-sensitive component of relaxation may be caused by impaired activity of the sarcoplasmic reticulum.

ATRIAL FUNCTION

The left atrium, in addition to its well-known function as a blood-receiving chamber, also acts as follows. First, by presystolic contraction and its booster function, it helps to complete LV filling (38). In LV diastolic dysfunction or failure, there is a compensatory increase in atrial contraction as reflected in the increased A wave in the Doppler mitral filling pattern. Second, the volume sensor of the heart releases atrial natriuretic peptide in response to intermittent stretch. Third, the atrium contains receptors for the afferent arms of various reflexes including mechanoreceptors that increase sinus discharge rate, thereby contributing to the tachycardia of exercise as venous return increases (Bainbridge reflex, Fig. 14-4).

The atria have a number of differences in structure and function from the ventricles (Table 12-7), having smaller myocytes with shorter action potential duration as well as a more fetal type of myosin (both in heavy and light chains). The more rapid atrial repolarization is thought to be caused by increased outward potassium currents, such as I_{to} and I_{KACh}. In addition, some atrial cells have the capacity for spontaneous depolarization. In general, these histologic and physi-

TABLE 12-7. Major differences between atria and left ventricle

Parameter	Atria	Left ventricle
Hemodynamic function	Receives venous blood and transmits it to ventricles	Ejects blood into aorta to maintain BP and CO
Blood volume control	Volume sensor	Volume ejector
Wall dimension	Thin	Thick
Myocyte size	20×5 μm	$75 \times (10-25)$ μm
Pressure generated	Low, 15–30 mm Hg	High, >100 mm Hg
Myosin phenotype, heavy[a]	Fetal, α (V_1)	Adult, α (V_3)[b]
Myosin phenotype, light	Fetal (A-LC1)	Adult (V-LC1)
ANP synthesis	Physiologic	Pathologic (also BNP)
Action potential	Prominent phase 1; short plateau; "triangular"	Small phase 1; long plateau; "square"

[a]See Table 8-3.
[b]For human isoforms, see Figure 13-10.
BP, blood pressure; CO, cardiac output; A-LC1, atrium-type myosin light chain 1; V-LC1, ventricle-type myosin light chain 1; ANP, atrial natriuretic peptide; BNP, brain natriuretic peptide.

ologic changes can be related to the decreased need for the atria to generate high intrachamber pressures, rather being sensitive to volume changes, while retaining enough contractile action to help with LV filling and to respond to inotropic stimuli (38).

LEFT VENTRICULAR COMPLIANCE

The diastolic volume of the heart is influenced by the loading conditions as well as the elastic properties of the myocardium. Elasticity means that the myocardium recovers its normal shape after removal of the systolic stress. Compliance is strictly defined as the relationship between the change in stress and the resultant strain (percentage of change in dimension or size). In clinical practice, it is taken as the ratio of dV/dP, i.e., the rate of volume change divided by the rate of pressure change. The relationship is curvilinear, and the initial slope of the change is gentle (highly compliant). As the pressure increases, the volume increases less and less (less compliant) so that there is a considerable increase in pressure for only a small increase in volume (Fig. 12-22).

The concept of diastolic distensibility is complementary to the more traditional term compliance. Distensibility refers to the diastolic pressure required to fill the ventricle to the same volume, not to the slope of the pressure–volume relationship. Thus, when compliance decreases, the distensibility is less, as seen at high filling pressures in the dilated failing heart (Fig. 12-23).

Whereas resting skeletal muscle is truly in a state of relaxation (so that the resting tension is close to zero), the heart has a very high resting tension. Resting stiffness may in part be attributed to the unique myocardial collagen network, thought to counter the high systolic pressure normally developed in the ventricles. Pathologic loss of compliance is usually caused by abnormalities of the

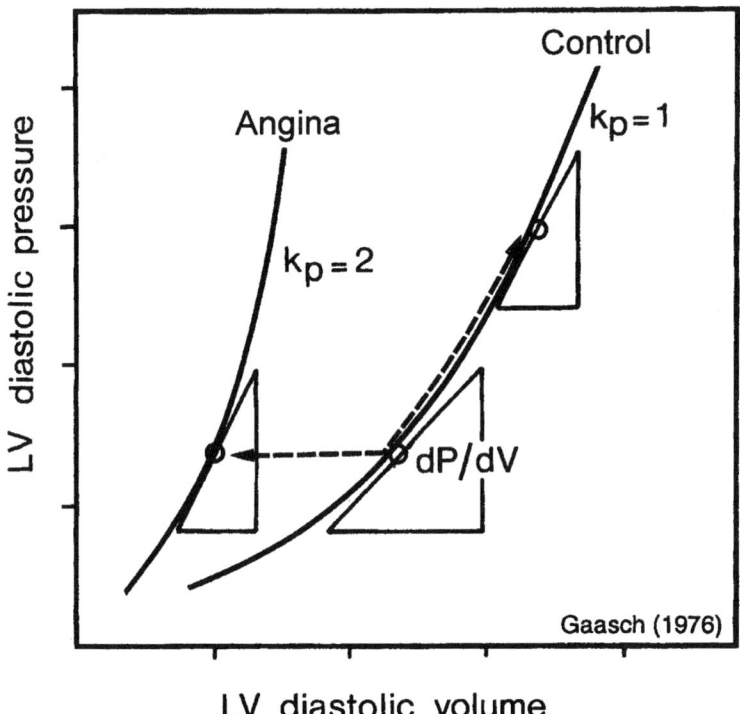

FIG. 12-22. Left ventricular (LV) stiffness and compliance. The volume stiffness reflects the relationship between the increase in heart volume and the increase in LV diastolic pressure (dP/dV). As seen on the left, the stiffness is increased because the modulus of chamber stiffness (K_p) is increased. Such a true increase in stiffness can occur in angina or myocardial infarction. As stiffness (dP/dV) increases, compliance (dV/dP, also called volume distensibility) decreases. (From Gaasch WH, Levine HJ, Quinones MA, et al. Left ventricular compliance: mechanisms and clinical implications. *Am J Cardiol* 1976;38:645–653, with permission.)

myocardium. For example, in myocardial hypertrophy, a greater pressure increase is required to achieve any given volume increase (the thicker the wall, the more intraluminal pressure is needed to make it stretch). When corrected for the increased mass, however, the muscular compliance in myocardial hypertrophy is close to normal.

A true loss of muscular compliance occurs because of a variety of causes, e.g., acute ischemia as in angina, fibrosis as after myocardial infarction, pathologic infiltrations (amyloidosis), causing a restrictive cardiomyopathy. In angina, the increased temporary stiffness probably is caused by a combination of an increase in intracellular calcium and of altered myocardial properties. In myocardial infarction, the connective tissue undergoes changes after 40 minutes of occlusion. Eventually, healing and fibrosis permanently increase stiffness. When muscle stiffness increases, so will chamber stiffness (the chamber being the ventricle). When the functioning of the chambers is indirectly impaired by an external

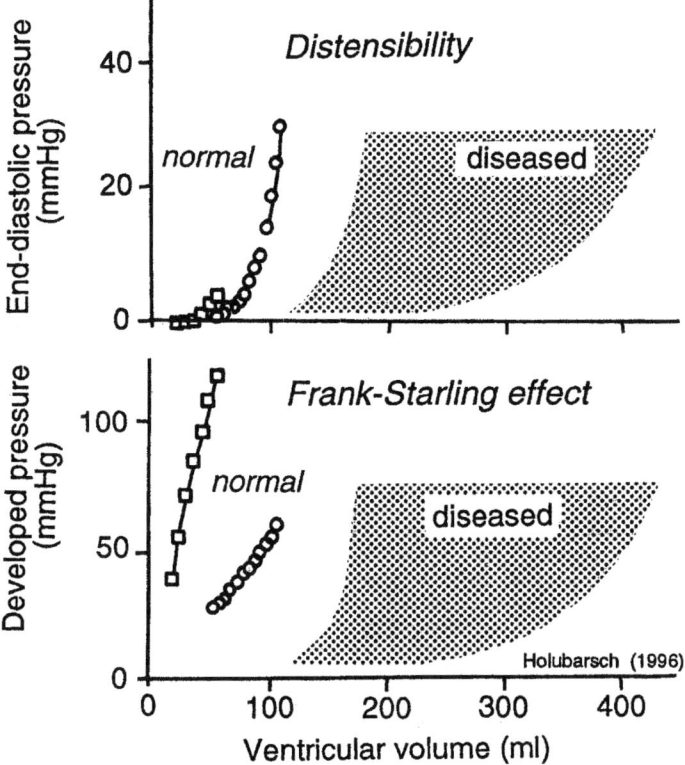

FIG. 12-23. Frank–Starling relationships in the failing human heart. The *open symbols* to the left show responses of two normal hearts to increased filling volumes. The *shaded areas* on the right are composites of pressure–volume relationships in five hearts afflicted with dilated cardiomyopathy. These dilated hearts function at much higher filling volumes to generate normal developed pressures (developed pressure = systolic pressure − diastolic pressure). The dilated hearts are more compliant at physiologic volumes but become less compliant at the higher filling pressures required for maintenance of cardiac output. For original data, see Holubarsch et al. (13).

constraint such as constrictive pericarditis, a hemodynamic situation similar to restrictive cardiomyopathy may arise. Extracardiac mechanical factors, such as those exerted by the pericardium and the lungs on the heart, also help to determine the diastolic pressure–volume relationship.

The compliance of the heart influences the Starling curve (when measured as stroke volume versus end-diastolic pressure) and the pressure–volume loop as well as the early diastolic filling rate of the heart. A stiffer (less compliant) heart will be on a lower Starling curve, and the baseline of the pressure–volume loop will increase upward more steeply, so that a higher left atrial pressure will be required for early diastolic filling (Fig. 12-24). For these reasons, compliance is a fundamental physiologic property of the heart.

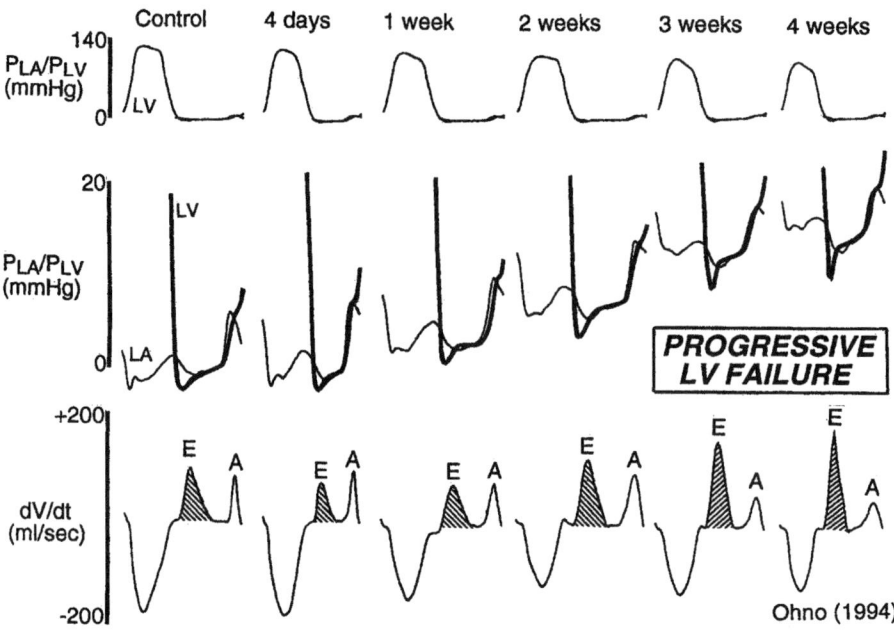

FIG. 12-24. Diastolic filling during progressive experimental heart failure. Note increasing left ventricular (LV) end-diastolic and left atrial pressures, at first with a normal E/A ratio, then A< E, then normalization, then E > A (pseudonormalization) as LV loses compliance. E indicates peak LV filling rate occurring early in diastole, and A indicates atrial contraction during late diastole. For A wave, see Color Plate 8-12. Analog record of left atrial (P_{LA}) and left ventricular (P_{LV}) pressures and the time derivative of LV volume (dV/dt) indicate the filling pattern. (Modified from Ohno M, Cheng CP, Little WC. Mechanism of altered patterns of left ventricular filling during the development of congestive heart failure. *Circulation* 1994;89:2241–2250.)

VENTRICULAR INTERACTION

Thus far, LV function has been discussed as if the left ventricle were working in isolation. In reality, its function is intimately linked to that of the right ventricle, both functionally and anatomically. Cardiac output of the left ventricle must equal that of the right ventricle unless there is a state of imbalance, as in conditions of acute LV failure when blood may accumulate in the lungs to cause pulmonary edema. In general, the right ventricle is working against a low resistance circuit, and afterload is not a major problem in physiologic conditions. What the right ventricle receives by means of its filling pressure in the venous system, it will empty in response to the Starling effect. The amount of pressure work generated by the right ventricle is relatively low, which explains the thinner right ventricular wall and the dominance of LV function in calculations of pressure work or of myocardial oxygen uptake.

Anatomically, the two ventricles are interlinked. They share a common septum. That septum constitutes part of the load against which each ventricle must work. In LV hypertrophy, which includes the septum, the right ventricle must, therefore, work harder and tends to become hypertrophied. This is systolic ventricular interaction. One type of diastolic ventricular interaction is the Bernheim effect, whereby a large left ventricle can compress the right ventricle, the volume on the left side being so great that the right side is unable to fill properly. A converse diastolic ventricular interaction can occur in severe heart failure, when the dilated failing right ventricle may impinge on the left (39). Under these circumstances, the measured LV end-diastolic pressure is not identical to the transmural pressure of the entire left ventricle (13). This explains the apparent descending limb of the Starling curve, demonstrated experimentally in failing hearts during acute volume loading experiments (Figs. 12-3 and 12-4). When the right ventricle is unloaded by the venodilator agent nitroglycerin, it can decrease in size and allow the LV function to improve.

PERICARDIUM AND ENDOCARDIUM

The normal pericardium has an important restraining effect on the diastolic properties of the ventricles, especially the right ventricle. Without the pericardium, the right ventricle would dilate by approximately 40% and the right atrium by approximately 70%. Therefore, the physical properties of the pericardium help to determine ventricular pressure–volume relationships and, indirectly, compliance. Normally LV diastolic pressure is greater than that in the other chambers by the amount of its transmural pressure (5 to 10 mmHg), the low pericardial pressure being equally applied to all chambers. During pericardial disease with cardiac tamponade, the pressure within the pericardial cavity increases as the volume increases, especially with acute increases in volume of more than 200 mL, so that the intrapericardial pressure equals or exceeds the normal diastolic filling pressure. When this happens, venous filling and therefore cardiac output are severely reduced.

TABLE 12-8. *Systolic and diastolic dysfunction of the myocardium*

	Systolic	Diastolic
Exertional dyspnea	Yes	Yes
Ejection fraction	Low	Normal (or increased in myocardial hypertrophy)
Mechanical parameter on pressure–volume loop	Impaired inotropic state	Impaired lusitropic state
PV[a] relationship	End-systolic PV altered	End-diastolic PV altered
Relaxation indices	Abnormal	Abnormal
(+)dP/dt$_{max}$	Abnormal	Normal
(−)dP/dt$_{max}$	Abnormal	Abnormal
Rapid filling phase	Abnormal	Abnormal
Atrial booster function	Responds to the associated diastolic failure	Increased early in course of development of failure; A-to-E ratio increased[b]

[a]PV, pressure–volume; see Figure 12-14.
[b]A-to-E ratio, see Figure 12-24.

CONTRACTILE PROPERTIES IN HUMAN HEART DISEASE

The failing human myocardium has impaired systolic and diastolic properties (Table 12-8) so that even when the venous filling pressure is adequate, the stroke volume is reduced when compared with normal, and blood pressure tends to decrease. An increased heart rate provides some compensation to help maintain cardiac output and, thereby, blood pressure. Nonetheless, the treppe effect is lost (Fig. 12-8), and work spent on generation of potential energy is increased relative to external work (Fig. 12-17). Homeostatic mechanisms that come into play sustain blood pressure (Fig. 16-14), but the severely failing myocardium does this at the cost of decreased efficiency of work (22). The faster heart rate is also oxygen inefficient, requiring more oxygen for less force development, as shown by the smaller differences between systolic and diastolic force development (Fig. 12-25).

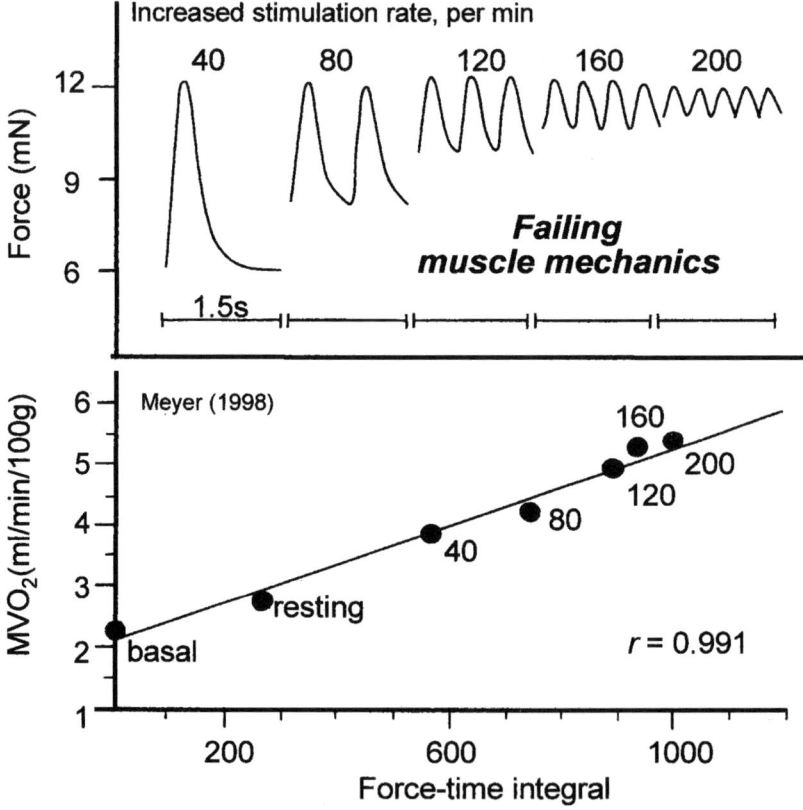

FIG. 12-25. Diastolic tension and failing muscle mechanics in human heart failure. Note the marked increase in diastolic tension during pacing of a muscle strip from advanced human heart failure. The linear relationship between increased myocardial oxygen uptake (MVO_2) and increased force (measured as the force–time integral) is shown at the bottom. The combination of decreased cardiac force development and increased oxygen uptake indicates decreased efficiency of cardiac work. (Modified from Meyer et al. *J Mol Cell Cardiol* 1998;30:1459–1470.)

Other defects include an impaired response to increased preload (Fig. 12-23), defective generation of cyclic adenosine 3′,5′-monophosphate in response to β-adrenergic stimulation and numerous defects of the patterns of handling of intracellular calcium (Fig. 6-12). In response to increased afterload, the intracellular calcium transient of trabecular myocardium from the severely failing human heart shows an abnormally prolonged and exaggerated pattern of increase, despite poor generation of force (40). It is controversial whether there is truly a defective Frank–Starling response, as claimed by Schwinger et al. (41) or whether apparent defects can be explained by the decreased distensibility of the dilated failing human heart, as claimed by Holubarsch et al. (13). According to the latter point of view, there still is some Starling response (Fig. 12-23) so that the LV filling pressure of patients with severe heart failure could be therapeutically set to be high enough to achieve an optimal Starling effect without being too high and causing pulmonary edema. For other methods of enhancing cardiac performance, see Table 12-9.

In aortic valve disease, the increased volume load of aortic regurgitation contrasts with the pressure load of aortic stenosis. In aortic stenosis, kinetic work increases sharply as the cross-sectional area narrows, whereas pressure work increases as the gradient across the aortic valve increases. Therefore, both types of work in aortic stenosis increase the myocardial oxygen demand. In aortic regurgitation, heart work and oxygen demand are increased by the increased wall stress resulting from the greater ventricular volume (Fig. 16-6) and by increased afterload. The latter results from associated systolic hypertension after the ejection of increased stroke volume into the arterial tree and increased wall stress from the volume load.

TABLE 12-9. *Stimuli to enhanced cardiac performance*

Stimulus	Physiologic mechanism
Rate-dependent effects	
Treppe phenomenon	"Sodium pump lag"; calcium entry exceeds rate of exit
Load dependency	
Preload increase	Length-dependent sensitization of contractile proteins to calcium
Afterload reduction	Failing myocardium is afterload dependent
Receptor stimulation	
β-Adrenergic (or similar drugs)	Positive inotropic and lusitropic effects; increased calcium entry; increased calcium-induced calcium release; increased uptake of calcium into sarcoplasmic reticulum
α-Adrenergic	Inconsistent effects on contraction
Angiotensin II[a]	Variably positive inotropic
Endothelin[a]	Positive inotropic (marked vascular effects)
Sodium pump inhibition	
Digoxin	Increased sodium–calcium exchange
Calcium sensitizers	
Levosimendan, others	Increased calcium sensitivity of troponin C

[a]Simultaneous increase in peripheral vascular resistance compromises inotropic effects.

SUMMARY

1. *The cardiac cycle.* LV contraction shuts the mitral valve so that the blood inside the left ventricle cavity is trapped for the duration of the isovolumic contraction phase until the aortic valve is forced open, and blood accelerates into the aorta during the phase of maximal ejection. LV relaxation follows. It results first in the phase of reduced ejection and then, after the aortic valve has closed, in isovolumic relaxation, until the pressure in the LV decreases below that in the left atrium, which opens the mitral valve. Rapid LV diastolic filling is followed by a slow phase (diastasis) before the atrial booster contraction, whereupon the heart is ready to reenter a new cycle.

2. *Preload and afterload.* Preload is the load on the ventricle before contraction starts, at the end of diastole. Afterload is that against which the left ventricle contracts.

3. *Acute effect of load on myocardial performance.* When either preload or afterload increases acutely, ventricular performance does as well. There are two major mechanisms. First, increased preload increases ventricular filling and hence the end-diastolic fiber length to enhance performance (Starling law) by the process of length-dependent activation. If afterload is increased, in addition to a transient increase in end-diastolic dimension, an alternative or proposed mechanism involves activation of stretch receptors to increase cytosolic calcium levels.

4. *Contractility or inotropic state.* This concept relates to changes in performance independently of the load, either because the cytosolic calcium level has increased (e.g., during β-adrenergic stimulation) or the myofibrils have become sensitized to calcium (e.g., in response to a calcium-sensitizing drug). In clinical practice, it is not easy to measure the inotropic state. Inaccurate but practical load-dependent indices include fractional shortening and the ejection fraction measured echocardiographically. More load-independent indices include end-systolic wall stress, much more difficult to measure, and measurement of pressure–volume loops

5. *Pressure–volume loops.* The inotropic state (contractility) is reflected in the end-systolic pressure–volume relationship, a linear function that is anchored on the x-axis at one end and the intercept with the end-systolic pressure of the pressure–volume loop on the other. It moves leftward and upward during inotropic stimulation. Conversely, the end-diastolic pressure–volume relationship is an index of the compliance (distensibility) of the myocardium, which is low at the high end-diastolic filling pressures seen in chronic congestive heart failure.

6. *Diastolic dysfunction.* Whereas decreased contractility is a classic feature of myocardial systolic failure, changes in the lusitropic state (ability to relax) are at least equally important in the development of pulmonary or systemic venous congestion and often occur in LV hypertrophy before overt systolic abnormalities. Tissue Doppler echocardiography is a new technique that detects such early systolic changes and challenges the concept of pure diastolic heart failure.

ACKNOWLEDGMENT

Professor Hiroyuki Suga, Director General of the National Cardiovascular Center Research Institute, Osaka, Japan, is thanked for advice on pressure–volume loops.

STUDENT QUESTIONS

1. The Starling law relates an increased diastolic fiber length to an increased force of contraction. How is this observation explained at a cellular level?
2. What role do calcium ions play in the regulation of cardiac contractility (inotropic state)?
3. Describe in detail the complete signal systems involved in the positive inotropic effect of β-adrenergic stimulation.
4. Distinguish between preload and afterload. Describe the effects of each on LV performance.
5. Give the major factors that increase myocardial oxygen demand and provide an example of how each operates.
6. What is contractility? Indicate difficulties that arise in its measurement.

CARDIOLOGIST-IN-TRAINING QUESTIONS

1. What is myocardial wall stress? Can it explain preload and afterload? How does it influence the myocardial oxygen demand?
2. Diastolic filling of the ventricles: describe the phases and diastolic dysfunction.
3. Is it really possible to distinguish between the effects of load independently from changes in contractility? List reasons for your answer.
4. Which classes of drugs increase myocardial cyclic adenosine 3′,5′-monophosphate levels, and what are the expected effects on myocardial performance? What is the role of calcium in these responses?
5. What is a positive lusitropic effect? Give the cellular mechanism and signal systems involved when this effect is obtained by adrenergic stimulation.
6. Heart failure: describe the contractile abnormalities (both at the cellular and the organ levels) in early and advanced heart failure.

REFERENCES

1. Henderson Y. Volume changes of the heart. *Physiol Rev* 1923;2:165–208.
2. Wiggers CJ. *Modern aspects of circulation in health and disease*. Philadelphia: Lea and Febiger, 1915.
3. Laniado S, et al. Temporal relation of the first heart sound to closure of the mitral valve. *Circulation* 1973;47:1006–1014.
4. Parisi AF, et al. Relation of mitral valve closure to the first heart sound in man. Echocardiographic and phonocardiographic assessment. *Am J Cardiol* 1973;32:779–782.
5. Hirschfeld S, et al. The isovolumic contraction time of the left ventricle. An echographic study. *Circulation* 1976;54:751–756.
6. Maier SE, et al. Evaluation of left ventricular segmental wall motion in hypertrophic cardiomyopathy with myocardial tagging. *Circulation* 1992;86:1919–1928.

7. Quinones MA, et al. Influence of acute changes in preload, afterload, contractile state and heart rate on ejection and isovolumic indices of myocardial contractility in man. *Circulation* 1976;53:293–302.
8. Ohno M, Cheng CP, Little WC. Mechanism of altered patterns of left ventricular filling during the development of congestive heart failure. *Circulation* 1994;89:2241–2250.
9. Starling EH. *The Linacre lecture on the law of the heart*. London: Longmans, Green, 1918.
10. Fuchs F. Mechanical modulation of the Ca2+ regulatory protein complex in cardiac muscle. *News Physiol Sci* 1995;10:6–12.
11. Rodriguez EK, et al. A method to reconstruct myocardial sarcomere lengths and orientations at transmural sites in beating canine hearts. *Am J Physiol* 1992;263:H293–H306.
12. Backx PH, et al. Fluorescent properties of rat cardiac trabeculae microinjected with fura-2 salt. *Am J Physiol* 1993;264:H1098–H1110.
13. Holubarsch C, Ruf T, Goldstein DJ, et al. Existence of the Frank-Starling mechanism in the failing human heart. Investigations on the organ, tissue and sarcomere levels. *Circulation* 1996;94:683–689.
14. Mulieri LA, Leavitt BJ, Martin BJ, et al. Myocardial force-frequency defect in mitral regurgitation heart failure is reversed by forskolin. *Circulation* 1993;88:2700–2704.
15. Schneider J, et al. Beat-to-beat ventricular performance in atrial fibrillation: radionuclide assessment with the computerized nuclear probe. *Am J Cardiol* 1983;51:1189–1195.
16. Strang KT, et al. β-Adrenergic receptor stimulation increases unloaded shortening velocity of skinned single ventricular myocytes from rats. *Circ Res* 1994;74:542–549.
17. Schweitzer NK, et al. Determinants of loaded shortening velocity in single cardiac myocytes permeabilized with α-hemolysin. *Circ Res* 1993;73:1150–1162.
18. Kannengiesser GJ, et al. Impaired cardiac work and oxygen uptake after reperfusion of regionally ischemic myocardium. *J Mol Cell Cardiol* 1979;11:197–207.
19. Pool PE, et al. Mechanochemistry of cardiac muscle. *Circ Res* 1968;23:465–472.
20. Suga H, et al. Mechanism of higher oxygen consumption rate: pressure-loaded vs volume-loaded heart. *Am J Physiol* 1982;242:H942–H948.
21. Gibbs CL. Cardiac energetics. In: Langer GA, et al., eds. *The mammalian myocardium*. New York: Wiley, 1974:105–133.
22. Asanoi H, et al. Energetically optimal left ventricular pressure for the failing human heart. *Circulation* 1996;93:67–73.
23. Chen C, et al. Noninvasive estimation of the instantaneous first derivative of left ventricular pressure using continuous-wave Doppler echocardiography. *Circulation* 1991;83:2101–2110.
24. Little WC, et al. Comparison of measures of left ventricular contractile performance derived from pressure-volume loops in conscious dogs. *Circulation* 1989;80:1378–1387.
25. Gandhi SK, et al. The pathogenesis of acute pulmonary edema associated with hypertension. *N Engl J Med* 2001;344:17–22.
26. Schiller NB, et al. Analysis of left ventricular systolic function. *Heart* 1996;75(suppl 2):17–26.
27. Yip G, et al. Left ventricular long axis function in diastolic heart failure is reduced in both diastole and systole: time for a redefinition? *Heart* 2002;87:121–125.
28. Gorcsan J, et al. Quantitative assessment of alterations in regional left ventricular contractility with color-coded tissue Doppler echocardiography. *Circulation* 1997;95:2423–2433.
29. Vogel M, et al. Noninvasive assessment of left ventricular force-frequency relationships using tissue Doppler-derived isovolumic acceleration. *Circulation* 2003;107:1647–1652.
30. Zhang R, et al. Cardiac troponin I phosphorylation increases the rate of cardiac muscle relaxation. *Circ Res* 1995;76:1028–1035.
31. Leite-Moreira AF, et al. Afterload induced changes in myocardial relaxation: a mechanism for diastolic dysfunction. *Cardiovasc Res* 1999;43:344–353.
32. Zile MR, Brutsaert DL. New concepts in diastolic dysfunction and diastolic heart failure: part 1. *Circulation* 2002;105:1387–1393.
33. Chen C, et al. Non-invasive measurement of the time constant of left ventricular relaxation using the continuous-wave Doppler velocity profile of mitral regurgitation. *Circulation* 1992;86:272–278.
34. Nagueh SF, et al. Doppler tissue imaging: a noninvasive technique for evaluation of left ventricular relaxation and estimation of filling pressures. *J Am Coll Cardiol* 1997;30:1527–1533.
35. Yu C-M, et al. Progression of systolic abnormalities in patients with "isolated" diastolic heart failure and diastolic dysfunction. *Circulation* 2002;105:1195–1201.
36. Bell SP, et al. Alterations in the determinants of diastolic suction during pacing tachycardia. *Circ Res* 2000;87:235–240.
37. Corey CR, et al. Role of sarcoplasmic reticulum in loss of load-sensitive relaxation in pressure overload cardiac hypertrophy. *Am J Physiol* 1994;266:H68–H78.

38. Hoit BD, et al. In vivo assessment of left atrial contractile performance in normal and pathological conditions using a time-varying elastance model. *Circulation* 1994;89:1829–1838.
39. Moore TD, et al. Ventricular interaction and external constraint account for decreased stroke work during volume loading in CHF. *Am J Physiol* 2001;281:H2385–H2391.
40. Vahl CF, et al. Intracellular calcium transient of working human myocardium of seven patients transplanted for congestive heart failure. *Circ Res* 1994;74:952–958.
41. Schwinger R, et al. The failing human heart is unable to use the Frank-Starling mechanism. *Circ Res* 1994;74:959–969.
42. Carabello BA. Aortic regurgitation in women. Does the measuring stick need a change. *Circulation* 1996;94:2355–2357.
43. Yamamoto K, et al. Analysis of left ventricular diastolic function. *Heart* 1996;75(suppl 2):27–35.
44. Frank O. Zur dynamik des Herzmuskels. *Z Biol* 1895;32:370–447.
45. McDonald KS, et al. Isometric and dynamic contractile properties of porcine skinned cardiac myocytes after stunning. *Circ Res* 1995;77:964–972.
46. Suga H, et al. Regression of cardiac oxygen consumption on ventricular pressure-volume area in dog. *Am J Physiol* 1981;9:H320–H325.

13

Overload Hypertrophy and Its Molecular Biology

"The hypertrophic response of cardiomyocytes is regulated by an enormously complex network of interacting cytosolic signaling pathways."

Force (1)

"Stretch him out longer."
King Lear, Shakespeare

When an excessive workload on the heart is sustained, ventricular myocytes grow in response to a complex series of events. A mechanical event, the hemodynamic load, must be translated into the biochemical signal for growth. Hypertrophy is the process by which each cell becomes larger (Fig. 13-1) as opposed to what happens when growth is achieved by an increased number of cells (hyperplasia). When hypertrophied, the initially excessive mechanical stress on the myocardium is corrected toward normal by operation of the Laplace law, whereby increased wall thickness decreases wall stress (Chapter 16). Nonetheless, the overall properties of the hypertrophied myocardium are by no means normal, and, in particular, diastolic function is often impaired as a relatively early event. There is now increasing, although still controversial, evidence that the myocardial cells can also, to a limited extent, undergo hyperplasia when the increased mechanical load is severe and especially in the failing heart (2). In contrast, there is no doubt that nonmyocardial cells of the heart, such as those of the coronary vascular tree and interstitial space, undergo both hypertrophy and hyperplasia, even as an early response to overload. Hypertrophy also sets in motion a complex reprogramming of cardiac gene expression, with the emergence of a more fetal phenotype.

PRESSURE VERSUS VOLUME LOAD

The adjustment of cardiac mass to hemodynamic load is a fundamental characteristic of the heart. Any sustained increase in the hemodynamic function

13. OVERLOAD HYPERTROPHY AND ITS MOLECULAR BIOLOGY

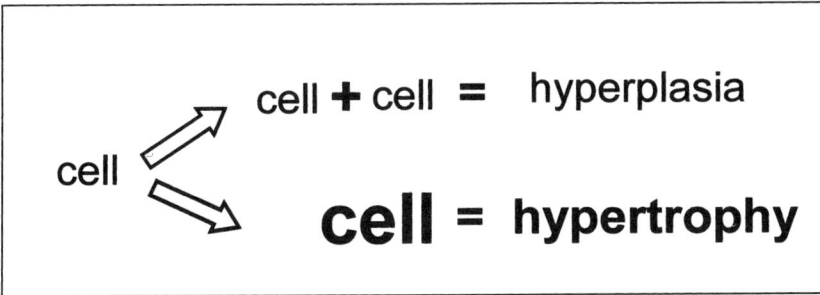

FIG. 13-1. **Cell growth.** Hypertrophy versus hyperplasia.

caused by either physiologic activity or pathologic alterations in the cardiovascular system eventually leads to changes in the heart/body weight ratio. This chapter focuses on the effects of a sustained pressure load and the differences from those of a volume load (Fig. 13-2).

A *pressure load* with increased left ventricular (LV) end-systolic pressure causes a thicker myocyte, greater mainly in volume but not in length. The mitochondria increase in number but decrease in relation to the overall cell volume, and the capillary network may be inadequate. A *volume load*, in contrast, increases end-diastolic pressure and causes the myocyte to elongate (but retains the same ratio of mitochondrial volume to the cell). Why pressure and volume

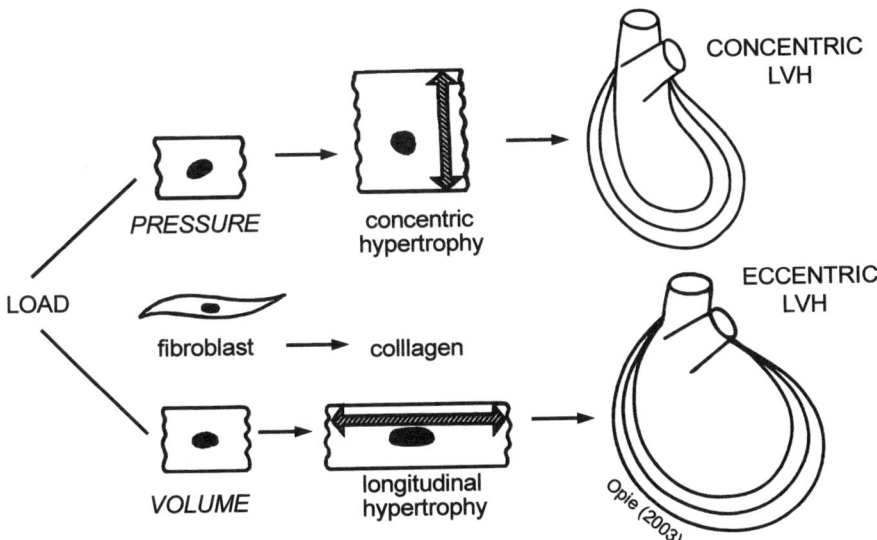

FIG. 13-2. **Pressure versus volume load.** Note cellular differences in response to pressure and volume load resulting in concentric and eccentric hypertrophy, respectively.

load should have different effects on the cell shape and contents is not fully known. Teleologically, however, during chronic pressure overload, increased cell thickness provides the greater force of contraction required to overcome the load. During a chronic volume load, longitudinal hypertrophy combines with "slippage" between myocytes to thin the walls to allow a greater cavity size, thereby increasing LV compliance despite increasing wall stress.

Meerson Three-Stage Model

Meerson (3) divided the development of pressure-induced hypertrophy into three stages of which only the first two are considered in this chapter.

Phase I: *Developing hypertrophy*, an acute period when the workload exceeds the work output that is normal for the initial mass of the heart. The pressure load initiates a series of growth signals.

Phase II: *Compensatory hypertrophy*, a period when the work-induced growth of the heart apparently compensates for the increased workload/cardiac mass ratio. Although gross mechanical function is often apparently normal, more subtle tests show a decreased rate of shortening velocity, delayed relaxation, and diminished coronary vascular reserve.

Phase III: *Heart failure*, when the work output per unit of cardiac mass decreases again due to the progressively decreasing ability of the heart to fill normally and to generate force. The transition from phase II to III is still poorly understood, as considered in Chapter 16. In contrast to the solid experimental data for this transition, the clinical evidence is still sparse even though the three-phase hypothesis had already been proposed almost one century ago by two great clinical cardiologists, Austin Flint and Sir William Osler.

MOLECULAR BASIS OF CARDIAC HYPERTROPHY

Hyperplasia is the increase in the number of cells by means of nuclear division and is the principal feature of cardiac growth during the fetal and neonatal periods. During the first 3 to 4 weeks of life, the number of cardiac myocytes in the heart doubles. As development progresses, particularly during the late gestation period, the number of dividing cells rapidly decreases. Thereafter, normal growth of the heart is accomplished solely or predominantly by the enlargement of existing myocytes, so that the diameter of myocytes increases from approximately 5 µm at birth to 12 to 17 µm in the adult heart. Interestingly, ventricular myocytes of various mammals appear to have the same diameter irrespective of animal size. The number of muscle cells thus varies directly with the size of the heart. A blue whale has about 10^5 more cells in its heart than does a rat. Cell death by apoptosis (Fig. 9-9), previously thought to be rare in the healthy heart, occurs increasingly with age and in diseased hearts. Although it remains true that most myocytes have the same life span as the entire organism, increasing,

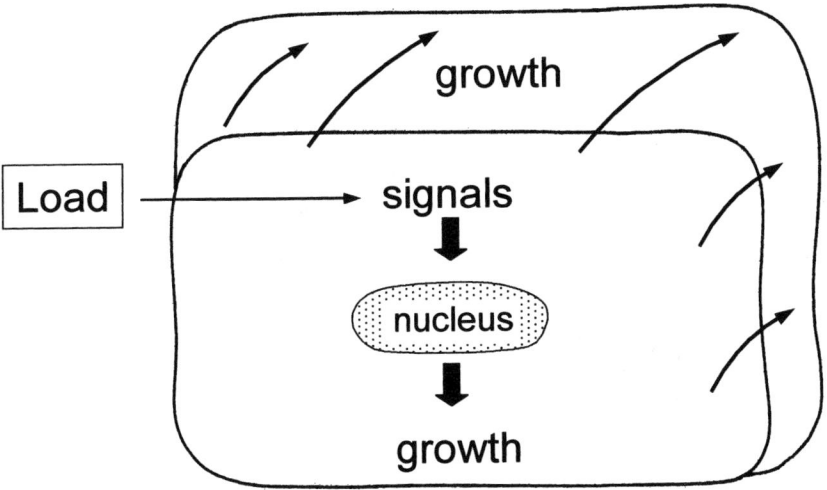

FIG. 13-3. Load leads to growth. A simplified model.

although contested, evidence shows that hyperplasia of cardiac myocytes can still occur in adult life (2).

The Road from Load to Hypertrophy

The mechanisms leading to myocardial hypertrophy and the many signals involved constitute extremely active areas of research. A simplified introduction to a complex situation is as follows (Fig. 13-3). An increased and sustained hemodynamic load is translated into a series of cell signals that cause the nucleus to initiate the formation of new proteins and cause subtle but important deformational changes in the microarchitecture. A host of signaling paths are activated, but two of special interest are the calcium–calcineurin path and the angiotensin path (Fig. 13-4).

Calcium-Calcineurin

Logically, if the heart has a greater load to overcome, then contractility should increase, and one way to achieve this is by increasing cytosolic calcium (4). The increased calcium may enter through two channels, the stretch-activated channels and L-type calcium channels (5,6). The key to this growth pathway is activation of calcineurin by calcium-calmodulin (Fig. 9-11). Most animal studies show that calcineurin is essential in the growth response to pressure overload (7,8). Persuasively, in human heart hypertrophy myocardial calcineurin activity is increased (9).

406   13. OVERLOAD HYPERTROPHY AND ITS MOLECULAR BIOLOGY

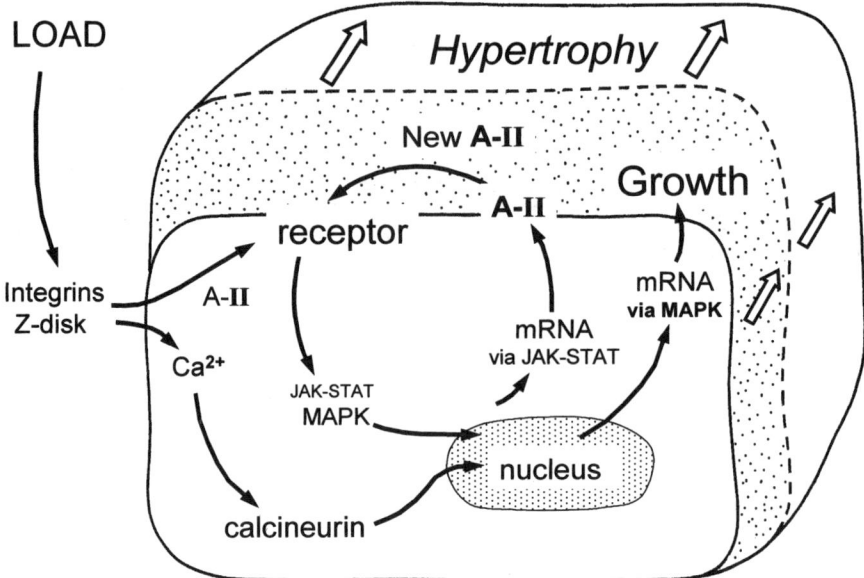

FIG. 13-4. Two major paths leading to hypertrophy. Load acts on the cytoskeleton including integrins and stretch channels (Fig. 13-6) to release preformed angiotensin II (*A-II*) that activates several pathways, including that leading to mitogen-activated protein kinase (*MAPK*) with at least three components (Fig. 9-3). A-II also cross-talks to other paths such as the nuclear factor κB path (Fig. 9-11). The Janus kinase–signal transducer and activator of transcription path (JAK-STAT) is involved in the autocrine loop whereby more A-II is made and growth is further promoted. Load also enhances cytosolic calcium, stimulating growth via calcineurin.

Angiotensin II

Mechanical strain also releases preformed angiotensin II (A-II) from the heart (7,8,10). A-II acts on its receptors to stimulate several paths, the major one being that leading to mitogen-activated protein (MAP) kinase, which contains components that promote both growth and apoptosis (Fig. 9-1). MAP kinase activates protooncogenes and nuclear stimulation of messenger RNA for various structural proteins, resulting in cell growth and hypertrophy.

Some specifics of the angiotensin response are as follows. In response to external pressure, synthesis and release of A-II are enhanced because the tissue renin–angiotensin system is up-regulated (11). Further enhancement occurs because A-II also stimulates the path leading to Janus kinase–signal transducer and activator of transcription (JAK-STAT) (Fig. 13-4), which promotes nuclear synthesis of A-II, thereby creating a self-augmenting autocrine A-II loop (12). The A-II AT_1-receptor subtype is upgraded, at least in response to stretch in neonatal myocytes (13). Clinical and experimental blockade of the AT_1 receptor is more effective than adrenergic β-blockade in regressing left ventricular hypertrophy (LVH) (14). Nevertheless, the AT_1-receptor is not essential for hypertrophy, as shown in knockout models (Chapter 9). Furthermore, in loaded cardiac myocytes, overall protein synthesis can be found even when there is blockade of A-II receptors (15). In brief, as important as A-II is in cardiac hypertrophy, it is dispensable, pointing to the existence of multiple growth-inducing pathways (Fig. 13-5). Mechanical factors acting on the cytoskeleton are crucial, whereas the anatomic site of major action of the several signaling systems varies to include not only the nucleus, but the mitochondria and the fibroblasts (Fig. 13-5).

Cytokines

Current research is helping to clarify the role of cytokine activity in hypertrophy. Graded mechanical stress releases increasing amounts of tumor necrosis factor-α (TNF-α) from the normal myocardium (16). TNF-α may be regarded as the director of the cytokine orchestra, with beneficial effects at physiologic levels and adverse proinflammatory effects at high levels of activity. TNF-α may interlink with other cytokines such as cardiotrophin-1 to promote prosurvival pathways that respond to stimulation of the gp130 receptor (Fig. 9-10) as occurs

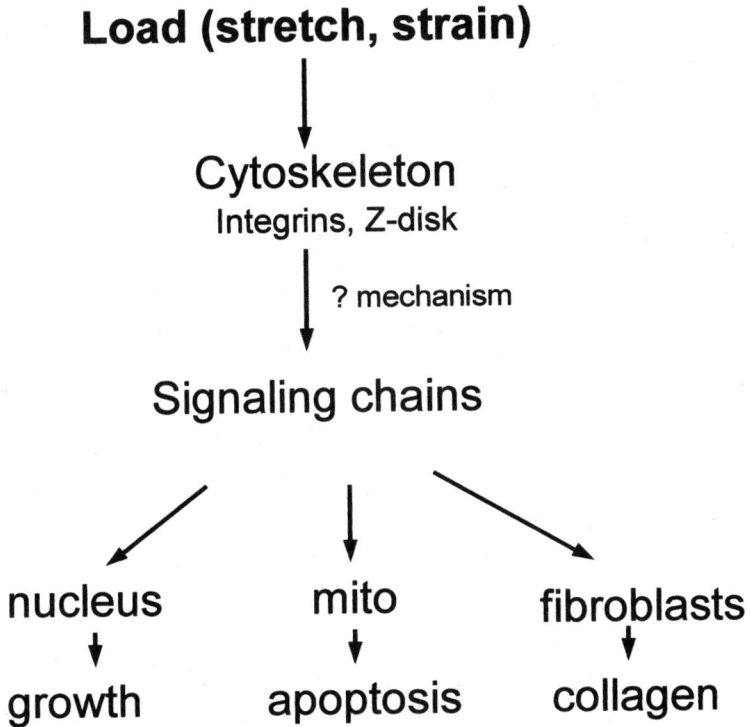

FIG. 13-5. Load transduction via signaling chains to cellular reactions. Note the crucial role of cytoskeleton (Fig. 13-7).

in a chronic volume load (17). In conformity with this concept, increased expression of myocardial TNF-α in mitral regurgitation is reversed when the volume overload is corrected by mitral valve surgery (18).

Systolic Versus Diastolic Signaling

There is no clear evidence that the different signaling paths explain different patterns of cell growth in pressure versus volume overload. Logically, pressure and volume should transmit different types of biomechanical stress and strain to the cytoskeleton. When strain is applied in systole, it activates several pathways including that leading to one component of the MAP kinase complex, extracellular signal-regulated kinase (ERK) (19). ERK activation by itself promotes fully compensated cardiac hypertrophy, with a result somewhat like the "large but good" heart of the athlete. This type of hypertrophy is accompanied by enhanced cardiac function, as shown in mice with genetic overactivity of ERK (Fig. 13-6). LV function in this model is superior to that in pressure-induced hypertrophy, perhaps because pressure also triggers proapoptotic paths (Fig. 9-1). Additionally, the systolic hypertrophic signal activates calcium-mediated pathways that involve calcineurin (Fig. 6-10).

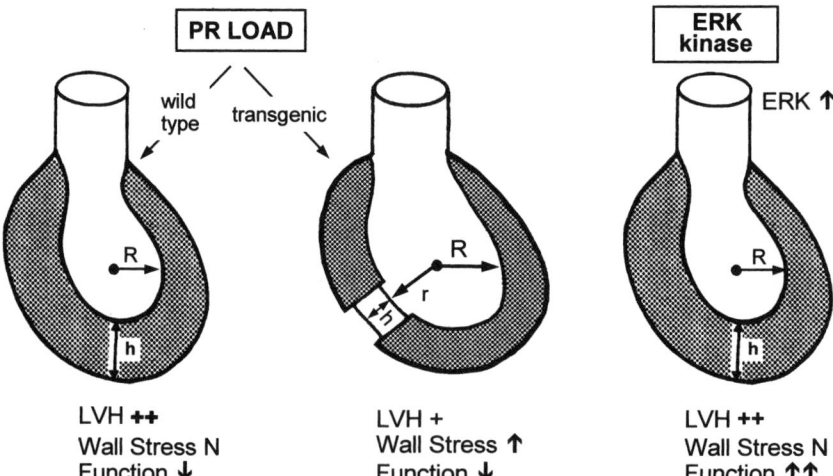

FIG. 13-6. "Compensated" hypertrophy is not necessarily compensated. **Left:** Left ventricular hypertrophy (*LVH*) in which wall stress is normalized (*N*) in response to sustained pressure load. Unexpectedly, LV mechanical function is reduced and not maintained. **Middle:** Response to pressure load in transgenic mice with inhibited G_q signaling so that the angiotensin and related receptor agonists such as endothelin are out of action. There is less LV hypertrophy, and wall stress remains increased. Nonetheless, mechanical function is less reduced than in the "compensated" heart shown on the left (23). **Right:** In a different transgenic model with increased extracellular signal–regulated kinase (Fig. 13-5), the ideal and truly compensated state is reached. Now the LVH normalizes wall stress and mechanical function is enhanced (52).

13. OVERLOAD HYPERTROPHY AND ITS MOLECULAR BIOLOGY

Note that stimulation of the MAP kinase family has mixed effects. Some components, such as ERK, have "pure" effects in growth promotion, whereas others have proapoptotic effects (Fig. 9-1). Furthermore, A-II stimulates fibrosis via transforming growth factor β (TGF-β) (20) and indirectly promotes growth via nuclear factor κB (NF-κB) (Fig. 9-11). Thus, when A-II promotes LVH, the overall effects are a mixture of potentially beneficial and harmful effects, in this sense arguing against the Meerson concept of "compensated" hypertrophy. Rather, the mixed molecular consequences could explain why LVH in humans has a poor prognosis.

LOAD EFFECTS ON SARCOLEMMA AND CYTOSKELETON

Biomechanical Strain

Biomechanical strain is an attractive but nonspecific term that covers the biologic response to a number of different mechanical forces that act on the heart cells to change the microarchitecture and cause deformation. Force, tension, and stress are fully defined in Chapter 12. *Force*, for example an increased intraventricular pressure, tends to pull the myocardium away from the resisting force of the cytoskeleton. *Tension* exists in the heart muscle as the result of two such forces pulling in different directions. *Mechanical stress* develops when tension is applied to a cross-sectional area of the ventricular wall and is defined by the Laplace law (Fig. 12-11). *Strain* is the change in cell shape produced by mechanical stress (19). *Stretch* is not the same as tension. When the external mechanical force causes elongation of the cell, it is stretched. Thus, the term stretch is more obviously applicable to a volume load than a pressure load. Experimentally, increased tension can be separated from increased stretch by varying the tension in isometric conditions. The distinction between tension and stretch could be important. Stretch may be the prime signal to cytokine expression (16) and elongation of the fibers in volume overload, whereas tension could be the signal in pressure overload.

Cytoskeletal Changes

These explain part of the response to stretch or tension. The microtubular network of the cell may be involved in linking mechanical stress on the sarcolemma to the formation of new proteins because increased density of the network follows acute mechanical overload (Fig. 13-7). Specifically, the mechanical stress signals act on integrin molecules that span the sarcolemma, transmitting forces to the cytoskeleton (Color Plate 8-11) and thereby spreading the signal throughout the cardiomyocyte to the nucleus (21). Thus, the whole cell is the "mechanosensor" (21). This pattern of signaling might best describe the effects of a pressure load. The Z disk–associated LIM protein may play a special role (Fig. 3-11).

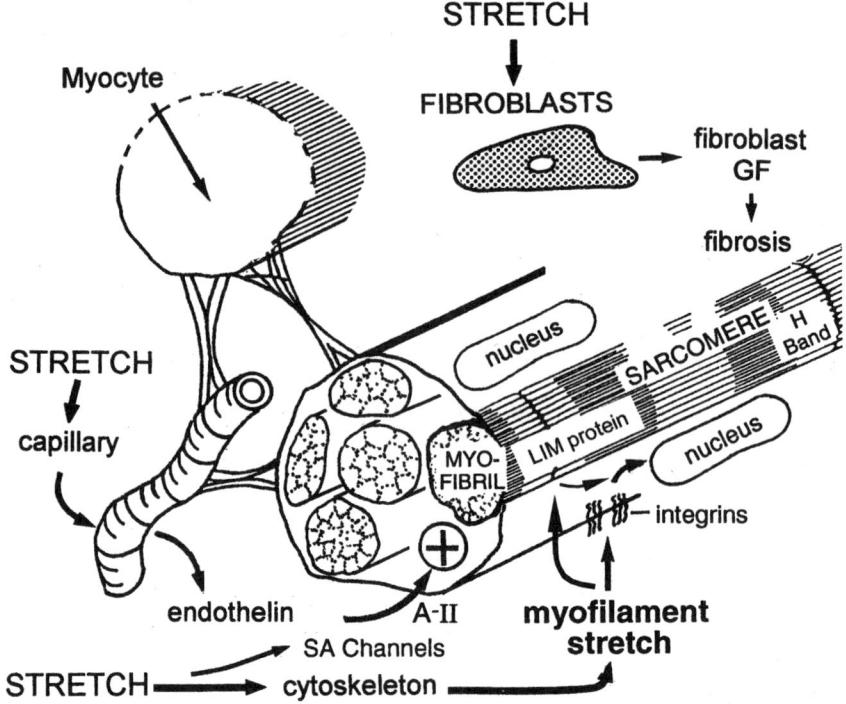

FIG. 13-7. Multiple effects of mechanical stretch signal on heart cells. Stretch acts at least three anatomic sites. First is via cytoskeleton and myofilament stretch, from where the signal is conveyed via integrins and LIM proteins in the Z disk that link mechanical stress on the sarcolemma to formation of new proteins in the nucleus. For LIM (*MLP*) protein, see Figure 3-11). Second, stretch releases endothelin, another growth factor, from the vascular endothelium. Third, stretch promotes the growth of fibroblasts and hence production of collagen. SA, stretch activated.

Stretch and Titin

Other sequences might better describe stretch effects as resulting from a chronic volume load. The putative role of the cytokine system has already been discussed. Some observations in mammals can be explained in part by the existence of *stretch-activated ion channels* (4). However, a better molecular explanation of the stretch effect is the newly described sensitivity of the Z disk to stretch (22). Sustained stretch is thought to act via titin to alter the molecular configuration of the Z disk–associated protein, the muscle LIM protein, and its associated T cap (Fig. 3-11). How these mechanical changes communicate with the growth paths is still not clear.

Strain and Nonmyocardial Cells

The extracellular A-II formed in response to deformation of myocytes both directly stimulates growth and releases other growth factors (Fig. 13-8). Thus,

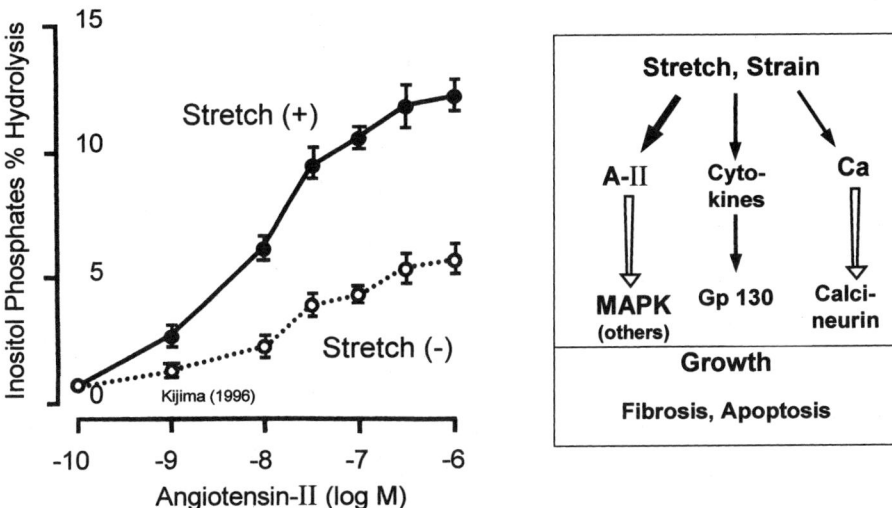

FIG. 13-8. Stretch and angiotensin II (*A-II*). **Left:** Effects of myocyte stretching on the inositol phosphate response to A-II. Cardiac myocytes were stretched for 12 hours. A-II–mediated inositol phosphate production, an index of the intracellular effects of A-II, was determined. (From Kijima K, et al. Mechanical stretch induces enhanced expression of angiotensin II receptor subtypes in neonatal rat cardiac myocytes. *Circ Res* 1996;79:887–897, with permission.) **Right:** A-II is one of several initiators of pathways that lead to growth and related effects such as fibrosis and apoptosis. For gp-130 receptor, see Figure 9-10. For calcineurin, see Figure 9-11.

endothelin, released from endothelial cells in response both to A-II and increased stretch, further promotes the activity of the protein kinase C system in vascular smooth muscle cells, already stimulated by A-II and stretch. Endothelin and A-II both release other growth factors, such as TGF-β from vascular smooth muscle cells, and fibroblast growth factor (FGF) from fibroblasts (Fig. 13-9). Myocardial TGF-β is increasingly expressed during cardiac hypertrophy (20). All these stimuli promote growth of matrix cells such as fibroblasts as well as cause myocytes to grow, beyond and in addition to the direct effects of stretch or tension on these cells. Therefore, the overall effects of mechanical deformation, both direct and indirect, help to explain the very complex yet dynamic picture of what happens in the heart in response to an increased load (Fig. 13-9).

Additional Factors in the Growth Response

Strikingly, the heart has several alternate growth factors and paths to nuclear stimulation at hand, apparently much in excess of what is essential. Such redundancy could mean that the response to an increased hemodynamic load is highly protected, so that when one path fails or is blocked, another can take over. Some of these supplementary growth factors or paths are now considered.

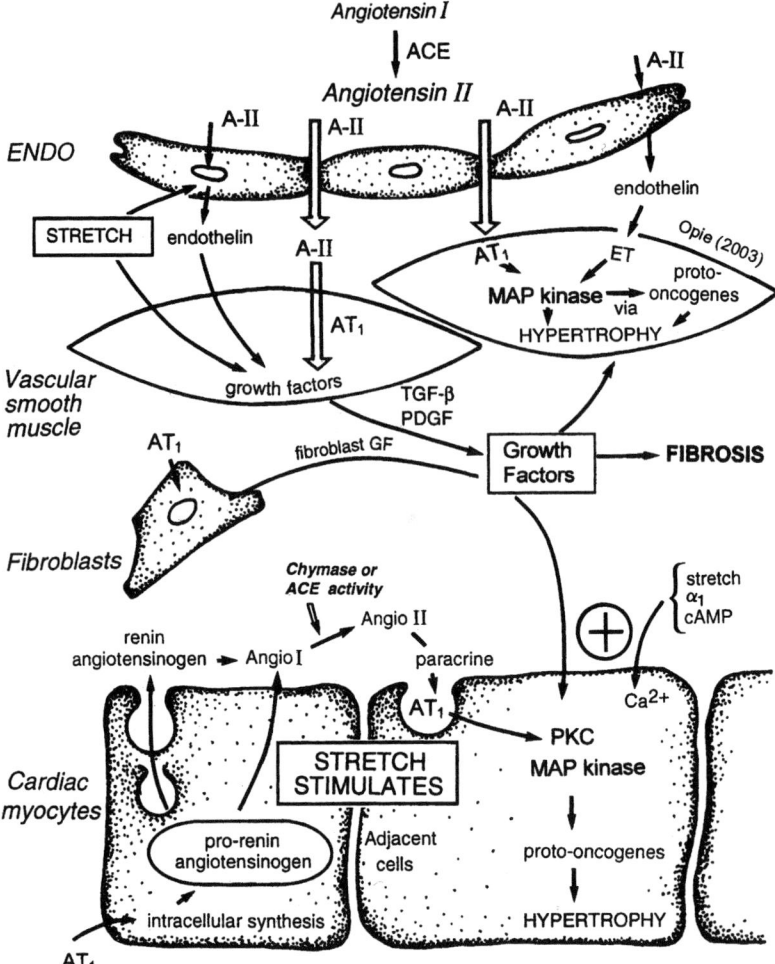

FIG. 13-9. Stretch and cardiac growth. Some proposals for a multicellular interactive renin–angiotensin system involving cardiac myocytes, fibroblasts, vascular smooth muscle, and endothelin. Stretch includes other forms of biomechanical strain. *PDGF*, platelet derived growth factor.

Endothelin

Agonists such as A-II, endothelin, and α_1-adrenergic activity that act on the G protein–coupled receptors that link to protein kinase C (PKC) via the G_q protein (Fig. 9-1), are all able to activate MAP kinase, transcription factors, and protooncogenes. The G protein G_q is an important part of this signaling chain, and its genetic ablation blocks the hypertrophic response to pressure overload (23). Of the three receptor agonists, A-II has attracted major attention for reasons already given. The other two agonists interacting with the PKC-MAP kinase system are α_1-adrenergic stimulation and endothelin. The endothelin response is complex, extending beyond the PKC-MAP kinase path. A-II, itself released by mechanical strain, releases endogenous endothelin (24), which in turn stimulates sodium–calcium exchange in the "reverse mode" to increase intracellular calcium (Fig. 6-7). Inhibition of this exchanger limits hypertrophic growth (25).

Adrenergic Stimulation

Cardiac enlargement results from chronic infusion of norepinephrine in doses that do not lead to hypertension. The mechanisms are complex and include activation of endothelin (26). Is the α_1-receptor specifically involved? Evidence from targeted overexpression of this receptor suggests no crucial role (27). Theoretically, by enhancing cell calcium, chronic β-adrenergic stimulation could indirectly promote growth by the calcium–calmodulin path (Fig. 6-10). In fact, β-adrenergic signaling is more likely to be involved in the acute fight-or-flight contractile response and in heart failure than in cardiac hypertrophy (28). Overall, adrenergic factors are less important in the hypertrophic process than A-II.

Growth Factors

When the fetal rat ventricle is transplanted into the anterior eye chamber and there is no hemodynamic workload, it is still possible, with the use of growth factors, to induce proliferation and differentiation of cells (29). The term growth factor is especially suited for those growth-promoting factors that do not link with PKC, such as insulin, insulinlike growth factor (IGF-I), TGF-β, platelet-derived growth factor, epidermal growth factor, and FGF. Such growth factors interact with membrane-associated growth factor receptors, similar to the insulin model, to stimulate intracellular transducers, such as kinases, which in turn phosphorylate a variety of intracellular proteins, thereby activating protooncogenes and various transcription factors.

Insulin and IGF-I interact with the insulin receptor (Fig. 9-5) to initiate a series of events linking via phosphatidylinositol 3-phosphate kinase and protein kinase B (Akt) to the mammalian target of rapamycin and from there to nuclear transcription and LVH (30). In human insulin resistance, there are high blood levels of insulin, which may help to explain why LVH develops even in some normotensive patients with diabetes. Some of the other growth factors such as TGF-β (31) and EGF (32) become active in response to A-II. Thus, in addition to promoting hypertrophy in its own right, A-II can recruit other growth factors that are directed away from myocytes and toward nonmyocyte cells such as fibroblasts and extracellular enzymes such as the metalloproteinases.

Growth hormone, secreted by the pituitary gland, promotes myocyte growth without fibrosis (33). The intracellular signaling paths are not established but presumably are similar to those of insulin. Growth hormone means something quite different from the term growth factors, despite the probable overlap in the intracellular signal systems. Clinically, the disease acromegaly is accompanied by cardiomegaly and LV dysfunction. Growth hormone does not play a role in stretch-induced hypertrophy.

Shared Signal Systems

At first sight, it would seem that there should be a clear separation between those agonists, such as A-II that link to PKC and MAP kinase via G_q and those linked to cytokine and growth receptors. Yet, starting from very different agonists, such as A-II and cytokines and their equally different receptors, there appear to be shared and interlinked signal systems (34), so that cross-talk between paths may be involved. For example, A-II links not only to MAP kinase but to NF-κB, hence acting on the same path that responds to calcineurin (Fig. 9-11). The cytokine gp130 receptor links to JAK-STAT, as shown in Figure 9-10, and to two more: ras-Raf-MAP kinase (35) and the phosphatidylinositol 3 kinase–Akt pathway that is part of the insulin response (Fig. 13-5) (36). Another proposal is that the stretch channel is linked to PKC and MAP kinase eventually to stimulate the production of protooncogenes and transcription factors.

Evaluation of Hypotheses

Although all these hypotheses represent reasonable interpretations of an impressive volume of experimental data, none of them fully explains all aspects of cardiac growth. The fact that the heart is able to translate the signals generated by hemodynamic activity into growth and that stretch appears to involve an ion channel puts the emphasis on mechanoreceptors. An attractive hypothesis is that stretch and tension induce the formation and secretion of A-II, which increases its own production. Of its many actions, A-II activates the paths leading to MAP kinase and, in addition, evokes the formation and release of other growth-promoting factors including endothelin and TGF-β. Other pathways appear to be independent of A-II such as the cytokine–JAK-STAT path and the calcium–calcineurin–NFAT path, but in reality cross-talk connects these signal systems. The apparent multiplicity, overlap, and redundancy of the growth-promoting signals and paths reflects Nature's need to ensure that heart cells can undertake one of their most basic functions, which is to grow when required. It is humiliating to think that after years of research, we are not yet certain why heart cells "thicken" in response to a pressure load but elongate and "thin" in response to a volume load.

ALTERED GENE EXPRESSION IN HYPERTROPHY

Immediate-Early Genes (Protooncogenes)

The cell hypertrophy of adult hearts and fetal cell division may have at least some features in common. Included in the early response to a hemodynamic load

TABLE 13-1. *Sequence of changes in growth controlling signals, protooncogenes, and genes in response to sustained pressure overload*

Time after onset of load	Response
30 min	Immediate early protooncogenes are induced (*c-fos, c-jun, C-myc, egr-1, HSP 70*)
6–12 hr	Induction of genes normally only expressed in fetus; contractile genes include β-myosin heavy chain, skeletal α-actin, β-tropomyosin; noncontractile genes include atrial and brain natriuretic peptides
12–24 hr	Up-regulation of constitutively expressed genes, such as myosin light chain 2, cardiac α-actin
>24 hr	General increase in protein and RNA content; increase in cell size but not number

Adapted from Glennon PE, Sugden PH, Poole-Wilson PA. Cellular mechanisms of cardiac hypertrophy. *Br Heart J* 1995;73:496–499.

are increases in the immediate-early genes, also called early response genes or protooncogenes, such as *c-fos*, *c-myc*, and *c-jun*, and the heat shock protein gene hsp 70. For example, in a transgenic model that overexpresses c-Myc, all the characteristic changes of cardiac hypertrophy are reproduced (37). During vascular collagen remodeling, A-II stimulates ERK, which phosphorylates transcription factors that induce the c-fos protooncogene to form a transcription complex, AP-1 (38). The protooncogene model explains early transitory changes in genes after cardiac overload (Table 13-1).

Growth Inhibition

This is not the same as apoptosis. Should myocytes "know" when to stop or to slow down the hypertrophic process? Clearly, this will inevitably happen when the signal to hypertrophy passes as when pressure overload stops or when there is blockade of the A-II receptors. A new proposal is that some early response genes, such as the calcineurin inhibitory protein and the suppressor of cytokine signaling, may negatively regulate hypertrophy (39). Additionally, glycogen synthase kinase, an unexpected inhibitor of hypertrophy at the level of transcription, may become active (40).

Isoenzymes: Isoforms of Contractile Proteins

Isoforms induced by the hypertrophic process have the same general function but with a slightly different molecular structure. This adaptation results from a shift of the type of myosin (isomyosin) from the α myosin heavy chain (α MHC or V_1) to the slow myosin isoform (β MHC or V_3). For example, the rate of shortening of the myofibril decreases through isoform replacement, which theoretically allows the heart to produce tension at a lower cost by reaching the required

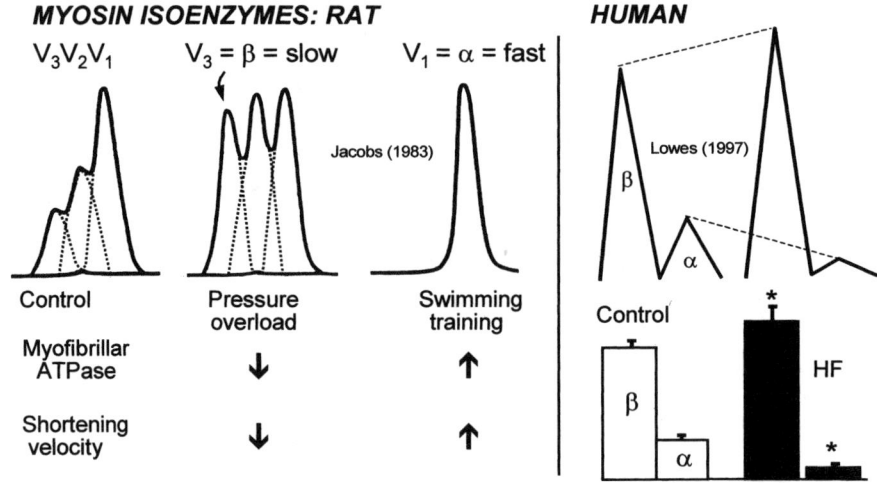

FIG. 13-10. **Pressure overload versus dynamic exercise; human heart failure. Left:** Contrasting effects of pressure overload and swimming training on myosin isoenzyme patterns of rat heart. Pressure overload increases slow type myosin V_3 (β). (Adapted from Jacob et al. *Adv Myocardiol* 1983;4:70.) **Right:** Percentage of expression of α versus β myosin heavy chain (*MHC*) in nonfailing heart and failing human heart (*HF*) in idiopathic dilated cardiomyopathy. Decreased α MHC could explain slower velocity of shortening, as in the rat heart. (Adapted from Lowes et al. *J Clin Invest* 1997;100:2315–2324.)

tension more slowly (Fig. 13-10). The cost of this benefit is decreased contractility and impaired maximal power production (41).

Fetal Phenotype during Hypertrophy

Chronic hemodynamic load results in quantitative changes in gene expression, so that there is the expression of a more fetal phenotype (Table 13-2). The fetal

TABLE 13-2. *Myocardial phenotype in adult, fetal, and hypertrophic failing rat hearts*

Phenotype	Adult	Fetal	Hypertrophy and failure
Cardiac α-actin	+++	+	+
Skeletal α-actin	+	+++	+++
Smooth muscle α-actin	+	+++	+++
α-Myosin heavy chain	+	+++	+
β-Myosin heavy chain	+	+++	+++
SERCA	+++	+	+
ANP, BNP	+	+++	+++
Fatty acid oxidation enzymes	+++	+	+
Glucose transporters	+	++	++

SERCA, sarco(endo)plasmic reticulum calcium–ATPase; ANP, atrial natriuretic peptide; BNP, brain natriuretic peptide. Also see Table 8-3 and Figure 16-22.

phenotype includes isoform changes (previous section), induction of growth factors such as TGF-β, early-response genes such as c-fos, increased β MHC, ventricular production of natriuretic peptides (atrial and brain) and of skeletal α-actin (7). These changes seem to occur especially in the failing heart, and, hypothetically, these changes could help the circulation to adapt to heart failure, for example, by increased sodium excretion as induced by atrial and brain natriuretic peptides (Fig. 16-24). Metabolic enzymes change so that fatty acid oxidation is down-regulated (42) and energy-sparing glycolysis is up-regulated. This mechanism of this *substrate switch* may be decreased expression of PPAR-α (43). As is discussed in Chapter 16, when this peroxisome proliferator–activated receptor is acutely reactivated by a specific agonist, then a reverse substrate switch occurs and the overloaded heart fails (Fig. 16-14). Thus, "increased glucose oxidation is essential for cardiac function in the face of pressure overload" (44). This concept has not been established for the human heart.

Isoforms in the Failing Human Heart

Atrial natriuretic peptide expression is up-regulated, but many of the other "fetal" changes result from down-regulation of the adult gene transcripts rather than up-regulation of fetal genes (45). MHC isoforms change, with either a relative decrease in α MHC and relative increase in β MHC (45) or down-regulation of α MHC with modest up-regulation of β MHC (Fig. 13-10). Regarding energy metabolism, the substrate switch from reliance on fatty acid to glucose dominance found in small animals cannot be directly be extrapolated to the human heart (45). Rather, in the failing human heart, key regulators of both glucose and fatty acid metabolism are reduced, which argues for a different concept, that of "energy starvation" (Fig. 16-7).

Changes in Action Potential and Ionic Currents

A constant finding during chronic mechanical pressure overload is the increase in the *action potential duration* (Fig. 13-11). This lengthening is not related directly to changes in the L-type calcium current, to the number of channels, or dihydropyridine receptors. Rather, decreased outward currents are largely responsible (46), such as an impaired outward repolarizing current, I_{to}, and an inward rectifier potassium current, I_{K1}.

Estrogens and Ryanodine Receptor

When the cardiac ryanodine receptor is damaged, there is a constant leak from the sarcoplasmic reticulum of calcium ions that promote hypertrophy, probably acting via the growth signal calcineurin. This process occurs in male, not female, mice, and estrogens may be cardioprotective by inhibiting hypertrophy (37).

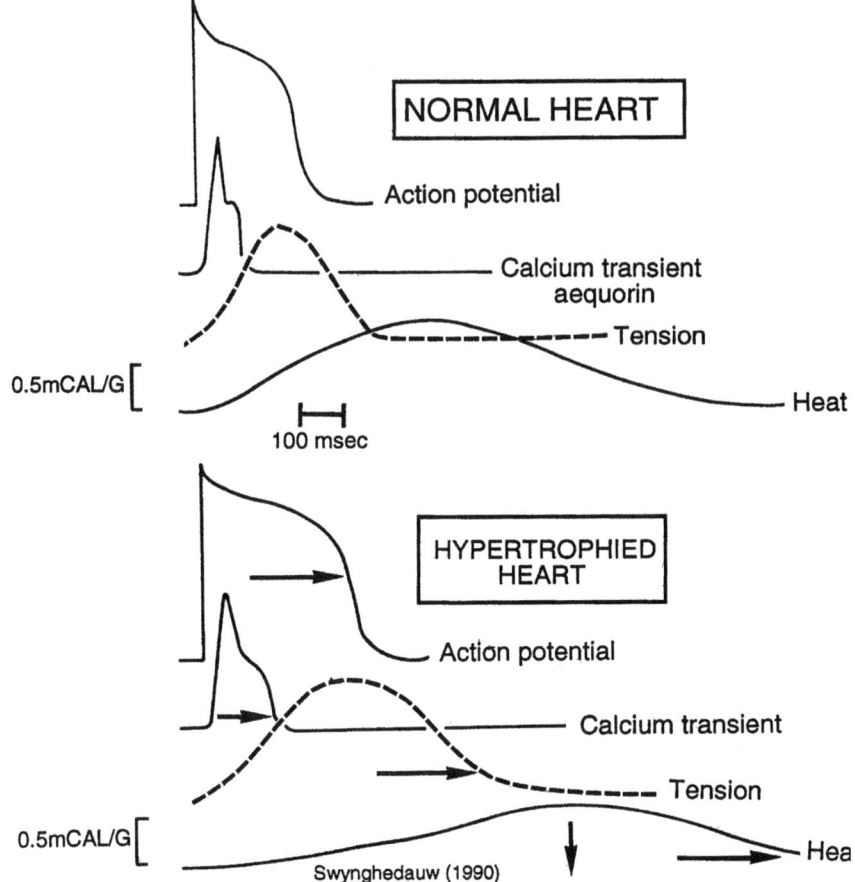

FIG. 13-11. Properties of hypertrophied heart. Excitation–contraction coupling and heat production in the hypertrophied heart compared with the normal heart. The lengthening of the action potential in the hypertrophied myocardium is not owing to any increase in the density of the inward calcium channels. Hypothetically, it is proposed that the hypertrophied heart works more economically (53), which can be seen from the reduced rate of heat production (53a).

ULTRASTRUCTURAL CHANGES IN HYPERTROPHIC HEART

When the myocardium undergoes hypertrophy, the myocytes increase considerably in size. Capillaries and interstitial cells, the latter containing collagen, increase to a lesser extent, by the process of hyperplasia. The myocyte increases basically by an increase in cell diameter and a much smaller increase in cell length, at least in response to pressure overload (Fig. 13-12). Several changes in the hypertrophic cell suggest a lower rate of calcium release and uptake (decreased β-receptor density, decreased sodium exchange, decreased density of the SERCA [sarco(endo)plasmic reticulum calcium–ATPase] pump and defects

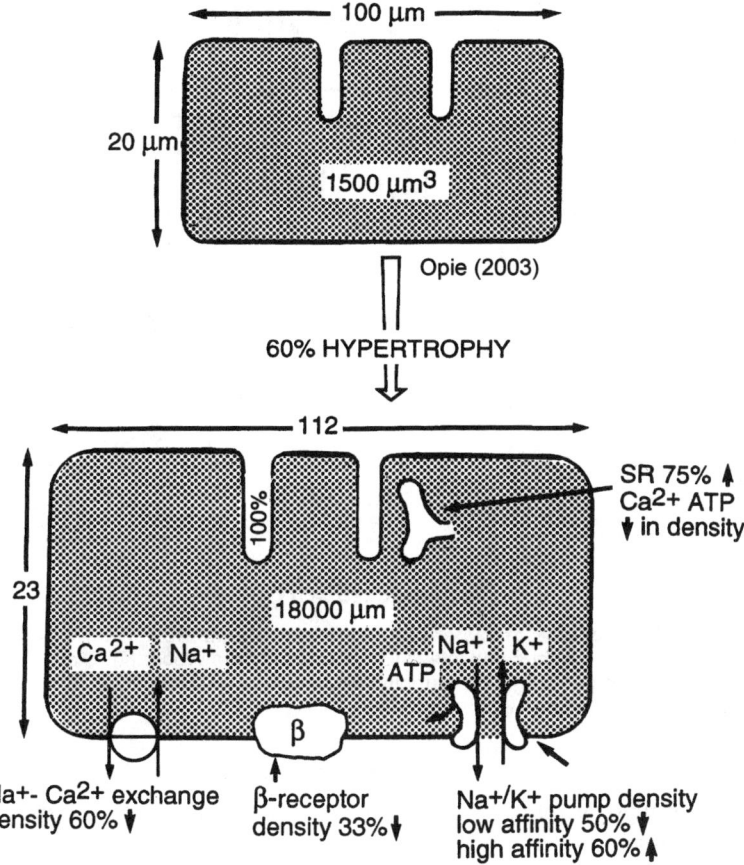

FIG. 13-12. Hypertrophic rat heart cell compared with normal. The data shown are for a 60% increase in cell volume. Note the decreased β-receptor density, decreased activity of sodium–calcium exchange, decreased sarcoplasmic reticulum (SR) calcium-ATPase activity, and increased density of the high-affinity sodium–potassium pump. For further details, see Swynghedauw (54).

in the ryanodine receptor. These changes add to the abnormalities of contraction associated with the decreased myosin ATPase activity.

Collagen and Interstitial Fibrosis

The myocardium is composed of cardiac myocytes and extracellular matrix, the latter being a three-dimensional collagen network (Fig. 3-13). Collagen turnover is controlled by metalloproteinases and the tissue inhibitors of metalloproteinases. An accumulation of collagen in the myocardium is termed fibrosis. Collagen exists in several genetically distinct types, of which types I and III are

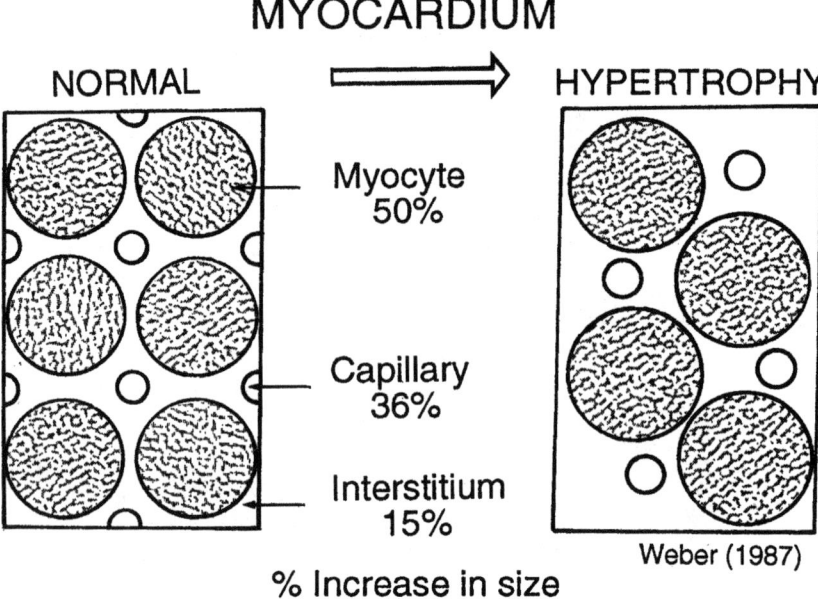

FIG. 13-13. Ultrastructure of hypertrophied myocardium. Note the increase in size of myocytes relative to capillaries and interstitium. (Adapted from Weber KT, Clark WA, Janicki, et al. Physiologic versus pathologic hypertrophy and the pressure-overloaded myocardium. *J Cardiovasc Pharmacol* 1987;10(suppl 6):S37–S49.)

found in the myocardium, type I being dominant and having a tensile strength greater than that of steel. The causes of the collagen increase during LV pressure overload are complex and in part relate to the blood supply. As the myocyte increases in cell diameter, the capillary surface area remains relatively unchanged, increasing by only a small amount (Fig. 13-13). Therefore, the distance between capillaries increases and the ratio of the capillary surface area to the total cell volume decreases. Furthermore, the coronary vascular reserve is impaired in the hypertrophic heart (Chapter 10). For these reasons, the blood supply to the thickened ventricle is potentially compromised, which is likely to increase fibrosis (47). Fibrosis is promoted by a variety of growth-promoting signals acting on the fibroblasts, including pressure and stretch, A-II (48), and its stimulation of TGF-β_1 (47), FGF, and aldosterone (49).

Vascular Remodeling

Just as the ventricles remodel and hypertrophy in response to a sustained pressure load, so do the arterial blood vessels in response to sustained blood pressure increases (for hypertension, see Chapter 14). Similar questions are posed: how much is caused by pressure (or stretch) and how much results from renin–

angiotensin activation? What role do the other growth factors play? What are the signal systems? In the aorta, an increased transmural pressure stimulates the local renin–angiotensin system, with net production of A-II (11). The angiotensin I (AT_1) receptors of the arterial tissue respond to both stretch and A-II. The fibrogenic effects of A-II appear to be mediated by two separate paths, the one leading via the ERK component of MAP kinase to activation of transcription factors and the other involving TGF-β (38). Both increased pressure and A-II act synergistically to induce the expression of *fibronectin*, one of the components of the extracellular matrix of the aorta (11). Complex remodeling takes place in response to hypertension, involving stretch, A-II and endothelin, and other factors all acting on vascular smooth muscle cells as well as on numerous extracellular matrix proteins (50). The peripheral arterioles stiffen, further increasing blood pressure.

CLINICAL APPLICATION: REGRESSION OF LEFT VENTRICULAR HYPERTROPHY

To review, the transduction of biomechanical stress and strain into growth signals travels along several or even many paths leading to enhanced transcription factors, resulting in overall growth of the contractile units. In this way, the myocardium becomes thicker in response to a pressure load, and wall stress or tension decreases, so that the oxygen demand per unit mass of the heart decreases despite the myocardium having to do the extra work of overcoming the increased afterload by the Laplace law (Fig. 12-11). There are also major changes in gene expression, so that the myocardium reverts to a more fetal phenotype. Glucose oxidation is protective to the hypertrophic myocardium, at least in rodents. Furthermore, myocyte growth is not a solitary event, and the complex signaling systems involved also result in a variety of potentially adverse companions such as fibrosis and possibly apoptosis. Overall, LVH is adverse, and if left untreated leads to deterioration of the structure and function of the heart as found in aortic stenosis in humans (47).

Not surprisingly, LVH is now recognized as an independent risk factor for cardiovascular disease, a logical proposition bearing in mind that LVH is a step on the way to heart failure. Thus, it makes sense to remedy those factors predisposing to pressure overload, such as hypertension or aortic stenosis, and those that cause volume overload, such as mitral or aortic valve regurgitation (Fig. 16-6).

Inhibition of Angiotensin II and Left Ventricular Hypertrophy

An additional question is whether there is any pharmacologic means of achieving regression of LVH after it exists. The basic data reviewed in this chapter show that A-II is crucial in the growth-promoting pathways, providing apparent logic for the clinical use of angiotensin-converting enzyme inhibitors or angiotensin receptor blockers to regress LVH. Do these agents act like any other antihypertensive agents to decrease stretch and thereby to reduce growth or do they have a unique role? If mechanical strain is the fundamental signal that in the first instance induces the up-regulation of tissue renin-angiotensin and the release of A-II, then any other antihypertensive agent (including a diuretic) that decreases blood pressure to relieve strain in the LV wall should also regress LVH, as is the case. However, inhibition of the renin–angiotensin system by the AT_1 blocker losartan is more effective in regressing human LVH than is β-blockade, even when the degree of blood pressure reduction is the same (14). This study (Losartan Intervention for Endpoint Reduction) argues for a specific role of the AT_1 receptor in the genesis of human LVH (Fig. 13-14). Other clinical studies, less extensive in nature, suggest an important role for calcium signaling and hence the significance of calcineurin.

The regression of fibrosis during the treatment of LVH is also desirable. That this can happen in patients is shown by serial measurements of a serum peptide derived from procollagen (48). LV chamber stiffness, the result of fibrosis, improves with A-II receptor blockade (51).

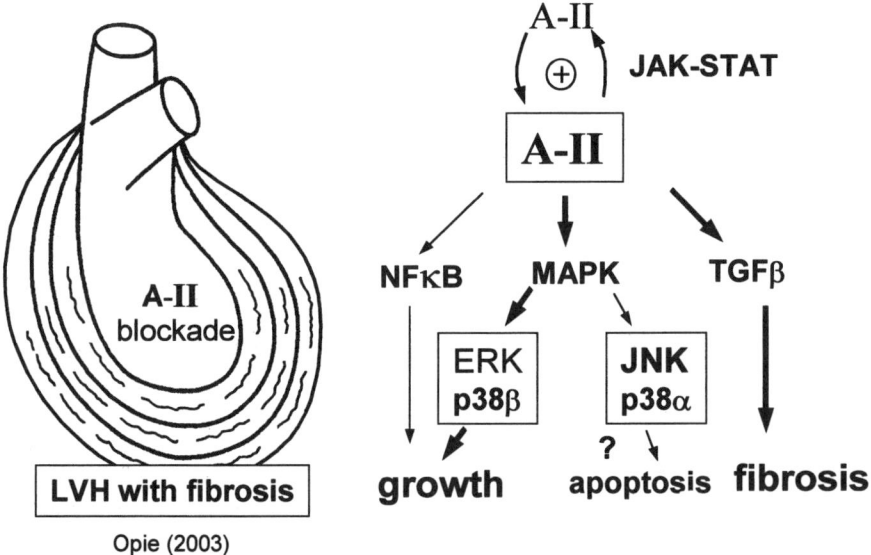

Opie (2003)

FIG. 13-14. Left ventricular hypertrophy with fibrosis in the human heart. **Left:** Proposed role of angiotensin II (A-II) blockade in achieving regression in Losartan Intervention for Endpoint Reduction study [see Kjeldsen et al. (56)]. **Right:** Proposed signaling paths resulting from increased activity of angiotensin II. Note autocrine loop via Janus kinase–signal transducer and activator of transcription that enhances formation of A-II. Major effects of A-II are probably by mitogen-activated protein kinase, with two of its components prosurvival and growth promoting (extracellular signal-regulated kinase and p38β) and two proapoptotic (c-Jun aminoterminal kinase and p38α). Growth may also be promoted via nuclear factor κB. Fibrosis is caused by transforming growth factor β, a cytokine increased by A-II. The overall effects of A-II would be left ventricular hypertrophy with several adverse aspects, as supported by transgenic studies in Figure 13-6.

It should not be forgotten that in hypertension the first essential is to reduce arterial pressure and that agents other than those inhibiting the renin–angiotensin system, such as the calcium channel blockers and diuretics, also achieve regression of LVH.

SUMMARY

1. *Biomechanical strain.* A pressure load must be distinguished from a volume load, the former leading to concentric and the latter to eccentric hypertrophy. The reason for these differences is not well understood, nor is it clear how biomechanical forces acting on the myocyte result in growth signals. Early distortions in the microarchitecture of extracellular matrix in response to mechanical forces activate signal systems that stimulate nuclear transcription so that synthesis of new messenger RNA takes place.
2. *Mechanosensors translate the mechanical signal,* such as a prolonged pressure overload, into growth signals. Stretch receptors are a specific subtype of mechanosensors that translate stretch signals into growth signals. The Z disk and its LIM protein are such sensors. In addition, calcium ions probably also enter the cells to stimulate calcineurin.
3. *Wall stress normalization.* The concept that LVH can normalize LV wall stress with benefit is challenged by genetic studies in mice.
4. *A-II is released from myocytes in response to biomechanical strain.* A-II is the most important of several G_q-protein linked receptor agonists that activate PKC and the associated growth cascade that leads to MAP kinases that phosphorylate transcription factors. A-II also acts in an autocrine manner to promote its own synthesis and cell growth. A-II releases other growth factors such as endothelin and TGF-β, the latter promoting growth of fibrous tissue.
5. *Stimulation of the MAP kinase family has mixed effects;* some components, such as ERK, have specific effects on growth promotion, whereas others have proapoptotic effects. Thus, when A-II promotes LVH, the overall effects (including fibrosis promoted by TGF-β) are mixed, explaining why LVH in humans has an adverse prognosis.
6. *Growth factors,* such as insulin, IGF-I, and others, link to a receptor group that includes the insulin receptor.
7. *MAP kinase and beyond.* MAP kinase is an important group of three or more enzymes, on which most but not all the growth-promoting pathways converge. MAP kinase phosphorylates transcription factors to activate protooncogenes to form transcriptional complexes. Protooncogenes are also called early-immediate genes.
8. *Fetal phenotype.* Especially in the failing hypertrophied heart, there is expression of the fetal phenotype with, for example, the capacity of the ventricles to manufacture atrial natriuretic peptide and brain natriuretic peptide. There is a protective substrate switch from reliance on fatty acid to glucose.

There are changes in the MHC isoforms that would help to explain decreased mechanical performance of the failing heart. Whether similar changes occur in human LVH is not known.

9. *Ionic changes.* The action potential duration is prolonged, possibly the result of inhibition of the repolarizing current I_{to}. T-type calcium channels are expressed in the hypertrophic ventricular myocardium, in which calcium transients have a low peak value with delayed recovery.
10. *Nonmyocytic cells.* In contrast to myocytes, the basic response of which is to undergo hypertrophy in response to a load, there is an early increase in the number of capillary cells and those of extracellular matrix. The increased collagen, formed in response to A-II, TGF-β, and other growth factors, induces the formation of collagen to cause fibrosis. This limits systolic and diastolic function.
11. *Vascular remodeling.* In response to increased intraluminal pressure, as in hypertension, there is a complex remodeling process mediated both by pressure and A-II. Thus, the peripheral arterioles stiffen and increase blood pressure further.
12. *Regression of LVH.* Mechanical strain such as pressure overload plays a key role in the cause of LVH. Hence, reduction of this load, for example, by blood pressure reduction, is essential to achieve regression of LVH. Angiotensin-receptor blockade is more effective than a beta-blocker in achieving regression, supporting experimental evidence that the renin–angiotensin system and A-II play a key role in the development and treatment of LVH in humans.

ACKNOWLEDGMENT

The constructive criticism of Dr. Clive Rosendorff, New York, is gratefully acknowledged.

STUDENT QUESTIONS

1. What are the three phases of pressure-induced hypertrophy that Meerson described? Does this progression fit with current concepts?
2. What is biomechanical strain? How may it influence cardiomyocyte growth?
3. Describe the major signal system linking A-II and occupancy of its receptor to stimulation of nuclear protooncogenes.
4. What other effects of A-II can lead to cardiac hypertrophy?
5. Why is insulin described as a growth factor? Describe how the signal systems that respond to insulin stimulation, leading from the receptor to nuclear transcription.

CARDIOLOGIST-IN-TRAINING QUESTIONS

1. What are the differences between hypertrophy and hyperplasia? When and why can cardiac myocytes undergo hyperplasia?

2. What are the differences in the growth response between pressure and volume overload?
3. Do you think that A-II has a specific role in the response to stretch? If so, is it mandatory to use angiotensin-converting enzyme inhibitors or angiotensin receptor blockers in the therapeutic management of LVH?
4. LVH in response to increased intraventricular pressure is compensatory because it returns the increased wall stress to normal according to the Laplace law. What are the problems with this concept?
5. Myocardial fibrosis is hypothesized as being a potentially irreversible step in the development of LVH. What are the major growth signals involved in the production of fibrosis, and how may these steps be interrupted by therapeutically active agents?

REFERENCES

1. Force T, et al. Apoptosis signal-regulating kinase/nuclear factor-κB. A novel signaling pathway regulates cardiomyocyte hypertrophy. *Circulation* 2002;105:402–404.
2. Anversa P, et al. Myocyte growth and cardiac repair. *J Mol Cell Cardiol* 2002;14:91–105.
3. Meerson FZ. The failing heart. In: Katz AM, ed. *Adaptation and deadaptation*. New York: Raven Press, 1983.
4. Sussman MA, et al. Dance band on the *Titanic*. Biomechanical signaling in cardiac hypertrophy. *Circ Res* 2002;91:888–898.
5. Crozatier B. Stretch-induced modifications of myocardial performance: from ventricular function to cellular and molecular mechanisms. *Cardiovasc Res* 1996;32:25–37.
6. Ruwhof C, et al. Mechanical stress stimulates phospholipase C activity and intracellular calcium ion levels in neonatal rat cardiomyocytes. *Cell Calcium* 2001;29:73–83.
7. Shimoyama M, et al. Calcineurin plays a critical role in pressure overload-induced cardiac hypertrophy. *Circulation* 1999;100:2449–2454.
8. Dorn II GW. Calcineurin inhibition in hypertrophy. Back from the dead. *Circulation* 2001;104:9–11.
9. Ritter O, et al. Calcineurin in human heart hypertrophy. *Circulation* 2002;105:265–2269.
10. Modesti PA, et al. Release of preformed Ang II from myocytes mediates angiotensingen and ET-1 gene overexpression *in vivo* via AT1 receptor. *J Mol Cell Cardiol* 2002;34:1491–1500.
11. Bardy N, et al. Pressure and angiotensin II synergistically induce aortic fibronectin expression in organ culture model of rabbit aorta. Evidence for a pressure-induced tissue renin-angiotensin system. *Circ Res* 1996;79:70–78.
12. Mascareno E, et al. Signal transduction and activator of transcription (STAT) protein-dependent activation of angiotensin promoter: a cellular signal for hypertrophy in cardiac muscle. *Proc Natl Acad Sci U S A* 1998;95:5590–5594.
13. Kijima K, et al. Mechanical stretch induces enhanced expression of angiotensin II receptor subtypes in neonatal rat cardiac myocytes. *Circ Res* 1996;79:887–897.
14. Dahlöf B. LIFE substudy: echo data show more LVH regression with losartan versus atenolol. http/www.theheart.org 2002.
15. Kent RL, et al. Passive load and angiotensin II evoke differential responses of gene expression and protein synthesis in cardiac myocytes. *Circ Res* 1996;78:829–838.
16. Wachtell K, et al. Change in diastolic left ventricular filling after one year of antihypertensive treatment. The Losartan Intervention for Endpoint Reduction in Hypertension (LIFE) Study. *Circulation* 2002;105:1071–1076.
17. Wollert KC, et al. Cardiotrophin-I activates a distinct form of cardiac muscle cell hypertrophy. Assembly of sarcomeric units in series via gp130/leukemia inhibitory factor receptor-dependent pathways. *J Biol Chem* 1996;271:9535–9545.
18. Oral H, et al. Myocardial proinflammatory cytokine expression and left ventricular remodeling in patients with chronic mitral regurgitation. *Circulation* 2003;107:831–837.
19. Sugden PH. Mechanotransduction in cardiomyocyte hypertrophy. *Circulation* 2001;13:1375–1377.

20. Kuwahara K, et al. Transforming cell growth factor-β function blocking prevents myocardial fibrosis and diastolic dysfunction in pressure-overloaded rats. *Circulation* 2002;106:130–135.
21. Ingber DE. Mechanical signaling and the cellular response to extracellular matrix in angiogenesis and cardiovascular physiology. *Circ Res* 2002;91:877–887.
22. Knoll R, et al. The cardiac mechanical stretch sensor machinery involves a Z disc complex that is defective in a subset of human dilated cardiomyopathy. *Cell* 2002;111:943–955.
23. Esposito G, et al. Genetic alterations that inhibit in vivo pressure-overload hypertrophy prevent cardiac dysfunction despite increased wall stress. *Circulation* 2002;105:85–92.
24. Aiello EA, et al. Autocrine stimulation of cardiac Na^+-Ca^{2+} exchanger currents by endogenous endothelin released by angiotensin II. *Circ Res* 2002;90:374–376.
25. Cingolani HE, et al. Na^+-H^+ exchanger inhibition. A new antihypertrophic tool. *Circ Res* 2002;90: 751–753.
26. Moser L, et al. Predominant activation of endothelin dependent cardiac hypertrophy by norepinephrine in rat left ventricle. *Am J Physiol* 2002;282:1389–1394.
27. Lin F, et al. Targeted α_{1A}-adrenergic receptor overexpression induces enhanced cardiac contractility but not hypertrophy. *Circ Res* 2001;89:343–350.
28. Du X-J. Sympathoadrenergic mechanisms in functional regulation and development of cardiac hypertrophy and failure: findings from genetically engineered mice. *Cardiovasc Res* 2001;50:443–453.
29. Bishop SP, et al. Morphological development of the rat heart growing *in oculo* in the absence of hemodynamic work load. *Circ Res* 1990;66:84–102.
30. Shioi T, et al. Rapamycin attenuates load-induced cardiac hypertrophy in mice. *Circulation* 2003; 107:1664–1670.
31. Schneider MD. Serial killer: angiotensin drives cardiac hypertrophy via TGF-β1. *J Clin Invest* 2002; 109:715–716.
32. Asakura M, et al. Cardiac hypertrophy is inhibited by antagonism of ADAM12 processing of HB-EGF: metalloproteinase inhibitors as a new therapy. *Nat Med* 2002;8:35–40.
33. Cittadini A, et al. Differential cardiac effects of growth hormone and insulin-like growth factor-1 in the rat. A combined in vivo and in vitro evaluation. *Circulation* 1996;93:800–809.
34. van Biesen T, et al. Mitogenic signalling via G protein-coupled receptors. *Endocr Rev* 1996;17: 698–714.
35. Yamauchi-Takihara K, et al. A novel role for STAT3 in cardiac remodeling. *Trends Cardiovasc Med* 2000;10:298–303.
36. Kuwahara K, et al. Cardiotrophin-1 phosphorylates Akt and BAD, and prolongs cell survival via a P13K-dependent pathway in cardiac myocytes. *J Mol Cell Cardiol* 2000;32:1385–1394.
37. Xiao G, et al. Inducible activation of c-Myc in adult myocardium in vivo provokes cardiac myocyte hypertrophy and reactivation of DNA synthesis. *Circ Res* 2001;89:1122–1129.
38. Tharaux P-L, et al. Angiotensin II activates collagen I gene through a mechanism involving the MAP/ER kinase pathway. *Hypertension* 2000;36:330–336.
39. De Keulenaer GW, et al. Identification of IEX-1 as a biomechanically controlled nuclear factor-κB target gene that inhibits cardiomyocyte hypertrophy. *Circ Res* 2002;90:690–696.
40. Hardt S, et al. Glycogen synthase kinase-3b. A novel regulator of cardiac hypertrophy and development. *Circ Res* 2002;90:1055–1063.
41. Herron T, et al. Loaded shortening and power output in cardiac myocytes are dependent on myosin heavy chain isoform expression. *Am J Physiol* 2001;281:H1217–H1222.
42. Sack MN, et al. Fatty acid oxidation enzyme gene expression is downregulated in the failing heart. *Circulation* 1996;94:2837–2842.
43. Taegtmeyer H, et al. Adaptation and maladaptation of the heart in diabetes: Part I. General concepts. *Circulation* 2002;105:1727–1733.
44. Young ME, et al. Reactivation of peroxisome proliferator-activated receptor α is associated with contractile dysfunction in hypertrophied rat heart. *J Biol Chem* 2001;276:44390–44395.
45. Razeghi P, et al. Metabolic gene expression in fetal and failing human heart. *Circulation* 2001;104: 2923–2931.
46. Hasenfuss G, et al. Calcium cycling in congestive heart failure. *J Mol Cell Cardiol* 2002;34:951–969.
47. Hein S, et al. Progression from compensated hypertrophy to failure in the pressure-overloaded human heart. Structural deterioration and compensatory mechanisms. *Circulation* 2003;107:984–991.
48. López B, et al. Usefulness of serum carboxy-terminal propeptide of procollagen type I in assessment of the cardioreparative ability of antihypertensive treatment in hypertensive patients. *Circulation* 2001;104:286–291.

49. Zannad F, et al. Limitation of excessive extracellular matrix turnover may contribute to survival benefit of spironolactone therapy in patients with congestive heart failure. Insights from the Randomized Aldactone Evaluation Study (RALES). *Circulation* 2000;102:2700–2706.
50. Intengan HD, et al. Structure and mechanical properties of resistance arteries in hypertension. Role of adhesion molecules and extracellular matrix determinants. *Hypertension* 2000;36:312–318.
51. Diez J, et al. Losartan-dependent regression of myocardial fibrosis is associated with reduction of left ventricular chamber stiffness in hypertensive patients. *Circulation* 2002;105:2512–2517.
52. Bueno OF, et al. The MEK1-ERK 1/2 signaling pathway promotes compensated cardiac hypertrophy in transgenic mice. *EMBO J* 2000;19:6341–6350.
53. Swynghedauw B, et al. The origins of cardiac hypertrophy. In: Swynghedauw B, ed. *Research in cardiac hypertrophy and failure*. London: INSERM/John Libbey Eurotext, 1990:23–50.
53a. Alpert NR, Mulieri LA. Increased myothermal economy of isometric force generation in compensated cardiac hypertrophy induced by pulmonary artery constriction in the rabbit. *Circ Res* 1982;50:491–500.
54. Swynghedauw B. Remodelling of the heart in response to chronic mechanical overload. *Eur Heart J* 1989;10:935–943.
55. Weber KT, et al. Physiologic versus pathologic hypertrophy and the pressure-overloaded myocardium. *J Cardiovasc Pharmacol* 1987;10(suppl 6):S37–S49.
56. Kjeldsen SE, et al. For the LIFE Study Group. Effects of losartan on cardiovascular morbidity and mortality in patients with isolated systolic hypertension and left ventricular hypertrophy. *JAMA* 2002;288:1491–1498.

PART V

The Circulation

14

Blood Pressure and Peripheral Circulation

Lionel H. Opie and David J. Paterson

"Most people will develop hypertension in their lifetime."
Kaplan (1)

Arterial blood pressure (BP) is a major regulator of cardiovascular function and, when chronically elevated, a leading cause of cardiovascular disease. Strictly speaking, BP is given by the peak and trough pressures found on direct arterial puncture. These are the systolic and diastolic values in millimeters of mercury (mmHg), yet they cannot be regarded as physiologic values because invasive monitoring is an impractical procedure in abnormal circumstances. Rather, less precise but widely available noninvasive determination of the brachial artery pressure is standard, using sphygmomanometer and stethoscope (Fig. 1-9). The systolic BP (SBP) value is taken as the level at which the first sounds start to come through as the pressure in the cuff is gradually reduced, and the diastolic BP (DBP) as the disappearance of all the sounds. These are often called the Korotkoff sounds, after the Russian physiologist who first described them. Even simpler is to use an accurately calibrated digital readout machine. Physiologically, although BP varies considerably from an early morning "high" to a nocturnal "low" (Fig. 1-9), specific limits are recognized. When BP is consistently too high, with the majority of daytime readings exceeding an arbitrary cut-off level of 140/90 mmHg, the condition is called hypertension. In young adults, values of approximately 120/80 mmHg are usual. With aging, BP often creeps up to become abnormal. Of note, there are large daily variations in BP in response to temporary events such as exercise or emotional stress.

PHYSIOLOGY OF BLOOD PRESSURE CONTROL

The control of BP is mediated through complex, overlapping mechanisms that interact to produce appropriate responses in a wide variety of circumstances. Arte-

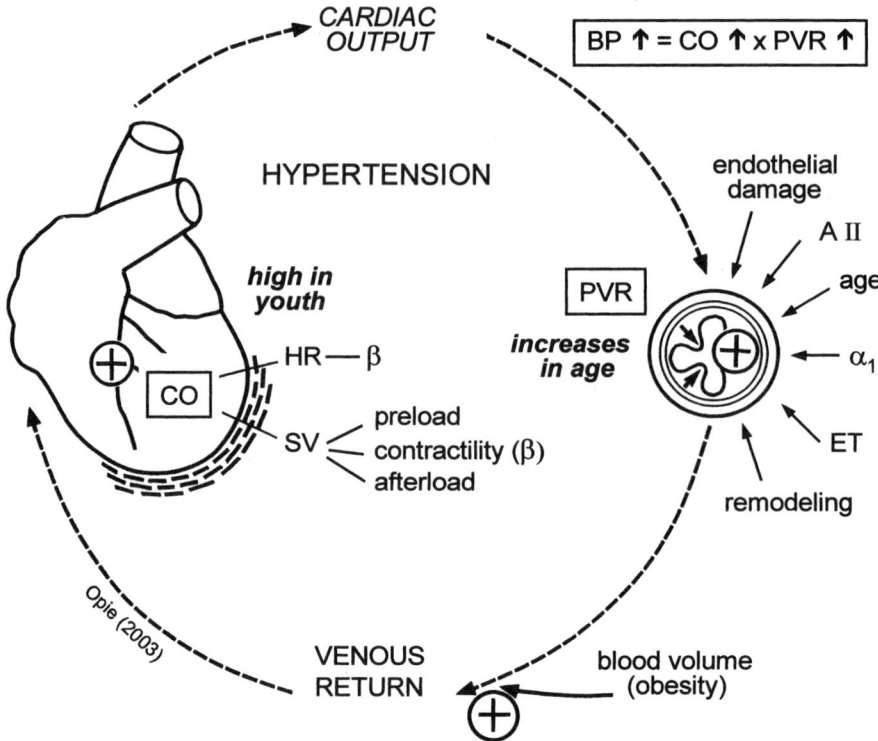

FIG. 14-1. Basic mechanisms in hypertension. In younger patients with hypertension, cardiac output (CO) is generally increased, whereas in older patients, peripheral vascular resistance (PVR) is increased. BP, blood pressure; SV, stroke volume; HR, heart rate; ET, endothelin; A II, angiotensin II; α_1, α-1 adrenergic.

rial BP, although subject to large diurnal variations, is relatively tightly controlled (Fig. 14-1); thus, mean BP = cardiac output × peripheral vascular resistance (PVR), where mean BP = DBP + 1/3 pulse pressure and pulse pressure = SBP − DBP.

The empirical formula for mean BP allows for the heart spending approximately twice as long in diastole as in systole. Note that the mean BP is not the arithmetical mean of SBP and DBP. During increasing exercise, cardiac output and SBP increase, but the mean BP is virtually unchanged. Mean BP is prevented from increasing excessively by β decreased PVR, also called total peripheral resistance. Such *acute regulation* of the PVR over minutes and hours is achieved largely by (a) autonomic control and baroreflexes, which provide rapid responses of the circulation to minute-by-minute BP variations, and (b) regulation of the peripheral arteriolar tone by both local metabolic factors such as nitric oxide and adenosine and by variable adrenergic or cholinergic signals. Long-term regulation of BP over days and weeks depends more on neurohumoral regulation of blood volume and renal factors, including the renin–angiotensin system, also with changes in the PVR.

Autonomic Control and Baroreflexes

The *vasomotor center* at the base of the brain coordinates autonomic control of the circulation by receiving incoming signals from the baroreflexes and then transmitting efferent impulses through vasoconstrictor or vasodilator fibers to the arterioles. The *nucleus solitarius* has a key role because it is the terminating site of the afferent stimuli coming from the baroreceptors in response to an increased or decreased arterial BP (Fig. 2-2). The afferent stimuli arrive from the baroreceptors via the vagus and glossopharyngeal nerves, and outgoing impulses go to the adrenergic and cholinergic vagal systems. In this way, the high-pressure side of the circulation is constantly monitored and BP is regulated.

Baroreceptors (high-pressure receptors) are situated on the arterial side of the circulation in the carotid sinus and aortic arch (Fig. 14-2). They play a key role in short-term regulation of BP. Despite their name (*baro*, pressure), these are stretch receptors that respond to arterial distention rather than to pressure. These mechanoreceptors form the first line of defense against acute hypertension or hypotension, adjusting both vagal tone and sympathetic outflow against the level

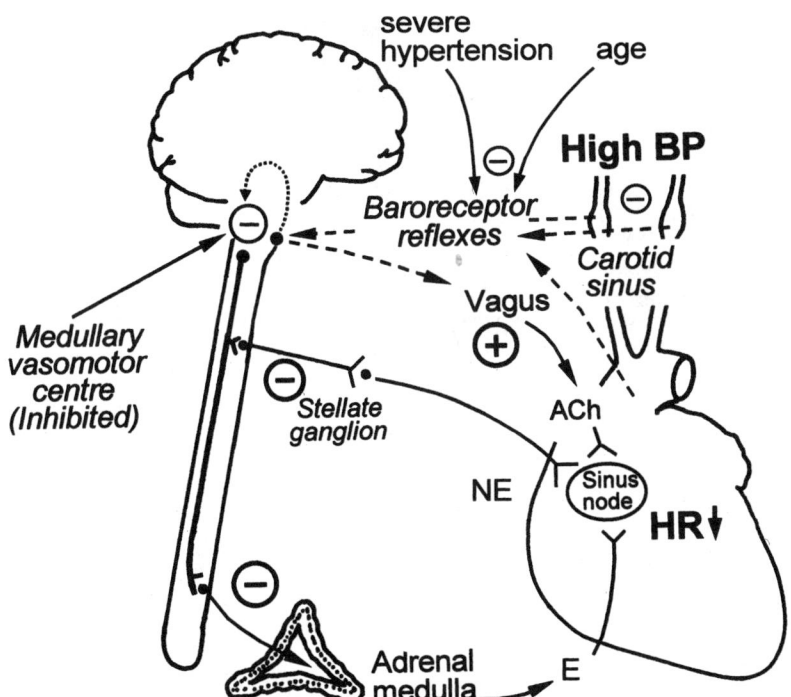

FIG. 14-2. High-pressure receptors and baroreflexes. In response to acute blood pressure (*BP*) elevation, there is inhibition of the sympathetic outflow and enhanced vagal activity that reduce heart rate (*HR*) and stroke volume (*SV*) to decrease BP toward normal.

of receptor input. The baroreceptors respond to both the rate of pressure-induced, stretch-mediated deformation and sustained BP changes.

In response to *acute hypertension*, the baroreflexes engender increased neuronal traffic to the vasomotor center, with consequent inhibition of sympathetic outflow and increase in vagal tone (Fig. 14-2). These changes in autonomic outflow decrease the heart rate, contractility, and cardiac output, as well as induce a decrease in PVR. Thus, the acute increase in BP induces self-correcting changes.

In response to acute hypotension or drug-induced vasodilation, there is a decrease in the distending pressure in the baroreceptors resulting in a decreased frequency of afferent stimuli with lessened signals to the nucleus solitarius, with a consequent increase in sympathetic outflow and inhibition of vagal tone (Fig. 14-3). The β-mediated reflex response will increase heart rate and contractility, so that cardiac output increases. Simultaneously, the α-mediated increase in

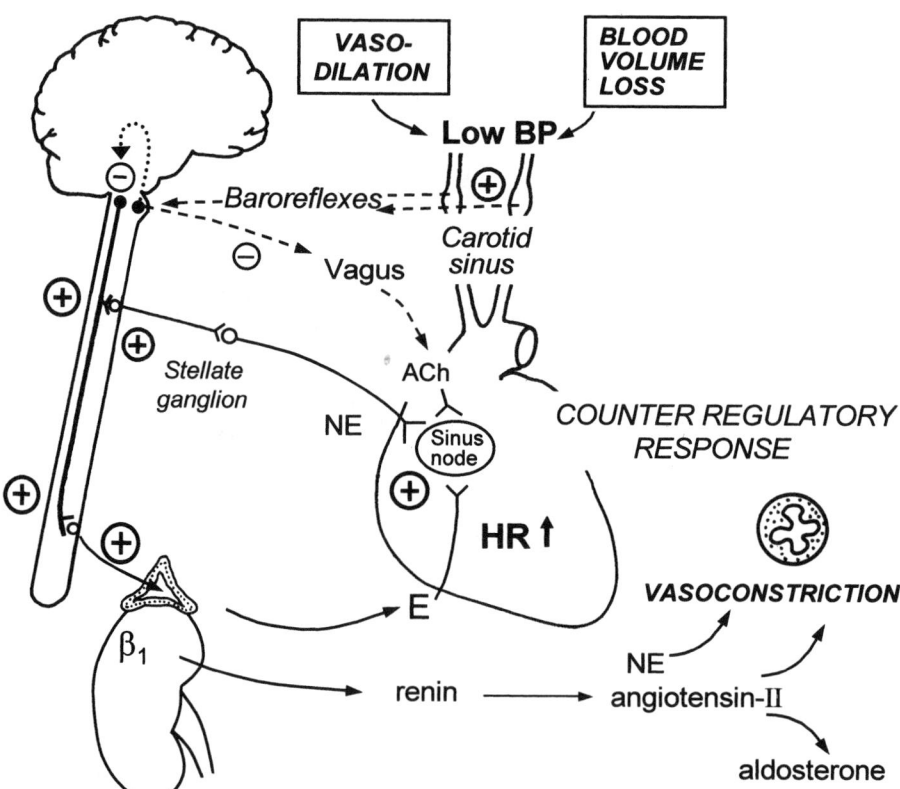

FIG. 14-3. **Baroreflex response to hypotension,** as induced by drug-induced vasodilation or loss of blood volume. Inhibition of vagal outflow and stimulation of adrenergic outflow mediate counterregulation and vasoconstriction.

PVR will also help to elevate BP. Similar self-corrective responses may occur when BP decreases abruptly after painful or psychological stimuli, probably in response to inhibitory input into the vasomotor center from higher centers such as the hypothalamus and cerebral cortex.

Low-Pressure Receptors

Distending volumes on the venous side of the circulation are sensed by *cardiopulmonary receptors*, which are stretch receptors in the atria, pulmonary arteries, and ventricular endocardium (Fig. 14-4). These receptors primarily respond to alterations in the filling volumes of the venous side of the heart (2). Thus, an increase in blood volume (e.g., by a transfusion) will send signals along vagal afferent fibers to the brain to inhibit the sympathetic outflow and to decrease the release of renin. Such inhibitory signals decrease PVR and lessen BP increase.

Bainbridge Reflex

This reflex increases the heart rate in response to increased atrial pressure (Fig. 14-4) and is mediated by stretch receptors in the atrium at the junction with

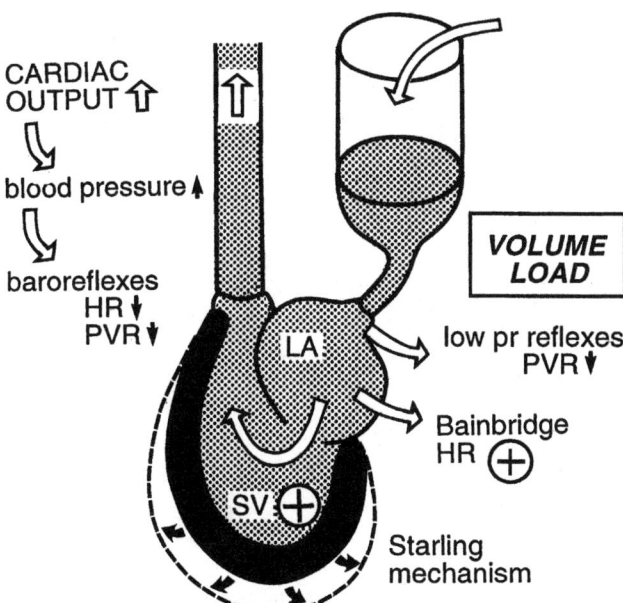

FIG. 14-4. Low-pressure and Bainbridge reflexes in response to volume load. Note that when blood pressure increases, high-pressure baroreflexes tend to reduce heart rate (*HR*) and peripheral vascular resistance (*PVR*).

the pulmonary veins (3). The result is that an increased venous return not only increases the stroke volume by the Frank–Starling mechanism but increases the heart rate further to increase the cardiac output. In some circumstances, such as in a recumbent resting conscious dog, the heart rate effect can account for the increase in cardiac output in response to a volume infusion (4). In humans, however, the Bainbridge effect is small.

Integrated Control of Peripheral Vascular Resistance

It must not be supposed that the baroreflexes and low-pressure receptors invoke only reflex autonomic changes. The response of the kidneys is also important (Fig. 14-5). Whenever there is decreased sympathetic outflow, the kidneys respond by less renin release, thereby attenuating angiotensin-mediated vasoconstriction. A converse sequence occurs with increased sympathetic outflow; for example, when standing, a reflex increase in PVR restores BP to the normal range. This increase is obtained by (a) reflex stimulation of the vasocon-

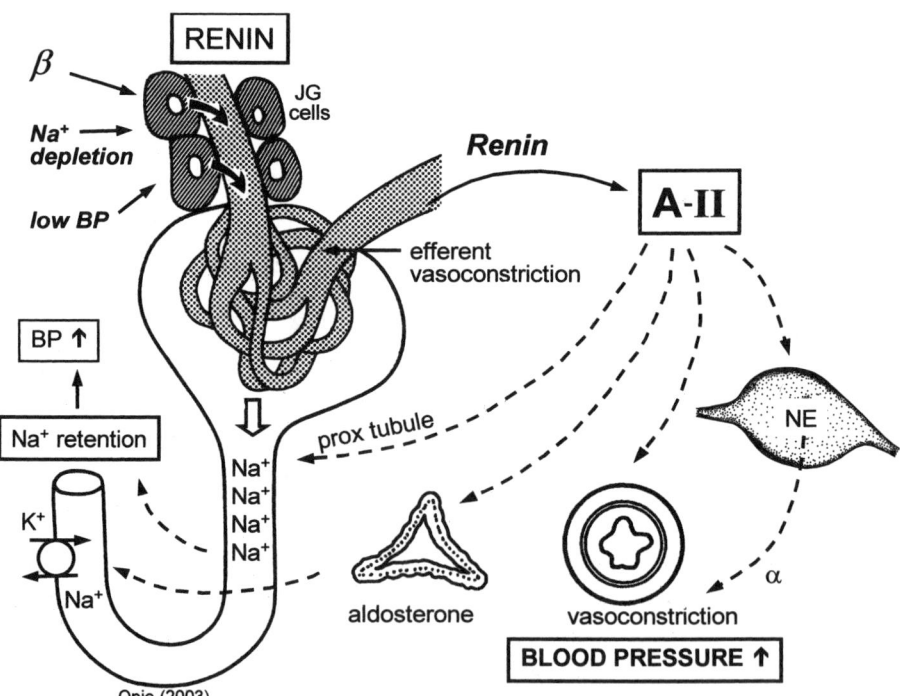

FIG. 14-5. Mechanisms for release of renin from juxtaglomerular (*JG*) cells of kidney: *1,* β$_1$-sympathetic activity; *2,* hypotension or decreased renal blood flow; and *3,* decreased tubular reabsorption of sodium as, for example, with a low-sodium diet or diuretic therapy. Note that renin, by forming angiotensin II, maintains efferent arteriolar vasoconstriction and, therefore, the intraglomerular pressure required for normal glomerular function.

strictive α_1-adrenergic receptors as a result of baroreflex activation and (b) stimulation of renin release from the kidneys, both by the low renal artery pressure and by a β_1-adrenergic–mediated effect, facilitated by the activity of the low-pressure reflexes. Conversely, if the BP increases too much, such as when cold evokes vasoconstriction, the protective mechanisms include baroreflex inhibition of the adrenergic system and endothelial regulation of BP. If the endothelium is normal, an increase in BP increases vascular shear forces that release vasodilatory nitric oxide. In the presence of damaged endothelium (repetitive elevation of BP), stimulation of the endothelium releases vasoconstrictive endothelin that increases PVR and further drives up BP.

Neurohumoral Control of Blood Pressure

Catecholamines

The endocrine functions of the catecholamines are primarily related to acute responses such as the fight-or-flight response. Whether, in addition, these agents are major factors affecting day-to-day or longer term BP control, as postulated by the neurogenic theory of hypertension, is still open to debate. Under normal circumstances, circulating norepinephrine does not exert significant vascular effects because the concentrations in plasma are too low, whereas epinephrine concentrations are within the active range. Nonetheless, norepinephrine released from the terminal neurons into the synaptic cleft is locally active to promote α_1-mediated vasoconstriction. A decrease in blood volume or BP evokes reflex β-adrenergic stimulation that releases renin from the kidneys, thereby helping to control blood volume.

Renin–Angiotensin System

Angiotensin II (A-II) is powerfully vasoconstrictive and the end product of a coordinated neurohormonal cascade that plays a central role in the control of fluid and electrolyte balance, blood volume, and BP regulation, as reviewed in Chapter 9 (Fig. 9-2). The key initial event is the release of *renin* from the juxtaglomerular (that is, lying next to the glomerulus) apparatus in the kidney (Fig. 14-5). Renin is released from the kidneys in response to three major stimuli: increased β_1-adrenergic stimulation, decreased renal artery pressure (hypotension), and decreased tubular reabsorption of sodium (e.g., in response to a low-sodium diet or diuretic therapy) (Fig. 14-5). Release of renin is inhibited by negative feedback from A-II. It also stimulates the release of aldosterone from the adrenal cortex, thereby increasing sodium reabsorption in the kidney and decreasing release of renin.

A-II has several other important effects besides vasoconstriction (Table 14-1). First, it regulates sodium and water balance at several levels. It promotes the release of the sodium-retaining hormone aldosterone from the adrenal cortex (Fig. 14-5). Next, it acts on the renal circulation to constrict the efferent renal

TABLE 14-1. *Role of angiotensin II in maintaining blood pressure during hypotension*

Site of action of A-II	Effect
Vascular smooth muscle	Constriction; increase of PVR
Renal efferent arteriole	Constriction; maintenance of GFR
Proximal renal tubule	Na⁺ reabsorption↑
Adrenal cortex	Aldosterone secretion↑
Central adrenergic activation	Increased release of NE
Ganglionic facilitation	Increased release of NE
Presynaptic receptors	Increased release of NE; decreased reuptake
Baroreflexes	Withdrawal of vagal tone

A-II, angiotensin II; PVR, peripheral vascular resistance; GFR, glomerular filtration rate; NE, norepinephrine.

arterioles, thereby increasing the intraglomerular pressure. Thus, during arterial hypotension, renal filtration function can be preserved. A-II also acts on the proximal renal tubules to stimulate the Na^+/H^+ exchanger to promote sodium reabsorption. In addition, A-II stimulates the thirst center in the hypothalamus, resulting in increased water intake while also increasing the secretion of water-retaining antidiuretic hormone (ADH). These effects have physiologic benefits when the body is threatened by sodium and water depletion but are clearly adverse in the context of heart failure.

A-II has an indirect, permissive adrenergic effect, stimulating the sympathetic nervous system at several levels (Fig. 14-6), by acting on (a) the brainstem to promote central adrenergic activation, (b) autonomic ganglia to facilitate neurotransmission, (c) presynaptic A-II receptors of sympathetic nerve terminal neurons to stimulate the release of norepinephrine and to lessen its reuptake, and (d) the endothelium to promote release of endothelin. By all these many actions, A-II helps to maintain blood volume and BP in the face of arterial hypotension.

A-II also interacts with the *baroreflexes*, which would normally set in motion a series of events that would tend to counteract all the multiple ways in which A-II increases BP. For example, it would be expected that the heart rate would decrease as BP increased. This does not happen because A-II acts on central A-II (subtype AT_1) receptors to reset the baroreflexes and to lessen the anticipated bradycardia (5).

Evidence of local tissue renin–angiotensin systems is that all components of the renin–angiotensin system can be identified in tissues such as heart and blood vessel walls. In arterioles, locally produced A-II is vasoconstrictive by increased intracellular Ca^{2+} concentrations. In the myocardium, the local renin–angiotensin system has a major role in the growth process that occurs during hypertrophy (Fig. 13-4).

Antidiuretic Hormone

This hormone is secreted by the posterior pituitary gland in response to stimulation of osmoreceptors located in the hypothalamus. For example, when a per-

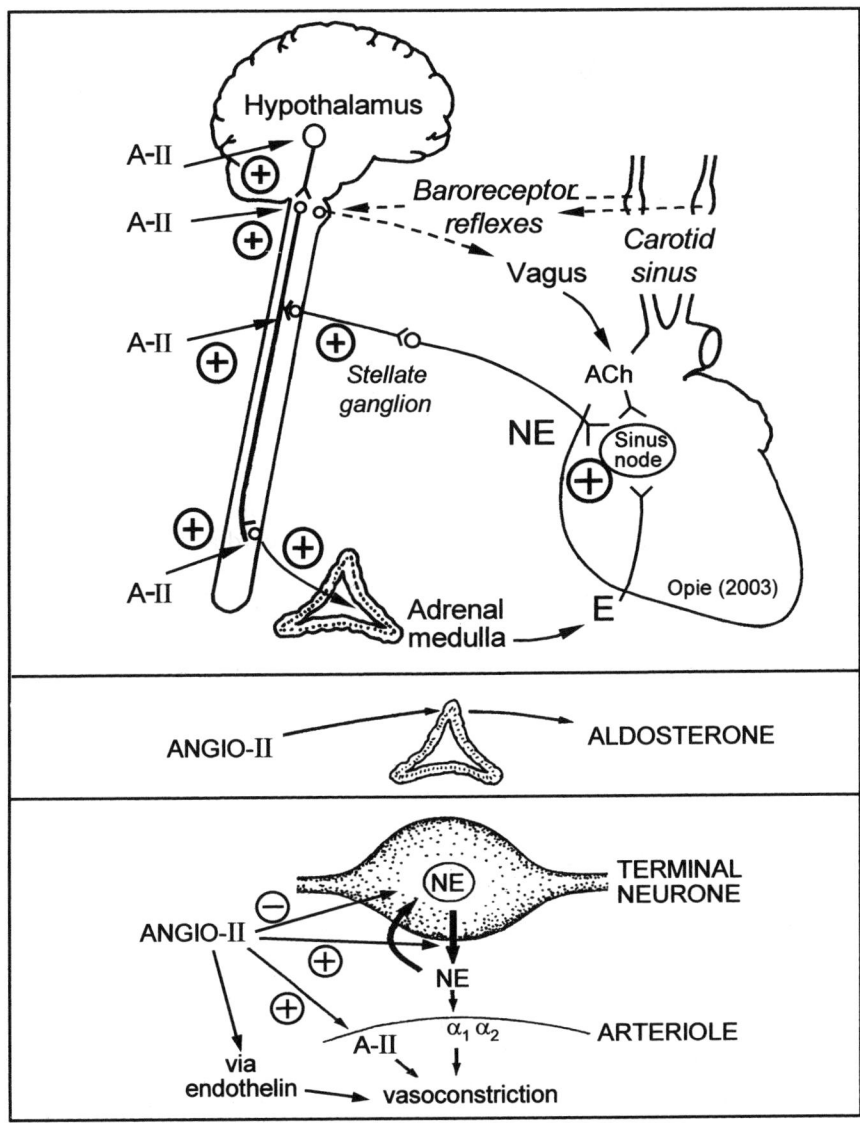

FIG. 14-6. **Multiple sites of action of angiotensin II (*ANGIO II, A II*)** including central activation, facilitation of ganglionic transmission, release of aldosterone from the adrenal medulla, release of norepinephrine (*NE*) from terminal sympathetic varicosities with inhibition of reuptake, and direct stimulation of vascular angiotensin II receptors. Angiotensin II also releases vasoconstrictive endothelin from the endothelium. The major net effect is powerful vasoconstriction. *Ach*, acetylcholine; *E*, epinephrine.

son in the desert lacks water to drink, the blood osmolality increases, and ADH is secreted to increase the reabsorption of water in the kidney. This action is via V_2-receptors located in the collecting duct of the nephron. ADH is also released in response to A-II, as in heart failure or when the low-pressure, volume-activated receptors in the atria sense a decrease in blood volume. These stimuli evoke, via ADH, a potent vasoconstrictor response at vascular V_1-receptors (hence the alternate name, *arginine vasopressin*).

Atrial Natriuretic Peptide

Atrial natriuretic peptide, also called atrial natriuretic factor, is released in response to atrial distention as in volume overload or left heart failure. It acts on vascular smooth muscle cells to promote vasodilation via the cyclic guanosine 3′,5′-monophosphate (cGMP) system (Fig. 16-22). In the sinus node, atrial natriuretic peptide promotes vagal-induced bradycardia by facilitating the release of acetylcholine (6). In the kidneys, atrial natriuretic peptide has diuretic actions by both a direct renal effect and inhibition of secretion of aldosterone.

Control of Peripheral Vascular Resistance

How is PVR generated? The high SBP and DBP in the aorta decrease abruptly at the level of the arterioles (Fig. 1-7). The diameter of the arterioles therefore controls PVR, according to the Poiseuille law (Fig. 2-14), which can be simplified as follows. *The resistance is inversely related to the fourth power of the radius.* Halving the radius will therefore increase PVR 16-fold. The major mechanisms controlling PVR are as follows.

1. *Vasoconstrictor receptors.* Three major vascular receptors increase cell calcium to promote arteriolar constriction (Fig. 7-15). These receptors respond to agonists that reflect neurogenic, neurohumoral, and endothelial function. First,

TABLE 14-2. *Contrasting regulation of contraction in myocardium and vascular smooth muscle*

	Myocardium	Vascular smooth muscle
Major agonists	β-Adrenergic	α-Adrenergic, A-II, ET, $β_2$
Major messengers	cAMP	IP_3 and cyclic nucleotides
Histology	Striated	Smooth, nonstriated
Metabolic rate	High	Low
Rate of contraction and relaxation	Fast	Slow; maintains tone, latch mechanism
Site of calcium regulation	Troponin C	Myosin light chain kinase
cAMP effects	Contract	Relax
cGMP effects	Inhibitory (modest effect)	Relax (powerful effect)

A-II, angiotensin II; ET, endothelin; $β_2$, $β_2$-adrenergic; cAMP, cyclic adenosine 3′,5′-monophosphate; IP_3, inositol triphosphate; cGMP, cyclic guanosine 3′,5′-monophosphate.

the α_1-adrenergic vasoconstrictor system operates via norepinephrine released from terminal neurons in response to adrenergic stimulation. Second, A-II, the end product of renin release, is a major constrictor in its own right in addition to its indirect actions via norepinephrine (Fig. 14-6). Third, endothelin is a powerfully vasoconstrictive peptide released from damaged endothelium.

2. *Cyclic nucleotide vasodilatory system.* Although the inhibition of vascular contraction by cyclic adenosine 3',5'-monophosphate and cGMP is complex in its mechanism, a useful simplification is that they both inhibit myosin light chain kinase that activates vascular contraction. Cyclic adenosine 3',5'-monophosphate increases in response to β-adrenergic vasodilation (Table 14-2). There are vasodilatory β-receptors (mainly $β_2$ in nature) in arterioles, especially in skeletal muscle but also in the coronary arterioles. These respond to circulating epinephrine released from the adrenal gland in reaction to severe stress or emotion. For reasons not well understood, norepinephrine released from the nerve terminals predominantly stimulates the vasoconstrictive α_1-receptors. cGMP increases in response to stimulation of the nitric oxide messenger system, as occurs during exercise. Therefore, the endothelium has potentially both vasoconstrictive and vasodilatory functions.

3. *Endothelial control of vascular resistance.* The established concept is that the healthy endothelium releases vasodilatory nitric oxide and the damaged endothelium releases vasoconstrictive endothelin (Fig. 10-3). Hence, endothelial integrity is important in the maintenance of coronary and peripheral vascular tone. Endothelin is so well known as a vasoconstrictor that it was surprising to find that, in a knockout mouse model, the total absence of endothelin led, not to hypotension, but to hypertension (7). The revised concept is that endothelin in low physiologic concentrations can vasodilate, acting on the vasodilatory ET_B receptors on the endothelium to release nitric oxide. In contrast, the vasoconstrictive receptors invoked by high-dose endothelin on the vascular smooth muscle cells are thought to be ET_A in nature, although these distinctions are not absolute.

In addition to nitric oxide, other vasodilators that are synthesized include prostacyclin and endothelium-derived hyperpolarizing factor, the latter still awaiting identification, although the "old-timer" potassium is a strong contender (8). Many other vasoactive substances act through endothelium-derived factors or metabolic activity of the endothelium. These include acetylcholine, bradykinin, arachidonic acid, histamine, 5-hydroxytryptamine (serotonin), substance P, and vasopressin. Hypoxia, thrombin, and oxygen-derived free radicals all inhibit the activity of vasodilator endothelial substances or increase the release of endothelin.

Shear stress mediates both physiologic and pathologic stimuli. Physiologically, shear stress, as during increased blood flow, leads to release nitric oxide and hence to flow-induced vasodilation. Excess shear stress, as in sustained arterial hypertension, can damage the endothelium with impaired release of nitric oxide and excess release of vasoconstrictive endothelin.

Myogenic Properties

Quite independently of the autonomic input, the arterioles respond to an increase in transmural pressure, as in hypertension or acute BP elevation, by contracting, which is to some extent a counterproductive response that will further increase PVR and hence BP. Nonetheless, this increase in the wall tension is mechanically required to offset the tendency of the increased intraluminal pressure to split the arteriole open (two halves forced apart).

Response of Skin to Heat and Cold

Vascular tone can be viewed as a balance between the vasoconstrictive and vasodilatory influences, the balance resulting in the degree of tone which in turn governs the arteriolar diameter and PVR. Nonetheless, vasoconstriction as an overall concept, includes three separate events, of which only one determines arteriolar tone: an increase in arteriolar tone (resistance vessels), an increase in venous tone (capacitance vessels), and increased cutaneous constriction as in response to cold. Not all these events may happen at the same time: the old adage recalls the combination of "warm heart, cold hands" in response to adrenergic stimulation, the cold hands resulting from constrictor cutaneous fibers.

By means of specific drugs (e.g., calcium channel blockers) or β_2-receptor stimulation, peripheral vasodilation can be obtained independently of exercise. Such vasodilation is not the same as heat-induced vasodilation, in which physiologic necessity diverts blood to the skin. In heat stress, arteriovenous shunts in the skin are sympathetically constricted to lessen heat loss through the skin. There may be such marked cutaneous vasodilation that blood can even be diverted from the muscles and the central blood volume can decrease, decreasing the left ventricular filling pressure (right atrial pressure) and making exercise in such conditions impossible. In contrast, in normal conditions in which an excessively increased ambient temperature is not the dominant factor and maintenance of central blood volume is possible, cutaneous vasodilation can occur without adverse redistribution of the circulation. Thus, the balance between PVR and cardiac output is maintained, so that BP is as close to normal as possible.

Autoregulation in Regional Circulations

Organs such as the brain, heart, and kidneys that need continuous perfusion have circulations that are relatively independent of circulatory control mechanisms, and autoregulation becomes more important (Fig. 10-10). This mechanism maintains the blood flow to the vital organ despite wide BP variations. In general, the lower limit of autoregulation is better studied than the upper limit. In the heart, the mean BP can decrease to 50 mmHg before the lower limit is reached (Fig. 10-10). In the brain, the lower limit is 73 mmHg, and with a further decrease to 43 mmHg, subjects develop symptoms of brain hypoperfusion (9). In the kidney, limits are less clearly defined because it is the intraglomerular pressure that matters, and this is regulated by changes in the resistance to blood flow exerted by both the afferent arterioles that carry blood to the glomerular and the efferent arterioles. Glomerular blood flow and filtration rates are constant over a very wide range of BPs because of compensatory changes in the tone of the afferent arterioles that regulate blood flow to the glomerulus (10). At low BPs, the efferent arterioles clamp down in response to increased A-II and thereby maintain the intraglomerular pressure.

In other circulations, autoregulation would be counterproductive. In skeletal muscle, prominent vasodilation is required during exercise, despite the increased SBP, because as much as 90% of cardiac output may be diverted to the working muscles. Thus, metabolic vasodilation comes into play. Conversely, the blood flow to the splanchnic circulation is not essential during exercise, so that vasoconstriction and diversion of blood to the exercising muscle and myocardium are achieved.

DIFFERENT BLOOD PRESSURE RESPONSES

Diurnal Blood Pressure Variations and Ambulatory Measurements

BP is not static over 24 hours but is highly variable. The nocturnal decrease in BP is associated with vagal activity. On wakening, withdrawal of vagal tone and an adrenergic "spurt" lead to transient early morning hypertension (Fig. 1-9). Thereafter, BP usually decreases gradually throughout the day but may increase during occupational or emotional stresses. Usually the heart rate and BP vary together, yet BP changes relatively less than the heart rate because of reflex compensatory mechanisms. The best way to detect these patterns of change is by monitoring BP noninvasively over 24 hours, placing an inflatable cuff in position around the upper arm. The cuff automatically inflates and deflates at preset intervals and digitally records the appearance and disappearance of the heart sounds. In general, the normal limits are approximately 5 to 10 mmHg lower than with ordinary "office" BP values. For example, in one study, the optimal ambulatory BP 24-hour values were 120 to 133 mmHg systolic and 65 to 78 mmHg diastolic, with values of 135/80mmHg or more indicating hypertension (11).

Mental Stress

There is a brisk adrenergic reaction to stress. β-Adrenergic stimulation considerably increases the heart rate. Perhaps unexpectedly, the extent to which BP increases is variable. In some subjects, there is rapid BP increase as uniquely captured by an ambulatory BP monitor during an earthquake (Fig. 14-7). The probable mechanism is excess α_1-adrenergic vasoconstriction as found in those likely to develop hypertension (prehypertensives). Stress also evokes a prolonged endothelin response, which impairs vasodilation (12). However, some subjects can withstand severe stress with only modest BP increases, for example, when selected medical students were subjected to a grueling test that con-

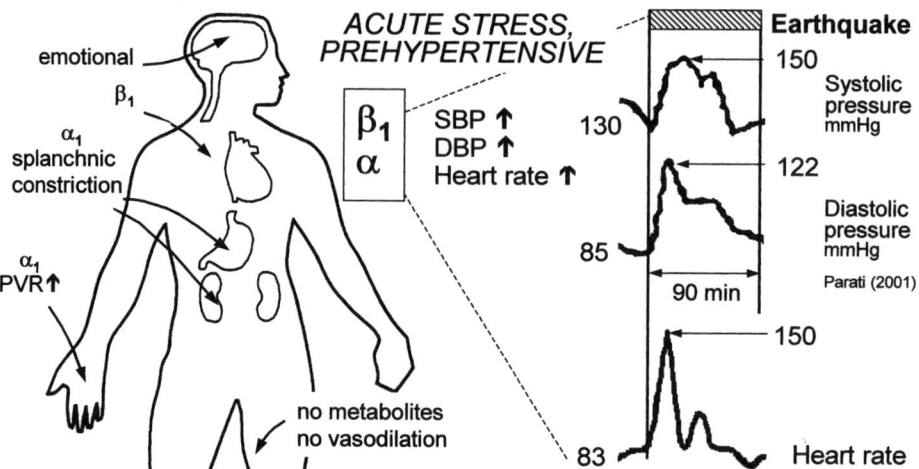

FIG. 14-7. Effect of earthquake on monitored blood pressure and heart rate (37). These marked surges are owing to increased sympathetic activity providing β_1-adrenergic stimulation to the heart. Normal β_2-adrenergic vasodilation in the periphery in this prehypertensive subject was probably overridden by α-adrenergic vasoconstriction (see text for variable blood pressure response to mental stress). *SBP*, systolic blood pressure; *DBP*, diastolic blood pressure.

sisted of a difficult oral examination in physiology with aggressive criticism even when correct answers were given (Fig. 14-8). There are several explanations for these differences. First, overall adrenergic activation variably induces α_1-adrenergic vasoconstriction and β_2-mediated peripheral arteriolar vasodilation, the latter especially found in those genetically endowed with more vasodilatory β_2-receptors in the arterioles (13). Second, sympathetic stimulation by mental stress evokes vasodilation, localized to the forearm, by poorly understood sympathetic cholinergic nerves that probably release nitric oxide (14).

White-Coat Syndrome

When doctors measure BP, it is usually higher than when nurses do. This is the "white-coat effect" and may occur in individuals who are usually normotensive as well as those already hypertensive. The mechanism of the white-coat effect is a temporary fear-induced increased sympathetic nerve activity that augments both BP and heart rate (Fig. 14-7). The risks of white-coat hypertension are twofold. First, in those who are basically normotensive, a false diagnosis of sustained hypertension can be made. Second, in those already hypertensive, the effects of drug therapy will be underestimated. The remedies for white-coat hypertension are also twofold. First, BP when taken by standard methods must only be measured when the subject is truly relaxed and rested. Repetitive values are often required. Second, if there is still doubt about the true BP value, a 24-hour ambulatory BP measurement must be performed.

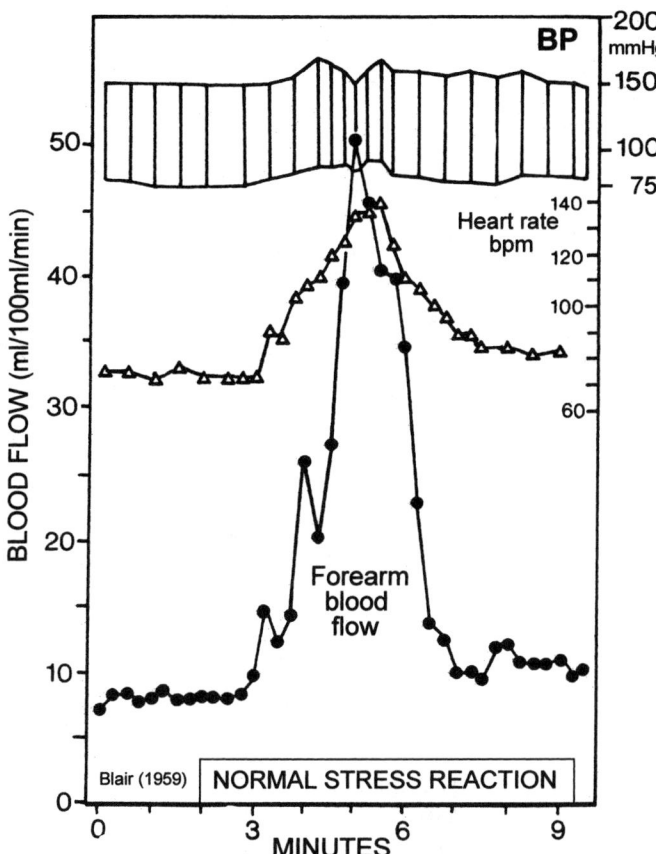

FIG. 14-8. Effect of severe emotional stress on blood pressure in a normal subject. This normal medical student was subjected to abnormal emotional and intellectual stress. His reward was that this recording lives on almost forever in textbooks of cardiovascular physiology. The marked increase in heart rate (Δ) is caused by increased sympathetic nerve activity to the sinus node and to circulating epinephrine released from the adrenal medulla. The striking increase in forearm blood flow (v) is caused by the circulating epinephrine stimulating vasodilatory $β_2$-adrenergic receptors in the skeletal muscle resistance vessels. The increase in blood pressure is caused by a greater increase in cardiac output than decrease in peripheral vascular resistance. (From Blair DA, Glover WE, Greenfield ADM, et al. Excitation of cholinergic vasodilator nerves to human skeletal muscles during emotional stress. *J Physiol* 1959;148:633–647, with permission.)

Orthostatic Stress

On standing up, between 500 and 800 mL of blood is trapped in the veins below the heart level (15). The decreasing venous return decreases cardiac output by the Frank–Starling mechanism; BP decreases and stimulates the baroreceptors and thereby evokes the sympathetic vasoconstrictive response (Fig. 14-9). Additionally, the vasoconstrictive renin–angiotensin system is activated. This

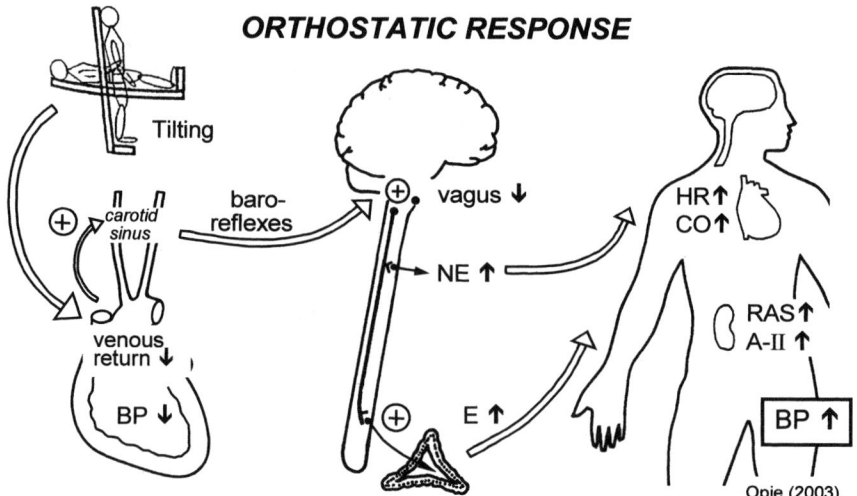

FIG. 14-9. Orthostatic response. An abrupt decrease in venous return decreases stroke volume by the Starling mechanism. The decrease in blood pressure stimulates reflex vagal inhibition and sympathetic activation, to increase heart rate (*HR*) and cardiac output (*CO*). Note ancillary role of the renin–angiotensin system (*RAS*) with increased vasoconstrictive angiotensin II (*A-II*).

is a rapid response so that normal subjects can stand up without fear of hypotension. As soon as there is even gentle contraction of the leg muscles, the venous return increases to restore the circulation to its prestanding state (16). Thus, standing still but not walking brings about the risk of excess decrease in the systolic pressure. *Postural hypotension* is defined as a decrease in SBP of 20 mmHg or more after 1 minute of standing quietly compared with values in the supine position. It occurs especially in elderly hypertensive subjects but also in others whose compensatory mechanisms are imperfect. When marked, the result is syncope, which is a transient loss of consciousness caused by cerebral hypoperfusion (15).

Acute Exercise

BP increases during exercise, with different patterns for static and dynamic exercise (Fig. 15-2). In normal subjects, it is mainly the SBP that increases during exercise because concomitant metabolism-driven peripheral vasodilation will decrease DBP, which would otherwise increase as the stroke volume increases. The result is that the mean BP increases little (Fig. 14-10).

Effects of Age on Arterial Blood Pressure

With increasing age, the SBP increases so that values greater than 140 mmHg become common. This physiologic pressure increase has adverse effects, as

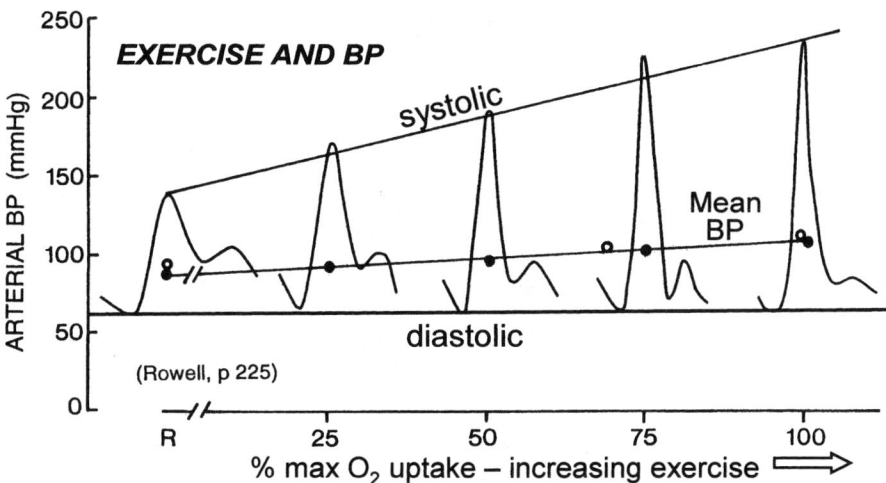

FIG. 14-10. Exercise and blood pressure (BP). Note increased systolic BP compared with little change in diastolic BP. Mean BP increases only slightly. (Modified from Rowell LB. *Human circulation, regulation during physical stress.* New York: Oxford University Press, 1986.)

shown by the beneficial clinical effects of reducing the excessively high SBP. The SBP is governed by the stroke volume and the elastic properties of the aorta (Fig. 1-8). During mid-systole, the aorta expands and at the end of systole and into diastole, the aorta exerts elastic recoil that maintains the DBP while the aortic valve is shut (Fig. 14-11). With age, as the aortic elasticity decreases, the buffer function of the aorta is progressively lost so that the DBP decreases. The stiffened aorta conducts the pulse wave faster in both directions, forward and backward, so that the characteristic abrupt increase and decrease of the pulse wave in the elderly can be explained (Fig. 14-12).

In a unique study, Lund-Johansen (17) followed a selected number of normal and hypertensive subjects for 20 years and studied them invasively during exercise. The striking feature was that in the younger hypertensive subjects, cardiac output and heart rate were higher than normal, in agreement with the increased adrenergic drive postulated by the neurogenic theory. With aging, PVR rose to increase the mean BP, and the stroke volume decreased (Fig. 14-13). Higher PVR was presumably owing to degenerative changes in the arterioles caused by loss of elasticity or endothelial damage and the decreasing stroke volume possibly owing to increasing myocardial fibrosis with age.

Pseudohypertension of the elderly is a condition in which BP as measured with the cuff overestimates the true arterial BP. Supposedly, this problem can be avoided if the Osler maneuver is used, which means that when the SBP is increased to 50 mmHg above the systolic value during the cuff procedure, if the wall of the artery stays palpable (Osler positive), then pseudohypertension may be suspected. However, this test has limited accuracy (18).

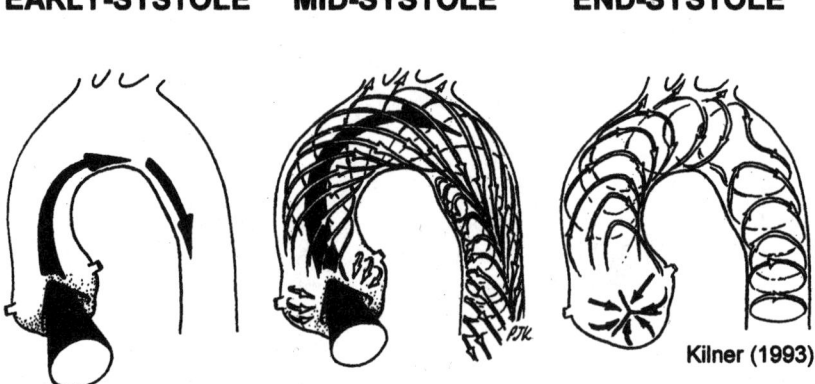

FIG. 14-11. Aortic hemodynamics during systole. Note the build up of forces in the aortic wall during mid-systole in preparation for later diastolic recoil. Aortic impedance is one important component of afterload, the other is arterial blood pressure. (From Kilner PJ, Yang GZ, Mohiaddin RH, et al. Helical and retrograde secondary flow patterns in the aortic arch studied by three-directional magnetic resonance velocity mapping. *Circulation* 1993;88:2235–2247, with permission.)

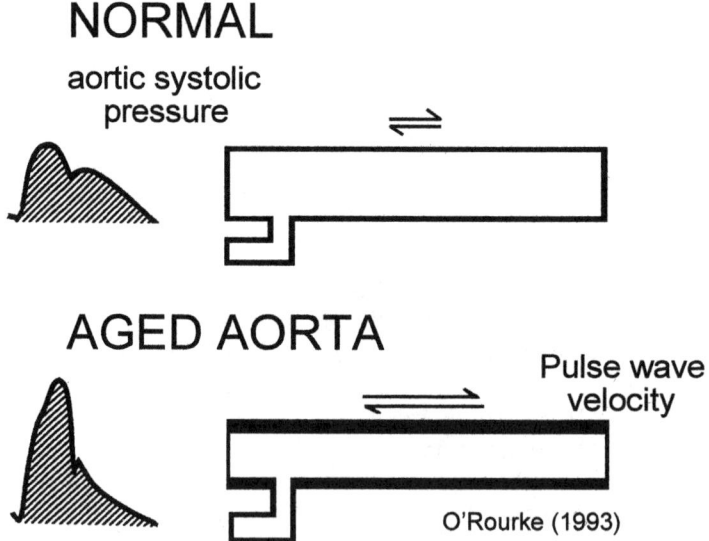

FIG. 14-12. The aged aorta. Effect on pulse wave velocity. (From O'Rourke. *Cardiovasc Res*, 1993, with permission.)

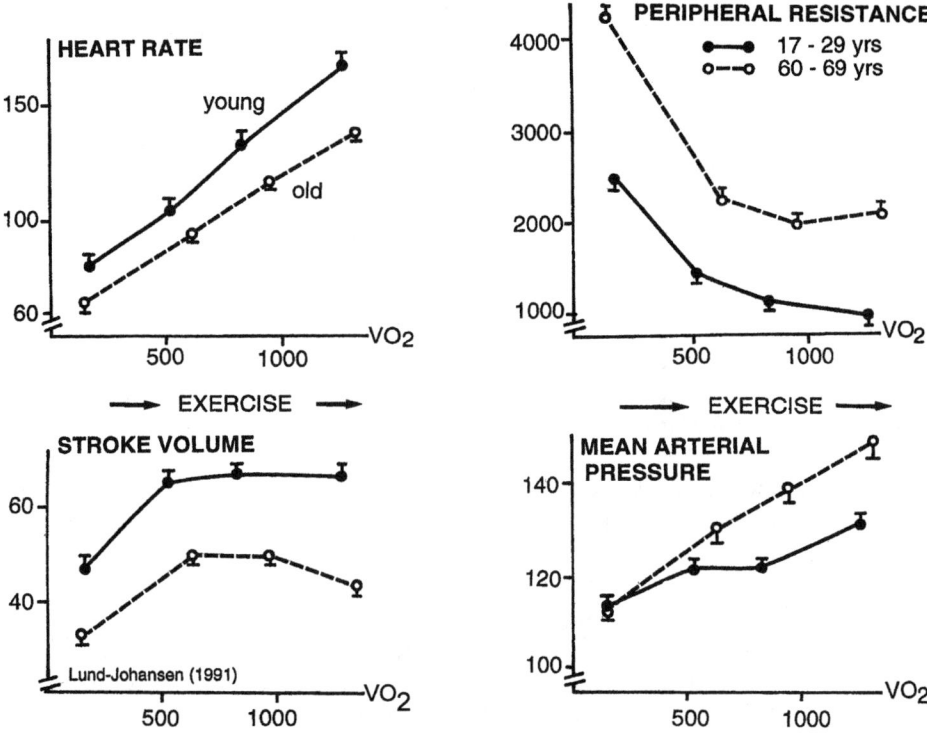

FIG. 14-13. Exercise effects on young and elderly patients with hypertension. Note increased stroke volume and heart rate in younger subjects and increased peripheral resistance in the group of elderly subjects. (From Lund-Johansen P. Twenty-year follow up of hemodynamics in essential hypertension during rest and exercise. *Hypertension* 1991;18:54–61, with permission.)

BLOOD PRESSURE AND AFTERLOAD

During systole, the left ventricle contracts against the afterload (the load after the onset of contraction, against which the left ventricle contracts during LV ejection. In the simplified model of the circulation, it is the PVR against which the heart contracts (Fig. 2-13). When this resistance increases, the BP and afterload increase. Generally, in clinical practice, it is a sufficient approximation to take the arterial BP as a measure of the afterload, provided there is neither significant aortic stenosis nor change in arterial compliance. Nonetheless, this approximation can be wrong, for example, when arterial compliance decreases in the elderly.

Wall Stress and Afterload

Afterload, being the load on the contracting myocardium, is also the wall stress after the onset of systole. Increased afterload means that increased intraventricular pressure has to be generated first to open the aortic valve and then to eject the blood during the ejection phase. These increases will translate themselves into an increased myocardial wall stress, which can be measured either as an average value throughout systole or at a given phase of systole, such as end-systole. Systolic wall stress reflects the two major components of afterload: arterial BP and arterial compliance. Decreased arterial compliance and increased afterload can be anticipated when there is aortic dilation, as in severe systemic hypertension or in the elderly.

Aortic Impedance

This gives another accurate measure of afterload. Aortic impedance is aortic pressure divided by aortic flow at that instance, so that this index of afterload varies at each stage of the contraction cycle. Factors reducing aortic flow, such as a high arterial BP, aortic stenosis, and loss of aortic compliance, will increase impedance and hence afterload. During systole, when the aortic valve is open, increased afterload will communicate itself to the ventricles by increasing wall stress. In left ventricular failure, aortic impedance is augmented not only by peripheral vasoconstriction but also by decreases in aortic compliance (19). The problem with the clinical measurement of aortic impedance is that invasive instrumentation is required. An approximation can be found by using transesophageal echocardiography to determine aortic blood flow at, for example, the time of maximal increase of aortic flow just after aortic valve opening.

Anrep Effect

When the afterload is abruptly increased by rapid elevation of the aortic pressure, a positive inotropic effect follows within 1 or 2 minutes. This change used to be called homeometric autoregulation (*homeo*, the same; *metric*, length) because it was apparently independent of muscle length and by definition a true inotropic effect. Then follows a reflex decrease of PVR mediated by the baroreflexes. A reasonable speculation would be that increased left ventricular wall tension could act on myocardial mechanical sensors to increase cytosolic calcium (Chapter 13). Thus, this effect would be different from that of an increase in preload (which acts by length activation).

HYPERTENSION: A GREATER THAN NORMAL BLOOD PRESSURE LEVEL

In systemic arterial hypertension, there is an upset of the complex regulation of the circulation so that the BP consistently runs higher than the normal range. Because BP is so variable and there is a spectrum of values from normal to abnormal, any cut-off point must be arbitrary. Taken in the standard way, the normal BP range is 120 to 129 mmHg systolic and 80 to 84 mmHg diastolic (20).

A sustained BP value of the resting seated subject exceeding 140/90 mmHg is generally regarded as too high because of vascular damage that leads to major cardiovascular complications, including stroke, myocardial infarction (heart attack), and heart failure. Lower BPs are, however, not free of risk of cardiovascular disease. For example, high normal (130 to 139 mmHg systolic and 85 to 89 mmHg diastolic) approximately doubles the 10-year risk of cardiovascular disease when compared with optimal BP, which is less than 120/80 mmHg (20).

Multifactorial Origin of Essential Hypertension

Only 5% of all hypertensives present with secondary hypertension caused by another abnormality such as an endocrine or renal disease. The remainder have *essential hypertension*, a complex condition of variable etiology. In most cases, several different factors acting over many years contribute to the development of essential hypertension, which is a heterogeneous disease that is multifactorial in origin (Fig. 14-14). The basic concept is a resetting of control mechanisms at a higher than normal BP level. For BP to increase requires a sustained increase in either cardiac output or PVR because BP = cardiac output × PVR. Normally, the baroreflexes would compensate for any increase in either cardiac output or PVR; therefore, there is impaired baroreflex sensitivity in hypertension (21). An increase in cardiac output is more commonly found in younger hypertensive patients and an increase in PVR in older patients (17).

Neurogenic Theory

This takes into account that the early phase of hypertension is often characterized by features suggestive of enhanced adrenergic activity, such as tachycardia and increased cardiac output (22). Over the years, there is a transition from high cardiac output to increased PVR, which could hypothetically be the result of several factors. A pivotal proposal of the neurogenic theory is increased adrenergic-induced peripheral arteriolar vasoconstriction with greater α-mediated constriction, whereas β_2-mediated vasodilation is unchanged or down-regulated (13).

Abnormalities of Sodium Handling

The normal pressure-induced excretion of sodium in the urine (natriuresis) is reset to a higher BP level in all forms of hypertension (23). An interesting hypothesis attempts to link decreased natriuresis by the kidney of patients with hypertension to excess retention of intracellular sodium in vascular smooth muscle (Fig. 14-14). The operation of sodium–calcium exchange then promotes increased cytosolic calcium and vasoconstriction. Alternatively or additionally, there may be a membrane defect in sodium transport so that vascular cells retain too much sodium. These hypotheses would also explain the antihypertensive

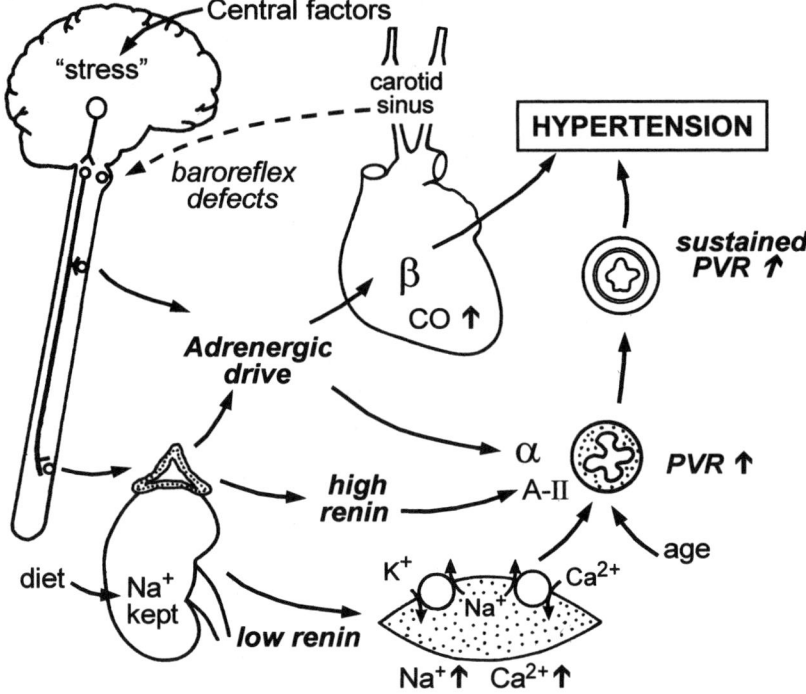

FIG. 14-14. **Multifactorial origin of hypertension.** Hypothetically, in the presence of minimal degrees of a genetically determined renal defect, small amounts of sodium are retained so that the extracellular fluid (*ECF*) volume is increased with release of the proposed natriuretic hormone natriuretic from the hypothalamus. This hormone inhibits sodium–potassium exchange in vascular smooth muscle. Cell sodium in the myocyte increases to increase calcium via the sodium–calcium exchange to enhance vascular tone. CO, cardiac output.

effect of a low-salt diet and diuretic compounds. Some but not all forms of hypertension are salt sensitive.

Salt-Sensitive Hypertension

Some individuals are more prone than others to develop hypertension when their diet is salt loaded, and there is a broad relationship between the salt intake of a population and mean BP levels. Patients with salt-sensitive hypertension are more prone to have a blunted nocturnal decrease in BP (nondipper pattern) and end-organ diseases such as left ventricular hypertrophy, proteinuria, and other adverse events, including sudden death (24). Logically, there should be abnormalities of renal handling of sodium in patients with salt-sensitive hypertension, with delayed salt excretion, as more commonly found in blacks and the elderly. Up-regulated renal epithelial sodium channel activity in black people with increased renal sodium reabsorption may explain the increased prevalence of hypertension in this population (25).

Obesity

Although obesity is commonly associated with hypertension, the mechanism remains ill defined. Because of the greater body mass of the obese, blood volume is also greater and cardiac output will tend to increase. For reasons that are not well understood, there may be activation of the adrenergic system in obesity (26), so that in some ways the circulation resembles that of the hyperkinetic younger hypertensives. Two other factors are involved: increased intraabdominal fat and pressure that impair renal function and insulin resistance.

Insulin-Resistance (Metabolic Cardiovascular Syndrome)

This condition is present when the ability of insulin to stimulate the uptake and metabolism of glucose by muscle is impaired (Fig. 14-15). Clinically, there are hypertension, obesity, maturity-onset type 2 diabetes, arteriosclerosis, and blood lipid disorders. The mechanisms are complex, including abnormal functioning of one of the peroxisome proliferator-activated receptors (PPAR-γ) (Fig. 9-13). As a group, patients with hypertension have insulin resistance, although the links are more marked in the obese than nonobese (27). Insulin resistance is also associated with increased adrenergic activity, either as the cause of the

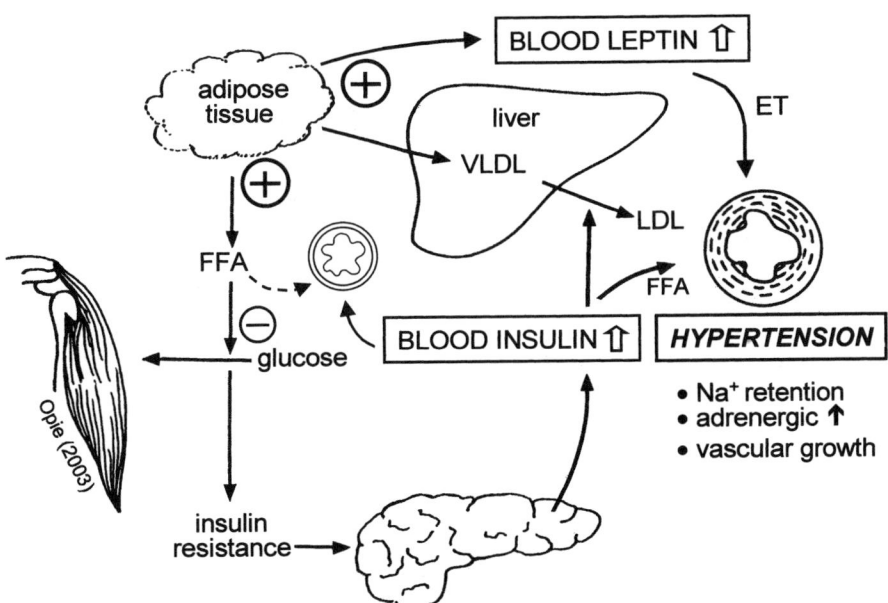

FIG. 14-15. Insulin resistance. Proposed sequence of events leading to insulin resistance. Based on inhibition of uptake of glucose by circulating free fatty acids (*FFA*). Note role of leptin. *ET*, endothelin; *LDL*, low-density lipoproteins; *VLDL*, very low density lipoproteins.

increase (28) or the consequence (29). Insulin resistance may be a step on the way to overt type 2 diabetes.

Low Renin Hypertension in Specific Population Groups

The elderly and black patients as a group are thought to have relatively low renin values and to be prone to salt-sensitive hypertension. Normally, salt loading leads to increased tubular reabsorption of sodium, with inhibition of renin release, less formation of A-II, and less constriction of the efferent renal arterioles (Fig. 14-5). In low renin groups, this compensatory mechanism is impaired. These observations have therapeutic implications because salt restriction and diuretics work best in low renin states.

Endothelium-Derived Factors in Hypertension

Does endothelial dysfunction play a role in hypertension? A current hypothesis is that increased intraluminal pressure damages the endothelium, thus allowing release of endothelin and inhibiting the release of nitric oxide. The ensuing vasoconstriction helps to perpetuate the hypertension (Fig. 14-16). In patients with hypertension, endothelin impairs endothelium-dependent vasodilation (30), which is indirect evidence that it could contribute to arteriolar constriction (31).

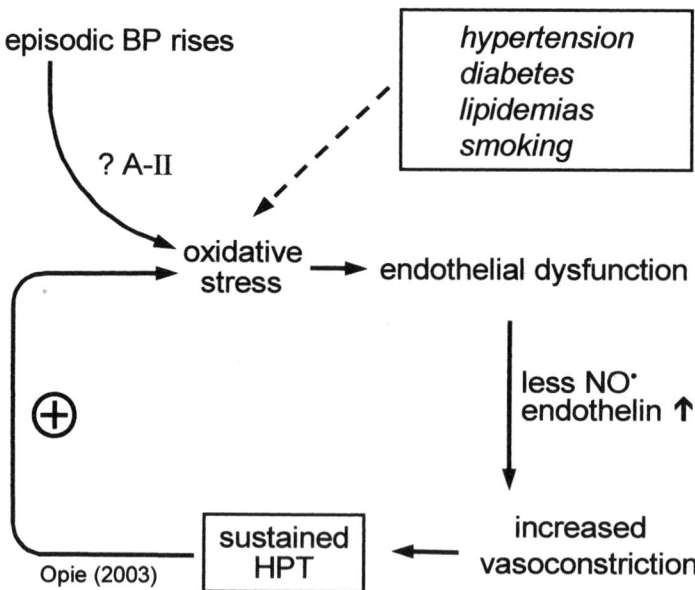

FIG. 14-16. Endothelial dysfunction and its hypothetical role in perpetuation of hypertension (*HPT*). *NO*, nitric oxide.

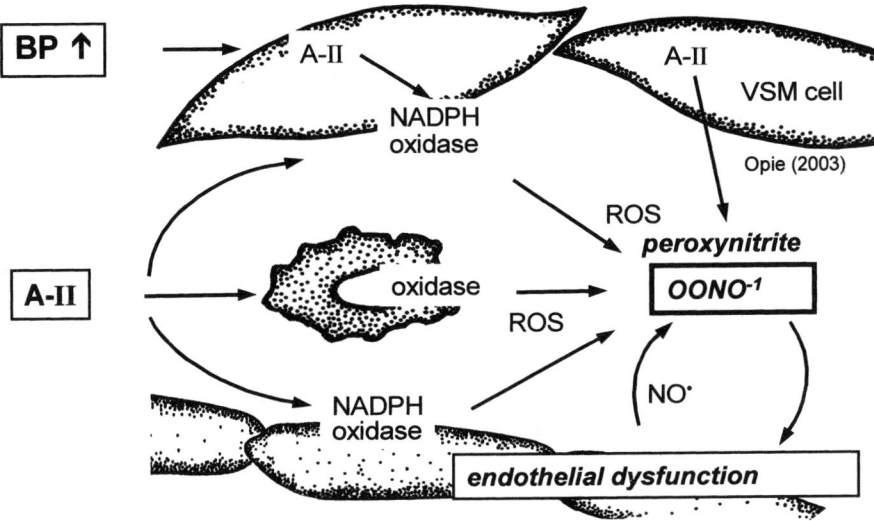

FIG. 14-17. Role of peroxynitrite in endothelial dysfunction. Reactive oxygen species (*ROS*) derived from several sources helps to convert nitric oxide (*NO*) to peroxynitrite, which promotes endothelial dysfunction. *A-II*, angiotensin II; *VSM*, vascular smooth muscle.

Regarding nitric oxide, a new concept is that oxidative stress promotes the formation of peroxynitrite, thereby consuming vasodilatory nitric oxide (32). The proposed major source of oxidative stress is the nicotinamide adenine dinucleotide phosphate (reduced form) oxidase system in vascular tissue (Fig. 14-17). This responds to both the enhanced formation of A-II (33), common in hypertension, and a direct mechanical effect of increased intravascular pressure (32). Hypothetically, either the hypertension could cause the endothelial dysfunction, or the latter could promote hypertension, so that there can be a vicious circle involving the endothelium and increasing BP (Fig. 14-16).

LIFESTYLE AND BLOOD PRESSURE

In addition to genetic and other predisposing factors, some aspects of the lifestyle can contribute to the development of hypertension. Obesity is often associated with essential hypertension, possibly acting through insulin resistance. In population studies, increasing dietary salt is associated with increasing BPs. Excess alcohol (more than two or three drinks per day) provokes hypertension, possibly by release of aldehydes that stimulate the adrenergic system. Although regular smoking does not alter resting DBP, ambulatory BP measurements show that smoking, via vasoconstrictive effects, is likely to increase BP swings. Emotional stress promotes temporary BP increases and could contribute to the development of hypertension. Stress may also act indirectly via excess smoking, especially with much caffeine, lack of exercise, and poor nutrition.

Conversely, endurance exercise training by regular isotonic aerobic exercise may help to reduce resting BP in addition to promoting weight reduction, a sense of well-being, and decreasing cardiovascular disease risk. Such training enhances vagal activity to produce the cardiac vagal phenotype (34), reducing heart rate and generally decreasing BP. A monastic environment also protects. Nuns living in a stress-free environment characterized by silence, meditation, and isolation from society avoid the otherwise inevitable increase of BP with age (35).

CARDIAC COMPLICATIONS OF HYPERTENSION

Whatever its cause, hypertension significantly increases both morbidity and mortality. The incidence of coronary artery disease, stroke, and renal dysfunction is increased. There is no simple relationship between arterial BP level and the complications of hypertension, except for BP and stroke. All vital organs can be affected except those protected by special circulations such as the liver and lungs. Cardiovascular complications are as follows.

Left ventricular hypertrophy is the consequence of a sustained pressure overload. It is often associated with diastolic dysfunction, which is not the same as systolic failure with congestive heart failure, which may be the result of sustained overload (Chapter 16). Another disadvantage of left ventricular hypertrophy is that the coronary vascular reserve is diminished, possibly the result of endothelial dysfunction. The complex signaling events underlying left ventricular hypertrophy are considered in Chapter 13.

Coronary artery disease is the most common cause of death in patients with hypertension in the Western world. BP lowering in trials has not given the expected reduction in coronary disease, perhaps because its multifactorial etiology would mandate simultaneous reduction of blood lipids and smoking cessation.

Coronary endothelial dysfunction can occur even in the absence of angiographically visible coronary disease as shown by the decreased coronary dilation in response to exercise in patients with hypertension (36).

Aortic aneurysm is often preceded by marked aortic unfolding. It presence indicates a marked loss of aortic elasticity and therefore increased afterload on the heart. Other vascular complications include the spectrum of cerebrovascular disease and renal artery stenosis.

SUMMARY

1. *Baroreflexes are high-pressure mechanoreceptors* that are important in the acute buffering of BP changes. For example, an acute increase in BP evokes a baroreflex-mediated decrease in cardiac output and decrease in PVR as a result of increased vagal and decreased sympathetic outflows.
2. *Low-pressure cardiopulmonary receptors* react to changes in blood volume by altering the autonomic discharge rate in such a way that fluid overload is

accompanied by decreased PVR, with converse changes when the blood volume is too low and the receptors are not normally stimulated.
3. *Renin–angiotensin system.* Both high- and low-pressure receptors couple to the renin–angiotensin system. During acute hypertension or fluid overload, the adrenergic discharge rate, PVR, and release of renin from the kidneys decrease. Conversely, during hypotension or when a circulating blood volume is too low, increased adrenergic discharge induces a β_1-adrenergic–mediated release of renin, which leads to increased A-II and peripheral vasoconstriction. A-II increases BP by multiple mechanisms beyond peripheral vasoconstriction, including adrenergic facilitation and baroreflex inhibition.
4. *PVR is an important regulator of BP.* Vasoconstriction or vasodilation by altering the PVR increases or decreases BP because BP = cardiac output × PVR. PVR is regulated by at least three factors: (a) autonomic control with α_1-adrenergic–mediated constriction in contrast to vagally or β_2- adrenergic–mediated vasodilation, (b) vasoconstrictive neurohormones such as A-II, and (c) endothelial control (vasoconstrictive endothelin versus vasodilatory nitric oxide).
5. *Hypertension is a state of chronically elevated BP,* usually multifactorial in origin, with increased cardiac output playing an important role in younger subjects and increased PVR being more important in the older group.
6. *The aorta has a dual role in relation to BP control.* First and physiologically, it is an important part of afterload, which is therefore not only composed of PVR and reflected in BP. Second, systolic hypertension in the elderly is the direct result of decreased compliance of the aorta.
7. *Role of endothelium.* Although no simple relationship exists between circulating endothelin levels and chronic hypertension, an attractive hypothesis is that the mechanical strains imposed by the high intravascular pressure could damage the endothelium to release more endothelin and less nitric oxide. This change may help to explain the progression of untreated hypertension with time.

STUDENT QUESTIONS

1. Outline the major differences in the regulation of the contraction in the myocardium and in vascular smooth muscle.
2. Describe the defense mechanisms of the body against hypotension.
3. What is the Poiseuille law? Describe how operation of this law could influence the BP.
4. Describe in detail how PVR increases in response to standing.
5. What changes may be found in afterload in chronic arterial hypertension?

CARDIOLOGIST-IN-TRAINING QUESTIONS

1. What is the neurogenic theory for hypertension? How can it explain the increase in PVR with age, as found in patients with hypertension?

2. When a subject enters a cold environment, the BP increases. Describe in detail the physiologic changes involved.
3. Why does the SBP increase with age, but the DBP tends to remain the same? What is the reason for the characteristic pattern of the peripheral pulse in the elderly?
4. In patients with hypertension, there may be impaired coronary vascular dilation. Why is this?
5. Describe the role of the renin–angiotensin system in BP control.

REFERENCES

1. Kaplan NM. *Clinical hypertension*, 7th ed. Baltimore: Williams & Wilkins, 1998.
2. Giles TD. Defining the role of atrial natriuretic factor in health and disease. *J Am Coll Cardiol* 1990;15:1331–1333.
3. Kappagoda CT, et al. The nature of the atrial receptors responsible for a reflex increase in heart rate in the dog. *J Physiol* 1979;291:393–412.
4. Vatner SF, Boettcher DH. Regulation of cardiac output by stroke volume and heart rate in conscious dogs. *Circ Res* 1978;42:557–561.
5. Reid IA. Angiotensin-II and baroreflex control of heart rate. *News Physiol Sci* 1996;11:270–274.
6. Herring N, et al. Natriuretic peptides, like NO, facilitate cardiac vagal neurotransmission and bradycardia via a cGMP pathway. *Am J Physiol* 2001;281:H2318–H2327.
7. Kurihara Y, Kurihara H, Suzuki H, et al. Elevated blood pressure and craniofacial abnormalities in mice deficient in endothelin-1. *Nature* 1994;368:703–710.
8. Edwards G, et al. K+ is an endothelium-derived hyperpolarizing factor in rat arteries. *Nature* 1998; 396:269–272.
9. Strandgaard S. Autoregulation of cerebral blood flow in hypertensive patients. The modifying influence of prolonged antihypertensive treatment on the tolerance to acute, drug-induced hypotension. *Circulation* 1976;53:720–727.
10. Blythe WB. Captopril and renal autoregulation. *N Engl J Med* 1983;308:390–391.
11. Ohkubo T, et al. Reference values for 24-hour ambulatory blood pressure monitoring based on a prognostic criterion. The Ohasama Study. *Hypertension* 1998;32:255–259.
12. Spieker LE, et al. Mental stress induces prolonged endothelial dysfunction via endothelin-A receptors. *Circulation* 2002;105:2817–2820.
13. Cockcroft JR, et al. β_2-Adrenoceptor polymorphism determines vascular reactivity in humans. *Hypertension* 2000;36:371–375.
14. Dietz NM, et al. Evidence for nitric oxide-mediated sympathetic forearm vasodilatation in humans. *J Physiol* 1997;498:531–540.
15. Mosqueda-Garcia R, et al. The elusive pathophysiology of neurally mediated syncope. *Circulation* 2000;102:2898–2906.
16. Rowell LB. *Human circulation, regulation during physical stress*. New York: Oxford University Press, 1986.
17. Lund-Johansen P. Twenty-year follow up of hemodynamics in essential hypertension during rest and exercise. *Hypertension* 1991;18:54–61.
18. Kuwajima I, Hoh E, Suzuki Y, et al. Pseudohypertension in the elderly. *J Hypertens* 1990;8:429–432.
19. Eaton GM, Cody RJ, Binkley PF. Increased aortic impedance precedes peripheral vasoconstriction at the early stage of ventricular failure int he paced canine model. *Circulation* 1993;88:2714–2721.
20. Vasan RS, et al. Impact of high-normal blood pressure on the risk of cardiovascular disease. *N Engl J Med* 2001;345:1291–1297.
21. Zanchetti A, Mancia G. Cardiovascular reflexes and hypertension. *Hypertension* 1991;18:III-13–III-21.
22. Julius S, Nesbitt S. Sympathetic overactivity in hypertension. A moving target. *Am J Hypertens* 1996; 9:113S–120S.
23. Stanley WC, Hall JL, Smith KR, et al. Myocardial glucose transporters and glycolytic metabolism during ischemia in hyperglycaemic diabetic swine. *Metabolism* 1994;43:61–69.

24. Weinberger MH, Fineberg NS, Fineberg SE, et al. Salt sensitivity, pulse pressure, and death in normal and hypertensive humans. *Hypertension* 2001;37:429–432.
25. Baker EH, et al. Transepithelial sodium absorption is increased in people of African origin. *Hypertension* 2001;38:76–80.
26. Hall JE, Zappe DH, Alonso-Galicia M, et al. Mechanisms of obesity-induced hypertension. *News Physiol Sci* 1996;11:255–261.
27. Reaven G, Lithell H, Landsberg L. Hypertension and associated metabolic abnormalities—the role of insulin resistance and the sympathoadrenal system. *N Engl J Med* 1996;334:374–381.
28. Meehan WP, Buchanan TA, Hsueh W. Chronic insulin administration elevates blood pressure in rats. *Hypertension* 1994;23:1012–1017.
29. Jamerson KA, Smith SD, Amerena JV, et al. Vasoconstriction with norepinephrine causes less forearm insulin resistance than a reflex sympathetic vasoconstriction. *Hypertension* 1994;23:1006–1011.
30. Cardillo C, et al. Improved endothelium-dependent vasodilation after blockade of endothelin receptors in patients with essential hypertension. *Circulation* 2002;105:452–456.
31. Schiffrin EL. Endothelin: potential role in hypertension and vascular hypertrophy. *Hypertension* 1995;25:1135–1143.
32. Sowers JR. Hypertension, angiotensin II, and oxidative stress. *N Engl J Med* 2002;346:1999–2001.
33. Griendling KK, et al. Angiotensin II stimulates NADH and NADPH oxidase activity in cultured vascular smooth muscle cells. *Circ Res* 1994;74:1141–1148.
34. Danson EJ, Paterson DJ. Enhanced neuronal nitric oxide synthase expression is central to cardiac vagal phenotype in exercise-trained mice. *J Physiol* 2003;546:225–232.
35. Timio M, Verdecchia P, Venanzi S, et al. Age and blood pressure changes. A 20-year follow-up study in nuns in a secluded order. *Hypertension* 1988;12:457–461.
36. Frielingsdorf J, Seiler C, Kaufmann P, et al. Normalization of abnormal coronary vasomotion by calcium antagonists in patients with hypertension. *Circulation* 1996;93:1380–1387.
37. Parati G, et al. Cardiovascular effects of an earthquake. Direct evidence by ambulatory blood pressure monitoring. *Hypertension* 2001;38:1093–1095.
38. Blair DA, Glover WE, Greenfield ADM, et al. Excitation of cholinergic vasodilator nerves to human skeletal muscles during emotional stress. *J Physiol* 1959;148:633–647.

15

Cardiac Output and Exercise

Lionel H. Opie and David J. Paterson

"The heart has a marvellous power of adjusting its output of mechanical energy...to the work which is imposed on it by the mechanical conditions of the circulation."

Starling (1)

Cardiac output is the volume of blood pumped by the heart. During dynamic exercise (e.g., running), the increase in cardiac output is obligatory, otherwise the exercising myocardium and skeletal muscle cannot obtain the required oxygen and nutrients. During emotional stress, the increase in cardiac output is not essential but a physiologic side effect of sympathetic stimulation.

The definition of cardiac output is the product of stroke volume (SV) and heart rate (HR): cardiac output $(\dot{Q})$ = SV × HR (units = liters per minute). The normal value is approximately 6 to 8 L/min, doubling or sometimes even tripling during peak aerobic exercise. An Olympic athlete might reach 25 L/min. Of the four major factors determining cardiac output (Fig. 15-1), the most important during exercise is the heart rate. The other three factors, i.e., preload, afterload, and contractile state of the myocardium, all influence stroke volume (for definitions, see Table 15-1).

During dynamic exercise, increased heart rate provides most of the adaptation (Fig. 15-2). In addition, there is increased venous return, which acts by the Frank–Starling mechanism, and increased contractility, which increases the stroke volume. Regarding afterload, systolic blood pressure (BP) increases during exercise despite peripheral vasodilation. Thus, the healthy heart can readily deal with all the hemodynamic changes occurring during exercise. In contrast, the failing myocardium cannot cope with increased peripheral resistance that results from angiotensin II and other vasoconstrictors.

There are important conceptual distinctions between increased cardiac output and increased work of the heart, although these two entities are easy to confuse. Increased cardiac output is the result of greater external cardiac work, whereas internal work can be greatly increased, as occurs with hypertrophied myocardium, without an obligatory increase in external work. When the work of the heart

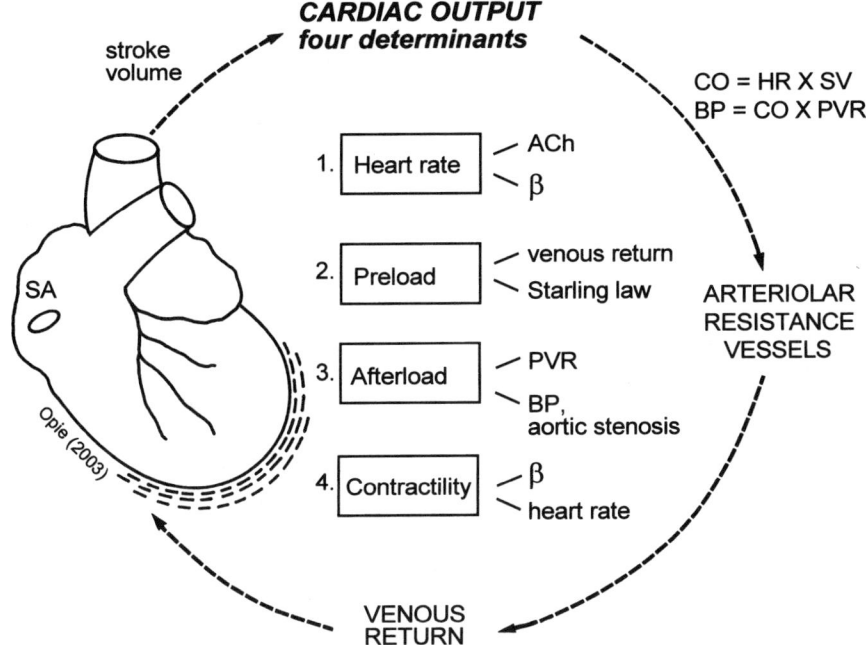

FIG. 15-1. Major factors regulating cardiac output (*CO*). Heart rate (*HR*) is regulated mainly by the relative input of cholinergic (*ACh*) and β-adrenergic (*β*) stimulation. Preload is regulated by venous return and also increases when the left ventricle fails to empty fully. Afterload increases when peripheral vascular resistance (*PVR*) increases or when there is aortic stenosis. Contractility increases with β-adrenergic stimulation or with increased fiber lengths. *SV*, stroke volume; *BP*, blood pressure; *PVR*, peripheral vascular resistance.

increases considerably during isometric exercise, cardiac output increases relatively little. Another conspicuous difference between heart work and cardiac output is found in the failing heart, which is afterload dependent (Chapter 16). In this serious situation, further increases in the peripheral resistance decrease cardiac output even though the work of the heart is increased. In other words, the oxygen

TABLE 15-1. *Definition of determinants of cardiac output*

Term	Definition
Heart rate	Number of heart beats per minute (complete cardiac cycle)
Preload	Left ventricular volume at the end of diastole; this is frequently approximated as the left ventricular end-diastolic pressure, assuming normal compliance and pressure–volume relationship
Afterload	Resistance against the ejection of blood, including the peripheral vascular resistance, any aortic valve stenosis, the aortic impedance, and the blood distending the left ventricle at the end of diastole
Contractility	Inherent capacity of the myocardium to contract independently of changes in preload and afterload

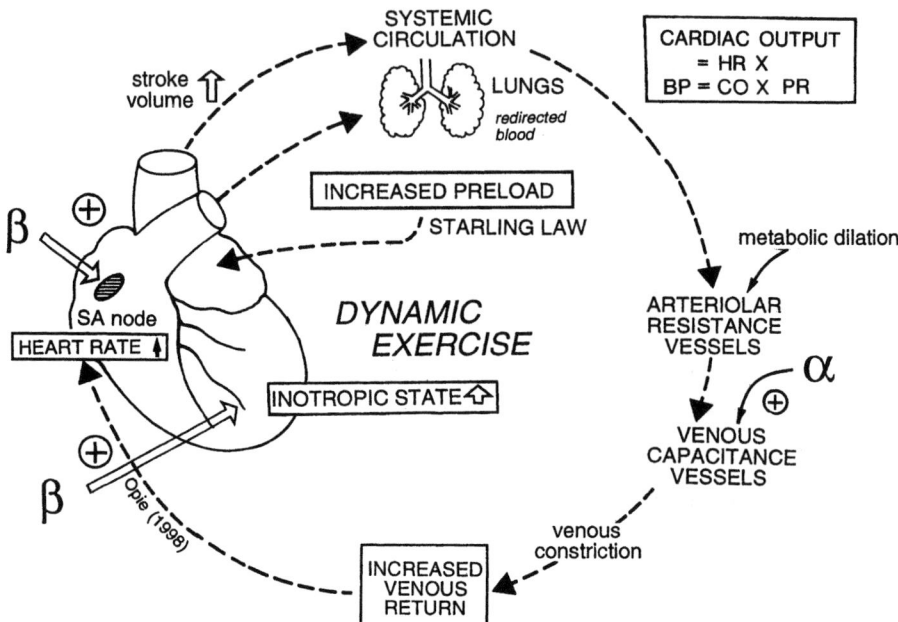

FIG. 15-2. Effects of dynamic exercise on circulation. The major factor in increased cardiac output of dynamic exercise is tachycardia, with contributions from increased preload (Starling mechanism) and increased inotropic state (contractility). β-Adrenergic stimulation (β) increases heart rate (HR) and the inotropic state. α-Adrenergic stimulation (α) contracts venous capacitance vessels to increase venous return and to redirect blood from the abdominal organs to the lungs (11). CO, cardiac output; PR, peripheral resistance.

demand increases even though cardiac output decreases. These distinctions emphasize the potential differences between the effects of increased cardiac output and increased heart work on the myocardial oxygen uptake.

HEART RATE AND CARDIAC OUTPUT

During dynamic exercise, the maximal heart rate that can be reached is given by the following arbitrary but widely used formula: maximal heart rate = 220 beats/min − age in years. Two other physiologic factors most consistently increasing heart rate and hence cardiac output are waking up in the morning and emotional stress, both of which are associated with increased β-adrenergic stimulation.

Each cycle of contraction and relaxation performs a specific amount of work and takes up a specific amount of oxygen. The faster the heart rate is, the greater the cardiac output and oxygen uptake are (Table 15-2). Exceptions occur (a) when the heart rate is extremely fast, as may occur during paroxysmal tachycar-

TABLE 15-2. *Factors increasing the heart rate, cardiac output, and the myocardial oxygen uptake*

β-Adrenergic stimulation
  Exercise
  Emotional stress
  Early morning increase in heart rate
Decreased vagal inhibition
  Early morning increase in heart rate
  Initiation of exercise
Disease states
  Cardiac conditions (cardiac output may not increase): congestive heart failure, arrhythmias, acute myocardial infarction
  Extracardiac conditions influencing the heart: thyrotoxicosis
  Fevers
Drug-induced tachycardia
  Sympathomimetic drugs such as bronchodilators (cardiac β_2-receptors)
  Vasodilators (reflex tachycardia, β_2-agonists)

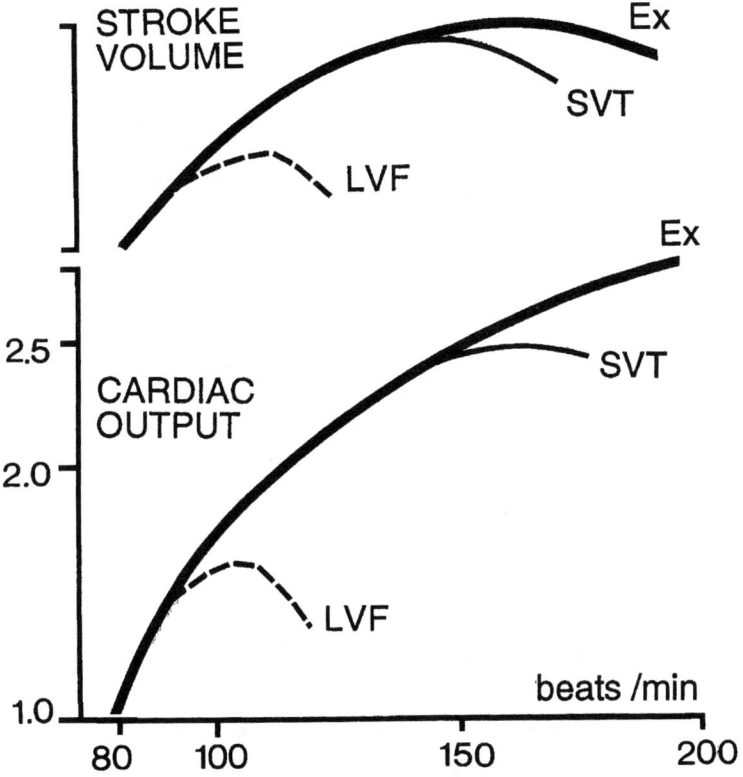

FIG. 15-3. Effect of heart rate on stroke volume and cardiac output. During dynamic exercise (*Ex*), an initial increase in stroke volume is followed by a near-plateau and then a small decline. Note the steep increase in cardiac output with only slight leveling off at maximal heart rates, despite the decrease in stroke volume, associated with a decreasing PVR (Fig. 15-2). In supraventricular tachycardia (*SVT*), in the absence of the adrenergic stimulation and peripheral dilation found in exercise, stroke volume and cardiac output both decrease because of decreased diastolic filling time. In subjects with left ventricular failure (*LVF*), there is a rapid decline in both stroke volume and cardiac output. Data for dynamic exercise adapted from Flamm et al. (11). Curves for SVT and LVF are hypothetical.

dia because an inadequate time for diastolic filling decreases cardiac output, (b) in the presence of coronary artery disease when less severe tachycardia decreases the stroke volume because of transient ischemic failure of the left ventricle, or (c) in left ventricular failure, when cardiac output increases only transiently before decreasing (Fig. 15-3).

Effects of Heart Rate on Cardiac Output

The heart rate can have both positive and negative influences on cardiac output (Fig. 15-3). In nonexercising normal subjects, an initial increase in heart rate by the sudden onset of supraventricular tachycardia yields the expected increase in cardiac output. Thereafter, the increase in heart rate is balanced by a decrease in stroke volume as the time for ventricular filling decreases, producing a flat, nearly plateau phase. As the heart rate increases even more, the diastolic filling time is even shorter and cardiac output decreases. In myocardial failure, the onset of the downward slope (Fig. 15-3) occurs much sooner, so that any plateau is lost. In dynamic exercise, in contrast, for any given heart rate, there is greater cardiac output, probably because of the accompanying adrenergic stimulation with an increase in contractility and with peripheral vasodilation (2). As the heart rate reaches extreme values (e.g., more than 170 beats per minute), cardiac output still increases but the stroke volume decreases.

Mechanism of Tachycardia of Exercise

During dynamic exercise in humans, increased heart rate provides most of the increased cardiac output. An initial withdrawal of vagal tone increases the heart rate from approximately 70 to approximately 110 beats per minute, and then augmented adrenergic drive develops so that the heart rate may double (Fig. 15-3). The signals for these changes come from the vasomotor center in the brainstem, which coordinates several types of input: the first is from a central command from the cerebral cortex (e.g., the runner's "readiness to go" at the start of exercise), the second arises from the exercising muscles (3), and the third is from the baroreceptors. The tachycardia-producing Bainbridge reflex (Fig. 14-4) is very weak in humans, theoretically stimulated by the increased venous return of exercise.

Adrenergic Outflow and Transplants

Increased β-adrenergic receptor stimulation is basic to the tachycardia of exercise. In dogs with cardiac denervation (4) or in humans after cardiac transplantation, the heart rate can still increase during vigorous exercise, although it does so more slowly and less than in controls because there is no vagal withdrawal. Increased circulating, rather than locally released, catecholamines are the major stimulus to the tachycardia. Overall, increased stroke volume is the major adaptation to exercise in those with transplants.

Force–Frequency Relationship

The tachycardia of exercise gives an added, albeit modest, positive inotropic effect by the Bowditch phenomenon (Fig. 12-8) whereby the force of ventricular contraction progressively increases even in an isolated papillary muscle preparation (Bowditch staircase phenomenon). In isolated human ventricular strips, increasing the stimulation rate from 60 to approximately 160 beats per minute enhances force development (Fig. 12-12). In samples from failing hearts, there is no such increase. Note that a persistently excessively high heart rate will decrease rather than increase force development, with eventual risk of tachycardiomyopathy (Chapter 16).

Other Major Determinants of Cardiac Output

Preload

During exercise, the left ventricular end-diastolic volume increases, which strongly suggests that the Frank–Starling mechanism also contributes to the increased cardiac output of dynamic exercise (5). Venous return must equal cardiac output, the latter increasing with the onset of exercise as the heart rate increases. Additional venous return may originate from redistribution of blood, for example, that squeezed out from the exercising skeletal muscles or redirected from the abdominal organs. As the venous return increases, the right atrial pressure increases and stroke volume increases in part by the Frank–Starling mechanism (5). Increased depth of breathing will reduce the intrathoracic pressure and help the venous return to flow to the right atrium.

Afterload

In general, when afterload decreases, cardiac output increases. Physiologic examples of this principle exist during peripheral vasodilation induced by a hot bath, sauna, or a meal (6). In these conditions, however, there is also accompanying tachycardia, such as during drug-induced vasodilation. Conversely, when afterload increases acutely, there is initially a compensatory mechanism to maintain the stroke volume, as originally described by Starling (Fig. 12-7). Presumably there is stretch-induced increased calcium entry into the myocytes. If the afterload is suddenly and excessively increased, then acute heart failure can be precipitated (e.g., during acute rupture of one of the cardiac valves). If afterload is chronically increased as in systemic hypertension, then compensatory ventricular hypertrophy will develop.

During dynamic exercise, there is marked peripheral arteriolar vasodilation with increased blood flow (exercise hyperemia) to the exercising muscles. Both autonomic and local metabolic factors are involved. Normally, α-mediated vasoconstriction contributes to the resting arteriolar tone. During exercise, the increased venous return acts via the low-pressure receptors (Fig. 14-4) to lessen

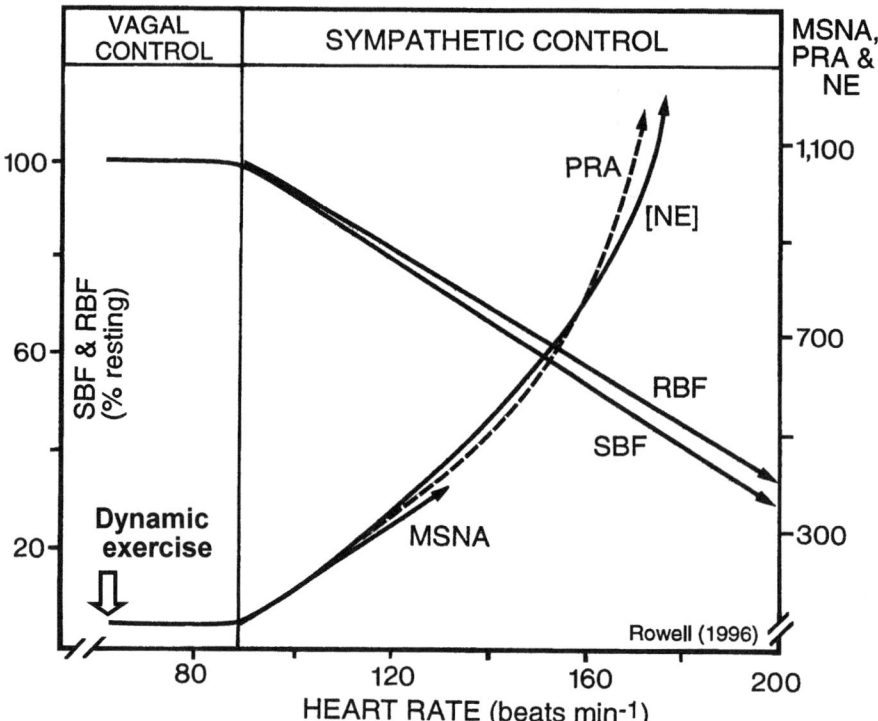

FIG. 15-4. Effects of dynamic exercise on vagal and sympathetic control. When the heart rate approaches 100 beats per minutes, vagal withdrawal is nearly complete and sympathetic effects start. There is an increase in circulating norepinephrine (*NE*) and plasma renin activity (*PRA*) and in directly measured muscle sympathetic nerve activity (*MSNA*). Concurrently, there are decreases in splanchnic blood flow (*SBF*) and renal blood flow (*RBF*). (Modified from Rowell LR, et al. Integration of cardiovascular control systems in dynamic exercise. In: Rowell LB, et al., eds. *Handbook of physiology. Section 12.* New York: Oxford University Press, 1996:730–838.)

peripheral vasoconstriction. As exercise increases in intensity, other vasoconstrictive factors such as angiotensin II and neuropeptide Y come into play (Fig. 15-4). Metabolic products of exercise lead first to inhibition of the distal α_2-mediated vasoconstriction in the smaller arterioles, and then at more intense levels of exercise to relief of α_1-mediated control of the larger arterioles (7).

Simultaneous β_2-mediated vasodilation, in response to increased circulating levels of epinephrine, probably also contributes. The magnitude of this vasodilator β-mediated response is determined by genetic polymorphism of the β-adrenoceptor (8). Vasodilation is also mediated by vasodilatory metabolites including formation of adenosine and others such as protons, carbon dioxide, and potassium. Vasodilatory nitric oxide is formed in vascular endothelium in response to increased blood flow. Nitric oxide also increases the glucose uptake of exercising skeletal muscle by activating the GLUT-4 transporter (Fig. 11-7) (9).

Cardiac Contractility

An enhanced β-adrenergic–mediated contractile state contributes to increased cardiac output during exercise, as shown by a decreased end-systolic volume (5). Conversely, during congestive heart failure or therapy with β-adrenergic blockade, decreased contractility means decreased stroke volume.

Measurement of Cardiac Output

The *Fick principle* has been the classic method for deriving cardiac output. The arteriovenous difference of oxygen is obtained by arterial puncture and a mixed central venous sample. The oxygen uptake is determined by spirometry. Cardiac output is the volume of blood needed to account for the oxygen uptake. The defect of this procedure is its invasive nature. Its advantage is its accuracy, especially in determining low cardiac outputs.

Thermodilution is part of the invasive technique of Swan–Ganz catheterization (Fig. 16-13). A known amount of ice-cold saline is injected into the central venous circulation. The rate of temperature decrease at the tip of the catheter further along depends on the cardiac output.

Angiographic techniques depend on determination of stroke volume (end-diastolic minus end-systolic image gives stroke volume, which, multiplied by heart rate, gives cardiac output).

Doppler determinations of cardiac output have the great advantage of being noninvasive, but not as accurate as invasive techniques. An ultrasound beam is directed at the stream of blood passing through the mitral valve. The signal returning to the sound-receiving crystal is shifted in frequency in response to the velocity of flow. The area of the mitral valve orifice is determined by two-dimensional echocardiography. Cardiac output is calculated from the mean velocity of the blood flow and the diastolic mitral valve area. Using such techniques, cardiac output during exercise can increase from the normal resting value of 6 to 7 L/min to 14 L/min during mild exercise and 25 L/min during severe exercise in the highly trained athlete. In congestive heart failure, cardiac output is low (Fig. 15-3), resulting in inadequate tissue perfusion during exercise. In cardiogenic shock (as in severe myocardial infarction), cardiac output is so low that the tissues are inadequately perfused even at rest, and life is threatened.

DYNAMIC VERSUS STATIC EXERCISE

In general, when the heart rate increases, so does cardiac output, the work of the heart, and myocardial oxygen uptake. The latter is governed by two major factors: heart rate and wall stress (reflecting preload and afterload) (Fig. 15-5). Metabolically, when the oxygen uptake is increased, the mitochondrial metabolic rate has increased with greater production of ATP, the latter being increasingly converted to adenosine 5′-diphosphate (ADP) as the

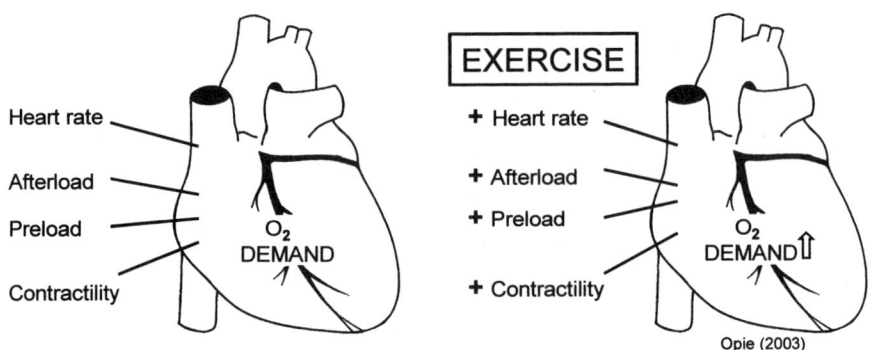

FIG. 15-5. Effect of exercise on myocardial oxygen demand. Determinants of the demand can be related to the load on the heart (wall stress), heart rate, and contractility.

heart work increases (Fig. 15-6). The greater amount of ADP drives the mitochondrial metabolism. Several clinical indices indirectly reflect the oxygen uptake (Table 15-3).

The two contrasting types of exercise, dynamic and static, have different consequences on these parameters (Fig. 15-7). Dynamic exercise (aerobic or isotonic) includes running, walking, and related sports, in which regular muscular activity occurs but against a light load. During dynamic running, the heart rate increases owing to an early withdrawal of the normal vagal inhibition followed by β-adrenergic stimulation. The latter also increases contractility. Cardiac output increases substantially because both heart rate and stroke volume increase (Fig. 15-8). The total peripheral resistance decreases as a result of exercise-induced metabolic dilation of arterioles in skeletal muscle, so that the diastolic BP decreases to a variable extent. In contrast, the systolic BP increases because increased contractility means that the blood is ejected more rapidly from the left ventricle to hit the elasticity of the major blood vessels, which expand more to accommodate the systolic pressure. There is concurrent splanchnic vasoconstriction, so that the distribution of cardiac output changes away from the abdominal viscera to the exercising muscles and the heart.

Static (isometric) exercise includes activities such as carrying a suitcase or weight lifting, in which muscle tension develops, but there is little or no displacement of the object worked against. Both systolic and diastolic BPs increase, with only a modest increase in heart rate (Fig. 15-8). Stroke volume is unchanged, so that cardiac output increases only in proportion to the heart rate. Peripheral vascular resistance (PVR) increases relatively little at low loads with increases at high loads. The increase in BP is accounted for by a combination of the increase in cardiac output and *pressor ergoreflexes* originating in the exer-

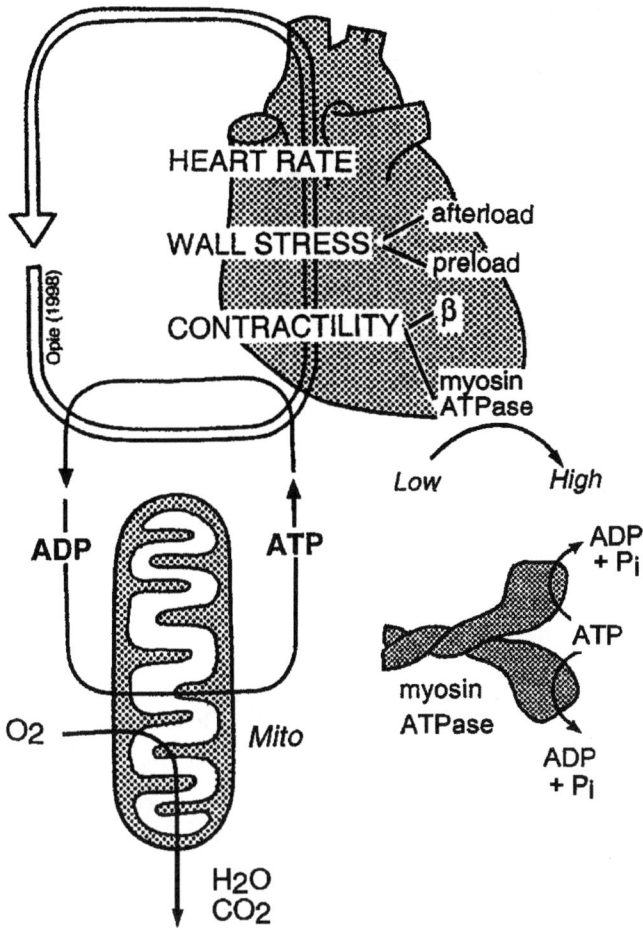

FIG. 15-6. Myocardial oxygen demand induces metabolic changes. Mitochondrial metabolism increases to augment oxygen uptake. The link between the determinants of oxygen demand and oxygen uptake by the mitochondria is the breakdown of adenosine 5′-triphosphate to adenosine 5′-diphosphate. The latter is an important signal for mitochondrial (*mito*) oxygen uptake.

cising muscles. The latter appear most active at higher intensities of static exercise (3). All these factors increase the myocardial oxygen demand during static exercise relatively more than the increase in the amount of external work performed. In contrast, during dynamic exercise, the large increase in heart rate causes both oxygen uptake and cardiac output to increase substantially, as does the external work.

TABLE 15-3. Some indices of myocardial oxygen uptake[a]

Index	Advantage	Comment
Heart rate	Extremely simple	Fairly good correlation[b]
Double product[b] Rate × pressure Systolic pressure × heart rate	Noninvasive, easy	No allowance for contractile state
Triple product[a] Above × systolic ejection time	Noninvasive, more difficult	Some allowance for contractile state
Time–tension index[a]	Little advantage, requires invasive methods	Should be called "time–pressure" index; little used
Pressure–volume area[c]	Direct from pressure–volume loop, requiring no assumptions	Clinically validated in humans but is invasive
Pressure–work index[d] of (SBP × HR × SV)	Noninvasive approximation	Should strictly be the integral pressure and flow during ejection period

[a]For cautions, see reference 9a.
[b-d]See references 9b–9d.
SBP, systolic blood pressure; HR, heart rate; SV, stroke volume.

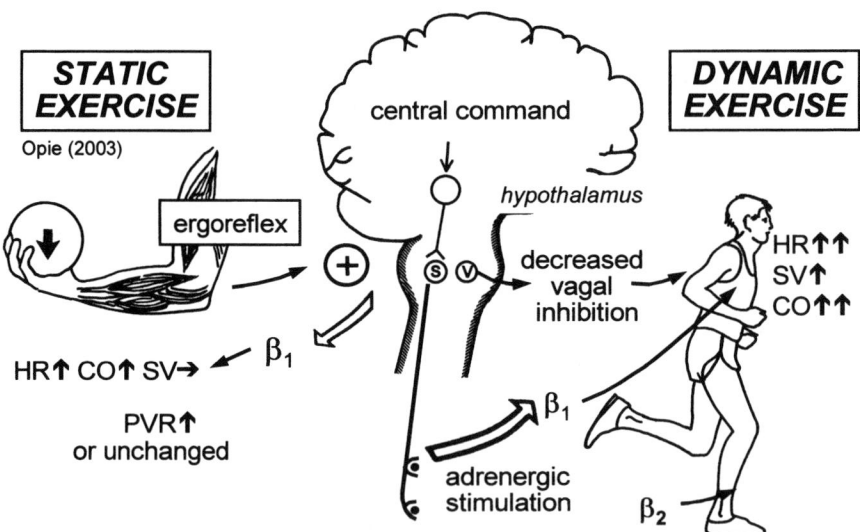

FIG. 15-7. Central integration and exercise-induced reflexes. Central command plays a major role in both dynamic and static exercise. During static exercise, ergoreflexes from the exercising muscle become more important. During dynamic exercise, central command leads to increased adrenergic and decreased vagal activity. The cartoon of static exercise (on the left) is modeled on Shepherd et al. (17). *HR*, heart rate; *CO*, cardiac output; *SV*, stroke volume; *PVR*, peripheral vascular resistance; β_1, β_1-adrenergic; *S*, sympathetic nucleus; *V*, vagal parasympathetic nucleus. For nucleus solitarius, see Figure 2-10.

15. CARDIAC OUTPUT AND EXERCISE   471

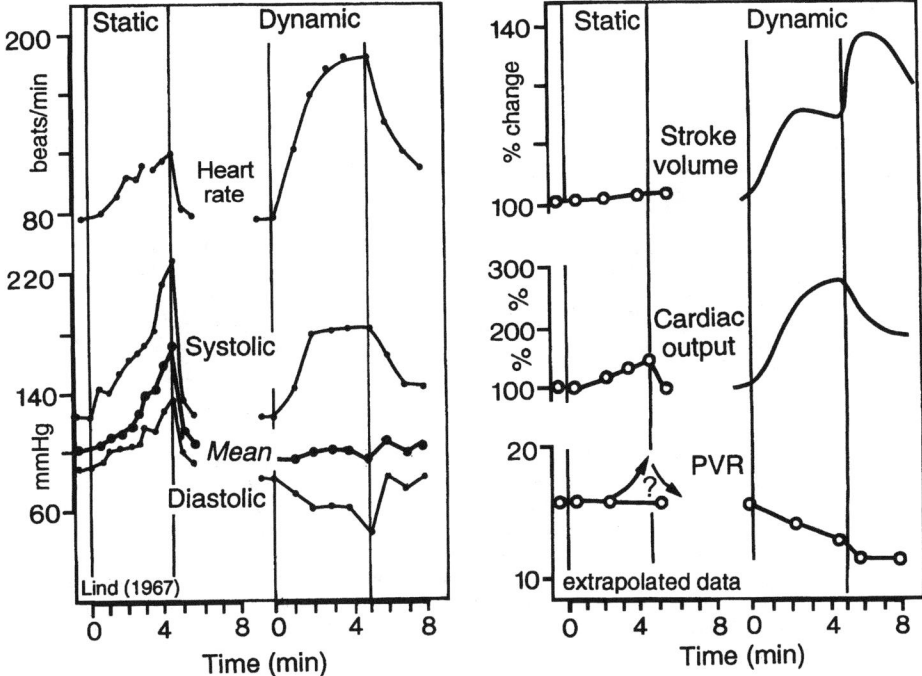

FIG. 15-8. Static versus dynamic exercise: hemodynamics. Static exercise at 30% of maximal voluntary contraction caused a much greater increase in systolic and mean blood pressures than did dynamic exercise, first at oxygen consumption values of 28.5 mL/kg/min and then at 43.8 mL/kg/min. Conversely, dynamic exercise increased heart rate much more. For original data, see Lind and McNicol (42). Data on stroke volume are extrapolated from Flamm et al. (11). Peripheral vascular resistance (*PVR*) for 0 to 2 minutes is based on Waldrop et al. (43) and for 2 to 4 minutes on Lind and McNicol (42), in which blood pressure increases markedly at 2 to 4 minutes of static exercise even when the increase in heart rate has leveled off; therefore, PVR must have increased.

Pressure–Volume Loops

Dynamic exercise and static exercise also have contrasting effects on the pressure–volume (PV) loop (Fig. 15-9). The greatly increased venous return of dynamic exercise increases the preload, whereas the increased contractility displaces upward the end-systolic point E_s. Thus, the increase in external work is great and that in internal work is small. Note that, as reviewed in Chapter 12, internal work is more correctly termed potential energy. Static exercise greatly increases afterload (see BP and PVR in Figure 15-8), so that inefficient internal work increases. Thus, static work is much more oxygen-demanding than might be expected. During dynamic exercise, the major adaptation is the increased heart rate. In addition, there are changes in the PV loop. Both systolic and diastolic components of the PV loop enlarge to increase the external work (Fig. 15-9). In

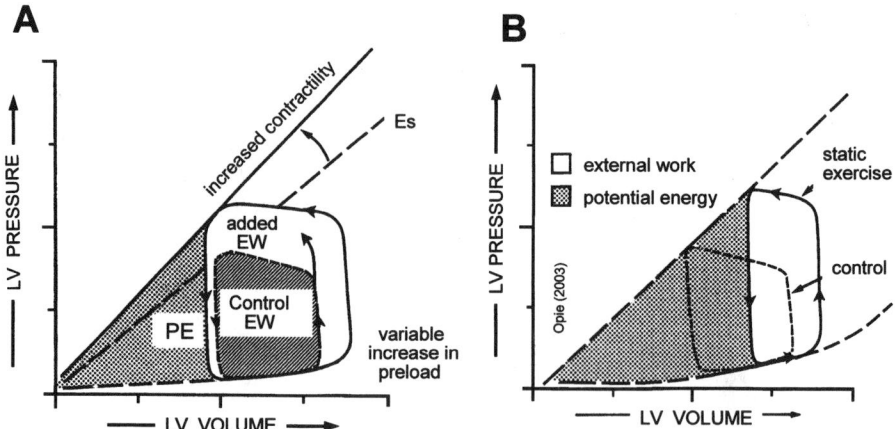

FIG. 15-9. Dynamic versus static exercise: effects on the pressure–volume loop. During dynamic exercise, sympathetic stimulation increases contractility to displace the end-systolic pressure–volume relationship (E_s). The much greater venous return increases preload to a variable extent, depending on the posture and the contractile response (for the horizontal dog, see Figure 15-10). The result is that external work is increased relatively more than work spent on potential energy (PE, *stippled area*). During static exercise, afterload greatly increases (see blood pressure and peripheral vascular resistance in Figure 15-8), so that more oxygen is inefficiently spent on generating potential energy. See also contrasting effects of volume and pressure work (Fig. 12-15).

addition, the early diastolic part of the PV loop moves downward (Fig. 15-10), so that in the exercising dog, left ventricular filling increases even without an increase in left atrial pressure (10). The mechanism involved is complex and associated with sympathetic stimulation and tachycardia. This exercise-induced change in the PV loop means that much more external work is being done during exercise, but slightly less internal work, which resembles the effects of β-adrenergic stimulation.

Posture

Thus, at really high rates of upright exercise, stroke volume begins to decrease even though cardiac output continues to increase, the latter as a result of heart rate increases (11). In congestive heart failure with a failing left ventricle, the stage at which stroke volume starts to decrease is much earlier than with the normal left ventricle (Fig. 15-3). The erect position, when compared with the supine, decreases venous return, so that at rest there is lower left ventricular end-diastolic pressure, lower stroke volume, and higher heart rate (12). In these circumstances, increased venous return could be expected to play a more major role than in recumbent exercise. In practice, the difference between upright and recumbent exercise is modest, and the major adaptation

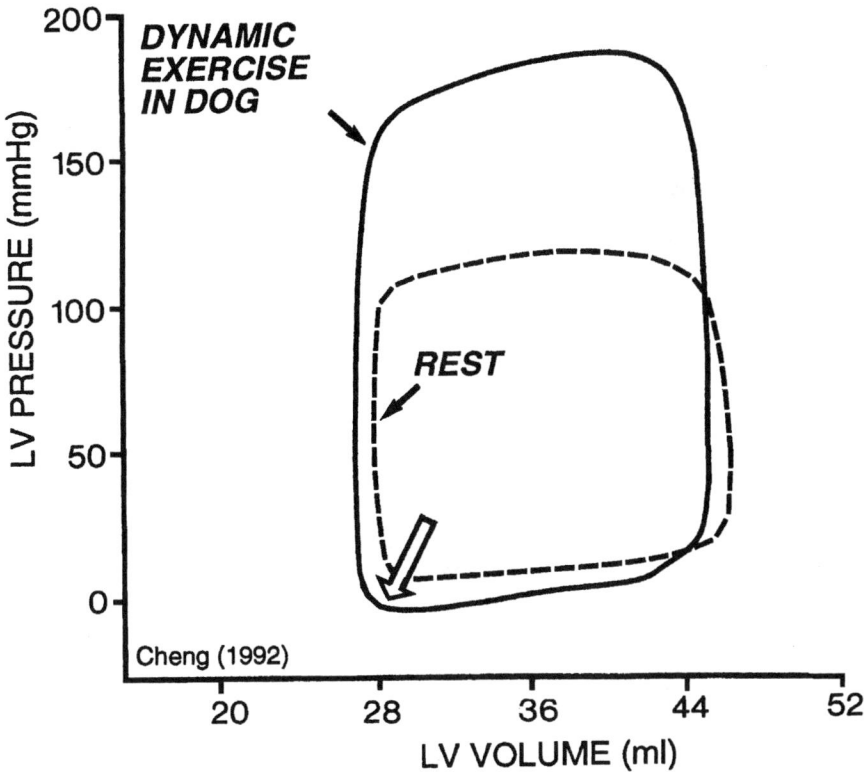

FIG. 15-10. Exercise in the dog promotes early left ventricular filling. During exercise in dogs, the early diastolic portion of the left ventricular pressure–volume loop moves downward (*arrow*). Speculatively, this may be caused by increased diastolic suction (Fig. 12-21). The decrease in early diastolic pressure increases the transmural filling pressure and flow to compensate for shortened diastole during exercise. (From Cheng C-P, et al. Mechanism of augmented rate of left ventricular filling during exercise. *Circ Res* 1992;70:9–19, with permission.)

remains that of increased heart rate with a lesser contribution from the Frank–Starling mechanism (12).

β-Adrenergic Blockade

Even when the β-adrenergic receptors are blocked by beta-blockers, the heart rate can still double during maximal exercise because of the principle of competitive antagonism whereby the enhanced adrenergic drive can displace the beta-blocker from the receptor. The absolute heart rates reached, however, are much reduced. Thus, the degree of exercise activity that can be reached is impaired, so that when normal subjects are exercised to their limit, cardiac output is approximately 25% lower after β-blockade (13).

Ergoreflexes and Central Integration

Ergoreflexes are initiated in the ergoreceptors of exercising muscles and lead to adrenergic stimulation (Fig. 15-7). Ergoreceptors are proposed as muscular receptors that respond to metabolic changes induced by skeletal muscle work, such as increased protons and potassium. During intense static exercise, when the muscle becomes ischemic because of the mechanical hindrance to blood flow, ergoreceptors initiate a reflex increase in the arterial BP. The elevated perfusion pressure helps to maintain blood flow to the exercising muscle. The afferent arm of this reflex travels along C fibers to convey stimuli to the nucleus solitarius (solitary tract nucleus) in the medulla, which coordinates the cardiovascular responses. Efferent stimuli then travel to the sympathetic vasomotor center and the vagal nucleus to mediate the increased BP and heart rate (Fig. 15-7).

Cardiovascular Control Centers

There are five centers concerned with central control: the insular cortex, hypothalamus, nucleus solitarius, vagal nucleus, and sympathetic vasomotor center. It must not be supposed that these centers act in isolation. Instead, there is a constant stream of messages between them. Details remain controversial, and these control centers are not as clearly defined as previously thought.

Central command is crucial for both static exercise and dynamic exercise. The chain of command goes from the insular cerebral cortex (14) to the hypothalamus (15) to the vasomotor centers in the medulla, from there stimulating the sympathetic and inhibiting the vagal outflow. For example, during total experimental paralysis of humans by neuromuscular blockade, attempted contraction of the paralyzed muscles still increases the heart rate and BP (16). This indicates that a central feed-forward mechanism alone can drive the cardiovascular system independently of any feedback from baroreflexes or muscle.

Autonomic Stimulation

Dynamic exercise differs from static exercise in that systemic hemodynamic changes are much more marked because increased cardiac output is needed to drive the blood to the many exercising muscles. Thus, striking differences from static exercise are the marked increases in heart rate, stroke volume, and cardiac output, together with vasodilation of the exercising muscles (Fig. 15-8). These can, for the most part, be explained by vagal withdrawal and adrenergic stimulation, the effects of the latter including splanchnic vasoconstriction to offset the decrease in PVR induced by muscle exercise. Vasodilation is best explained by the liberation of nitric oxide and other vasodilators in response to increased phasic muscle activity and physiologic shear stress on the endothelium. Baroreflexes must be down-regulated to avoid a decreased heart rate as systolic BP increases.

Thus, during dynamic exercise, the overall picture that emerges is a major role for "straight-down" feed-forward control of the heart and circulation starting centrally. During static exercise, by contrast, the risk is that the muscles become ischemic because of sustained muscular contraction, in response to which ergoreflexes increase BP and muscle perfusion pressure (Fig. 15-7). PVR remains unchanged or even increases while the exercising muscle mass is small, but as the mass increases and PVR decreases, a more "dynamic pattern" emerges (17).

Cardiac Energy Metabolism in Exercise

Patterns of substrate metabolism of the human heart during exercise can be defined by the use of coronary sinus catheterization. There is a marked increase in the contribution of lactate to the oxidative metabolism of the heart during a short burst of exercise. Thus, the heart takes up and oxidizes the lactate that is being produced by the peripheral muscles. During prolonged exercise when blood lactate is used up and the levels of free fatty acids increase, the latter become the dominant fuel. At the onset of severe exercise, when the heart is not receiving enough external substrate, glycogen is broken down and is preferentially used as glucose (18).

During exercise, the oxygen uptake of the myocardium must increase as each of the determinants increases: heart rate, contractility, and wall stress (Fig. 15-5). Wall stress increases in response to increased afterload as BP increases. Cellular metabolic signals are set off by increased work to ensure that an adequate flow of substrates is ultimately metabolized by the citrate cycle to produce enough adenosine 5'-triphosphate (ATP). As cytosolic ATP is rapidly converted by contraction to ADP, mitochondrial oxygen uptake and ATP formation are stimulated, nicotinamide adenine dinucleotide (reduced form) ($NADH_2$) is converted to nicotinamide adenine dinucleotide, the citrate cycle is stimulated, and the uptake of glucose, lactate, and free fatty acids is enhanced (Fig. 11-16).

The mechanism whereby increased heart work stimulates glucose uptake is not fully known, although it involves increased translocation of glucose transporters to the sarcolemma. An increase in cyclic adenosine 3',5'-monophosphate in response to nitric oxide may contribute to increased glucose uptake (9). Lactate uptake increases because transfer of pyruvate into mitochondrial pathways is enhanced after increased availability of nicotinamide adenine dinucleotide and activation of pyruvate dehydrogenase. The mechanism of increased uptake of free fatty acids is linked to increased mitochondrial metabolism and increased removal of acetyl-CoA and $NADH_2$ to stimulate the β-oxidation spiral. The stimulus to increased mitochondrial respiration is a not fully understood but appears to be a combination of increased ADP from increased myocardial work and increased mitochondrial calcium levels.

EXERCISE TRAINING AND THE HEART

Exercise Phenotype

Repetitive exercise training results in the exercise phenotype (Fig. 15-11). With dynamic aerobic training, the resting heart rate decreases (19) as a result of an alteration of the balance between the sympathetic and parasympathetic neural stimulation to the heart and changes in the intrinsic pacemaker currents. Two of the basic signs of exercise training are (a) a reduction in resting heart rate and heart

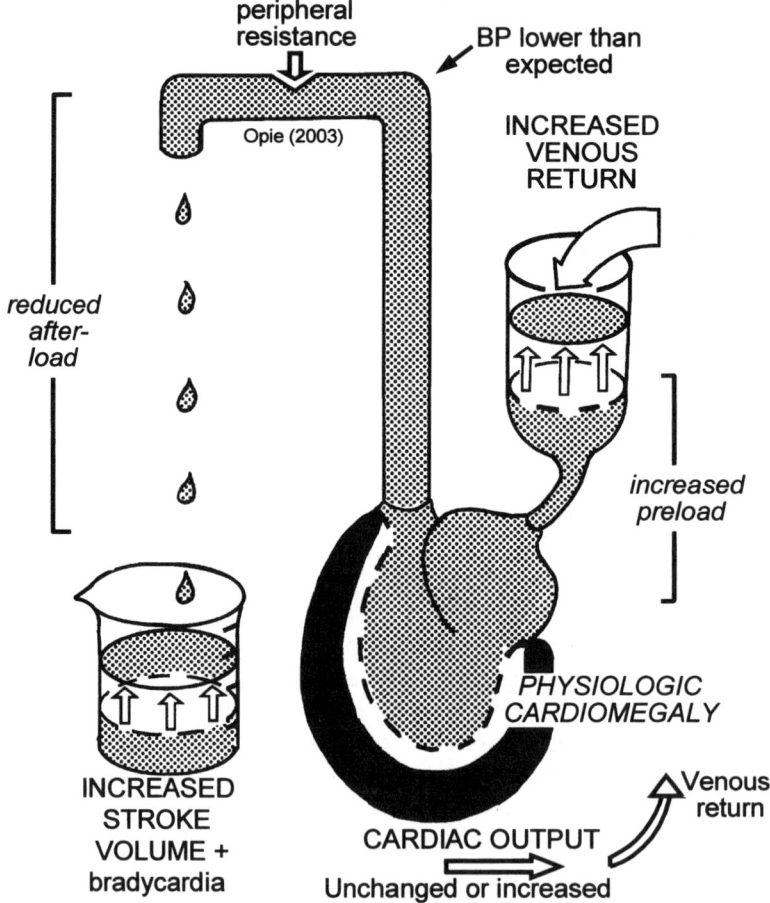

FIG. 15-11. The athlete's heart. As a simplification, the adaptations involved in dynamic exercise training may be regarded as compensatory responses to a chronic volume load, including physiologic cardiomegaly. BP, blood pressure.

rate response to submaximal exercise and (b) a more rapid recovery of the resting heart rate after exercise ends. Exercise training up-regulates neuronal nitric oxide synthase with the local production of nitric oxide in the vagal ganglia and nerve terminals (20). Nitric oxide acts presynaptically to increase the release of acetylcholine and to antagonize the sympathetic nervous system (Fig. 7-17). Thus, exercise training has some effects similar to those of β-adrenergic blockade (21) except that the level of exercise reached is much higher in trained than in β-blocked individuals. This phenotype of exercise training must be distinguished from that of extremely strenuous training, such as in world-class, high-performance athletes in whom there is sympathetic rather than vagal dominance (22), thereby aiding their peak performance but with unknown effects on long-term health.

The Athlete's Heart

True *physiologic hypertrophy* occurs (23) and must be distinguished from pathologic hypertrophy as in hypertrophic cardiomyopathy, which can cause sudden death in young athletes. It is not known whether the stimulus to hypertrophy in endurance athletes is intermittently prolonged workloads or stimulation by catecholamines. Physiologic left ventricular hypertrophy differs from pathologic left ventricular hypertrophy by the setting in which it occurs, the accompanying bradycardia, and improved rather than impaired early diastolic filling on Doppler echocardiography. Thus, it is a "balanced enlarged heart" (23). Pathologic hypertrophy impairs myocardial relaxation, whereas physiologic hypertrophy allows the heart to contract and relax better. Both physiologic and pathologic hypertrophy regress, at least to some extent, when the initiating stimulus is removed (24).

The increased vagal tone (either absolute or relative) of the athlete can give rise to *excess bradycardia* with prolonged conduction between atria and ventricles (prolonged PR interval) and abnormalities of repolarization. In rare cases, sinus node function is suppressed, some heartbeats fail to develop, and even hypotensive episodes result. Occasionally, conduction through the atrioventricular node is so delayed that the *Wenkebach phenomenon* develops (Fig. 5-21). Such diseases of overtraining can be cured by less exercise.

Exercise as Prophylaxis for Cardiac Protection

Lack of exercise is now recognized as a major independent risk factor for cardiovascular disease. Conversely, exercise training is associated with a lower all-cause mortality and reduced risk for coronary heart disease in middle-aged and older men (25). Explanations for the apparent beneficial effect of dynamic exercise in preventing ischemic heart disease are as follows.

1. Exercise training could act in a nonspecific way to modify the risk factors, such as by favorably altering blood lipoprotein patterns or by decreasing BP (25).

2. Exercise training may decrease the release of catecholamines from the heart, thereby reducing the arrhythmogenic effect of coronary artery occlusion (26).
3. Exercise training promotes baroreflex sensitivity and overall vagal activity (27) that is protective against ischemia and cardiac ventricular arrhythmias. A slow heart rate at rest is in general a sign of greater longevity than a faster rate.
4. Exercise training may increase coronary collateral blood flow after coronary occlusion (28).
5. Exercise training may augment the degree of coronary vasodilation in response to testing by nitroglycerin, suggesting improved endothelial function (29).
6. Regular exercise delays age-associated "stiffening" of the arteries (30).
7. Exercise by enhancing the rate of glucose transport across the muscle membranes helps to lessen insulin resistance and thereby lessens obesity and reduces the risk of maturity-onset diabetes, both of which predispose to cardiovascular disease.

Exercise and Age

With age, cardiovascular capacity declines so that maximal oxygen uptake decreases. However, in five intensively studied males subjects, 3 weeks of bed rest at age 20 gave a greater decline in physical work capacity than did 3 decades of aging (31). Looking into the next age group (50 to 76 years of age), there is an age-associated loss of endothelial function that can be prevented by regular aerobic exercise, approximately 45 minutes daily for 5 to 6 days per week (32).

Exercise-Induced Arrhythmias

One concern is that exercise may precipitate arrhythmias. In a majority of cases, such arrhythmias are related to coronary heart disease in which exercise amplifies the negative cardiac effects of ischemia. In addition, systemic circulatory changes could play a role. Blood catecholamine levels may increase as much as 15-fold during exercise, plasma potassium can double, and the blood pH may decrease by 0.4 units (33). Each of these exercise-induced changes could induce arrhythmias at rest, yet in normal subjects they are paradoxically well tolerated. The proposal is that adrenergic stimulation offsets the harmful effects of an increased external potassium level and vice versa. This principle of mutual antagonism is explained by the capacity of adrenergic stimulation to increase the inward calcium current despite K^+-induced depolarization and for a high external K^+ to shorten the action potential and thereby lessen the risk of calcium-induced afterdepolarizations (33).

EMOTIONAL STRESS, BRAIN, AND HEART

Emotional stress, like exercise, is a potent source of catecholamine discharge. The effects of intense cerebral activity, such as forced fast mental arithmetic, are closely related. Central distress, acting via the hypothalamus and medullary centers, leads to enhanced activity of the adrenergic system, including increases in circulating epinephrine, so that β-adrenergic activity is enhanced. The increased β-adrenergic discharge also leads to a series of events that enhance myocardial oxygen uptake: tachycardia, increased contractility, and increased cardiac output (34).

Hemodynamics during Emotional Stress

Psychological stress generally causes the PVR to decrease (34,35), with an increase in splanchnic vasoconstriction (Fig. 15-12). There can even be a marked increase in forearm blood flow, reflecting brisk peripheral vasodilation, and a rel-

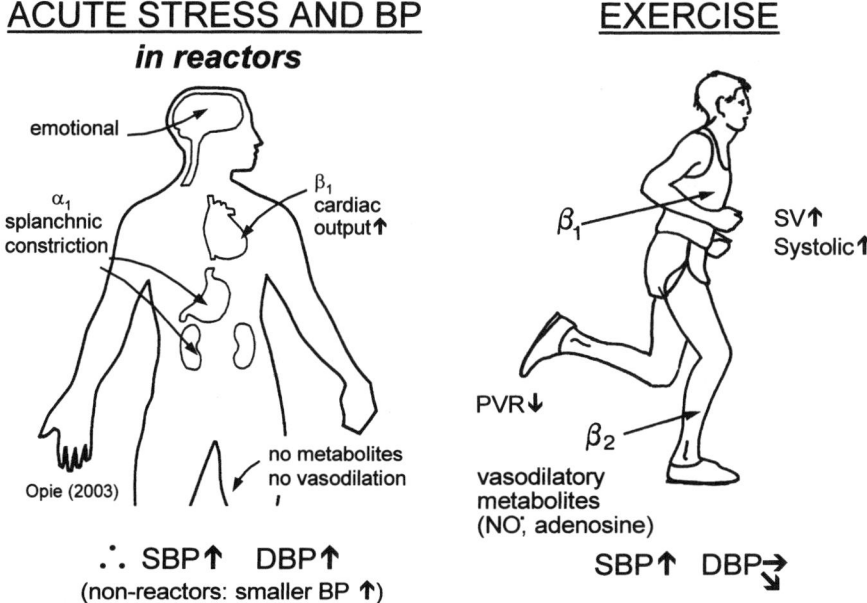

FIG. 15-12. Contrasting circulatory effects of acute emotional stress and dynamic exercise. One of the major differences is the production of vasodilatory metabolites by rhythmically exercising muscle, which in turn means that diastolic blood pressure (*BP*) does not increase. Emotional stress causes less marked BP increase in nonreactors (Fig. 14-8). According to the neurogenic theory, episodes of emotional stress might, by repetitively increasing the BP in those genetically susceptible to excess vasoconstriction, lead to sustained hypertension (Fig. 14-16). *SBP*, systolic BP; *DBP*, diastolic BP; *NO*, nitric oxide; α, α-adrenergic; β, β-adrenergic.

TABLE 15-4. *Comparative effects of exercise, mental stress, volume and pressure loading on hemodynamic parameters*

	HR	SV	CO	PVR	BP
Volume load	++	0 or +	++	0 or −	0
Pressure load (hypertension)	+	0	+	++	++
Exercise, dynamic erect	+++	+	+++	−	+ SBP −DBP
Exercise, static	+	0	+	0	++
Mental stress	++	+	++	−	+
Epinephrine infusion	++	+	++	−	+SBP −DBP
Norepinephrine infusion	±	±	±	++	++
Acetylcholine	−	−	−	−	−

Data sources: erect bicycle (35a), static exercise (17, 42), mental stress (34, 35b), infusion of epinephrine (35c), infusion of norepinephrine (35d).

HR, heart rate; SV, stroke volume; CO, cardiac output; PVR, peripheral vascular pressure; BP, blood pressure; +, increased effect; −, decreased effect; SBP, systolic blood pressure; DBP, diastolic blood pressure; ±, little effect.

atively small increase in BP (Fig. 14-8). These responses partly resemble those of dynamic exercise (Table 15-4). It seems likely that in some individuals there is a tendency to increased PVR, perhaps through excess α_1-adrenergic–mediated vasoconstriction or a genetic deficiency of the vasodilatory β_2-adrenoceptors (8). Such persons might be at greater risk of the development of subsequent hypertension. In normotensive persons, mainly plasma epinephrine increases during mental stress, epinephrine being predominantly vasodilatory by β_2-adrenergic stimulation (34,36). Borderline hypertensives, however, experience an increase in both epinephrine and norepinephrine secretion, the latter being vasoconstrictive. Hypothetically, repeated episodes of elevated BP can damage the vascular endothelium and facilitate the development of chronic hypertension (Fig. 14-16). In true hypertensives, peripheral resistance increases rather than decreases during mental stress (35).

Sudden Death and Stress

Psychological stress may play a role in the precipitation of sudden cardiac death. For example, on the day of an earthquake in Los Angeles, there was a sharp increase in the number of sudden deaths from cardiac causes (37). The mechanism very probably involves sympathetically mediated increases in heart rate and BP (Figs. 14-7 and 14-8). Emotional upset may trigger acute myocardial infarction in approximately 20% of cases (38). A hypothetical chain of events starts with central distress and arousal and leads through the hypothalamus and medulla (39) to cardiovascular adrenergic activation and a potentially lethal increase in myocardial levels of the arrhythmogenic second messenger cyclic adenosine $3',5'$-monophosphate (40).

Sudden Death and Exercise

Although regular exercise protects the heart in several ways, as already noted, in rare cases, vigorous exercise causes sudden death. In the majority, the explanation in almost all cases is underlying cardiac disease such as coronary artery disease or hypertrophic cardiomyopathy. The likelihood is that the increased myocardial oxygen demand of severe exercise cannot be met so that severe myocardial ischemia precipitates fatal ventricular arrhythmias (41).

SUMMARY

1. *Cardiac output*. This is the product of stroke volume and heart rate. The dominant factor governing cardiac output during dynamic exercise is heart rate. Other factors include preload, afterload, and contractility. Cardiac output is an important component of the external work of the heart. In general, the same factors that increase cardiac output increase myocardial oxygen uptake, but there are important differences depending on the amount of internal work done, which is much increased during a pressure load including static exercise. In contrast, during a volume load (similar to dynamic exercise), internal work increases little and external work and oxygen uptake increase in proportion to the heart rate.

2. *Dynamic versus static exercise*. Exercise is an example of a physiologic increase in oxygen uptake. There are important contrasting differences between dynamic and static exercise. Increased cardiac output of dynamic exercise is mediated by a combination of increased venous return, increased heart rate (the dominant factor), and increased contractility. In addition, the systolic but not diastolic pressure increases. In contrast, in static exercise, both systolic and diastolic pressures increase, probably as a result of reflexes arising in the muscles and conveyed by C fibers to cardiovascular centers in the medulla and hypothalamus. During dynamic exercise, the prime control mechanisms are increased cortical command and feed-forward signaling that increase sympathetic adrenergic activity and decrease vagal inhibition.

3. *Myocardial response to exercise*. As heart rate and BP increase, more external work and more oxygen uptake are required. A higher rate of myocardial oxygen uptake reflects increased ATP production. Mitochondrial metabolism is driven by a greater rate of formation of ADP and an increased mitochondrial calcium concentration. Glycogen may play a special role in the energy metabolism of the exercising heart, especially at the onset of increased heart work.

4. *Athlete's heart*. In this condition, bradycardia and physiologic left ventricular hypertrophy go together. It is distinguished from pathologic left ventricular hypertrophy by the setting in which each occurs and by the improved diastolic filling in the physiologic variety.

5. *Endurance training by repetitive aerobic exercise* counters lack of exercise, which is an independent risk factor for cardiovascular disease. The mechanisms involved are multiple, including enhanced vagal tone.

6. *Emotional stress.* In this case, the increased myocardial oxygen demand is mediated by a combination of β- and α-adrenergic activity. In normal individuals, secretion of epinephrine dominates, and the tachycardia is accompanied by an increased stroke volume, peripheral vasodilation, and surprisingly modest changes in BP. However, in individuals with hypertension or borderline hypertension, emotional stress can induce substantial BP increases.

STUDENT QUESTIONS

1. List and define each of the major determinants of cardiac output.
2. What differences do you expect between static (isometric) exercise and dynamic (isotonic or aerobic) exercise in relation to (a) heart rate, (b) cardiac output, and (c) BP?
3. What is the relationship between wall stress and myocardial oxygen uptake?
4. During static exercise, both systolic and diastolic BPs increase. Trace the reflex pathways involved.
5. How do exercise and emotional stress, both of which increase catecholamine discharge, differ in their hemodynamic effects?

CARDIOLOGIST-IN-TRAINING QUESTIONS

1. What determines myocardial oxygen uptake in (a) dynamic exercise in a normal subject, (b) static (isometric) exercise, (c) tight aortic stenosis, and (d) left ventricular failure?
2. Can heart work be increased without major changes in myocardial oxygen uptake? If so, describe the mechanisms involved and speculate on any therapeutic potential.
3. Exercise (endurance) training may have beneficial cardiovascular effects. What are they and which mechanisms may be involved?
4. What is the athlete's heart? How can it be distinguished from pathologic left ventricular hypertrophy?
5. During an earthquake, a man of 65 dies suddenly after a brief period of a central chest pain diagnosed as acute myocardial infarction. Speculate on the mechanisms involved.

REFERENCES

1. Starling EH. *The Linacre lecture on the law of the heart.* London: Longmans, Green, 1918.
2. Pierard LA, et al. Left ventricular function at similar heart rates during tachycardia induced by exercise and atrial pacing: an echocardiographic study. *Br Heart J* 1987;57:154–160.
3. Gandevia SC, et al. Cardiovascular responses to static exercise in man: central and reflex contributions. *J Physiol* 1990;430:105–117.
4. Donald DE, et al. Response to exercise in dogs with cardiac denervation. *Am J Physiol* 1963;205:393–400.

5. Rowell LR, et al. Integration of cardiovascular control systems in dynamic exercise. In: Rowell LB, et al., eds. *Handbook of physiology. Section 12*. New York: Oxford University Press, 1996:730–838.
6. Yi JJ, et al. Effects of food on the central and peripheral haemodynamic response to upright exercise in normal volunteers. *Br Heart J* 1990;63:22–25.
7. Anderson KM, Faber JE. Differential sensitivity of arteriolar α_1- and α_2-adrenoreceptor constriction to metabolic inhibition during rate skeletal muscle contraction. *Circ Res* 1991;69:174–184.
8. Cockcroft JR, et al. β_2-Adrenoceptor polymorphism determines vascular reactivity in humans. *Hypertension* 2000;36:371–375.
9. Young ME, et al. Nitric oxide stimulates glucose transport and metabolism in rat skeletal muscle in vitro. *Biochemistry* 1997;322:223–228.
9a. Gobel FL, Nordstrom LA, Nelson RR, et al. The rate-pressure product as an index of myocardial oxygen consumption during exercise in patients with angina pectoris. *Circulation* 1978;57:549–556.
9b. Takaoka H, Takeuchi M, Odake M, et al. Comparison of hemodynamic determinants for myocardial oxygen consumption under different contractile states in human ventricle. *Circulation* 1993;87:59–69.
9c. Rooke GA, Feigl EO. Work as a correlate of canine left ventricular oxygen consumption and the problem of catecholamine oxygen wasting. *Circ Res* 1982;50:273–286..
10. Cheng C-P, et al. Mechanism of augmented rate of left ventricular filling during exercise. *Circ Res* 1992;70:9–19.
11. Flamm SD, et al. Redistribution of regional and organ blood volume and effect on cardiac function in relation to upright exercise intensity in healthy human subjects. *Circulation* 1990;81:1550–1559.
12. Poliner LR, et al. Left ventricular performance in normal subjects: a comparison of the responses to exercise in the upright and supine positions. *Circulation* 1980;62:528–534.
13. Epstein SE, et al. Effects of beta-adrenergic blockade on the cardiac response to maximal and submaximal exercise in man. *J Clin Invest* 1965;44:1745–1753.
14. Williamson JW, et al. Activation of the insular cortex during dynamic exercise in humans. *J Physiol* 1997;503:277–283.
15. Eldridge FL, et al. Exercise hypernea and locomotion: parallel activation from the hypothalamus. *Science* 1981;211:844–846.
16. Gandevia SC, et al. Respiratory sensations, cardiovascular control, kinaesthesia and transcranial stimulating during paralysis in humans. *J Physiol* 1993;470:85–107.
17. Shepherd JT, et al. Static (isometric) exercise. *Circ Res* 1981;48(suppl 1):179–188.
18. Goodwin GW, et al. Preferential oxidation of glycogen in isolated working rat heart. *J Clin Invest* 1996;97:1409–1416.
19. Blumenthal JA, et al. Aerobic exercise reduces levels of cardiovascular and sympathoadrenal responses to mental stress in subjects without prior evidence of myocardial ischemia. *Am J Cardiol* 1990;65:93–98.
20. Danson EJ, et al. Enhanced neuronal nitric oxide synthase expression is central to cardiac vagal phenotype in exercise-trained mice. *J Physiol* 2003;546:225–232.
21. Brundin T, et al. Effects remaining after withdrawal of long term beta-receptor blockade. *Br Heart J* 1976;38:1065–1072.
22. Iellamo F, et al. Conversion from vagal to sympathetic predominance with strenuous training in high-performance world class athletics. *Circulation* 2002;105:2719–2724.
23. Scharhag J, et al. Athlete's heart. Right and left ventricular mass and function in male endurance athletes and untrained individuals determined by magnetic resonance imaging. *J Am Coll Cardiol* 2002;40:1856—1863.
24. Pelliccia A, et al. Remodeling of left ventricular hypertrophy in elite athletes after long-term deconditioning. *Circulation* 2002;105:944–949.
25. Sesso HD, et al. Physical activity and coronary heart disease in men. *Circulation* 2000;102:975–980.
26. Posel D, et al. Exercise training after experimental myocardial infarction increases the ventricular fibrillation threshold before and after the onset of reinfarction in the isolated rat heart. *Circulation* 1989;80:138–145.
27. Iellamo F, et al. Effects of a residential exercise training on baroreflex sensitivity and heart rate variability in patients with coronary artery disease. A randomized, controlled study. *Circulation* 2000;102:2588–2592.
28. Griffin KL, et al. Endothelium-mediated relaxation of porcine collateral-dependent arterioles is improved by exercise training. *Circulation* 2001;104:1393–1398.
29. Haskell WL, et al. Coronary artery size and dilating capacity in ultradistance runners. *Circulation* 1993;87:1076–1082.

30. Tanaka H, et al. Aging, habitual exercise and dynamic arterial compliance. *Circulation* 2000;102: 1270–1275.
31. McGuire DK, et al. A 30-year follow-up of the Dallas Bed Rest and Training study. I. Effect of age on the cardiovascular response to exercise. *Circulation* 2001;104:1350–1357.
32. DeSouza CA, et al. Regular aerobic exercise prevents and restores age-related declines in endothelium-dependent vasodilation in healthy men. *Circulation* 2000;102:1351–1357.
33. Paterson DJ. Antiarrhythmic mechanisms during exercise. *J Appl Physiol* 1996;80:1853–1862.
34. Freyschuss U, et al. Cardiovascular and sympathoadrenal responses to mental stress: influence of β-blockade. *Am J Physiol* 1988;255:H1443–H1451.
35. Schmieder RE, et al. Disparate hemodynamic responses to mental challenge after antihypertensive therapy with beta-blockers and calcium entry blockers. *Am J Med* 1987;82:11–16.
35a. Iskandrian AS, Hakki AH, DePace NL, et al. Evaluation of left ventricular function by radionuclide angiography during exercise in normal subjects and in patients with chronic coronary heart disease. *J Am Coll Cardiol* 1983;1:1518–1529.
35b. Schulte W, Neus H. Hemodynamics during emotional stress in borderline and mild hypertension. *Eur Heart J* 1983;4:803–809.
35c. Stratton JR, Pfeifer MA, Ritchie JL, et al. Hemodynamic effects of epinephrine: concentration-effect study in humans. *J Appl Physiol* 19845;58:1199–1206.
35d. Barcroft H, Swan HJC. In: *Sympathetic control of human blood vessels*. London: Edward Arnold, 1953.
36. Grossman E, et al. Disparate hemodynamic and sympathoadrenergic responses to isometric and mental stress in essential hypertension. *Am J Cardiol* 1989;64:42–44.
37. Leor J, et al. Sudden cardiac death triggered by an earthquake. *N Engl J Med* 1996;334:413–419.
38. Tofler GH, et al. Analysis of possible triggers of acute myocardial infarction (The MILIS Study). *Am J Cardiol* 1990;66:22–27.
39. Skinner JE. Regulation of cardiac vulnerability by the cerebral defense system. *J Am Coll Cardiol* 1985;5:88B–94B.
40. Lubbe WH, et al. Potential arrhythmogenic role of cyclic adenosine monophosphate (AMP) and cytosolic calcium overload: Implications for prophylactic effects of beta-blockers in myocardial infarction and proarrhythmic effects of phosphodiesterase inhibitors. *J Am Coll Cardiol* 1992;19: 1622–1633.
41. Lampert R, et al. Emotional and physical precipitants of ventricular arrhythmia. *Circulation* 2002; 106:1800–1805.
42. Lind AR, McNicol GW. Muscular factors which determine the cardiovascular responses to sustained and rhythmic exercise. *CMAJ* 1967;96:703–713.
43. Waldrop TG, et al. Central neural control of respiration and circulation during exercise. In: Rowell LB, et al., eds. *Handbook in physiology, section 12*. New York: Oxford University Press, 1996: 333–380.

16

Heart Failure: Neurohumoral Responses

A big heart is bad heart.
The Egyptian Book of the Dead

There are basically three myocardial mechanisms that lead to heart failure (Table 16-1): pressure overload, volume overload, and primary myocardial disease (cardiomyopathy). A fourth and common cause of heart failure is coronary artery disease with postinfarction remodeling. In each case, through different mechanisms, the myocardium attempts to compensate for the primary defect before the stage of overt myocardial failure develops. In addition, there are complex neurohumoral changes in the circulation that attempt to maintain normal organ perfusion in the face of decreasing myocardial function. These changes involve activation of the renin–angiotensin system and a hyperadrenergic state. This chapter first discusses the specific conditions that lead to heart failure, the mechanism of progression from left ventricular hypertrophy (LVH) to failure, and the clinical problem of what heart failure is and what it does to the patient.

HEART FAILURE INDUCED BY PRESSURE OR VOLUME OVERLOAD

To review: the consequences of mechanical overload, pressure, or volume overload involves two different cellular mechanisms and two different results, as outlined in Chapter 13 (Fig. 13-2). Eventually each type of load may change into a dilated failing heart (Fig. 16-1). Taking the example of pressure overload, the increase in myocardial performance required to overcome increased afterload has the disadvantage of greatly increasing LV wall stress. In other words, the transmural force acting on the left ventricle will tend to dilate the heart, which further increases wall stress, and LV failure rapidly becomes increasingly inevitable. Thus, with a sustained pressure load, the myocardium adapts by concentric hypertrophy, which means that it becomes thicker with-

TABLE 16-1. *Causes of left-sided heart failure*

Excessive pressure load
  Aortic stenosis
  Hypertrophic obstructive cardiomyopathy
  Arterial hypertension
Excessive volume load
  Aortic or mitral regurgitation
  High-output states (thyrotoxicosis)
  Some types of congenital heart disease
Primary myocardial disease
  Hypertrophic (nonobstructive) cardiomyopathy
  Hypertrophic obstructive cardiomyopathy
  Dilated cardiomyopathy
  Cardiomyopathy of the elderly
  Myocarditis
  Metabolic heart disease
  Endocrine heart disease
Impaired left ventricular filling
  Tight mitral stenosis
  Constrictive pericarditis
  Restrictive cardiomyopathy

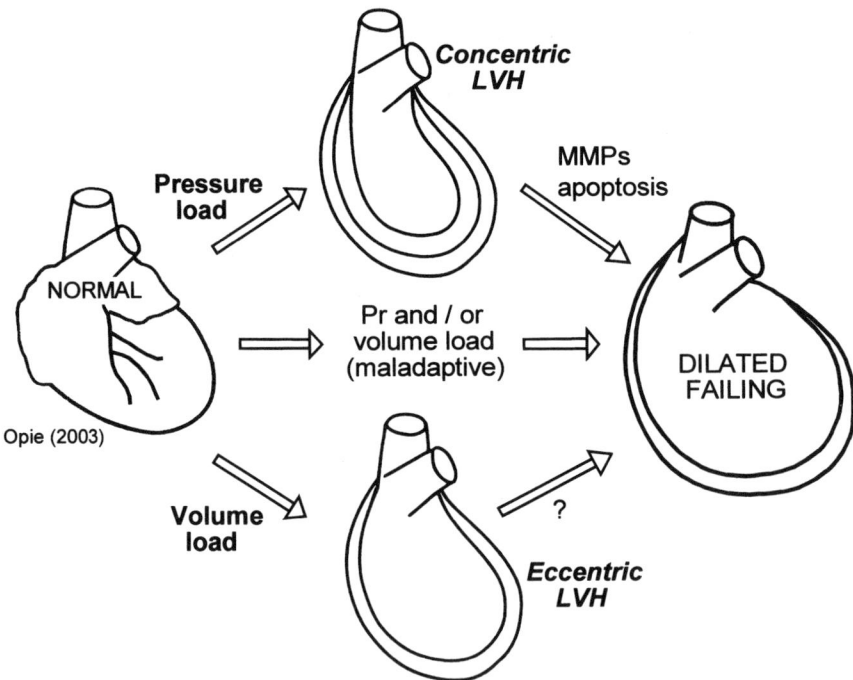

FIG. 16-1. Hypertension and the heart. Chronically elevated blood pressure causes compensatory concentric hypertrophy, thereby lessening the effect of increased afterload on wall tension (Fig. 12-15). Concentric remodeling, without increase in left ventricular (LV) mass but with a smaller than normal LV cavity size, may reflect combined pressure loading and volume unloading. Eccentric hypertrophy might reflect combined pressure and volume loading. Different types of hypertension have different circulating volumes, which might hypothetically account for these ill-understood differences in the LV response. *LVH*, left ventricular hypertrophy.

out increasing in radius, and wall stress normalizes. Such LVH is often called compensatory hypertrophy.

How "compensatory" is LVH? It is clear from the discussion in Chapter 13 that many processes are occurring at the same time, including concurrent stimulation of fibroblasts that increases collagen to impair myocardial mechanical function. Furthermore, myocardial blood supply is compromised. Locally synthesized angiotensin II (A-II) is evoked in response to mechanical overload, and downstream signals leading to mitogen-activated protein kinase are important in promotion of growth. However, such signals might have mixed prosurvival and proapoptotic effects (Fig. 9-1). The inevitable conclusion is that pressure overload induces both beneficial adaptive changes (normalization of wall stress) and adverse maladaptive changes. The latter may account for the adverse remodeling that contributes to the development of heart failure in pressure overload (1).

Left Ventricular Dysfunction and Failure in Hypertrophy

LVH is characterized by increased LV wall thickness and mass, with abnormal diastolic properties. There are loss of distensibility (so that the ventricle is stiffer), impaired relaxation, and decreased early diastolic filling. Additionally, early subtle systolic dysfunction becomes more obvious as the disease progresses so that in reality starting from a portion of dominant diastolic failure, there evolves combined systolic and diastolic failure (2). Characteristically, the patient experiences exertional shortness of breath (dyspnea), and the echocardiogram shows a decrease or reversal of the normal E/A (early filling/atrial contraction) ratio (Fig. 12-24). These abnormalities of relaxation result in part from the mechanical properties of the hypertrophied ventricle, such as increased interstitial connective tissue (3) in which type I collagen is increased. *Diastolic heart failure* refers to the combination of diastolic dysfunction with clinical evidence of fluid retention. Among the elderly, in whom most heart failure occurs, diastolic heart failure commonly occurs in the absence of overt systolic failure (defined by a depressed ejection fraction of less than 50%) (4).

The greater the aortic pressure is against which the myocardium must work, the thicker the ventricular wall becomes, at the cost of impaired LV function yet with an efficiency of external work comparable with that in patients with hypertension without LVH (5). Thus, despite impaired systolic function, LVH can in this sense be "compensatory," as postulated by many. Whether LVH is "good," "bad," or "mixed" may depend on the predominant signal systems that generated the hypertrophy, whether predominantly those that promote cell survival or those that promote adverse events such as fibrosis or apoptosis (see earlier comments).

Volume Overload and Left Ventricular Function

The initial event in a volume load is hemodynamic, being valvular regurgitation (incompetence) of either the mitral or aortic valve. Some authors include the effects of severe and prolonged exercise training as a volume load, but it seems better to distinguish between a pathologic origin and a physiologic origin for the load. Exercise training can in no true sense be equated with an organic regurgitant valve lesion. *Regurgitation* means that with every contraction, more of the stroke volume is recycled, so that a greater volume of blood must be dealt with per beat. To deal with this volume load, there are both changes in the loading conditions and in ventricular size. First, the volume load means that preload increases and the heart would be functioning at the limit of the end-diastolic volume (Fig. 12-15). Second, Grossman et al. (6) proposed that a volume load could cause "longitudinal hypertrophy" (Fig. 13-2), thereby increasing the size of the LV cavity that in turn could increase the chamber size without increasing the wall thickness. Some increase in chamber volume may also be attained by slippage of cells (same number of cells, wall is thinned). The result of volume overload is that there is enhanced early diastolic filling and decreased LV stiffness, so that diastolic function improves rather than deteriorates as in pressure overload. Nonetheless, as the chamber size increases, wall tension must increase. The inevitable consequence is some pressure-induced hypertrophy, which allows the LV cavity to decrease but not fully to normalize wall stress (Fig. 16-1).

Volume Versus Pressure Load

Extremely severe degrees of hypertrophy, 100% or more, as found in marked concentric hypertrophy, do not occur in volume-induced hypertrophy, possibly because the greater systolic wall stress of the pressure load is a more potent stimulus to myocyte hypertrophy with thickening rather than elongation of the myocytes (Fig. 16-2). Because of less increase in the thickness of the LV free wall and less internal work (potential energy) with a volume load, the oxygen supply/demand ratio is likely to be better maintained than in a pressure load (Fig. 12-17). Also, diastolic function improves in a volume load and deteriorates in a pressure load.

Hypertensive Patterns

Although often thought of as imposing a pure pressure load on the myocardium and therefore causing concentric LVH, other patterns such as eccentric LVH are more common (Fig. 16-2). The causes for these differences are poorly understood. An associated volume load (increased blood volume found in some hypertensives) might explain eccentric hypertrophy. In others, associated coronary artery disease could contribute to ventricular dilation. In *concentric remodeling*, the LV mass is normal, the cavity size is reduced, the wall thickness is increased, and the stroke volume is decreased. These findings are "surprising and counterintuitive from the vantage point of most clinical cardiologists" (7) but could possibly result from the combination of pressure overload and volume "underload." Of the three patterns of hypertrophy, the concen-

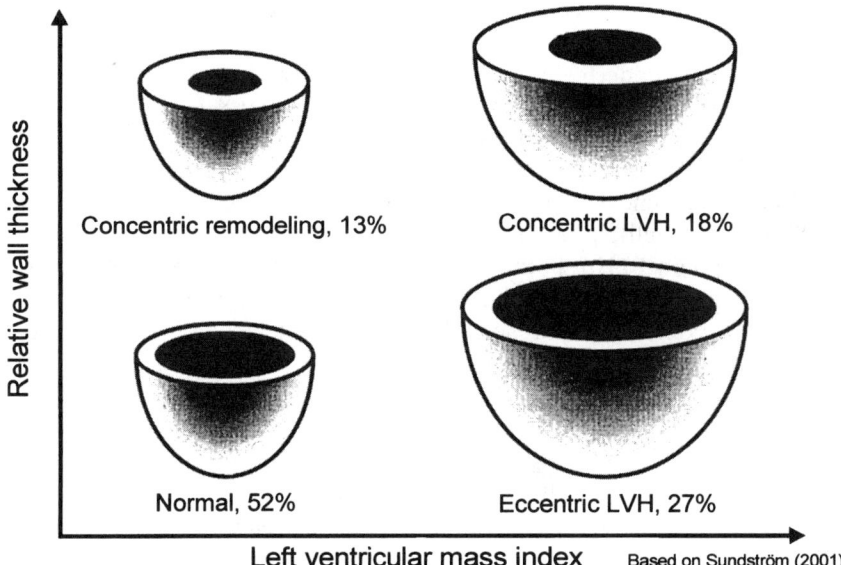

FIG. 16-2. Four patterns of left ventricular hypertrophy found in hypertension. The causes of these different types of left ventricular hypertrophy are not well understood. Based on Sundstrom (55).

tric type carries the worst prognosis, possibly because the thickened ventricle has a greater risk of potential ischemia and because of cellular changes such as increased cell death (8).

PRIMARY MYOCARDIAL FAILURE: CARDIOMYOPATHY

In primary myocardial failure, there is no initial defect in the loading conditions of the left ventricle, so that both volume and pressure loads are initially normal. For a given end-diastolic volume (and therefore sarcomere length), tension generation is inadequate because of the primary myocardial disease or cardiomyopathy (*myopathy*, muscle degeneration). Sometimes the cause of the disease is known (secondary cardiomyopathy), and sometimes it is unknown (primary cardiomyopathy). For practical purposes, whenever the origin of the myocardial disease is obscure, it is useful to consider a state of primary cardiomyopathy.

In *hypertrophic cardiomyopathy*, not really an example of heart failure, the ventricular wall is abnormally thick and the cavity is small. There are some similarities between the early stages of compensated concentric hypertrophy of this type of cardiomyopathy and the first phase of hypertrophy in response to a pressure load. The state of marked concentric hypertrophy found in primary hypertrophic cardiomyopathy causes a high systolic ejection fraction, and diastolic dysfunction predominates. Here the major problem lies in the small size of the

LV cavity, virtually obliterated by the hypertrophy, with consequent inability to fill normally during diastole.

Genetic defects underlie hypertrophic cardiomyopathy, which is often but not always a disease of the sarcomere (Color Plates 8-9 and 8-10). The muscle cells undergo excess growth in response to a genetic abnormality of the contractile proteins (Fig. 16-3). The growth factors concerned may be similar to those evoked in aortic stenosis (9). Nine abnormal genes have been found, encoding for different contractile proteins such as β myosin heavy chain, α tropomyosin, or cardiac troponin T (10). In the familial disease, there are links to mutations in the genes for adenosine 5′-monophosphate–activated protein kinase, a key enzyme in the control of adenosine 5′-triphosphate levels in the heart. Thus, the suggestion is that energy depletion may underlie the myocardial dysfunction (10). Of interest but difficult to explain is that some of these patients also experience preexcitation, i.e., the Wolff–Parkinson–White syndrome. The latter may account for the high incidence of sudden death.

In primary *dilated cardiomyopathy*, the initial event is myocardial failure of an unknown cause, sometimes an occult viral infection (Fig. 16-4). An enlarged heart with increased end-systolic and end-diastolic volumes characterizes the condition. Poor systolic pressure generation causes the ejection fraction to decrease, causing a self-induced volume overload to take place, accompanied by a marked increase in wall stress. There is usually some degree of compensatory hypertrophy, inadequate to normalize wall stress. Dilated cardiomyopathy can also develop as a secondary phenomenon, whenever a large mass of

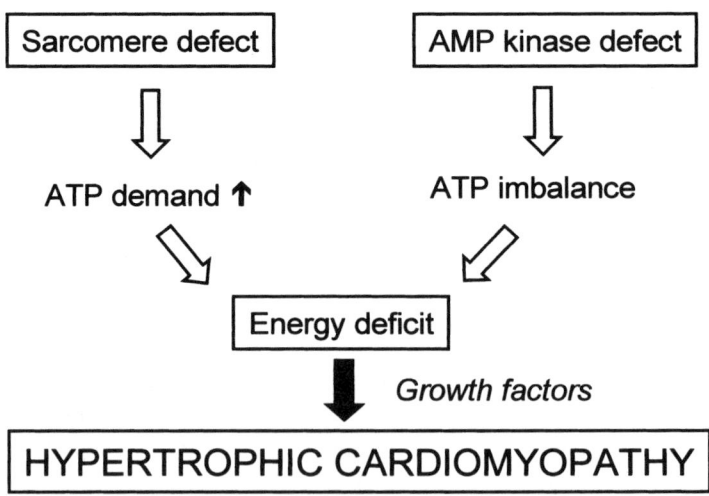

FIG. 16-3. Hypertrophic cardiomyopathy. Proposed role of sarcomere defects and adenosine 5′-monophosphate–activated protein kinase in generating the energy deficits that may explain some types of this condition.

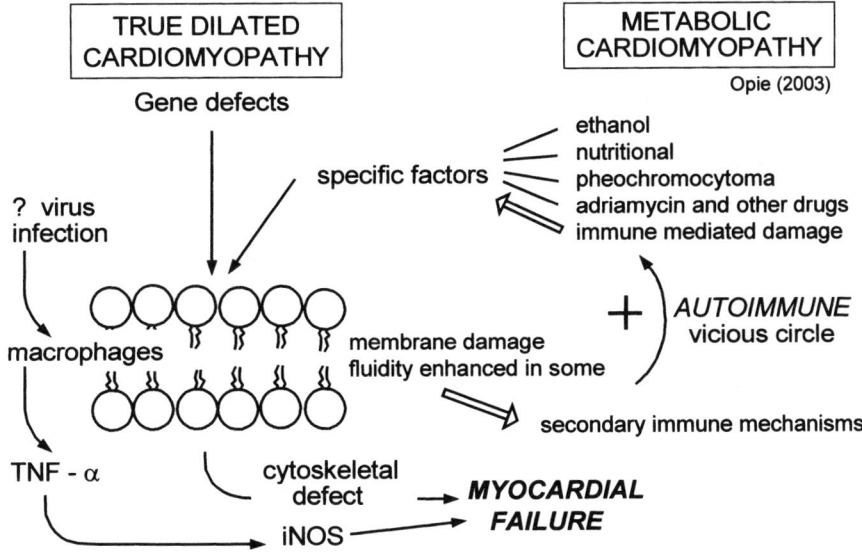

FIG. 16-4. Postulated cellular mechanisms in dilated cardiomyopathy. Note the role of tumor necrosis factor-α (*TNF-α*), thought to induce nitric oxide synthase (*iNOS*), to produce excess negatively inotropic nitric oxide (*NO*), thereby increasing the degree of myocardial failure.

myocardium is damaged, as in alcoholic damage, after a large myocardial infarction, or with severe generalized coronary artery disease. Increasingly, abnormalities of the cytoskeleton are regarded as basic in dilated cardiomyopathy. For example, *dystrophin defects* are common and may result from a viral infection or hereditary causes. There are now many transgenic models affecting both the contractile proteins and the chaperone molecules that guard protein folding. Taking the current experimental data together, there is a strong case for proposing that defects in the cytoskeleton are the predominant cause of dilated cardiomyopathy.

The *cardiomyopathy of the elderly* is the result of fewer myocytes. Starting with approximately 10^9 myocytes in the heart of a young adult, the cells decrease at the rate of 38 million per year (11). In compensation, there is modest hypertrophy of the remaining cells, without being able to maintain a normal myocardial mass. Therefore, there is an overall loss of contractile power.

Tachycardiomyopathy is the condition induced in animals by prolonged pacing-precipitated tachycardia. The human counterpart is a dilated failing heart resulting from incessant ventricular tachycardia or persistent fast atrial fibrillation. The mechanisms are not fully understood but include up-regulation of the myocyte renin–angiotensin system with excess production of A-II, promoting both myocyte hypertrophy and death (12). Eventually, the myocytes become smaller and contract poorly.

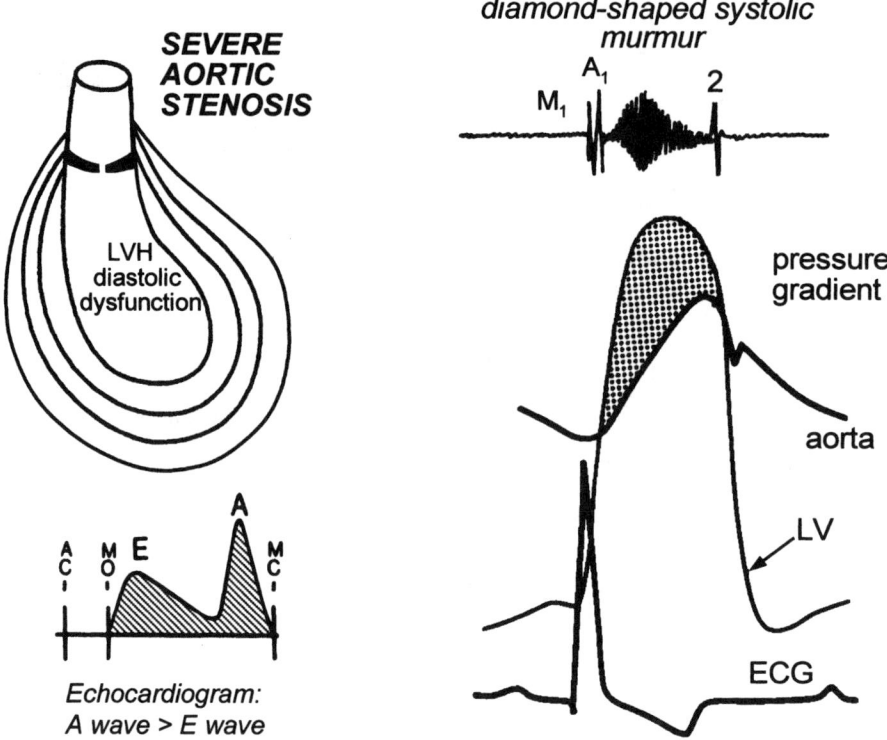

FIG. 16-5. Severe aortic stenosis. The thickened stiff aortic valve that causes left ventricular hypertrophy (*LVH*) and diastolic dysfunction (at top on left). The characteristic systolic murmur (at top on right). The pressure gradient between the left ventricle (*LV*) and the aorta (at bottom on right). The echocardiographic features of LV diastolic dysfunction, as blood flows past the mitral valve into the left ventricle (at bottom on left) (Fig. 12-24). *E*, early filling; *A*, atrial contraction, increased in the left atrial hypertrophy caused by diastolic dysfunction.

COMMON VALVE LESIONS

Prototypical valve lesions are aortic stenosis and regurgitation and mitral stenosis and regurgitation (Figs. 16-5, 16-6, and 16-7). Each of these causes a specific hemodynamic lesion, i.e., a pressure load in the case of aortic stenosis and a volume load in the regurgitant lesions. Tight mitral stenosis limits the flow from the left atrium to the left ventricle and causes a clinical picture resembling heart failure even in the presence of normal LV myocyte function because it restricts both the inflow and hence the outflow of blood from the left ventricle.

Specific Effects of Aortic Stenosis

Aortic stenosis is an example of a very gradually developing pressure overload to which the human heart can adapt over years via LVH. Despite severe

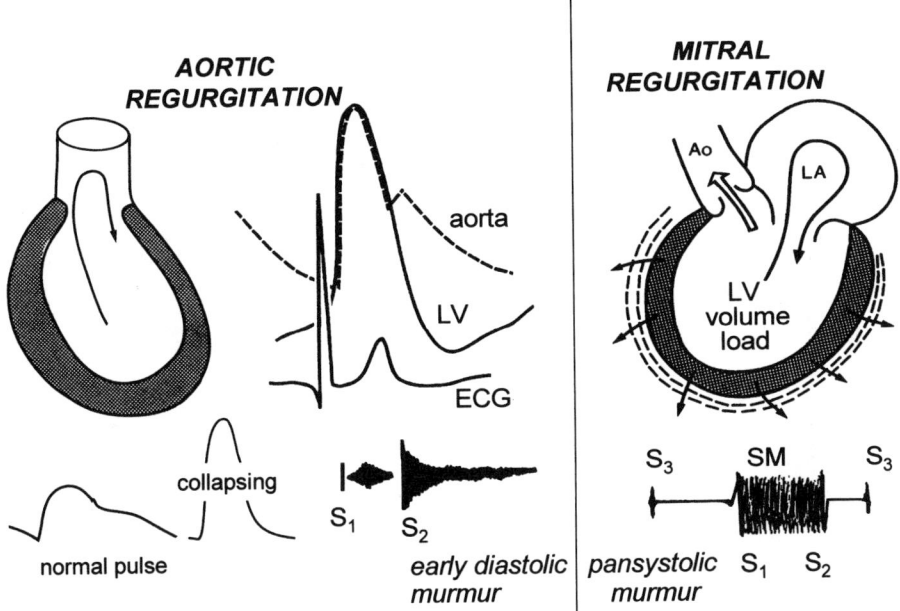

FIG. 16-6. Aortic and mitral regurgitation. Left: Diastolic aortic regurgitation with characteristic collapsing pulse and prominent early diastolic murmur after the second heart sound (S_2). **Right:** Systolic leak through the mitral valve with mitral regurgitation. During systole, a regurgitant jet of blood enters the left atrium (*LA*), causing a loud systolic murmur (*SM*) stretching from the first to the second heart sounds (S_1 to S_2).

obstruction, the patient may initially have predominant diastolic dysfunction. With time, systolic function decreases. The growth response is mediated, at least in part, through renin–angiotensin activation and A-II, which accounts for the increased expression of messenger RNA for collagen (types I and III), transforming growth factor β (TGF-β$_1$), and fibronectin (8). These changes explain increased myocardial fibrosis in aortic stenosis. The greater the fibrosis is, the greater the LV end-diastolic pressure (an indication of diastolic heart failure) is and the lower the ejection fraction (an indication of systolic failure) (8). Increasing myocyte degeneration is a broader concept that includes, besides fibrosis, cellular atrophy and myocyte death (8). Taken together, these changes also correlate with the degree of LV dysfunction in aortic stenosis.

Specific Aspects of Aortic and Mitral Regurgitation

These do not produce similar hemodynamic effects, although both are examples of volume overload. In aortic regurgitation, the volume overload leads to eccentric hypertrophy with enough increase in wall thickness to restore the wall stress to normal. When this balance fails and the extent of expansion of the LV

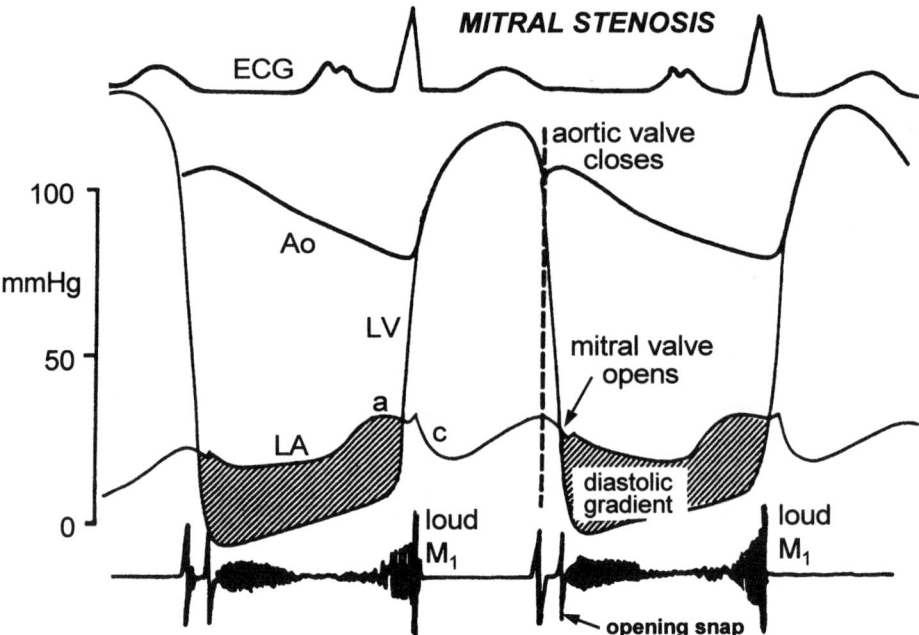

FIG. 16-7. Hemodynamics of mitral stenosis. Compare with Wiggers cycle (Color Plate 8-12). *Ao*, aortic pressure; *LA*, left atrium; *a* and *c*, components of atrial pressure wave; M_1, mitral component of first heart sound.

cavity exceeds the compensatory increase in wall thickness (13), the left ventricle fails. The electrocardiogram may show an interesting progression from the pattern of "diastolic volume overload" (Fig. 16-6) to that of LV "strain" with repolarization changes (Fig. 5-26), presumably reflecting the change from compensated to decompensated eccentric hypertrophy.

In *mitral regurgitation*, part of the stroke volume is ejected into the atrium during systole, thereby decreasing rather than increasing afterload. This may be why mitral regurgitation may be so well tolerated for so long and why it often seems a less serious lesion than aortic regurgitation. These apparent benefits of mitral regurgitation (improved diastolic function and reduced afterload) revert toward normal if mitral valve repair is performed promptly. The crucial benefit of surgical repair or replacement of the mitral valve is that the enlarged ventricular cavity becomes smaller. The postoperative prognosis worsens with more severe preoperative systolic dysfunction.

PROGRESSION FROM HYPERTROPHY TO FAILURE

Overload with overt systolic failure traditionally develops when either pressure or volume overload is no longer "compensated" for by the appropriate degree of hypertrophy and the radius increases excessively with increasing wall stress. Several reservations are noteworthy. First, in hypertensive hearts, concentric hypertrophy has a worse prognosis than the dilated eccentric type. Second, animal knockout models can delineate conditions in which LV function is better sustained in the dilated than in the more hypertrophic state, although only the latter has normalized wall stress (Fig. 13-6). Third, compensation is only apparent in that LV function in patients is depressed when carefully tested. Fourth, some overloaded hearts progress directly to failure (1), perhaps because of predisposing genetic abnormalities. Finally, the established experimental sequence from pressure overload to compensatory LVH to the dilated failing heart has not been directly established in humans, although there is good indirect evidence (8). The mechanisms by which apparently compensated hypertrophy may develop into failure have been troubling experimentalists for decades. Some proposals follow.

The Myocardium Outstrips Its Blood Supply

Linzbach (14) considered concentric hypertrophy the normal myocardial response to a pressure load that persisted until a critical limit was reached, at which point the hypertrophied heart would outstrip its blood supply, leading to focal necrosis and myocardial failure. His proposed critical limit was approximately 500 g, which is approximately twice the normal heart weight. During myocardial hypertrophy, the capillary surface area decreases in relation to the myocyte volume and the distance between the capillaries increases (Fig. 13-3). Even today, vascular defects are considered crucial to myocardial deterioration in heart failure (8).

Impaired Coronary Vascular Reserve and Endothelial Defects

Coronary reserve is the ratio of coronary resistance at rest to that after maximal coronary dilation (e.g., by the vasodilator dipyridamole) (Fig. 10-5). Such dilation is greatly decreased in the presence of coronary artery disease. The major mechanism is endothelial dysfunction, which impairs the normal coronary vasodilator response. Coronary reserve is decreased in LVH, even in the absence of coronary artery disease, especially in the subendocardial zones that are subject to the greatest wall stress. Thus, especially during exercise, when the much thicker hypertrophied muscle mass requires a much higher myocardial oxygen uptake, the coronary vasodilation is inadequate. Repeated bouts of exercise-induced ischemia could eventually lead to fibrosis by stimulation of collagen synthesis. When fibrosis sets in, it tends to "strangulate" the normal myocardial cells (15).

Role of Angiotensin II and Aldosterone

A-II, acting via TGF-β, is potentially a major stimulus to fibrosis (8), as is aldosterone. Thus, the renin–angiotensin system may not only play a crucial role in the hypertrophic process but also in irreversible damage. In the peripheral arterioles (and the coronary vessels), A-II promotes formation of reactive oxygen species with endothelial dysfunction and increased vasoconstriction (Fig. 9-11).

Increased Collagen Tissue and Matrix Remodeling

In physiologic amounts, collagen may help to limit ventricular dilation when it is increased in proportion to the degree of myocardial hypertrophy. In contrast, when there is an excessive collagen response to ischemia or metabolic signals such as A-II, compliance decreases with an increase in *chamber stiffness* or a decrease in *distensibility*. Experimentally, at least in some models, the nonelastic type I collagen increases more (16). Clinically, this promotes poor diastolic relaxation and, hence, diastolic failure. In the pressure–volume loop, the pressure increases more than it should for any given volume increase because the thicker the ventricle wall is, the more the intraluminal pressure required to make it stretch is. Thus, the wall tension increases more than expected, with a corresponding increase in the oxygen demand. This in turn contributes to relative ischemia of the hypertrophied myocardium and further promotes interstitial fibrosis.

However, for LV chamber enlargement to occur, *myocyte slippage* is required. This in turn means weakening of the excess collagen network, the result of the activity of the matrix metalloproteinases (MMPs) (Fig. 16-8). A critical result may be decreased collagen cross-linking with weakening of the matrix, thereby allowing *matrix remodeling* with myocyte slippage and LV chamber enlargement (16). Exactly how the MMPs and the counterbalancing enzymes that inhibit them (tissue inhibitors of MMPs) are regulated remains unclear. Presumably, the balance between their activities governs the stability of the collagen network.

Controversial: Apoptosis

The left ventricle undergoes progressive dilation and thinning during the development of severe heart failure. Hypothetically, apoptosis may contribute to the attrition. Apoptosis, as more fully described in Chapter 18, is a gene-directed process that results in predictable cell death. There is new gene expression, for example, of the *Fas* gene and inactivation of the antiapoptotic gene *bcl-2*. Only a low incidence of apoptotic cells is found in severe heart failure. However, if only 0.2% of the entire population of cells were lost per day, then, because the apoptotic cycle is so short, as much as 50% of the total pool of myocardial cells could be lost over 1 year (17). A current hypothesis emphasizes mitochondrial damage in response to adenosine 5′-triphosphate depletion, excess cytosolic calcium, or excess oxidative stress. The damaged mitochondria then liberate cytochrome c to set apoptosis in motion (Fig. 9-9). Others fail to find significant apoptosis in heart failure or LVH developing into failure or invoke paths resembling those of apoptosis but without the diagnostic nuclear findings (8). These

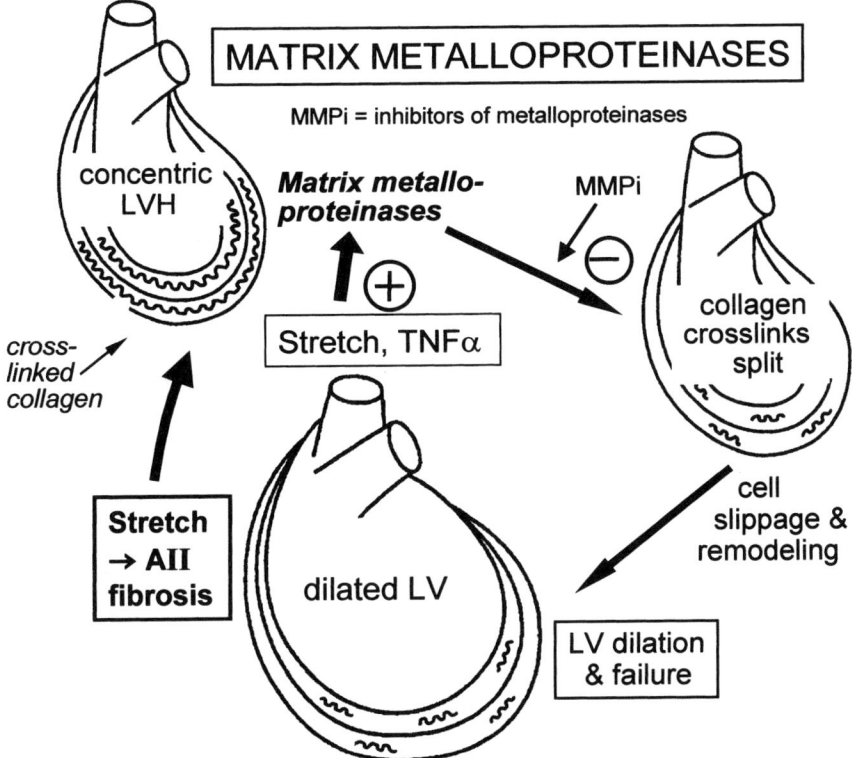

FIG. 16-8. Proposed role of matrix metalloproteinases in progression from concentric left ventricular hypertrophy (*LVH*) to dilated left ventricle. The primary stimulus to the increased collagen is pictured as stretch-induced formation of angiotensin II (*A-II*). The latter probably stimulates fibrosis by transforming growth factor β (*TGFβ*) (Fig. 13-14) The metalloproteinases split the collagen cross-links with cell slippage and LV dilation. The role of tissue inhibitors of metalloproteinases (*TIMPs*) is not clear.

workers also find cell death by necrosis or autophagic ("self-eating") death by lysosomes to be more common (8).

IS THERE A BASIC BIOCHEMICAL DEFECT?

Apart from the proposed consequences of oxygen imbalance, a more fundamental biochemical defect has been suspected since at least 1913, when Clark found that the hypodynamic frog's heart "loses its power of combining with calcium." Since then, studies too numerous to analyze have delineated defects in oxidative phosphorylation, high-energy phosphate metabolism, calcium ion movements, contractile proteins, protein synthesis and breakdown, and catecholamine metabolism. It is apparent, however, that there is no simple unifying hypothesis to explain divergent findings. One problem is that congestive failure is the end product of numerous different chronic processes, such as ischemic heart disease, valvular heart disease, hypertension, cardiomyopathy, and high-output states such as thyrotoxicosis. Nonetheless, studies on heart tissue removed at the time of transplantation or insertion of an LV assist device, together with data from increasingly sophisticated animal models, suggest that Clark was right and that calcium abnormalities are fundamental in the defective systolic function of the left ventricle.

Abnormal Calcium Transients

Typically in failing hearts, there are multiple abnormalities of calcium cycling (Table 16-2). In terminal human heart failure, there is a decreased increase of internal calcium, followed by prolonged, slowly decreasing calcium transient (Fig. 16-9). Particularly when the heart rate is fast, there is not enough time for the internal calcium to decrease to baseline levels (18), which may explain why tachycardia is so badly tolerated in heart failure. The impaired calcium transients reflect at least two defects in the sarcoplasmic reticulum (SR) and one in the Na^+/Ca^{2+} exchanger. First, in failing human hearts, the calcium uptake pump SERCA [sarco(endo)plasmic reticulum calcium–ATPase] is expressed at a lower level (19); second, calcium-induced calcium release is impaired (20). As SERCA 2a, the specific isoform involved, is down-regulated, the relative abundance of phospholamban in its unphosphorylated form progressively inhibits calcium uptake by the SR (21). Regarding calcium release by the ryanodine receptor (RyR) 2, that too is faulty in heart failure in that the receptor is hyperphosphorylated, probably in response to excess β-adrenergic stimulation (20). An alternate view is that there is only one basic defect, the reduced net uptake of calcium by the SR, that leads to decreased calcium stores within the SR and thus to decreased release of calcium by the RyR (22). In addition to these defects of calcium handling by the SR, there is increased calcium entry into the failing myocytes via the up-regulated Na^+/Ca^{2+} exchanger, also thought to result from enhanced sympathetic activity (23). The overall result is cellular calcium overload that exaggerates the already impaired contractile function and threatens serious arrhythmias (Fig. 20-14).

Energy Starvation

Experimentally, there can be enhanced uptake of oxygen per gram of active tension developed, which is a variety of oxygen wastage (24). The mechanism for this is not known. A speculative cause could be cytosolic calcium overload. The corresponding situation in patients may be the increased oxygen consumption per unit. In patients with LVH, increased internal work (potential energy) explains the abnormal increase in myocardial oxygen uptake (Fig. 12-15). Based on this change and the reduced coronary vascular reserve, the myocardial oxy-

TABLE 16-2. Pathophysiologic mechanisms in congestive heart failure

Change	Mechanism	Advantages	Disadvantages
Hypotension	Depressed inotropic state	Conserves oxygen	Evokes adrenergic activation supply MVO_2 increased
Tachycardia	Baroceptor mediated, reflex adrenergic	Helps to maintain cardiac output as stroke volume↓	Cardiac output decreased
Arteriolar vasoconstriction	Adrenergic drive increased; renin-angiotensin↑; endothelin release	Helps to maintain blood pressure	
LV volume increased	Mitral regurgitation, fiber slippage	Helps to maintain stroke volume by the Starling mechanism	MVO_2↑; Wall tension↑
Atrial stretch	ANP secretion	Vasodilatory and diuretic	Promotes atrial fibrillation
Myosin ATPase↓	Gene reprogramming; altered isoenzymes in animals	High pressure, low speed work	Slower rate of contraction inotropic state↓
Catecholamine depletion of heart	Unknown; decreased uptake and synthesis	Protects myocardium from calcium overload	May contribute to inotropic state↓
Liver enlargement	Hepatic congestion	None	May cause hepatic failure
Renal congestion	Poor renal perfusion	None	May precipitate prerenal failure
Congested lungs	Increased pulmonary wedge pressure; LV diastolic dysfunction	Limits exercise; conserves MVO_2	Dyspnea, pulmonary edema
Gene resetting neonatal phenotype	Chronic LV failure	LV makes ANP, BNP, adrenomedullin	Fatty acid enzymes↓; energy production↓

MVO_2, myocardial oxygen uptake; LV, left ventricular; ANP, atrial natriuretic peptide; BNP, brain natriuretic peptide; ↓, decreased; ↑, increased.

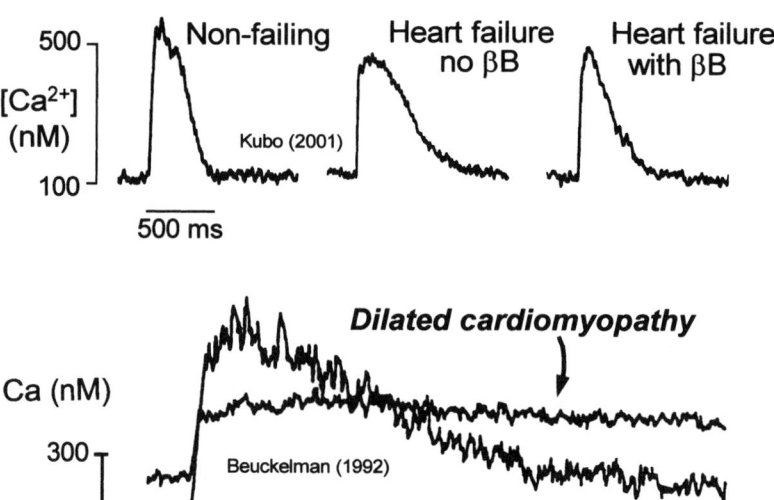

FIG. 16-9. Calcium transients in heart failure cells. Top: Effect of β-blockade (βb) in improving calcium transients in severe human heart failure. Data from Kubo et al. Circulation 2001;104: 1012. **Bottom:** In cells from severe dilated cardiomyopathy, the calcium transients increase less than in controls and then stay abnormally elevated. From Beuckelman et al., Circulation 1992; 85:1046.

gen supply/demand is more likely to be imbalanced, giving rise to foci of myocardial ischemia that promote fibrosis and consequences and impair myocardium compliance. This oxygen imbalance, depressed internal energy transfer (25) and other metabolic abnormalities in the failing heart (Fig. 16-10) lead to a state of energy starvation according to the Katz hypothesis (26).

Substrate Switching

In rat hearts subject to pressure overload hypertrophy, the fetal gene program is reexpressed, which leads to a substrate switch with increased dependence on glycolysis for contractile work. If there is a forced switch to fatty acids, then the heart fails (Fig. 16-11). In contrast, in severe human heart failure, both fatty acid and glucose pathways appear to be down-regulated (27). These human heart data are more in support of the energy starvation proposal than of the substrate switch hypothesis.

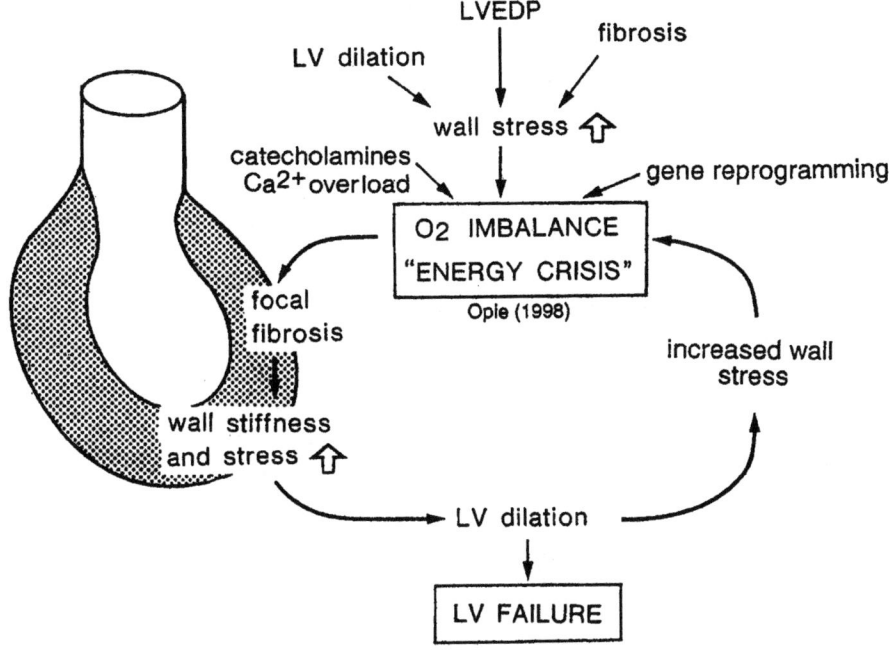

FIG. 16-10. **Proposed energy crisis in the failing heart.** Note the role of oxygen imbalance. The onset of focal fibrosis by collagen growth impairs mechanical function, which in turn may promote the progression from the apparently compensated hypertrophic state to the dilated failing myocardium. *LV*, left ventricle, *LVEDP*, left ventricular end-diastolic pressure.

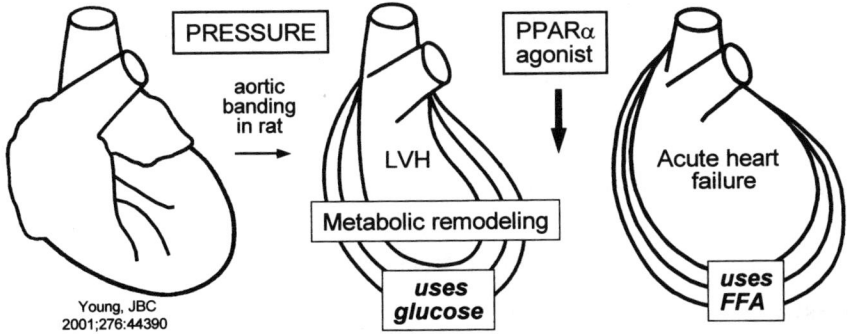

FIG. 16-11. **Metabolic remodeling.** Aortic banding in the rat produces left ventricular hypertrophy (*LVH*) with a myocardium that preferentially uses glucose as its major fuel. Adding a peroxisome proliferator–activated receptor-α agonist (see Figure 9-15) increases the use of free fatty acids (*FFA*) by the heart, which then acutely fails. Based on Young et al. *J Biol Chem* 2001; 276:44390.

Myosin Isoforms and ATPase Activity in Heart Failure

Abnormal myosin isoenzymes are formed in experimental congestive heart failure and in the failing human heart (Fig. 13-10). The increased expression of the slow isoform of myosin heavy chain is associated with decreased ATPase values and depressed mechanical function.

Sarcomere Overstretch?

It was thought that in congestive heart failure, the sarcomeres were overstretched, thereby removing myosin cross-bridges from their interactive sites on the actin. However, this concept has been laid to rest by direct measurements of sarcomere length in human heart failure (Fig. 16-12). Sarcomere length does not exceed approximately 2.3 μm. Nonetheless, during systole, the sarcomere length is shorter. There still is some Starling response, but greater end-diastolic pressures and volumes are required to achieve an adequate developed pressure (Fig.

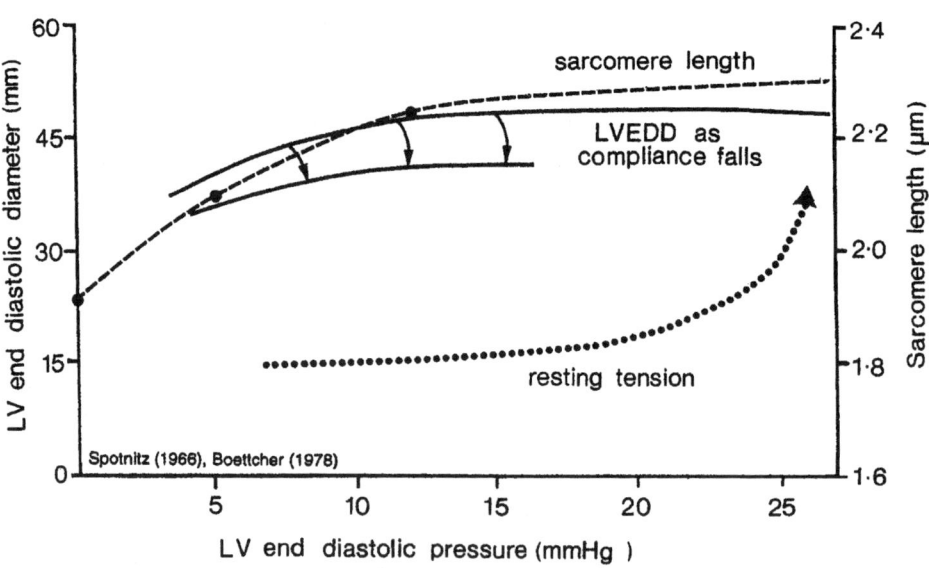

FIG. 16-12. Sarcomere length in heart failure. As left ventricular (*LV*) end-diastolic pressure increases, the LV end-diastolic volume [measured here as LV end-diastolic diameter (*LVEDD*)] increases over low pressures but rapidly reaches a maximum. Similarly, sarcomere length also reaches a maximum. If the LV end-diastolic pressure is increased beyond the physiologic limit of approximately 12 mmHg, resting tension starts to increase and will impair subendocardial myocardial perfusion. If the compliance of the ventricle is decreased, as after myocardial infarction, dV/dP decreases, and there is less volume increase for a given pressure increase (Fig. 12-25). These relationships can explain some aspects of the Frank–Starling curve in heart failure. Data based on Spotnitz et al. *Circ Res* 1966;18:49 and Boettcher et al. *Am J Physiol* 1978; 234:H338.

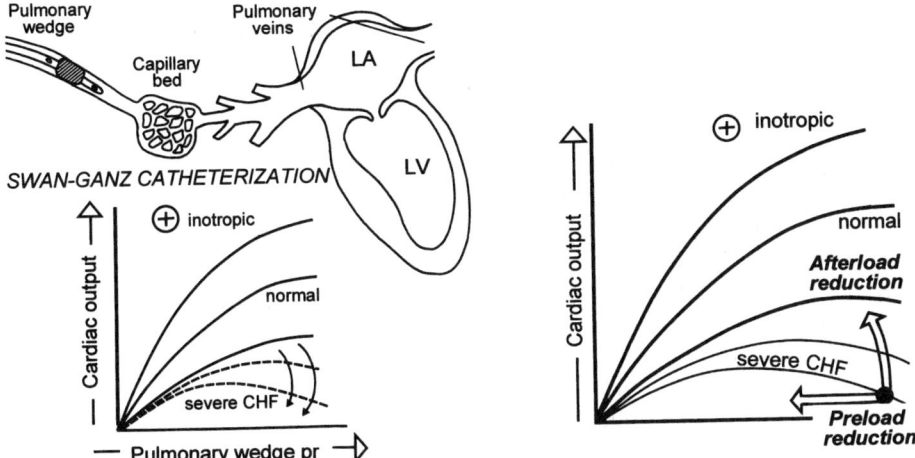

FIG. 16-13. Swan–Ganz catheterization and load reduction in heart failure. **Left:** Insertion of catheter into a pulmonary capillary bed into the pulmonary wedge position, thereby indirectly measuring left atrial (*LA*) and therefore left ventricular filling pressure. Theoretical Starling curves are shown for severe congestive heart failure (*CHF*) and for positive inotropic intervention. **Right:** Effects of therapeutic preload and afterload reduction on cardiac output. For example, nitrates reduce preload, and angiotensin-converting enzyme inhibitors reduce both preload and afterload, whereas digitalis compounds have a positive inotropic effect.

12-23). The greater subendocardial wall stress implies risk of relative ischemia and further fall-off in LV performance.

The Descending Limb of the Frank–Starling Curve

Because of the impaired LV contractile state, the heart is on a lower than expected Starling curve (Fig. 16-13). Further elevation of venous pressure fails to increase cardiac output as expected. To explain this "descending limb," ventricular interaction may be invoked. Heart failure increases the *central blood volume*, which is the total blood volume in heart and lungs. The associated increase in venous return increases right atrial filling pressure, which is right ventricular preload. This tends to dilate the right ventricle, which in turn presses on the left ventricle, a process called *ventricular interaction* (28). Thus, LV function decreases, which explains the descending limb of the Frank–Starling curve found in severe heart failure.

THE CLINICAL SYNDROME OF CONGESTIVE HEART FAILURE

There is no entirely satisfactory definition of heart failure. The clinical and physiologic definitions do not always match. The clinical picture of fully developed congestive heart failure is an admixture of three separate components.

First, as a result of *diastolic failure*, there is imperfect emptying of the left atrium and filling of the left ventricle, so that features of pulmonary congestion and increased venous pressure develop. Second, there is *systolic failure* with impaired contractile behavior of the heart and decreased force development, so that the myocardium is on a lower Frank–Starling curve than normal (Fig. 16-13). Stroke volume and cardiac output increase less than they should during exercise, peripheral perfusion is impaired, and muscular fatigue develops. Third, there are important *neurohumoral changes* that increase peripheral vascular resistance and afterload; sympathetic tone is increased, the renin–angiotensin–aldosterone system is activated, and there is fluid retention with peripheral congestion and edema so that preload is further increased.

Definitions of congestive heart failure are often tautologically flawed. Some authors hold that heart failure may be defined as a state in which the heart fails to maintain adequate circulation for the needs of the body despite a satisfactory venous pressure. In brief, heart failure is then illogically defined as a state in which the heart fails. Another defective definition dates back to Lewis (29) who, in 1933, wrote: "There is but one meaning to the term cardiac failure—it signifies the inability of the heart to discharge its contents adequately." However, except during the phase of increasing pulmonary edema, the left ventricle must be discharging as much blood as enters, and, therefore, this definition is far from perfect.

For clinical purposes, heart failure is a clinical syndrome characterized by exertional symptoms and caused by heart disease. This simple definition, verbally proposed by Packer some years ago, is supported by the European Society of Cardiology (30) and allows the bedside diagnosis of heart failure. *Congestive heart failure* is the term that encompasses fluid and sodium retention ("congestion") sufficiently severe to cause an increased jugular venous pressure, pulmonary fluid retention, systemic edema, or liver enlargement. The New York Heart Association proposed a widely used classification of heart failure into four classes based on the severity of dyspnea, thus emphasizing the clinical relevance of the diastolic failure and the fluid retention that cause such symptoms.

What are the differences between LV dysfunction and failure? LV dysfunction exists when there are abnormalities of relaxation or contraction, so that the heart cannot fill or empty properly (31). LV failure occurs when either of these abnormalities results in fluid retention or exercise intolerance.

Vicious Circle of Heart Failure

Heart failure begets heart failure (Fig. 16-14). The neurohumoral response to heart failure leads to increased baroreflex-mediated adrenergic activity, associated with enhanced activity of renin and A-II. These changes result in greater vascular resistance and afterload. Thus, the left ventricle must work against a greater load, and LV function deteriorates further. This sequence explains why there is such a poor prognosis in untreated heart failure.

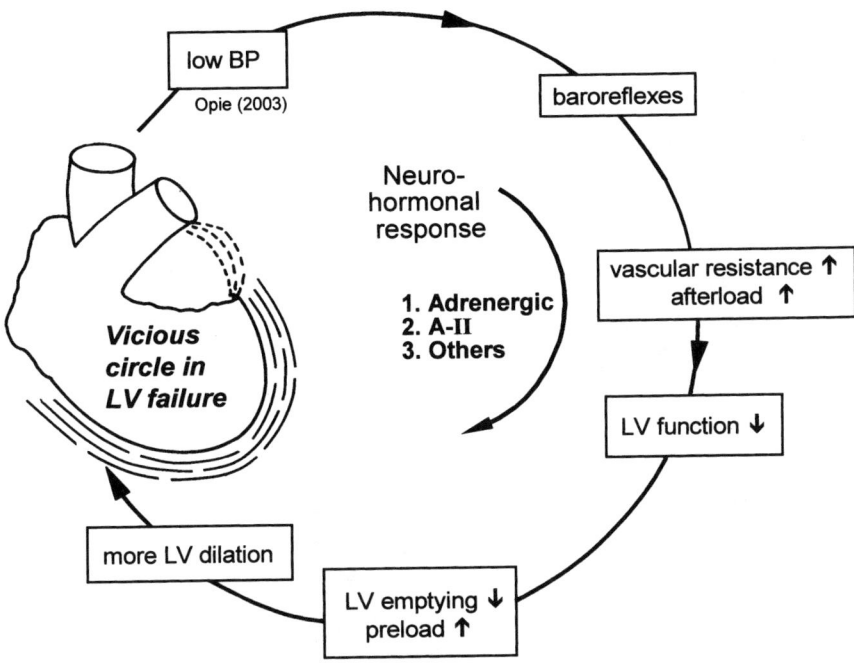

FIG. 16-14. **Neurohormonal vicious circle** in heart failure. *A*-II, angiotensin II.

Diastolic and Systolic Heart Failure: Possibly Outmoded But Still Relevant

The distinction between the forward and backward aspects of congestive heart failure extends over many years. Even today, with our sophisticated understanding of hemodynamic and neurohumoral abnormalities, this division is useful, albeit often artificial. The preferred current terms are systolic and diastolic failure (Figs. 16-15 and 16-16). Basically, the critical hemodynamic events are (a) backward or diastolic failure with an increased pulmonary capillary pressure, (b) forward or systolic failure from depressed myocardial contractility, and (c) the hemodynamic vicious circle with increased systemic vascular resistance and increased afterload with worsening of LV function and exaggeration of forward failure (Fig. 16-16). Whereas diastolic failure may occur without overt systolic failure, the latter is always accompanied by diastolic failure.

Diastolic failure has the following clinical consequences (Table 16-3): increased pulmonary wedge pressure (Fig. 16-16), pulmonary crackles, a tendency to pulmonary edema, pulmonary arterial hypertension, right ventricular failure, jugular venous pressure elevation, hepatic distention and dysfunction, and increased renal vein pressure and renal dysfunction. Of all these features, breathlessness, or dyspnea, is the most sensitive index of backward failure. "The first indication of cardiac failure is to be found in diminished tolerance to exer-

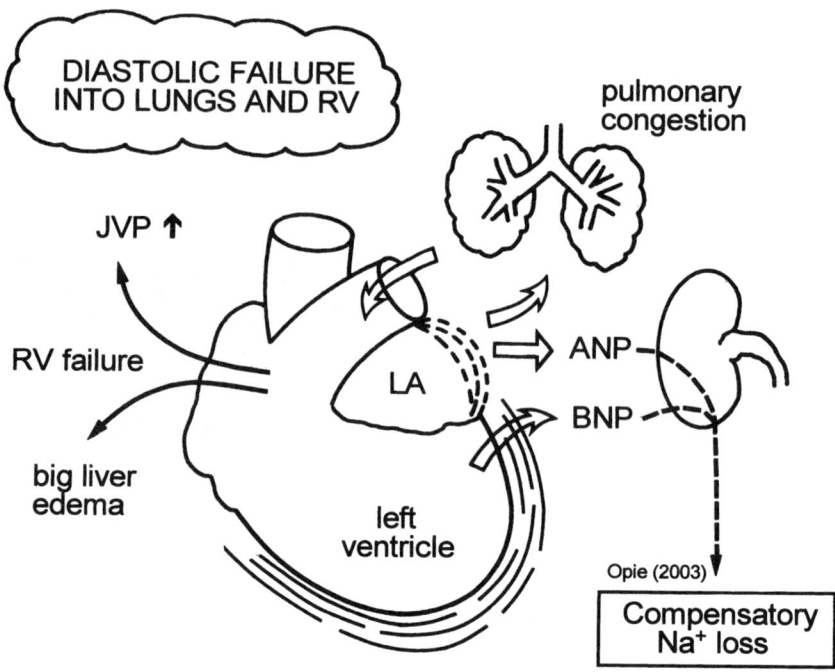

FIG. 16-15. Backward or diastolic failure. The differentiation into backward and forward failure is didactic; in reality, these two patterns often occur together. Note the association with pulmonary congestion and abnormalities of left atrial emptying or left ventricular relaxation. *RV*, right ventricle; *LA*, left atrium; *JVP*, jugular venous pressure; *ANP*, atrial natriuretic peptide; *BNP*, brain natriuretic peptide.

cise. Of the very numerous tests of cardiac efficiency...there is none that approaches in delicacy the symptom breathlessness" (29).

Such breathlessness can best be related to an increased pulmonary capillary wedge pressure, which in turn signifies either abnormal LV filling or decreased left atrial emptying. In other words, backward failure and diastolic dysfunction result from the same basic abnormality in diastolic filling patterns of the left ventricle. Both effort intolerance and diastolic dysfunction can be early features of LVH, and both have the same hemodynamic explanation.

Systolic failure is best explained by poor systolic ejection. It is consistently associated with backward failure. Poor muscle perfusion causes impaired exercise capacity with muscle fatigue on exertion. The onset of tachycardia, increased peripheral vasoconstriction, and sodium retention with edema all result from forward failure. Sodium retention results from increased aldosterone secretion, impaired glomerular filtration rate, and renal dysfunction (the latter resulting in part from decreased renal perfusion and also from backward failure). Aldosterone is a sodium-retaining hormone secreted by the adrenal gland. A critical event in the progression of forward failure is the activation of the neurohu-

16. HEART FAILURE: NEUROHUMORAL RESPONSES

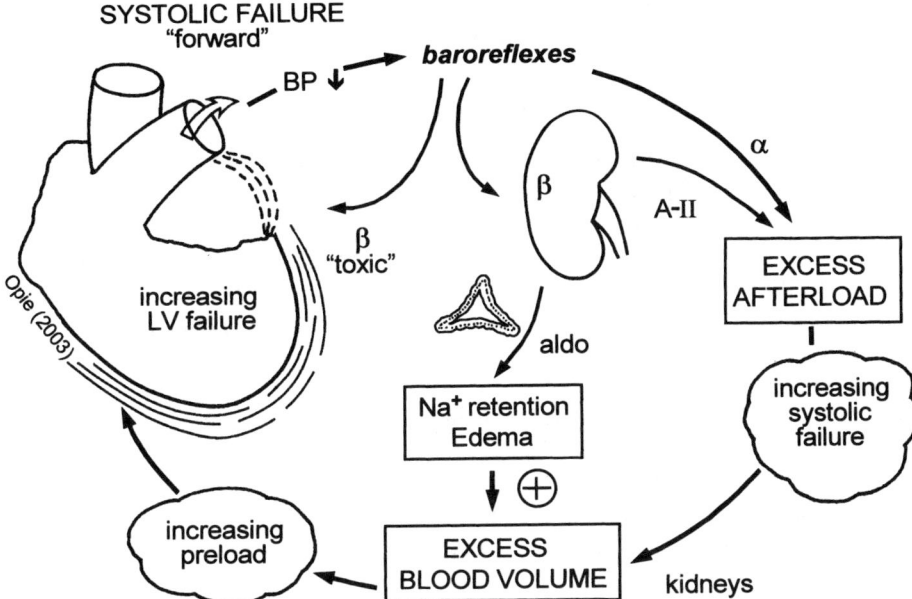

FIG. 16-16. Forward or systolic failure. Note the association of forward failure with hypotension and neurohumoral activation with consequent afterload increase to which increased angiotensin II (*A-II*) and endothelin (*ET*) contribute. α_1, α-adrenergic; β, β-adrenergic; *aldo*, aldosterone.

TABLE 16-3. *Common symptoms and signs of congestive heart failure and their mechanisms*

Symptoms/signs	Mechanism
Backward failure	
Exertional dyspnea	Increased back pressure with exercise; impaired diastolic relaxation
Pulmonary crepitations (crackles, extra lung sounds)	Increased left ventricular end-diastolic pressure with back pressure
Right ventricular failure, elevated jugular venous pressure,[a] distended liver	Features of increasing back pressure
Forward failure	
Exertional limb fatigue	Forward failure with low cardiac output
Cold extremities	Peripheral vasoconstriction; sympathetic and renin–angiotensin activation
Tachycardia	Sympathetic activation; Bainbridge reflex
Edema and fluid retention	Aldosterone activation
Metabolic-endocrine	
Impaired renal function	Backward and forward failure
Oliguria (low urine volume)	Severe fluid retention; poor renal perfusion
Low serum sodium	Aldosterone and vasopressin secretion
Low serum potassium	Usually drug induced (diuretics, sympathomimetic agents), sometimes effect of excess aldosterone

[a]Correlates with pulmonary wedge pressure, see Butman et al. (31a).

moral abnormalities (so-called because the adrenergic nervous system is closely associated with the renin–angiotensin humoral response).

CATECHOLAMINES AND β-RECEPTORS IN HEART FAILURE

It is not clear exactly at what point in the development of congestive heart failure *sympathetic adrenergic stimulation* starts. Experimentally, it is closely associated with failure of myocardial contractility (32). We know that in severe heart failure, plasma norepinephrine is elevated, that the degree of elevation bears a relation to the severity of heart failure, and that the plasma level of norepinephrine is powerfully related to the prognosis (33). Therefore, it is reasonable to suppose that myocardial failure results in sympathetic activation and that such activation has adverse consequences. A possible mechanism is that impaired myocardial function results in relative hypotension that stimulates the baroreceptors to activate the sympathetic nervous system.

Excess catecholamine stimulation adversely affects the myocardium, as already outlined in Chapter 7. As β_1-adrenergic receptors are downgraded (Fig. 16-17), and β_2-adrenergic receptors become more prominent and may even

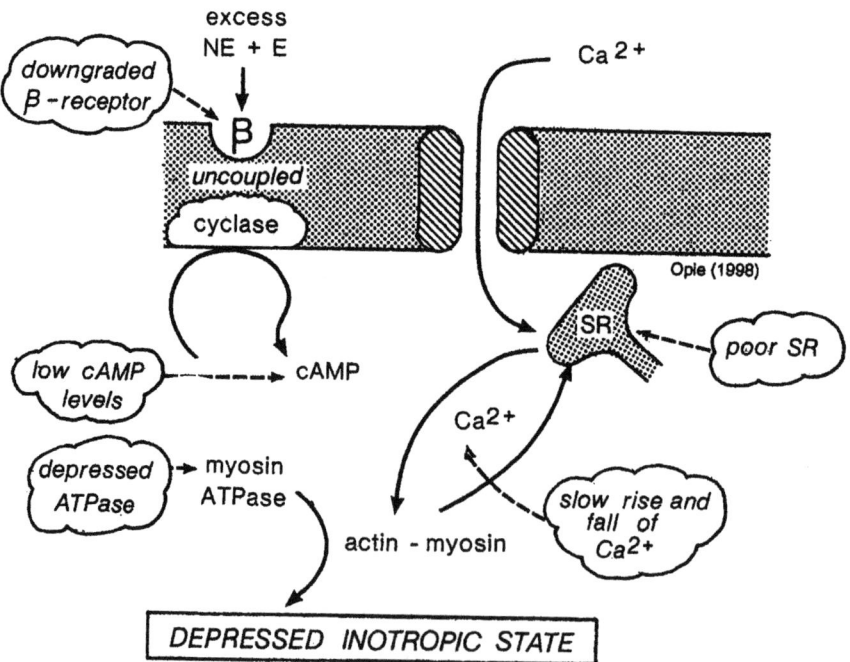

FIG. 16-17. Calcium cycling in severe heart failure. Note the multiple mechanisms for the depressed inotropic state. *NE*, norepinephrine; *E*, epinephrine; *SR*, sarcoplasmic reticulum; *β*, β-adrenergic; *cAMP*, cyclic adenosine 3′,5′-monophosphate.

inhibit formation of cyclic adenosine 3′,5′-monophosphate (cAMP) via G_i signaling (Fig. 16-18). The total of the potential harm of excess catecholamine stimulation is serious and includes (a) enhanced sarcolemmal permeability, (b) intracellular calcium overload and a delayed diastolic decrease in calcium, (c) arrhythmogenic mechanisms that follow excess cAMP or calcium stimulation, (d) impaired mechanical function, possibly with impaired diastolic relaxation, (e) increased apoptosis (17), and (f) myocardial oxygen wastage (34). The ultimate effects of excess catecholamines and calcium overload are likely to be harmful and contribute to the process of accelerating myocardial failure. In addition, excess sympathetic stimulation releases renin from the kidneys, leading to the adverse effects of A-II, including cardiac remodeling.

The major hemodynamic consequences of sympathetic stimulation include (a) β-adrenergic–mediated sinus tachycardia and α-adrenergic–mediated peripheral vasoconstriction (Table 16-2), both of which have potentially harmful effects on the failing myocardium, the former by decreasing the diastolic filling time and the latter by increasing afterload and (b) a potential positive inotropic effect, which

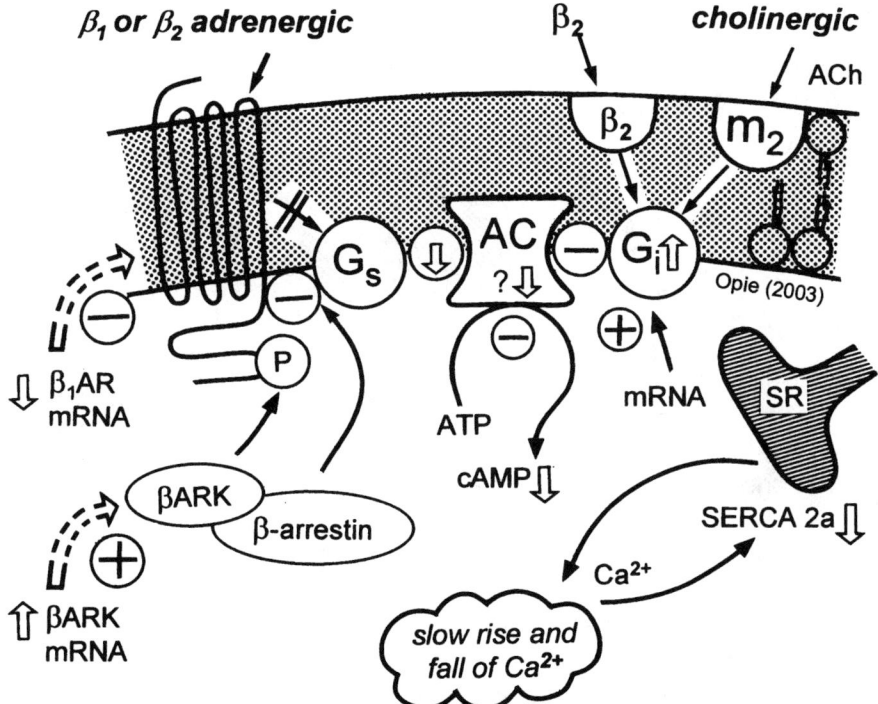

FIG. 16-18. Mechanisms of β-adrenergic receptor desensitization and internalization. Note the links between internalized receptor complex and stimulation of growth via mitogen-activated protein (*MAP*) kinases. This sequence might contribute to abnormal ventricular growth in heart failure. (Modified from Hein et al. *Trends Cardiovasc Med* 1997;7:137.)

only in part compensates for decreased stroke volume and the inherent contractile failure of the myocardium because of down-regulation of the β-adrenergic messenger system (Fig. 16-18). It is not clear whether such excessive and prolonged myocardial sympathetic stimulation leads directly to $β_1$-adrenergic receptor downgrading or whether genetic reprogramming is involved; the result is less inotropic response to catecholamines (35,36). This impaired response to catecholamines is relatively specific to the myocardium, so that increased sympathetic stimulation of the kidneys leads to the expected increase in renin release with consequent formation of vasoconstrictive A-II.

$β_1$-Adrenergic Receptor Down-regulation

During the development of congestive heart failure, circulating catecholamine levels increase, especially during exercise. Long-term, high-level exposure to such catecholamines should lead to a marked decrease in myocardial responsiveness through the process of desensitization (Fig. 16-18). The rate of development of such changes is not known, but the whole process extends over hours or even longer (Fig. 7-6). β-Adrenergic–induced desensitization requires the

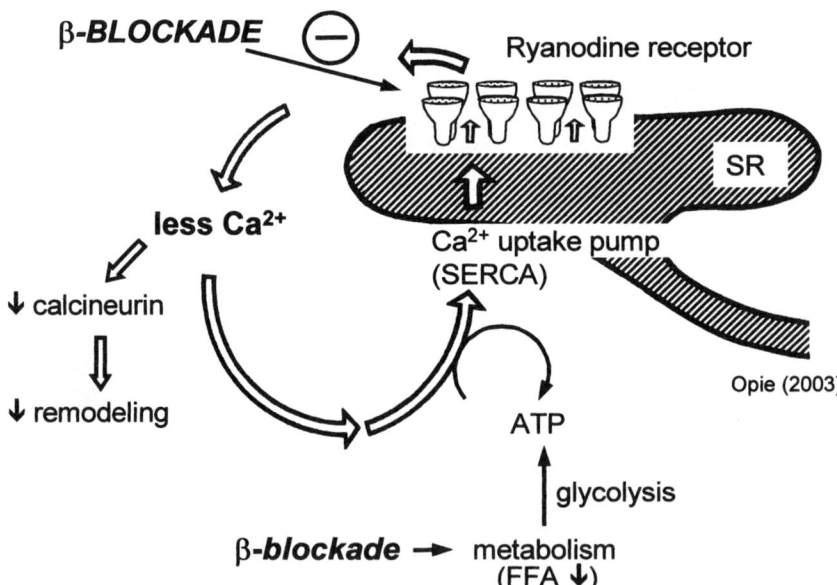

FIG. 16-19. **Hypothetical effects of β-blockade on ryanodine receptors.** By decreasing hyperphosphorylation (Fig. 6-12), there is less calcium leak from the sarcoplasmic reticulum (*SR*). Cytosolic calcium decreases, with less stimulation of the growth factor calcineurin. Calcium uptake by the SERCA (sarco(endo)plasmic reticulum calcium–ATPase) pump may hypothetically be improved as result of increased production of adenosine 5′-triphosphate by glycolysis.

activity of the β-adrenergic receptor kinase that phosphorylates and thereby inactivates the β- adrenergic receptor (Fig. 16-19). Inhibition of the activity of the β-adrenergic receptor kinase prolongs survival and enhances the effects of beta-blocker therapy in a transgenic mouse model of severe heart failure (37), thus emphasizing the overall adverse effects of excess β-adrenergic stimulation on the β-adrenergic messenger system.

Compensatory Role of β_2-Adrenergic Receptors

Sizable amounts of β_2-adrenergic receptors are found in the nonfailing human ventricle, amounting to approximately 15% of the combined β_1 plus β_2-adrenergic receptor population. These β_2-adrenergic receptors may physiologically help to sustain the full and maximal inotropic response to catecholamine stimulation and pathologically come into greater prominence as the β_1-adrenergic receptors are downgraded. Nonetheless, the β_2-adrenergic receptors also do not function normally in that they are partially uncoupled from the G proteins (Table 16-4). Thus, β_2-agonist stimulation does not have the full expected inotropic result. In fact, β_2-agonist activity may be linked via the inhibitory G protein G_i to a negative inotropic antiapoptotic effect (38).

TABLE 16-4. Receptors and signaling systems in severe congestive heart failure[a]

Receptors
  β_1-Adrenergic receptors downgraded, i.e., density and activity decreased[b]
  β_2-Adrenergic receptor density unchanged; functional uncoupling[b]
  α_1-Adrenergic receptors relatively increased in density[b]
  VIP receptors decreased in density but affinity considerably more[c]
G proteins
  G_i increased with inhibition of adenylate cyclase[d–f]
  G_s normal[g] or decreased[h]
Adenylate cyclase
  Decreased cyclase activity with less production of cAMP, related to G_i increase[e]; still responds directly to forskolin[i]
cAMP
  Production impaired, presumably owing to adenylate cyclase inhibition[j]
Calcium transients
  Impaired transients with low peak and delayed decrease in diastole[i]
  Calcium uptake by SR unchanged[j] or decreased in situ[j,k]
  Calcium release by SR decreased[l]
  Single calcium channel activity normal[k, m]
  Amount of calcium entry via calcium channel may be abnormal[l]

[a]References 37a, 37b.
[b–h]See references 37c–37i.
[i]Reference 18.
[j–m]See references 37j–37m.
VIP, vasoactive intestinal peptide; cAMP, cyclic adenosine 3′,5′-monophosphate; SR, sarcoplasmic reticulum.

Cyclic Adenosine 3′,5′-Monophosphate Generation in Heart Failure

Another serious abnormality in end-stage heart failure is poor generation of cAMP (Fig. 16-17) in response to β-adrenergic agonist agents (18). When cardiac cAMP is increased by adenovirus transfer of adenyl cyclase, contractility of the failing myocardium increases (39).

$β_3$-Adrenergic Receptors

In addition to their important role in adipose tissue, these receptors may have a cardiac function. The proposal is that they respond to adrenergic stimulation by an unexpected negative inotropic response, so that their relative overexpression in the failing heart could exaggerate the already poor mechanical function (40).

Benefit of β-Adrenergic Blockers in Heart Failure

If given in high doses to a patient with severe heart failure, circulatory collapse can occur, whereas when given in low doses that are cautiously increased to patients already stabilized by other agents for heart failure, there is a striking reduction in mortality. The mechanisms are complex (Fig. 16-19). Besides an antiarrhythmic effect, β-blockade is able to reverse remodeling (41) and improve to internal calcium cycling (42). A recent proposal is that the cardiac RyR that controls the release of calcium ions from the SR is hyperphosphorylated in heart failure, so that there is excess release of calcium from SR with cytosolic calcium overload (20,42). This process is inhibited by β-blockade, so that the control of calcium is restored toward normal. Second, β-blockade decreases the uptake and use of free fatty acids by the failing human heart (43). Fatty acids adversely influence the failing heart (Fig. 16-11). Hypothetically, increased glycolysis could improve the availability of adenosine 5′-triphosphate for the calcium-uptake pump of the SR. Other mechanisms include (a) bradycardia, thereby decreasing myocardial energy demand and the energy deficit (Fig. 16-10); (b) protection from catecholamine-induced fatal ventricular arrhythmias; (c) improved β-adrenergic signaling; (d) antiapoptosis; and (e) decreased activation of renin–angiotensin inhibition because β-stimulation releases renin from the kidneys. β-Blockade consistently improves cardiac output of patients with heart failure and abnormal patterns of gene expression revert toward normal (44).

ANGIOTENSIN II AND OTHER VASOCONSTRICTIVE PEPTIDES

In severe heart failure, both myocardial tissue and circulating levels of A-II are increased. Besides acting as a local myocardial growth factor (Fig. 13-14), angiotensin-mediated vasoconstriction adds to that resulting from the sympathetic activation (Fig. 16-20). Both a low renal perfusion pressure and increased β-adrenergic stimulation contribute to renin release (Fig. 16-21). The A-II thus formed both directly constricts the peripheral vessels and enhances the degree of sympathetic activation. A-II also evokes the release of aldosterone that retains sodium and water to increase body fluid volume. The latter process is clinically manifest as excess volume in the legs, detected by pitting in response to finger pressure (edema). Sodium and water retention resulting from aldosterone secretion tends to reverse the low renal perfusion pressure but provokes pulmonary edema. The causes of increased renin secretion are, therefore, subject to feedback, which may explain why in nearly half of untreated patients with severe cardiac edema, the renin and aldosterone levels are normal (45). In some severe cases, the low blood sodium resulting from excess volume retention sends out the wrong signals to the pituitary gland (at the base of the brain) and causes an inappropriate secretion of the *antidiuretic hormone* (Fig. 2-12). Antidiuretic hormone is also called *vasopressin* (*vaso*, vessels; *pressin*, pressure) and may further increase afterload by peripheral vasoconstriction. It also decreases renal loss of water, with more retention of extracellular fluid and an

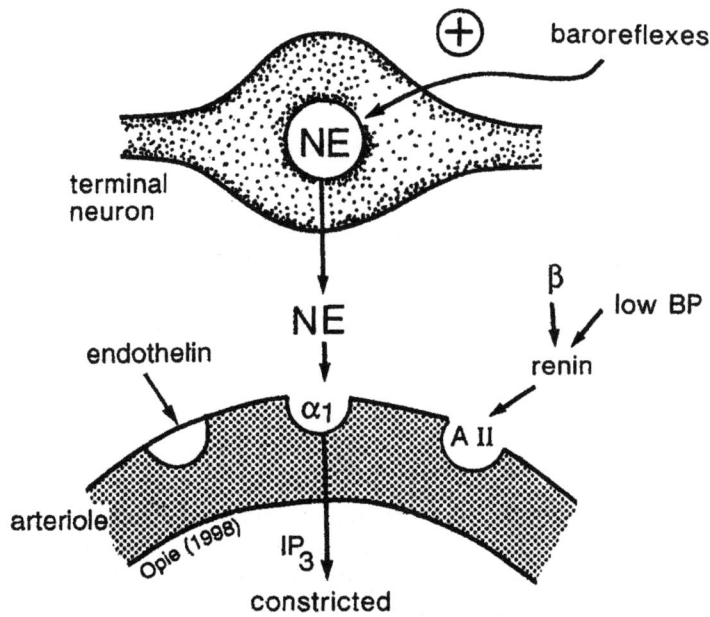

FIG. 16-20. Afterload increase in heart failure. *NE*, norepinephrine; *β*, β-adrenergic; *BP*, blood pressure; *IP₃*, inositol trisphosphate; α_1, α_1-adrenergic; *A-II*, angiotensin II.

514   *16. HEART FAILURE: NEUROHUMORAL RESPONSES*

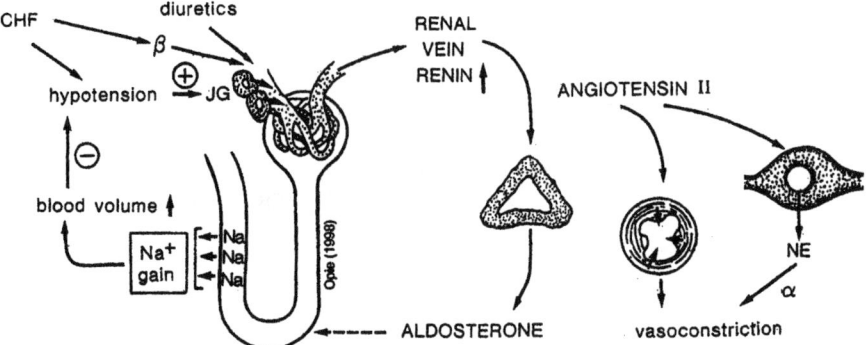

FIG. 16-21. Renin–angiotensin system in congestive heart failure (*CHF*). In congestive heart failure, renin secretion from the juxtaglomerular (*JG*) cells in the kidney increases by two mechanisms: hypotension and increased β-adrenergic stimulation (*β*). Circulating renin then stimulates a plasma substrate to convert circulating angiotensinogen to angiotensin I, which is converted to angiotensin II in the tissue to cause vasoconstriction. Angiotensin II also increases release of norepinephrine (*NE*) to further promote vasoconstriction. Angiotensin II releases aldosterone from the adrenal glands, thereby causing sodium and water retention, which helps to maintain blood pressure and renal perfusion. There is thus a feedback loop on the kidney to decrease renin secretion. Note the role of diuretic therapy in promoting renin release. α, α-adrenergic.

exaggeration of the low blood sodium (hyponatremia), which contrasts with overall sodium retention.

Sodium Retention and Edema

Increased secretion of aldosterone leads to overall retention of water (fluid) and sodium, which is termed edema and is a characteristic of congestive heart failure (Fig. 16-21). The overall retention of sodium is the combined result of excess aldosterone secretion and poor renal blood flow. It should be stressed that there can be a combination of low serum sodium together and marked overall sodium retention, reflecting the respective consequences of vasopressin and aldosterone secretion.

Endothelin in Heart Failure

Circulating levels of endothelin are greatly increased in severe heart failure. The source of the endothelin is at least in part the myocardium in which there are increased levels of preproendothelin-1 (46). Increased A-II, both circulating and in the tissue, promotes the synthesis of increased endothelin. Endothelin may also be formed independently of A-II, for example, by damage to endothelial cells, and such endothelin may play a role in the transition from LVH to heart failure (47). Endothelin in excess has a direct toxic myocardial effect, perhaps by promoting calcium overload (46).

Cytokines in Heart Failure

Cytokines are locally acting autocoid polypeptide mediators (Greek, *autos*, self; *akos*, remedy). Cytokines act locally in one of several manners: autocrine (active on the cells of origin), paracrine (acting on neighboring cells), or juxtacrine (acting on adjacent cells). Examples are the inflammatory cytokines, such as the interleukin-1 and -6, derived from macrophages and leukocytes. Such cells are especially found in the myocardium in infective cardiomyopathies but also after myocardial infarction and reperfusion. The concept of beneficial adaptive cytokine effects at their physiologic concentrations contrasts with adverse maladaptive effects of excess cytokines, as already discussed in Chapter 9.

The importance of cytokines in heart failure is still not fully elucidated, but it is often proposed that increased formation of tumor necrosis factor-α (TNF-α) in the heart and increased circulating levels have adverse effects. The mechanism of increased formation of TNF-α in the heart may be related to enhanced activity of A-II (48). Such overexpression of TNF-α may accelerate apoptosis to increase the severity of heart failure (Fig. 9-9). Induction of TNF-α in the hypertrophic heart may activate the metalloproteinases, thereby promoting remodeling with LV dilation and LV pump failure (49). In support of the adverse effects of TNF-α, overexpression of TNF-α in mice leads to dilated cardiomyopathy (48). Furthermore, increased expression of myocardial TNF-α in mitral regurgitation is reversed when the volume overload is corrected by mitral valve surgery (reference 18 in Chapter 13).

ATRIAL AND BRAIN NATRIURETIC PEPTIDES

Thus far, many of the adaptations discussed have been potentially harmful to the failing myocardium, either directly or by increasing afterload and preload. However, release of atrial natriuretic peptide (ANP) from the atria and brain natriuretic peptide (BNP) from the ventricles have properties beneficial for the circulation in heart failure (Fig. 16-22). Both have diuretic activity (increased urine flow), vasodilate, and inhibit aldosterone secretion. Why are these beneficial effects not apparent? The increased levels of ANP in congestive heart failure are overcome by the drives to vasoconstriction and sodium retention resulting from renin–angiotensin–aldosterone activation. ANP does have potentially beneficial effects in congestive heart failure as shown by the worsening of signs when monoclonal anti-ANP antibodies are given in experimental heart failure (50).

Atrial and Brain Natriuretic Peptide Release from the Failing Ventricle

Besides being secreted from the atria, ANP can also be formed and secreted from hypertrophic and diseased ventricles. *ANP gene reprogramming* occurs in LVH. Volume or pressure overload promotes the release of ANP or its precur-

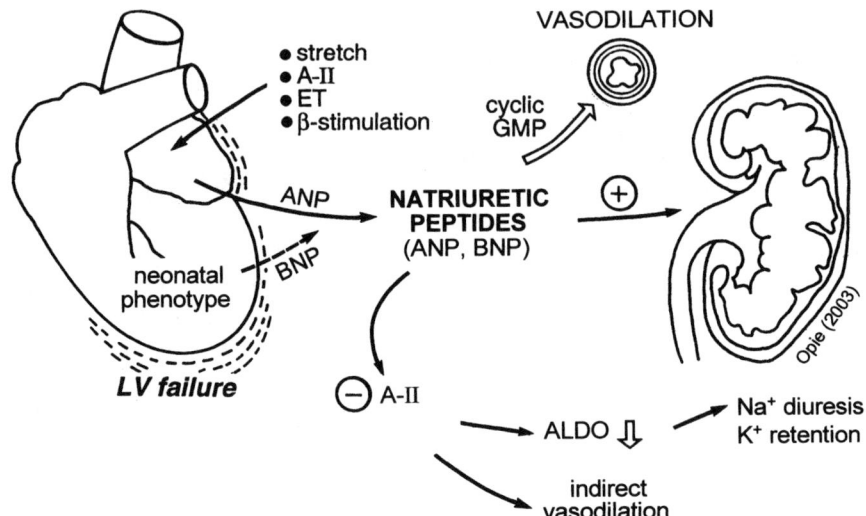

FIG. 16-22. Atrial (*ANP*) and brain (*BNP*) natriuretic peptides. ANP is released from the atria in response to stretch or β-adrenergic (*β*) stimulation, angiotensin II (*A II*), or endothelin (*ET*). In congestive heart failure, there is increased release with increased blood levels of ANP. In congestive heart failure, some of the circulating ANP comes from the ventricles, as does BNP. ANP and BNP have effects that oppose those of renin–angiotensin activation (Fig. 16-20) and compete with angiotensin II for receptors. Generally, the beneficial effects of ANP and BNP secretion are outweighed by vasoconstrictive stimuli and excess sodium retention. *ALDO,* aldosterone secretion from the adrenal cortex.

sors, especially from the endocardial layer where the wall tension is higher. In severe human heart failure, nuclear RNA for ANP is greatly increased (51). Physiologically, it remains true that the atria and not the ventricles are the major source of ANP. BNP is also released from the atria and especially from failing ventricles. BNP has become important to clinical cardiologists. It is a diagnostic test for a wide range of LV problems, including diastolic dysfunction and congestive heart failure, and is a predictor of sudden death in those with severe heart failure (52).

Adrenomedullin

This newly identified peptide, first found in extracts of human pheochromocytoma, has potent vasorelaxing and natriuretic properties and in this way resembles ANP. In severe human heart failure, it is found in the circulation and secreted by the heart. When infused into patients with heart failure, it increases urine volume and sodium excretion (53). Presumably, it joins ANP and BNP as self-protecting peptides made by the failing myocardium.

PRINCIPLES OF THERAPY FOR CONGESTIVE HEART FAILURE

Conventional therapy has five major principles. First, diuretic therapy, by increasing urine and sodium output, relieves the fluid retention and pulmonary congestion, thereby reducing the preload on the heart (Fig. 16-14) and greatly easing the symptoms of the patient. Unfortunately, diuretic therapy promotes the secretion of renin, which helps to cause angiotensin-induced vasoconstriction. Second, angiotensin-converting enzyme inhibition has several benefits. Most obviously, it relieves the vasoconstriction and excess afterload resulting from excess activation of the renin–angiotensin system. More hidden benefits might lie in the inhibition of the myocardial renin–angiotensin system and lessening of fibrosis with improvement of diastolic function. These compounds improve exercise capacity, probably in part through improving diastolic properties. In patients with severe congestive heart failure, added therapy by angiotensin-converting enzyme inhibition decreases mortality. Besides the angiotensin-converting enzyme inhibitors, other vasodilators decrease preload by dilating the venous system or decrease afterload by acting on the arterial dilators. Third, β-blockade, cautiously introduced to those already treated as previously described, decreases mortality by mechanisms already discussed. Fourth, positive inotropic agents, such as digitalis, stimulate the myocardium to contract and move it to a higher Frank–Starling curve (Fig. 16-13). In general, inotropes act by either increasing cytosolic calcium or increasing the sensitivity of the contractile proteins to calcium. Such agents have not decreased mortality, and in some cases have decreased survival, perhaps because of the adverse effects of an increased cytosolic calcium level (Fig. 20-15). Nonetheless, digoxin also acts in a neurohumoral manner to decrease sympathetic outflow, which may explain why it decreases hospitalization of patients with heart failure, which is an important end point. Fifth, spironolactone also decreases mortality, in part by decreasing myocardial fibrosis. Finally, vasodilators, such as nitrates and hydralazine, relieve preload and afterload, respectively.

Novel therapies are being developed. Biventricular pacing is now established. For example, the antioxidant agent allopurinol improves endothelial function in heart failure. The idea of adding more cardiomyocytes (e.g., by direct injection of neonatal cell) is very exciting (54). In the near future, gene therapy is likely, for example, using the adenovirus technique to insert the mRNA for SERCA, thereby helping to overcome defective calcium handling.

Surgical Procedures

These have expanded the possibilities of symptom relief in severe heart failure. The first and best known major advance was the initial cardiac transplantation in Cape Town, South Africa, by Christiaan Barnard in 1967. This technique is still limited by problems of immune-based rejection of the donor heart and currently by a lack of donors. LV assist devices unload the dilated ventricle by pumping blood from the ventricle to the aorta. Myocyte function and size improve, there is better uptake of calcium by the SR, and LV remodeling is reversed. Collagen cross-linking improves, suggesting decreased destruction of the extracellular matrix by MMPs. Thus, mechanical assistance to the ailing left ventricle allows it to recover as the load is lessened, thereby providing a bridge to recovery.

SUMMARY

1. *An excessive pressure load* is initially compensated for by concentric hypertrophy. Hypertension is an example of an excess pressure load and may lead to LVH, impaired LV diastolic function, and eventually LV dilation. The mechanism of the change from the compensated hypertrophic to the dilated myocardium is still under evaluation, but impaired coronary vascular reserve with focal hypoxia and fibrosis may be a crucial factor.
2. *An excessive volume load* causes the myocardial chamber to enlarge by mechanisms not fully understood, possibly by longitudinal hypertrophy and fiber slippage. Some radial hypertrophy also takes place. The resulting compensated state can exist for a long time. However, the longitudinally enlarged cell appears not to compensate well for demands for further hypertrophy, and eventually failure occurs.
3. *In primary myocardial disease* (cardiomyopathy), the cause of the defect is unexplained. In dilated cardiomyopathy, the diseased myocardium causes the cavity to enlarge, thereby increasing wall tension. In hypertrophic cardiomyopathy, the cause of the hypertrophy is genetic. The extreme degree of hypertrophy sensitizes the myocardium to a series of abnormalities that eventually cause myocardial fibrosis and thus myocardial failure.
4. *The coronary vascular reserve* of the hypertrophied myocardium is impaired, which makes it especially sensitive to the possibility of an oxygen supply/demand imbalance, most notably in the subendocardial zones.
5. *Focal fibrosis* may be the consequence of focal hypoxia and causes increased chamber stiffness and permanent damage. Excess circulating catecholamines, as found in patients with established congestive heart failure, can have further adverse effects on the myocardium through calcium overload, thereby increasing myocardial oxygen demand and decreasing myocardial mechanical performance.
6. *The sarcomere lengths* are at or close to a maximum in myocardial failure, and any increase in LV end-diastolic pressure leads to increased endocardial wall tension, with a defect in the oxygen supply/demand ratio. Increasingly, the myocardium functions at the limits of the Starling curve, and any further increase in LV end-diastolic pressure is not matched by an increase in performance. Rather, as subendocardial wall tension and afterload increase, LV performance fails to increase despite the increase in the LV diastolic pressure.
7. *Diastolic dysfunction* is closely linked to abnormalities of LV filling and LV relaxation. The result is increased left atrial and pulmonary wedge pressure, closely linked to the severity of the shortness of breath.

8. *The clinical picture of severe heart failure* is intimately associated with the concomitant development of a series of myocardial metabolic and circulatory neurohumoral abnormalities, including renin–angiotensin–aldosterone activation. These abnormalities serve to aggravate the severity of heart failure by increasing myocardial mechanical impairment and by systemic effects, such as sodium retention, volume overload as a result of fluid retention, and increased afterload on the heart by virtue of increased peripheral vascular resistance.
9. *Cytokines* such as interleukin-1 and -6 and TNF-α may contribute to adverse outcomes in heart failure.
10. *ANP* is released by increased pressure acting on the atria and, to a lesser extent, on the ventricles. ANP stimulates vascular guanylate cyclase to cause vasodilation and, by an unknown mechanism, increases diuresis. Part of the molecule is similar to A-II, and ANP antagonizes effects of A-II, including vasoconstriction and release of aldosterone. BNP is also released from the failing left ventricle and has properties similar to those of ANP.
11. *Adrenomedullin* is another recently identified vasodilating and natriuretic peptide. In established heart failure, these benefits of the three vasodilating peptides are overcome by opposing vasoconstrictive and sodium-retaining stimuli, such as A-II, endothelin, vasopressin, and aldosterone.
12. *Novel therapies* include mechanical assist devices that relieve the excessive wall stress on the left ventricle and thereby unload the heart. Stem-cell therapy is vigorously being explored. Established therapy includes β-adrenergic blockade, angiotensin-converting enzyme inhibition, diuretics, and now, biventricular pacing.

STUDENT QUESTIONS

1. Describe the molecular mechanisms governing myocardial growth in the development of LVH.
2. Describe typical calcium transients in advanced heart failure. How do these patterns come about?
3. What is the role of the renin–angiotensin–aldosterone system in the evolution of congestive heart failure?
4. What are cytokines and how might they play a role in heart failure?
5. What are the physiologic function and role of ANP and BNP in heart failure?

CARDIOLOGIST-IN-TRAINING QUESTIONS

1. What are the patterns of LV response in chronic hypertension? Specifically describe how these conditions differ with respect of LV wall thickness and cavity size. What differences in wall stress do you expect?
2. Is "compensated LVH" really compensated? Give reasons for your answer.
3. In which types of cardiomyopathy are molecular mechanisms involved in the etiology?

4. Can the Starling relationship explain the changes in contractile function of the dilated failing left ventricle? Include an evaluation of the changes of sarcomere length found in this condition.
5. What roles do catecholamine stimulation and β-adrenergic receptors have in the evolution of the syndrome of advanced heart failure?

ACKNOWLEDGMENT

Professor P. J. Commerford, Cape Town, South Africa, provided constructive criticism.

REFERENCES

1. Norton GR, et al. Heart failure in pressure overload hypertrophy. *J Am Coll Cardiol* 2002;39:664–671.
2. Yu C-M, et al. Progression of systolic abnormalities in patients with "isolated" diastolic heart failure and diastolic dysfunction. *Circulation* 2002;105:1195–1201.
3. Cuocolo A, et al. Left ventricular hypertrophy and impaired diastolic filling in essential hypertension. Diastolic mechanisms for systolic dysfunction during exercise. *Circulation* 1990;81:978–986.
4. Zile MR, et al. New concepts in diastolic dysfunction and diastolic heart failure: part 1. *Circulation* 2002;105:1387–1393.
5. Nitenberg A, et al. Left ventricular mechanical efficiency in hypertensive patients with and without increased myocardial mass with normal pump function. *Am J Hypertens* 2001;14:1231–1238.
6. Grossman W, et al. Wall stress and patterns of hypertrophy in the human left ventricle. *J Clin Invest* 1975;56:56–64.
7. Reichek N. Patterns of left ventricular response in essential hypertension. *J Am Coll Cardiol* 1992;19:1559–1560.
8. Hein S, et al. Progression from compensated hypertrophy to failure in the pressure-overloaded human heart. Structural deterioration and compensatory mechanisms. *Circulation* 2003;107:984–991.
9. Ritter O, et al. Calcineurin in human heart hypertrophy. *Circulation* 2002;105:265–2269.
10. Blair E, et al. Mutations of the g_2 subunit of AMP-activated protein kinase cause familial hypertrophic cardiomyopathy: evidence for the central role of energy compromise in disease pathogenesis. *Hum Mol Genet* 2001;10:1215–1220.
11. Olivetti G, et al. Cardiomyopathy of the aging human heart. Myocyte loss and cellular hypertrophy. *Circ Res* 1991;68:1560–1568.
12. Barlucchi L, et al. Canine ventricular myocytes possess a renin-angiotensin system that is upregulated with heart failure. *Circ Res* 2001;88:298–304.
13. Starling M, et al. Mechanisms for left ventricular systolic dysfunction in aortic regurgitation: importance for predicting the functional response to aortic valve replacement. *J Am Coll Cardiol* 1991;17:898–900.
14. Linzbach AJ. Heart failure from the point of view of quantitative anatomy. *Am J Cardiol* 1960;5:370–382.
15. Jalil JE, et al. Fibrosis-induced reduction of endomyocardium in the rat after isoproterenol treatment. *Circ Res* 1989;65:258–264.
16. Woodiwiss AJ, et al. Reduction in myocardial collagen cross-linking parallels left ventricular dilatation in rat models of systolic chamber dysfunction. *Circulation* 2001;103:155–160.
17. Colucci WS. Apoptosis in the heart. *N Engl J Med* 1996;335:1224–1226.
18. Morgan JP, et al. Abnormal intracellular calcium handling, a major cause of systolic and diastolic dysfunction in ventricular myocardium from patients with heart failure. *Circulation* 1990;81(suppl III):III-21–III-32.
19. Hasenfuss G, et al. Calcium cycling in congestive heart failure. *J Mol Cell Cardiol* 2002;34:951–969.
20. Marks AR. Cardiac intracellular calcium release channels. Role in heart failure. *Circ Res* 2000;87:8–11.

21. Minamisawa S, et al. Chronic phospholamban-sarcoplasmic reticulum calcium ATPase interaction is the critical calcium cycling defect in dilated cardiomyopathy. *Cell* 1999;99:313–322.
22. Piacentino III V, et al. Cellular basis of abnormal calcium transients of failing human ventricular myocytes. *Circ Res* 2003;92:651–658.
23. Schillinger W, et al. Importance of sympathetic activation for the expression of Na^+-Ca^{2+} exchanger in end-stage failing human myocardium. *Eur Heart J* 2002;23:1118–1124.
24. Gunning JF, et al. Myocardial oxygen consumption during experimental hypertrophy and congestive heart failure. *J Mol Cell Cardiol* 1973;5:25–38.
25. Ye Y, et al. High-energy phosphate metabolism and creatine kinase in failing hearts. A new porcine model. *Circulation* 2001;103:1570–1576.
26. Katz AM. Cardiomyopathy of overload. A major determinant of prognosis in congestive heart failure. *N Engl J Med* 1990;322:100–110.
27. Razeghi P, et al. Metabolic gene expression in fetal and failing human heart. *Circulation* 2001;104:2923–2931.
28. Moore TD, et al. Ventricular interaction and external constraint account for decreased stroke work during volume loading in CHF. *Am J Physiol* 2001;281:H2385–H2391.
29. Lewis T. *Diseases of the heart*. London: Macmillan, 1933.
30. Remme WJ, et al. Task Force Report. Guidelines for the diagnosis and treatment of chronic heart failure. Task Force for the Diagnosis and Treatment of Chronic Heart Failure, European Society of Cardiology. *Eur Heart J* 2001;22:1527–1560.
31. Cohn JN. The management of chronic heart failure. *N Engl J Med* 1996;335:490–498.
31a. Butman SM, Ewy GA, Standen JR, et al. Bedside cardiovascular examination in patients with severe chronic heart failure: importance of rest or inducible jugular venous distension. *J Am Coll Cardiol* 1993;22:968–974.
32. Legault F, et al. Functional and morphological characteristics of compensated and decompensated cardiac hypertrophy in dogs with chronic infrarenal aorto-caval fistulas. *Circ Res* 1990;1990:846–859.
33. Cohn JN, et al. Plasma norepinephrine as a guide to prognosis in patients with chronic congestive heart failure. *N Engl J Med* 1984;311:819–823.
34. Opie LH, et al. Adrenaline-induced "oxygen-wastage" and enzyme release from working rat heart. Effects of calcium antagonism, beta-blockade, nicotinic acid and coronary artery ligation. *J Mol Cell Cardiol* 1979;11:1073–1094.
35. Bristow MR, et al. Decreased catecholamine sensitivity and beta-adrenergic receptor density in failing human hearts. *N Engl J Med* 1982;307:205–221.
36. Ogletree-Hughes ML, et al. Mechanical unloading restores β-adrenergic responsiveness and reverses receptor downregulation in the failing human heart. *Circulation* 2001;104:881–886.
37. Harding VB, et al. Cardiac βARK 1 inhibition prolongs survival and augments β blocker therapy in a mouse model of severe heart failure. *Proc Natl Acad Sci U S A* 2001;98:5809–5814.
37a. Lohse MJ. G-protein-coupled receptor kinases and heart. *Trends Cardiovasc Med* 1995;5:63–68.
37b. Brodde OE, Daul A, Michel-Rehner M, et al. Agonist-induced desensitization of β-adrenoceptor function in humans. Subtype-selective reduction in $β_1$- or $β_2$-adrenoceptor-mediated physiological effects by xamoterol or procaterol. *Circulation* 1990;81:914–921.
37c. Bristow MR, Port JD, Gilbert EM. The role of adrenergic receptor regulation in the treatment of heart failure. *Cardiovasc Drugs Ther* 1989;3:971–978.
37d. Hershberger RE, Anderson FL, Bristow MR. Vasoactive intestinal peptide receptor in failing human ventricular myocardium exhibit increased affinity and decreased density. *Circ Res* 1989;65:283–294.
37e. Eschenhagen T, Mende U, Nose M, et al. Increased messenger RNA level of the inhibitory G protein α subunit $G_{iα-2}$ in human end-stage heart failure. *Circ Res* 1992;70:688–696.
37f. Böhm M, Eschenhagen T, Gierschik P, et al. Radioimmunochemical quantification of Giα in right and left ventricles from patients with ischaemic and dilated cardiomyopathy and predominant left ventricular failure. *J Mol Cell Cardiol* 1994;26:133–149.
37g. Feldman AM, Cates AE, Veazey WB, et al. Increase of the 40,000-mol wt pertussis toxin substrate (G-protein) in the failing human heart. *J Clin Invest* 1988;82:189–197.
37h. Schnabel P, Bohm M, Gierschik P, et al. Improvement of cholera toxin-catalyzed ADP-ribosylation by endogenous ADP-ribosylation factor from bovine brain provides evidence for an unchanged amount of G in failing human myocardium. *J Mol Cell Cardiol* 1990;22:73–82.
37i. Feldman AM, Tena RG, Kessler PD, et al. Diminished beta-adrenergic receptor responsiveness and

cardiac dilation in hearts of myopathic Syrian hamsters (BIO 53.58) are associated with a functional abnormality of the G stimulatory protein. *Circulation* 1990;81:1341–1352.
37j. Böhm M, Reiger B. Schwinger RH, et al. cAMP concentrations, cAMP dependent protein kinase activity, and phospholamban in non-failing and failing myocardium. *Cardiovasc Res* 1994;28: 1713–1719.
37k. Movsesian MA, Bristow MR, Krall J. Ca^{2+} uptake by cardiac sarcoplasmic reticulum from patients with idiopathic dilated cardiomyopathy. *Circ Res* 1989;65:1141–1144.
37l. D'Agnolo A, Luciani G, Mazzucco A, et al. Contractile properties and Ca^{2+} release activity of the sarcoplasmic reticulum in dilated cardiomyopathy. *Circulation* 1992;85:518–525.
37m. Holmberg SRM, Williams AJ. Single channel recordings from human cardiac sarcoplasmic reticulum. *Circ Res* 1989;65:1445–1449.
38. Singh K, et al. Adrenergic regulation of myocardial apoptosis. *Cardiovasc Res* 2000;45:713–719.
39. Lai NC, et al. Intracoronary delivery of adenovirus encoding adenylyl cyclase VI increases left ventricular function and cAMP-generating capacity. *Circulation* 2000;102:2396–2401.
40. Moniotte S, et al. Upregulation of beta$_3$-adrenoreceptors and altered contractile response to inotropic amines in human failing myocardium. *Circulation* 2001;103:1649–1655.
41. Groenning BA, et al. Antiremodeling effects on the left ventricle during beta-blockade with metoprolol in the treatment of chronic heart failure. *J Am Coll Cardiol* 2000;36:2072–2082.
42. Doi M, et al. Propranolol prevents the development of heart failure by restoring FKBP 12.6-mediated stabilization of ryanodine receptor. *Circulation* 2002;105:1374–1379.
43. Wallhaus TR, et al. Myocardial free fatty acid and glucose use after carvedilol treatment in patients with congestive heart failure. *Circulation* 2001;103:2441–2446.
44. Lowes BD, et al. Myocardial gene expression in dilated cardiomyopathy treated with beta-blocking agents. *N Engl J Med* 2002;346:1357–1365.
45. Anand IS, et al. Edema of cardiac origin. Studies of body water and sodium, renal function, hemodynamic indexes, and plasma hormones in untreated congestive cardiac failure. *Circulation* 1989; 80:299–305.
46. Sakai S, et al. Inhibition of myocardial endothelin pathway improves long-term survival in heart failure. *Nature* 1996;384:353.
47. Iwanaga Y, et al. Differential effects of angiotensin II versus endothelin-1 inhibitions in hypertrophic left ventricular myocardium during transition to heart failure. *Circulation* 2001;104:606–612.
48. Kalra D, et al. Angiotensin II induces tumour necrosis factor biosynthesis in the adult mammalian heart through a protein kinase C-dependent pathway. *Circulation* 2002;105:2198–2205.
49. Bradham WS, et al. Tumor necrosis factor-alpha and myocardial remodeling in progression of heart failure: a current perspective. *Cardiovasc Res* 2002;53:822–830.
50. Ruskoaho H, et al. Regulation of ventricular atrial natriuretic peptide release in hypertrophied rat myocardium. Effects of exercise. *Circulation* 1989;80:390–400.
51. Lowes BD, et al. Changes in gene expression in the intact human heart. *J Clin Invest* 1997;100: 2315–2324.
52. Maisel A. B-type natriuretic peptide levels: diagnostic and prognostic in congestive heart failure. What next? [Editorial]. *Circulation* 2002;105:2328–2331.
53. Nagaya N, et al. Hemodynamic, renal and hormonal effects of adrenomedullin infusion in patients with congestive heart failure. *Circulation* 2000;101:498–503.
54. Müller-Ehmsen J, et al. Rebuilding a damaged heart. Long-term survival of transplanted neonatal rat cardiomyocytes after myocardial infarction and effect on cardiac function. *Circulation* 2002;105: 1720–1726.
55. Sundstrom J. Left ventricular hypertrophy and the insulin resistance syndrome. *Comprehensive summaries of Uppsala dissertations from the Faculty of Medicine, Uppsala, Sweden.* Uppsala: Acta Universitatis Upsaliensis, 2001.

PART VI
Pathophysiology

17

Lack of Blood Flow: Ischemia and Angina

Lionel H. Opie and Gerd Heusch

"Motion will soon be lost in the part thus deprived of blood."
Erichsen (1)

Although there still is some debate about the definition of myocardial ischemia, in the end, the concept is simple: ischemia means that the blood supply to the myocardium is inadequate to maintain normal oxidative metabolism. The Greek *ischo* means to hold back, and *haima* means blood. The word ischemia was apparently first used by Rudolf Virchow in 1858: *"so habe ich den neuen Ausdruck der Ischaemie vorgeschlagen, um damit die Hemmung der Blutzufuhr, die Vermehrung der Widerstände des Einströmens zu bezeichnen"* (2).

The approximate translation is that the word ischemia describes the limitation of the blood supply with an increased resistance to flow. The fundamental concept of supply/demand imbalance as a cause of ischemia came from observations on an exercising limb (3).

> In health when we excite the muscle action to more energetic action than usual, we increase the circulation in every part. If, however, we call into vigorous action a limb around which we with a moderate degree of tightness applied a ligature, we find then that the member can only support its action for a very short time; for now its supply of energy and its expenditure do not balance each other.

Myocardial ischemia therefore exists when the reduction of coronary flow is so severe that the supply of oxygen to the myocardium cannot meet the oxygen demands of the tissue (Fig. 17-1). How can the myocardium survive such a severe insult? A current biologic concept, based on general biologic principles derived from liver and brain cells, proposes two phases of adaptation: short-term "defense" and longer term "rescue" (4). Applying these proposals to the oxygen-deficient heart, the aim of short-term defense is to achieve a new balance between the oxygen demand and supply by a combination of down-regulation of contraction and up-regulation of anaerobic energy production by glycolysis. The aim of defense

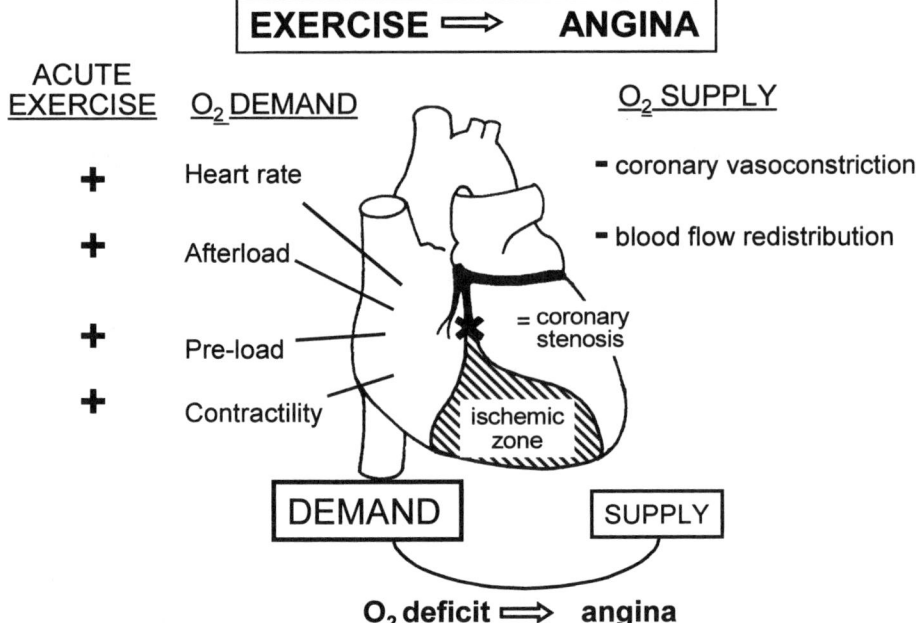

FIG. 17-1. Myocardial oxygen demand during exercise. The major determinants in the normal heart are heart rate, afterload, preload, and contractility. When the myocardial oxygen demand increases and blood flow is not concomitantly increased or is even reduced, as in exercising patients with coronary stenosis, the result is the chest pain called angina pectoris. Clinically, the heart rate increase during exercise is one of the major determinants of myocardial oxygen uptake.

and rescue is to avoid cell death (Chapter 18), otherwise inevitable when the ischemia is overwhelmingly severe and prolonged. Long-term rescue is still poorly understood, but increasingly it seems that ischemia, perhaps acting through hypoxia, is able to induce a series of cellular signals that both bring into play otherwise dormant protective paths, as in short-term preconditioning, and lead to protective genetic reprogramming as in delayed preconditioning (Chapter 19).

ACUTE ADAPTATION TO ISCHEMIA

Perfusion–Contraction Match and Mismatch

The major adaptation to a sudden decrease in blood flow is a corresponding decrease in contraction (Fig. 17-2). Because of the linearity of the response, this is an example of perfusion–contraction match. On reperfusion, there is delayed mechanical recovery or stunning, an example of perfusion–contraction mismatch (Fig. 17-3) (5). The decreased work during ischemia proportionately decreases the oxygen demand and helps to conserve the underperfused myocardium.

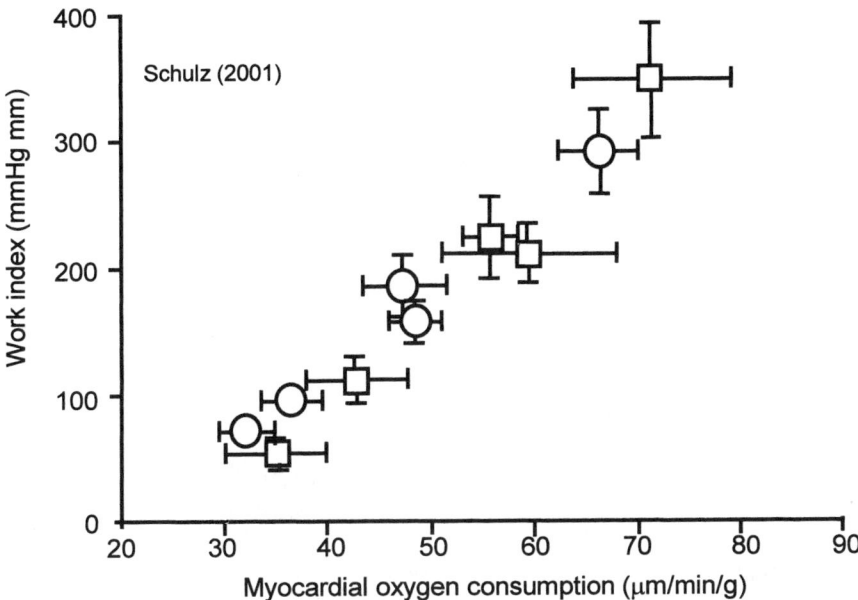

FIG. 17-2. Perfusion–contraction matching. As the coronary perfusion pressure decreases in pigs with coronary stenosis, there is a linear decrease in the myocardial oxygen consumption and the work of the heart. (Adapted from Schulz R, et al. Progressive loss of perfusion-contraction matching during sustained moderate ischemia in pigs. *Am J Physiol* 2001;280:H1945–H1953.)

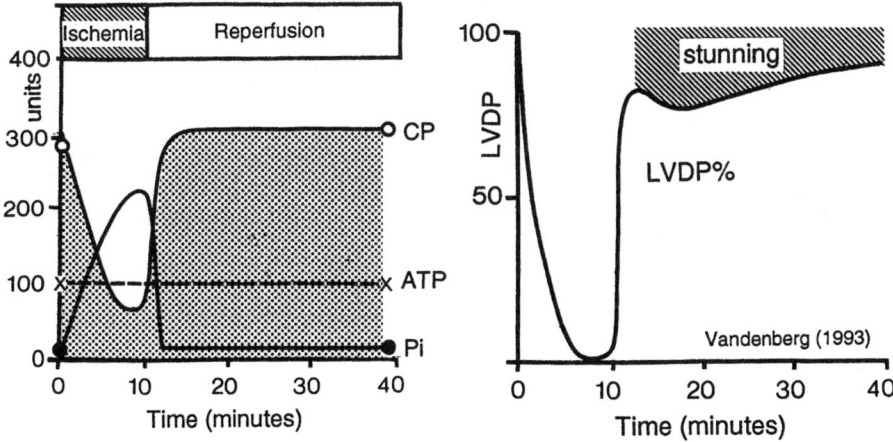

FIG. 17-3. Transient ischemia followed by reperfusion. Ten minutes of ischemia at 30°C results in a rapid decrease in creatine phosphate (*CP*) and increase in inorganic phosphate (*Pi*), whereas adenosine 5'-triphosphate (*ATP*) is buffered. Left ventricular developed pressure (*LVDP*) decreases abruptly. Arbitrary concentration units for CP, ATP, and Pi. (Modified from Vandenberg JI, et al. Mechanisms of pHi recovery after global ischemia in the perfused heart. *Circ Res* 1993;72:993–1003.)

Protective Metabolic Changes

Very rapidly after the onset of ischemia, there is an energy imbalance (Fig. 17-3) with a decline of high-energy phosphate compounds, particularly phosphocreatine, which protects the level of adenosine 5'-triphosphate (ATP) as long as possible, with an increase in intracellular inorganic phosphate. This change is one of the main signals to the down-regulation of contraction, which decreases within a few beats of the onset of coronary artery ligation. Simultaneously, the decline in the energy status is probably the major signal to the increase in anaerobic glycolysis, which occurs within 8 seconds of coronary occlusion in the dog heart (6). The latter has as its initial source the acute onset of glycogen breakdown, quickly followed by an increase in glucose transport. Intracellular acidosis develops quickly, contributing to the decreased contraction. Thus, the ischemic myocardium can survive for a limited time, for as long as 15 minutes of severe ischemia (6) by a combination of inhibition of contraction and initiation of anaerobic glycolysis. The result is that on reperfusion, there are rapid recovery of mechanical function (albeit to a somewhat lower level because of stunning) and reversal of the metabolic abnormalities (Fig. 17-3). The potential danger is that the ischemic decrease in contractile power may seriously threaten the well-being of the body as a whole because cardiac output will decrease if the ischemia involves enough myocardium.

Ischemic Contractile Failure

The major adaptation to ischemia is an abrupt decrease in the oxygen demand as contraction rapidly decreases. Many theories have been advanced for such contractile failure (Table 17-1). The two basic mechanisms most frequently advanced relate to either the effects of poor oxygen delivery or the accumulation

TABLE 17-1. *Possible causes of early impairment of contractility in severe ischemia*

Proposed mechanism
Accumulation of metabolites
Intracellular acidosis with displacement of Ca^{2+} from intracellular binding sites on contractile proteins
Accumulation of inorganic phosphate with an interaction with calcium
Accumulation of neutral lactate
Changes in high-energy phosphate levels or availability
Decreased turnover of ATP
Decreased level of cytosolic phosphocreatine with impaired phosphocreatine shuttle[a]
Decreased ATP in a contractile subcompartment
Decreased free-energy change (Δ_G) of ATP hydrolysis
Mechanical effects of decreased coronary flow
Loss of tissue turgor by reversed "garden hose" or "erectile" effect

[a]Phosphocreatine = creatine phosphate (7).
For other references, see reference 59.
ATP, adenosine 5'-triphosphate.

of inhibitory metabolites. The first factor results in depletion of high-energy phosphate compounds, including ATP and creatine phosphate. Many experiments have shown that contractile failure occurs before there is a major depletion of ATP, which is initially conserved because of the buffer function of creatine phosphate (7). Such data cast doubt on the solitary role of the lack of ATP in contractile failure. Rather, the decrease in cytosolic creatine phosphate is sufficiently severe to suggest that the phosphocreatine (creatine phosphate) shuttle may be inhibited (7) so that the problem may lie with energy transfer from the mitochondria. Cytosolic ATP is required to regulate movement of sodium and hence calcium ions at the sarcolemma (8,9).

The second hypothesis, more than 50 years old and still much favored, is that the accumulation of products of ischemia causes pump failure. In 1935, Tennant (10) related early contractile failure to a build up of lactic acid. In 1969, Katz and Hecht (11) expanded this hypothesis in an influential editorial that proposed that intracellular acidosis decreased contractility because protons displaced calcium from binding sites on the thin contractile filaments. A similar proposal stresses the retention of carbon dioxide during ischemia (Fig. 17-4), also acting by the production of intracellular acidosis. Nonetheless, intracellular acidosis can account for only approximately half the total decrease in contractile activity (12). An alternate hypothesis is that the build up of inorganic phosphate released especially from creatine phosphate is crucial, acting in a still poorly understood manner (13,14).

Whatever the mechanism (possibly a combination of the suggested proposals), the important point is that marked contractile failure and compensatory metabolic changes can occur within 10 to 120 seconds of the onset of severe ischemia (15). When contractile failure is very severe but localized, the ischemic myocardium actually bulges in systole (*dyskinesia*).

Effects of Poor Oxygen Delivery during Ischemia

The lack of adequate oxygen supply to the mitochondria rapidly decreases the energy available to the cytoplasm. The rapid decline of high-energy phosphates, especially of creatine phosphate, stimulates glycolysis and glycogenolysis, and glycolytic flux is promoted to a greater extent than its end products [pyruvate and nicotinamide adenine dinucleotide, reduced form ($NADH_2$)] can enter the oxygen-deprived mitochondria. Potassium also escapes from ischemic cells, in part because of activation and opening of the potassium channels that are normally inhibited by ATP. Oxidation of fatty acids is reduced, and there is an accumulation of lipid metabolites with adverse detergent properties. There are important metabolic and mechanical differences between mild and severe ischemia (Table 17-2).

Lack of Adenosine 5'-Triphosphate

Ultimately, all ion gradients depend on the availability of ATP. Activity of the ATP-dependent potassium channel may be influenced specifically by the avail-

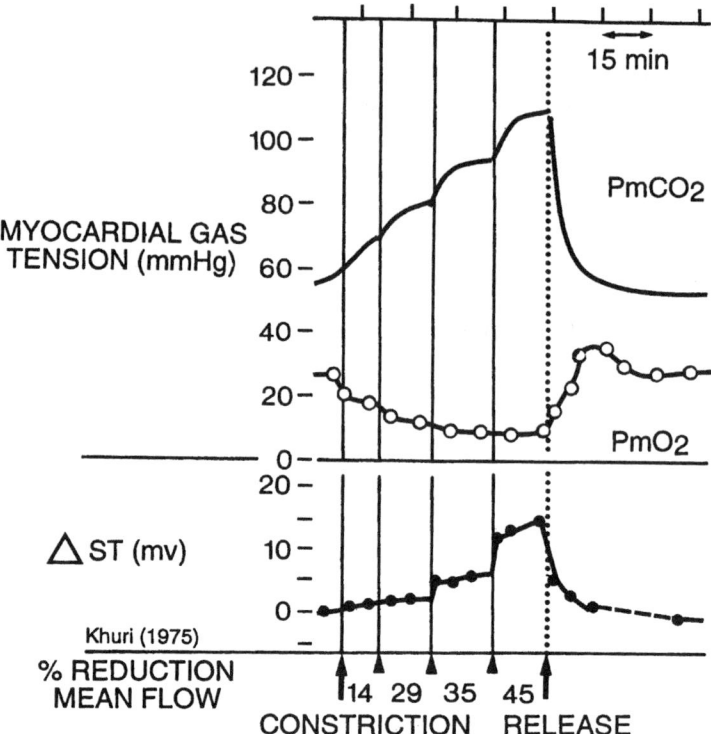

FIG. 17-4. Effects of progressive myocardial ischemia. Extent of reduction of mean coronary flow resulting from increasing coronary artery constriction is shown at bottom of figure, together with effects on ST segment changes and myocardial CO_2 tension ($PmCO_2$) and myocardial oxygen tension (PmO_2). (From Khuri SF, et al. The significance of the late fall in myocardial Pco_2 and its relationship to myocardial pH after regional coronary occlusion in the dog. Circ Res 1985;56:537–547, with permission.)

ability of glycolytic ATP. Likewise, provision of glycolytic ATP may play a role in the regulation of the sodium pump and hence of intracellular sodium and calcium levels. Lack of oxygen is not the only cause of ATP depletion. Another cause lies in a variety of metabolic cycles that are ATP wasting, which have no apparent benefit for the ischemic myocardium and yet need ATP. An example is the excess internal cycling of excess levels of calcium found in the ischemic-reperfused myocardium, in and out of the sarcoplasmic reticulum, a process that needs ATP for the uptake cycle. Other metabolic cycles, provoked by ischemia and wasting ATP involve the breakdown of triglyceride and glycogen and their resynthesis. These processes may contribute to proton production in ischemia (Table 17-3).

TABLE 17-2. *Mechanical and metabolic differences between mild and severe ischemia*

	Mild ischemia	Severe ischemia
Prototype	Demand ischemia with metabolic washout	Supply ischemia without metabolic washout
Animal model[a]	Low-flow global ischemia	Coronary artery ligation with added pacing
Human condition	Angina of effort or pacing	Coronary occlusion; acute myocardial infarction, balloon inflation
Diastolic stiffness[b]	Increases	Decreases
Cytosolic calcium	Increases	Increases
Cause of increased cytosolic calcium	? Inhibited glycolysis ?$Na^+/H^+/Ca^{2+}$ exchange	Tissue acidosis + $Na^+/H^+/Ca^{2+}$ exchange
Factors opposing effect of increase in cytosolic calcium	None	Tissue acidosis, increased tissue inorganic phosphate
Coronary arteries in ischemic zone	Arteries normally distended, may contribute to stiff heart	Collapsed; loss of turgor with reversed garden hose effect
Pressure–volume loop	End-diastolic point moves up	End-diastolic point may move rightward
Left ventricular systolic performance[c]	Moderately reduced	Markedly reduced
Reperfusion	Diastolic failure[d]	Systolic and diastolic failure

[a]Reference 40. [b]Reference 15a. [c]Reference 41. [d]Reference 15b.

TABLE 17-3. Sources of proton formation and acidosis in the myocardium in anoxia-ischemia

Process	Mechanism of generation	Comment
Inhibition of mitochondrial oxidation of $NADH_2$	Inhibition of mitochondrial metabolism	$NADH_2$ formed by anaerobic glycolysis is regenerated to NAD by conversion of pyruvate to lactate; other processes must be responsible for increased cytosolic $NADH_2$/NAD ratio in ischemia
Anaerobic glycolysis	ATP breakdown	Anaerobic glycolysis results in no proton production; protons form during breakdown of ATP
Increased tissue CO_2	Continued residual respiration; poor washout	Only in ischemia, not in anoxia
Triglyceride–FFA cycle	Continued breakdown and resynthesis of TG; ATP lost with proton production	3 ATP used per cycle, 6–7 protons produced per cycle
Glycogen turnover	Excess recycling uses ATP and produces protons	1 ATP, 1 UTP, and 1 proton per cycle
Mitochondrial uptake of calcium	Counter transport of protons with calcium ATP breakdown	Uptake of calcium by mitochondria uses ATP and therefore produces protons

$NADH_2$, nicotinamide adenine dinucleotide (reduced form); NAD nicotinamide adenine dinucleotide; ATP, adenine 5'-triphosphate; FFA, free fatty acid; TG, triglyceride; UTP, uridine 5'-triphosphate.

Anaerobic Glycolysis

Ischemia has a biphasic effect on glycolysis depending on its severity (Fig. 11-3). First, there is stimulation. Then, as the severity of ischemia increases, delivery of glucose decreases, glycogen becomes depleted, and inhibitory metabolites accumulate, so that the glycolytic rate decreases. During mild ischemia, glycolysis is stimulated at several levels, including translocation of the glucose transporters GLUT-1 and -4 to the sarcolemma (16), while the activity of the key enzyme phosphofructokinase increases so that the glycolytic rate increases as the energy status declines (Fig. 11-23). The major beneficial consequence of such anaerobic glycolysis is increased production of glycolytic ATP, quite inadequate in amount to replace the total energy needs of the contracting myocardium (Fig. 11-24), yet probably crucial in providing ATP strategically located near the sarcolemma and thus maintaining ion gradients. Although the existence of such a pool of membrane-related ATP is still controversial, the concept is useful in explaining some of the effects of the benefit of the provision of glucose to the ischemic myocardium.

Fatty Acid Metabolism in Ischemia

There are two major changes in fatty acid metabolism. First, ischemic inhibition of fatty acid oxidation (basically by deprivation of blood flow and oxygen) leads to an accumulation of lipid metabolites, including intracellular free fatty acids, acyl-CoA, and acylcarnitine. As the tissue contents of the metabolites increase, they are thought to inhibit various aspects of membrane function, such as the mitochondrial translocase, the sodium pump, and phospholipid cycles. Second, membrane phospholipids are broken down by the action of phospholipases, activated by an accumulation of calcium within the ischemic cell. High concentrations of the breakdown products accumulate to form micelles, which are highly membrane active. Such events may in part explain early ischemic ventricular arrhythmias (Chapter 20).

Cytosolic Calcium in Ischemia

Concordant data, obtained by several different methods, provide substantial evidence that cytosolic calcium can increase in ischemia (17–19). Experimentally, within seconds of complete arrest of coronary flow, left ventricular pressure decreases abruptly toward zero as cytosolic calcium increases rapidly and substantially (20). During prolonged or simulated ischemia, there is a consistent increase in cytosolic calcium either before (21), concurrently with the onset of ischemic contracture (17), or just after the maximal depletion of ATP (19). The proposed adverse consequences of the increased calcium level include damage to contractile proteins, activation of phospholipases, increased depolarization, ischemic contracture, and mitochondrial damage (Figs. 19-2 through 19-5).

Cytosolic Magnesium

The affinity of ATP for magnesium is higher than that of adenosine 5′-diphosphate, so that cytosolic magnesium increases during ATP hydrolysis (19). By loading isolated myocytes with the magnesium-sensitive dye magnesium green, it is possible to establish a relationship between the depletion of ATP and other consequences of ischemia such as contracture and the opening of the ATP-sensitive sarcolemmal potassium channel (K_{ATP}).

Sodium and Sodium/Proton Exchange

Internal sodium increases rapidly at approximately the time of onset of ischemic contracture, and the mechanism may be twofold. First, as the ATP supply by anaerobic glycolysis becomes insufficient, the supply of "membrane" ATP is too low for the sodium pump, which then slows down with an increase in internal sodium and loss of potassium. Second, as acidosis develops, the sodium–proton exchange operates to eject protons and to gain sodium. Proof of the role of the exchanger is that administration of the inhibitor cariporide lessens ischemic injury (22). An accumulation of sodium is potentially serious, leading to mitochondrial damage (23) and eventually to increased osmotic pressure that can rupture the cell membrane with irreversible damage.

Effects of Poor Washout of Metabolites during Ischemia

The close links and an inverse relationship between the decrease in myocardial O_2 tension and the increase in CO_2 tension (Fig. 17-4) after the onset of ischemia mean that there is simultaneous onset of both poor oxygen delivery and poor metabolite washout. CO_2 accumulates in the ischemic zone partially as a result of continued residual respiration with formation of CO_2 and partially as the result of liberation of CO_2 from bicarbonate by protons. When the perfusate of an isolated heart is given an excessively high P_{CO_2}, there is a rapid decrease in left ventricular pressure, which can be reversed by an increase in calcium in the perfusion fluid (24). The tissue P_{CO_2} does not stay elevated indefinitely during prolonged myocardial ischemia. There is a late decrease in myocardial tissue P_{CO_2} and in the hydrogen ion concentration, probably a reflection of progressive irreversible cellular damage and loss of mitochondrial function (25), so that the production of CO_2 by residual mitochondrial oxidative metabolism decreases.

Benefit Versus Harm of Acidosis

The combination of accumulation of CO_2 and protons decreases the pH of the ischemic tissue considerably from the normal value of approximately 7.0 to 6.5 (26,27) or even lower. The consequent decrease in contractility should, theoretically, self-protect against ischemia by decreasing the oxygen demand. Furthermore, development of calcium-dependent ischemic contracture could be counteracted by acidosis. Direct evidence of protection by acidosis is that during ischemia, a low pH inhibits the enzyme 5'-nucleotidase, which breaks down adenosine 5'-monophosphate, so that during reperfusion, there is a more rapid rate of resynthesis of ATP (28). Because of the heterogeneity of ischemia, the pH in some severely ischemic cells might decrease enough to activate lysosomes, with irreversible tissue destruction. Thus, mild acidosis may be beneficial (29) and severe acidosis may be harmful to the survival of the ischemic myocardium.

Lactate Accumulation

Increased neutral lactate in severe ischemia may have the following effects: decreased contractile activity in the ischemic zone (10), promotion of mitochondrial damage (30), decrease in the action potential duration (31), and inhibition of glycolysis at the level of glyceraldehyde 3-phosphate dehydrogenase (32). Are these really the effects of neutral lactate, or could it be that with the formation of large amounts of lactate, lactic acid could also be formed? Cairns et al. (33) showed that 20 mmol/L external neutral lactate decreased the internal myocyte pH by only 0.24 pH units, probably because of inhibition of the outward transport of protons by the lactate/proton cotransporter. The decrease in internal pH could, by Na^+/H^+ and Na^+/Ca^{2+} exchange, substantially increase cytosolic calcium with adverse consequences. Tissue lactate levels can increase to very high levels after coronary ligation with adverse effects, so that lactate could contribute to the overall mechanism of ischemic damage (26).

Nicotinamide Adenine Dinucleotide (Reduced Form) and Malate–Aspartate Shuttle

For glycolysis to proceed requires disposal of the $NADH_2$ ($NADH + H^+$) that is continuously generated. During normal oxygenation, cytoplasmic $NADH_2$ is removed by the malate–aspartate cycle, which depends on continued mitochondrial respiration and therefore slows or stops in ischemia (Fig. 11-12). In hypoxia or ischemia, $NADH_2$ is converted to nicotinamide adenine dinucleotide (NAD) as pyruvate forms lactate, so that the expected accumulation of $NADH_2$ is prevented. Nonetheless, the cytoplasmic $NADH_2/NAD$ ratio will be forced toward $NADH_2$ as the tissue lactate increases in relation to the pyruvate level because of the equilibrium relationship. $NADH_2$ accumulation in the cytosol means more protons so that intracellular acidosis is promoted. Pyruvate dehydrogenase, located on the mitochondrial membrane, is inhibited by $NADH_2$ so that entry to the citrate cycle is inhibited, more lactate forms, and the ratio $NADH_2$ to NAD increases further. $NADH_2$ also accumulates in the mitochondria with adverse effects: (a) there is inhibition of dehydrogenase enzymes at several sites, so that any residual activity of the citrate cycle is decreased and (b) intramitochondrial calcium increases, as proposed (34), probably because increased intramitochondrial H^+ influences exchange systems across the mitochondrial membrane in such a way that the internal calcium increases.

CLINICAL CONSEQUENCES OF ACUTE ISCHEMIA

Myocardial ischemia may be clinically manifest in at least four different ways: (a) mechanical: contractile failure that may cause left-sided heart failure and shortness of breath, (b) subjective: chest pain, (c) electrical: characteristic electrocardiographic changes and arrhythmias, and (d) morphologic: prolonged ischemia progressing to irreversible infarction. The severity and duration of the flow reduction govern the response pattern (Table 17-4). Importantly, patients often have varying degrees of collateral blood flow that variably alleviate the effect of the stenosis-related flow decrease. Furthermore, vessels to the ischemic zone may be able to dilate in response to the release of vasodilators such as adenosine (Fig. 10-5) and bradykinin that are released from the ischemic myocardium. When ischemia is transient, events occur in a well-defined order, as follows.

The Ischemic Cascade

When deliberate ischemia is induced by therapeutic coronary occlusion during balloon angioplasty, adverse events develop (35). Impaired contractile function (hypokinesia progressing to dyskinesia) starts within approximately 20 seconds, ST segment shifts come after 20 seconds, and chest pain after approximately 40 seconds. Wall motion recovers quickly after reperfusion if the ischemia is of short duration. The overall pattern, called the ischemic cascade (36), is similar to that which a patient experiences during an attack of angina pectoris, as typically induced by walking (Fig. 17-5). However, the earlier onset of diastolic than systolic dysfunction is not certain. In addition, postischemic recovery can take as long as 60 minutes, an example of stunning in humans.

TABLE 17-4. *Relationship between severity of coronary flow restriction and reported effects in ischemia*

Flow reduction (%)	Effect
15	Midzone P_{CO_2} increase, P_{O_2} decrease[a]
20	Endocardial TQ-ST changes.[b] Transmural ATP relatively constant; after 5 hr drops by ~20%[c]
20–30	Mid-zone external potassium increases, pH decreases TQ-ST changes[d]
30–40	Subepicardial external potassium increases[c]
40–50	Segmental shortening impaired[d]
60–70	Epicardial activation delay and TQ-ST changes[d]
80–85	Epicardial action potential duration shortening[d]
90	Transmural ATP reduced to 6% after 5 hr[c]

[a]Reference 25.
[b–d]See references 34a–34c.
ATP, adenosine 5′-triphosphate.

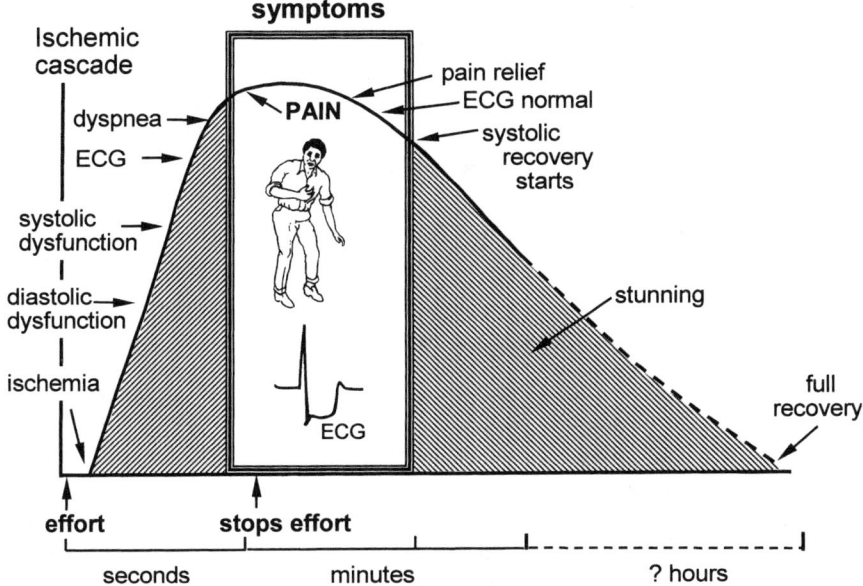

FIG. 17-5. The ischemic cascade. With the onset of exercise in a person subject to the chest pain known as angina, the myocardial demand of oxygen is increased and the blood supply is unchanged or even reduced. Rapidly thereafter, there is mechanical dysfunction, followed by electrocardiographic changes and shortness of breath (dyspnea) and only then pain. On stopping effort, there is pain relief. Full recovery of cardiac function is delayed, an example of stunning (Fig. 17-11).

Oxygen Balance in the Ischemic Zone

An intuitively plausible hypothesis is that angina pectoris can be caused whenever the myocardial oxygen demand exceeds the supply to cause myocardial ischemia (e.g., when exercise increases the myocardial oxygen demand). However, a close matching of perfusion (supply) and function (demand) occurs during exercise-induced myocardial ischemia (37). The effects of some therapeutic agents, such as the β-adrenergic blocker *propranolol*, can be explained by alterations in the demand/supply ratio (Fig. 17-1) because β-blockade reduces the increased heart rate normally found during exercise. However, β-blockade also improves the blood flow to the ischemic myocardium (38). Factors likely to precipitate angina of effort are all those that increase the oxygen demand in the face of a supply limited by coronary artery disease. During exercise, the increase in heart rate and blood pressure precipitates effort angina, whereas an increase in heart rate (together with some increase in systolic blood pressure) is probably the major factor in emotion-provoked angina. The role of catecholamine-induced oxygen wastage as a factor increasing the oxygen demand has not been defined, nor has it been searched for, apart from a specific experimental situation in which low-dose catecholamine infusion given to patients with coronary artery disease was able to evoke an increased oxygen uptake independently of hemodynamic changes (39).

The overall metabolic changes in angina pectoris are well described. The occurrence of lactate production during angina attacks produced by pacing shows that angina is accompanied by anaerobic glycolysis. There is no reason to believe that the basic metabolic patterns found in human myocardial ischemia differ in any way from those in animal preparations. The release of inorganic phosphate and potassium proves that there is breakdown of high-energy phosphates and loss of potassium from ischemic cells in humans and in animals.

Supply Versus Demand Ischemia

Ischemia, thus, can be linked to myocardial contractile failure through a series of events that result ultimately from a decreased blood supply. As the severity of coronary constriction increases, the myocardial O_2 tension decreases (Fig. 17-4). This condition is termed supply ischemia by Apstein and Grossman (40). In contrast, when demand ischemia is produced by an increase in oxygen demand, as occurs when the heart rate is increased during angina induced by exercise or pacing, the consequences for myocardial contraction are different with regard to the contractile defect. In demand ischemia, there is increased diastolic tension rather than systolic failure (41), possibly owing to increased cytosolic calcium (Fig. 19-2). The crucial event in supply ischemia is the accumulation of metabolites, such as inorganic phosphate and protons, leading to contractile failure with relaxation of the myofibrils. The distinction between supply and demand ischemia may not be as clear-cut because of variations in the duration and severity of ischemia and because matching of perfusion and contraction is eventually operative. Subendocardial blood flow is also decreased, even in demand ischemia by a transmural and collateral redistribution of flow (37).

In angina of effort, demand ischemia with excess cytosolic calcium would be expected. If so, recovery from angina should be delayed while the stiffened myocardium reverts to normal. Some evidence supports this proposal because effort angina is accompanied by predominant diastolic heart failure with accelerated recovery if a calcium channel blocker is given (42).

Anginal Chest Pain and Silent Ischemia

The origin of chest pain typical of angina pectoris is still not fully understood. Years ago, the legendary British cardiologist Lewis postulated the formation of the pain substance P. The P substance of Lewis must be distinguished from the current concept of substance P (peptidergic), which is a powerful vasodilator acting by release of nitric oxide (43). The metabolite causing the pain must be formed readily in ischemia, must disappear as ischemia eases, and must be present for some hours in patients developing acute myocardial infarction. A more recent postulate is that the pain is caused by adenosine, derived from ATP breakdown (Fig. 10-5), as shown by the effects of adenosine infusion, which causes both an ischemic-like chest pain and forearm ischemic pain (44). In addition, adenosine exerts protective effects such as coronary vasodilation and negative inotropism and is a trigger to preconditioning (see later in this chapter).

Ischemia in humans is not necessarily accompanied by pain. Painless or *silent ischemia* is shown by the development of typical electrocardiographic changes of ischemia as well as contractile failure on the echocardiogram in patients with coronary artery disease who at that time do not have any chest pain. Postulates are that (a) the ischemia is relatively mild and therefore does not stimulate the pain receptors and (b) the patients are less sensitive to painful stimuli than normal (perhaps because of a defect of the sensory nerves, as in persons with diabetes).

ELECTROCARDIOGRAPHIC FEATURES OF ISCHEMIA

Potassium Loss and Depolarization

Potassium changes are fundamental in explaining the early electrocardiographic features of ischemia. Potassium is released into the local venous blood within seconds of the coronary artery ligation in a dog model, together with an increase in CO_2, lactate, and inorganic phosphate and a decrease in pH. Because there is ischemia, the potassium ions are not washed away but accumulate on the outside of the ischemic cells. Thus, the transsarcolemmal gradient of potassium ions progressively decreases with membrane depolarization. The simultaneous loss of potassium can be linked to that of inorganic phosphate by the postulated role of the ATP-dependent potassium channel. It is proposed that depletion of cytosolic ATP leads to opening of the potassium channel normally inhibited by the intracellular level of ATP (Fig. 17-6). Breakdown products of ATP, such as adenosine 5'-diphosphate and adenosine, also help to open the channel. In isolated myocytes studied with the technique that controls the voltage of a small patch of the sarcolemma (patch-clamp technique), continued glycolysis is more effective than oxidative phosphorylation in preventing ATP-sensitive potassium channels from opening (45). Other mechanisms also mediate the loss of potassium from the ischemic cells. Some proposals are (a) co-ionic loss as the positively charged potassium cation leaves the myocardial cell in company with the negatively charged lactate and phosphate ions (Fig. 17-7), (b) inhibition of the sodium–potassium pump as the local availability of ATP decreases sufficiently to inhibit the pump (Fig. 11-20), and (c) increased flow of the background potassium current (46).

Changes in Action Potential and ST Segment

If an exploring electrode is placed directly on the epicardial surface of the ischemic myocardium soon after coronary artery ligation, the action potential

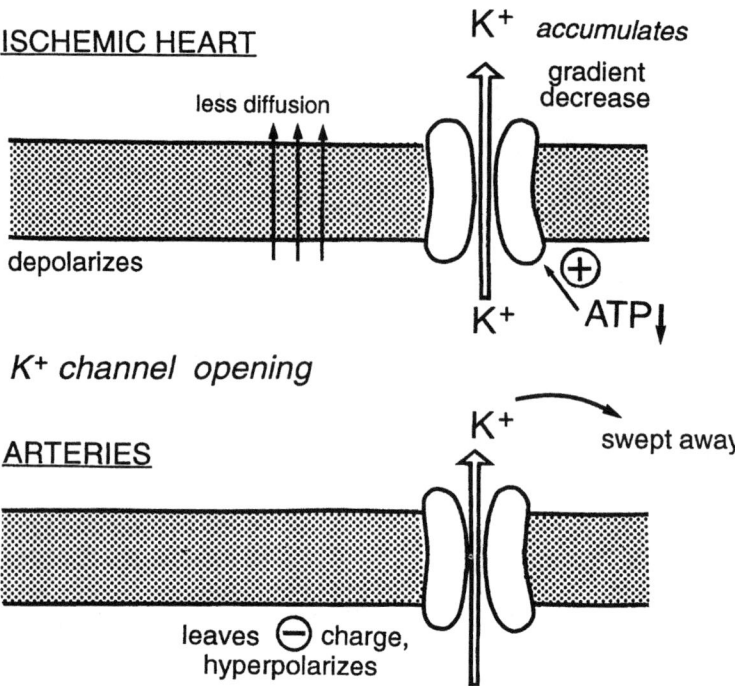

FIG. 17-6. Role of adenosine 5′-triphosphate (ATP)–sensitive potassium channel in ischemia. In ischemia (top), the poor blood flow leads to loss of membrane-related ATP and opening of the ATP-dependent potassium channels with an accumulation of extracellular potassium ions, which cause depolarization. Note major difference from arteries (bottom) where this channel has a vasodilatory role that depends on hyperpolarization as potassium ions are removed from the extracellular site by the circulation.

pattern undergoes characteristic changes largely caused by potassium ion loss from ischemic cells (Fig. 17-8). Topical applications of hyperkalemic solutions to the epicardium or intracoronary infusions provoke changes very similar to those of acute ischemia. The loss of only 1% of extracellular potassium, increasing the intracellular potassium from 4.0 to 9.6 mmol/L, can markedly decrease the resting membrane potential and the action potential duration (47). Potassium loss of this magnitude and rapidity occurs almost entirely through the sarcolemmal ATP-sensitive potassium (K_{ATP}) channels, as shown in a mouse knockout model in which this channel is genetically inactivated (48).

Current of Injury

During ischemia, a current of injury develops as depolarization causes the negative transmembrane potential found in diastole to decrease and become

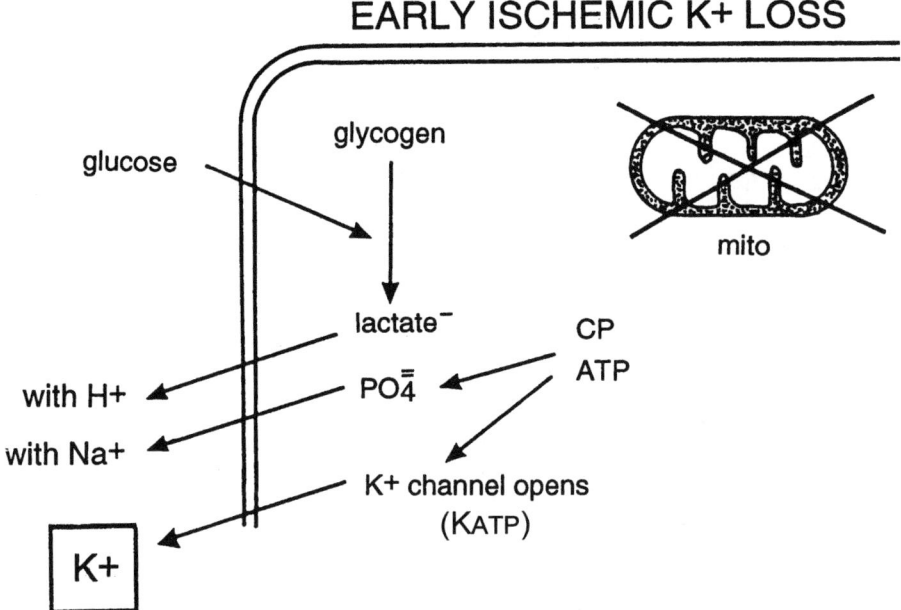

FIG. 17-7. Early ischemic potassium loss. Early potassium ion loss soon after the onset of myocardial ischemia is largely owing to opening of the adenosine 5'-triphosphate–dependent potassium channel, with co-ionic loss of K+ by which the positively charged potassium ions exit with negatively charged inorganic phosphate and lactate ions. The inhibition of the sodium pump follows later.

more positive than the surrounding normal tissue (Fig. 17-9). Therefore, in diastole, the current flows from ischemic to normal tissue. This change appears to start with only a very modest reduction in coronary flow of approximately 20% (Table 17-4). If an electrode were to be placed directly on the ischemic zone (epicardial electrode), the current flowing away from the ischemic zone would produce baseline TQ depression. The net effect is elevation of the ST segment relative to the rest of the complex (ST elevation, Fig. 17-9). Ischemia also decreases the amplitude of the action potential and shortens the action potential duration (possibly by enhanced K^+ channel activity), so that the ischemic zone is less negative in systole than is the normal myocardium. Hence, in systole, current flows from the normal myocardium to the ischemic zone, and some true ST elevation is produced to add to the apparent elevation (produced by the diastolic, K^+-induced current). Exact measurement of the isoelectric line in patients show that approximately 70% of the ST change is explained by diastolic currents and a lesser component by systolic currents (49).

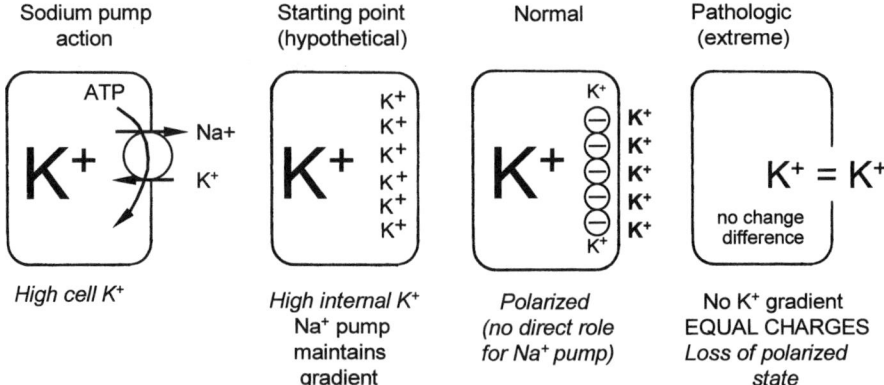

FIG. 17-8. **Schematic of role of potassium ions in membrane polarization.** In the normal cell **(left)**, the activity of the sodium pump increases cell potassium (K^+). This means that potassium ions are distributed along the inner aspect of the sarcolemma (next panel). These potassium ions tend to migrate outward because of the high permeability of the sarcolemma for potassium ions (next panel). Large negatively charged molecules such a proteins are left without the "balancing" positive potassium ions. The high external K^+ causes a layer of positive charges just outside the cell. The combination with the internal negative charges causes the cell to be polarized. During extreme pathology such as severe ischemia, several mechanisms including loss of sodium pump activity remove the potassium gradient from inside to outside the cell, which is now fully depolarized **(right)**.

Epicardial Versus Endocardial Electrocardiogram

Whether ischemic depolarization will be evident as ST segment elevation or ST segment depression on the surface electrocardiogram depends on whether the ischemic zone is epicardial or endocardial. Apparent ST segment elevation occurs in some clinical conditions, such as epicardial ischemia or transmural ischemia, which may result from Prinzmetal variant angina with severe spasm or early-phase myocardial infarction. In contrast, in effort angina, the subendocardial zone is mainly rendered ischemic, and the direction of current flow is away from the electrode that causes apparent ST segment depression on the surface electrocardiogram.

ST Changes and Severity of Ischemia

To summarize, ST deviations, largely but not entirely, reflect extracellular potassium ion accumulation as a result of acute ischemic injury. Thus, not surprisingly, attempts have been made to relate the degree of precordial ST deviation in early myocardial infarction to the magnitude of extracellular potassium accumulation and the severity of myocardial ischemia. There are, however, complex geometric factors that influence how a flow of current is recorded by an electrode (47). At best, measurements of early ST segment deviations will give only an approximation of the severity of ischemia. Nonetheless, ischemic ST

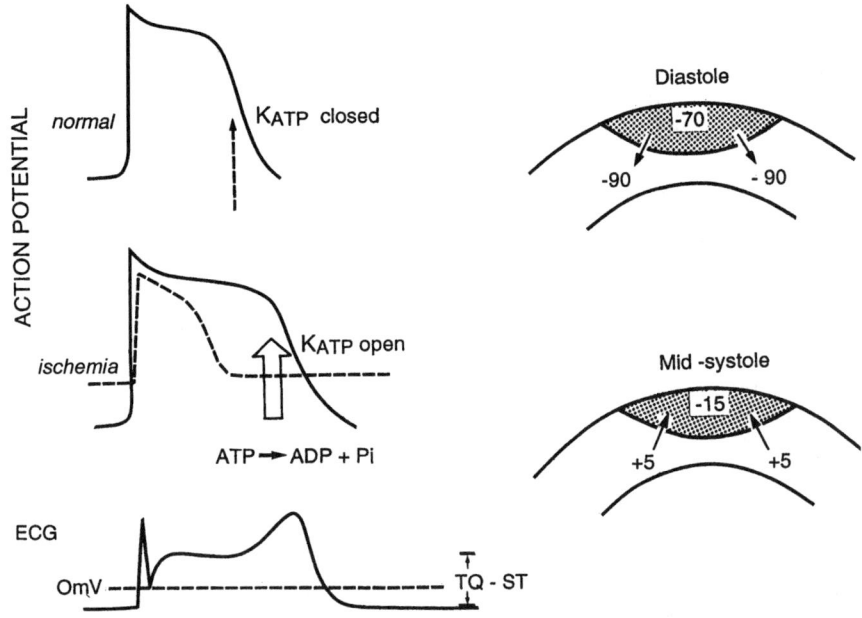

FIG. 17-9. Ischemic changes in action potential pattern and epicardial electrocardiogram. During the normal action potential (at top on left), the adenosine 5'-triphosphate (ATP)—sensitive potassium channel is closed. During ischemia, the resting membrane potential is less negative, with a slow rate of depolarization and an early return to a higher resting level. Thus, there is shortening of the action potential duration and plateau. During diastole (at top on right), ischemic depolarization causes a less negative value in the ischemic zone (*dotted area*). Current therefore flows from the ischemic to the nonischemic zone causing depression of the TQ segment. During mid-systole, however, the changes in the action potential duration mean that the ischemic zone is more negative than the nonischemic zone (compare *dashed* and *solid lines* at left in middle). Therefore, during systole current flows from the nonischemic to the ischemic tissue, which is reflected as ST segment elevation. Thus, there are two components for the apparent ST segment elevation of the epicardial electrocardiogram (at bottom on left): true TQ depression (which is dominant) and true ST elevation.

segment depression during effort testing is a very reliable end point if it is found. Generally, a horizontal depression of at least 1 mm of the ST segment is required for a positive effort test (Fig. 17-10). With 2-mm depression, there are fewer false positives. Only approximately two-thirds of patients with coronary artery disease have a positive effort test, and sometimes features other than ST depression are the end point (chest pain, blood pressure decrease instead of the normal increase, arrhythmias, shortness of breath, fatigue).

T-Wave Inversion and Ischemia

Particularly confusing is the difference between acute metabolic ischemia, characterized by ST segment deviation (as already discussed), and the ischemia of

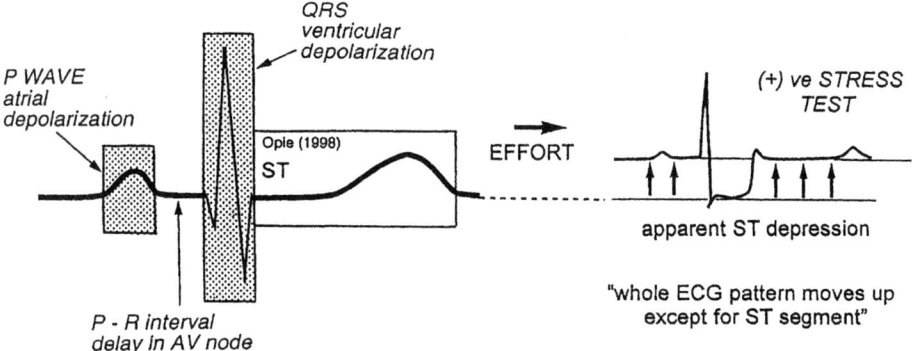

FIG. 17-10. Electrocardiogram in effort angina. The horizontal decrease in the ST segment of 1 mm or more is defined a positive stress test. The quotation is the perceptive remark of a junior medical student.

some clinical electrocardiologists, who also include a chronically inverted T wave as part of the picture of ischemia. An acutely inverted T wave is thought to be a reflection of variations in the rate of repolarization throughout the myocardium and variations in the action potential duration, shortened by ischemia, possibly as a result of inadequate production of ATP at the cell membrane. Such ischemic T wave changes generally are associated with ST segment changes (Fig. 5-29). However, a permanently inverted T wave in isolation usually does not indicate true metabolic ischemia. Rather, focal ischemia has probably progressed to fibrosis, so that the epicardium is repolarized differently from the endocardium.

RECOVERY FROM ISCHEMIA

Experimentally, there is rapid recovery from ischemia that is not accompanied by contracture. For example, low-flow ischemia can be withstood for hours if the ischemic myocardium is supplied with external glucose. Clinicians have, however, often found delayed recovery from exercise-induced angina, with systolic wall motion in ischemic segments taking 60 minutes to recover (Fig. 17-11) (42, 50), despite the return of coronary flow within 5 to 14 minutes (51). This delayed mechanical recovery is, therefore, a form of stunning, and one of the important metabolic derangements responsible could be an increase in cytosolic calcium levels (Fig. 19-2). If so, it is important to track the metabolic events in the recovery period.

Normalization of Ions

At the end of a period of potentially reversible ischemia, there is an intracellular accumulation of protons and sodium and calcium ions. Numerous studies with inhibitors of sodium–proton exchange have shown a more rapid recovery

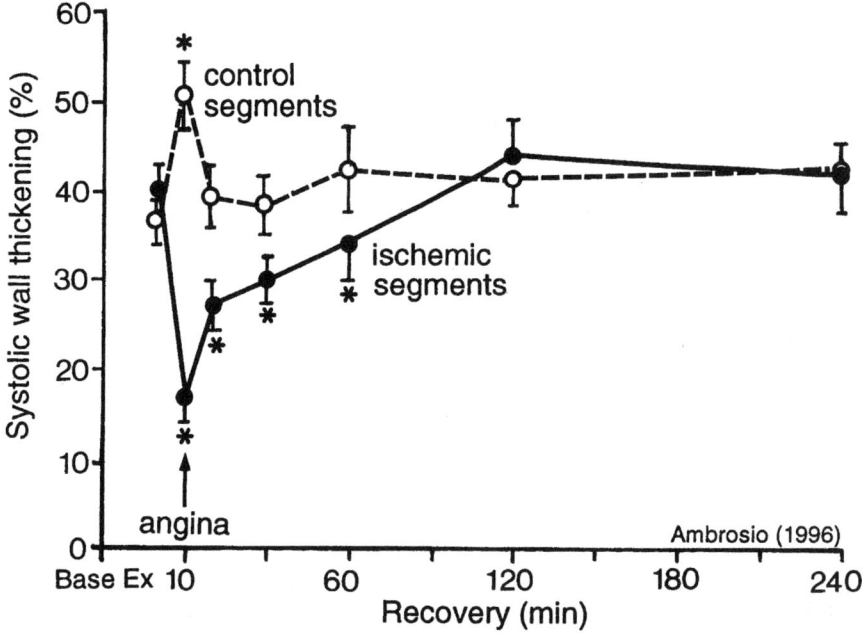

FIG. 17-11. Delayed postanginal recovery of systolic wall motion. Note that after the cessation of angina, the previously ischemic segments take 60 minutes or more to recover when compared with controls. For further details, see Ambrosio et al. (50).

from ischemia in the presence of these agents, suggesting that the operation of this exchanger helps to normalize the cell pH. The resultant decrease in the proton load during early reperfusion promotes recovery (52). In addition, protons are extruded with lactate by the lactate proton cotransporter (53).

Energy Metabolism during Recovery from Ischemia

Several complex changes, not yet fully defined, occur. A current hypothesis is that glycolysis is harmful because there is uncoupling of glycolysis from glucose oxidation during recovery from ischemia (54). Increased rates of glycolysis during postischemic recovery are accompanied by inhibition of glucose oxidation (54), the latter probably resulting from a relative increase in fatty acid metabolism. Overall, the rates of mitochondrial metabolism are depressed (55), and fatty acids appear to compete better than glucose for this residual metabolism. Measures to enhance glucose oxidation include replenishment of the citrate cycle intermediates by pyruvate (Chapter 11), the agent dichloroacetate, which promotes pyruvate oxidation (52), and steps to decrease fatty acid oxidation. When there is an adequate amount of pyruvate from glycolysis that is useful for stimulation of mitochondrial respiration, glycolysis is beneficial and not harmful, presumably by supplying energy for the calcium uptake pump of the sarcoplasmic reticulum, thereby decreasing internal calcium (56).

THERAPEUTIC MODIFICATION OF ISCHEMIA

Classical Antianginal Agents

Both beta-blockers and calcium channel blockers act beneficially to increase the blood supply and to decrease the oxygen demand. β-Adrenergic blockers act by decreasing the heart rate and contractile state of the myocardium, whereas calcium blockers act, at least in part, by relief of exercised-induced coronary vasoconstriction. Both types of agent also reduce the afterload by decreasing blood pressure.

Nitric Oxide Donors

Nitrates are thought to act in part as coronary dilators and in part as venodilators, thereby reducing the venous return to the heart and lessening wall stress and associated compression of subendocardial blood vessels. Because nitrates are nitric oxide donors, it is of interest that a further possible mechanism of action is as follows. Several studies have now shown that nitric oxide appears to inhibit mitochondrial metabolism, which will decrease the oxygen demand (57). Agents indirectly producing nitric oxide, such as the angiotensin-converting enzyme inhibitors, which decrease the breakdown of bradykinin and stimulate the endothelium to form nitric oxide, may also reduce myocardial oxygen demand.

Heart Size

An enlarged heart means that ventricular wall stress is increased according to the Laplace law (Fig. 12-13), so that the oxygen demand increases. Thus, treatment of cardiac failure becomes important because it will, in general, reduce the size of the ventricles. Thus, in addition to conventional antianginal therapy, both diuretics and angiotensin-converting enzyme inhibitors may be required in this situation.

Metabolic Mechanisms

Ischemia is basically a metabolic problem. Therapies include infusion of glucose-insulin that promotes glycolysis and reduces blood fatty acid levels (Fig. 11-25). The metabolism-modifying drugs ranolazine and trimetazidine have no hemodynamic effects but act by inhibiting myocardial fatty acid oxidation and thereby promote protective glucose oxidation.

Revascularization

In the long run, myocardial ischemia can often be best decreased by coronary artery bypass grafting or interventions aimed at dilating the culprit stenosis. Balloon angioplasty, previously popular, is now being replaced and complemented by insertion of a stent, a device that keeps the diseased artery physically open. This procedure, like balloon angioplasty, entails the risk of restenosis. A major advance is the realization that much of the restenosis is caused by stimulation of the protein kinase B (Akt) growth path (Fig. 9-1). This path can be inhibited by the antibiotic rapamycin, also called sirolimus, which is implanted in the stent. The problem of restenosis is now disappearing (Fig. 17-12). Another problem of angioplasty and stenting is plaque rupture and microembolization of atheroscle-

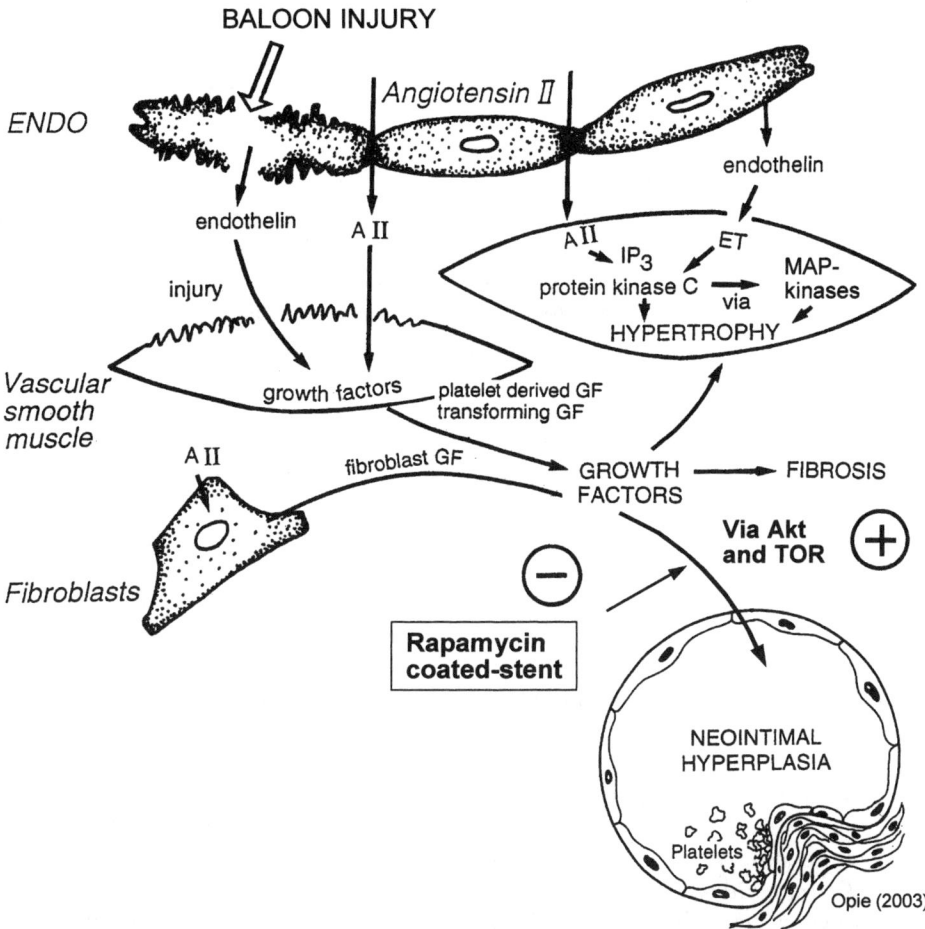

FIG. 17-12. Molecular events in restenosis and prevention by rapamycin. Note the role of balloon-induced endothelial injury, with release of endothelin (*ET*) and angiotensin II (*A II*) and stimulation of growth factors (*GF*). For protein kinase B (Akt) and target of rapamycin (TOR), see Figure 9-5. IP_3, inositol 1,4,5-trisphosphate.

rotic debris into the distal microcirculation resulting in microinfarction and an inflammatory response (58).

SUMMARY

1. *Perfusion–contraction matching during ischemia.* As the blood flow decreases, myocardial contraction proportionally decreases.
2. *Acute adaptation to ischemia.* The two major processes are (a) inhibition of the energy demand by decreased myocardial contraction and (b) an increase in anaerobic glycolysis to compensate in part for the decrease in oxidative metabolism.
3. *Metabolic consequences of myocardial ischemia.* These can be divided into those caused by inadequate oxygen supply and those caused by inadequate washout of metabolites. Common to both processes is an increase in cytosolic calcium.
4. *Supply versus demand.* Myocardial ischemia exists when the blood supply is impaired and/or when the demand is too great.
5. *Demand ischemia.* When there is increased oxygen demand in the face of fixed blood inflow (as occurs during effort-induced angina), the myocardium becomes stiffer (decreased compliance). The proposed explanation is that increased cytosolic calcium impairs relaxation.
6. *Survival of ischemic tissue.* This depends on both the severity and duration of the ischemia.
7. *The ischemic cascade.* In humans during angina of effort, myocardial mechanical failure precedes electrocardiographic changes, which in turn precede symptoms. Although systolic recovery starts soon after cessation of exercise, full recovery may take much longer and is an example of stunning.
8. *Effects of ischemia on the cardiac action potential.* Fundamental in the cause of ischemic changes is potassium loss from the ischemic zone, with accumulation of potassium ions in the extracellular space. The result is ischemic depolarization and shortening of the action potential duration. The underlying mechanism of such early potassium loss and the clinical electrocardiographic ST segment changes are largely the opening of the ATP-sensitive potassium channel K_{ATP}.
9. *Effort electrocardiography test.* These changes in the action potential are reflected in ST segment depression on the surface electrocardiogram, and during exercise, a sufficient degree of horizontal depression of 1 mm or more indicates a positive stress test.
10. *Therapeutic procedures.* Established treatment is to conserve the myocardial oxygen supply by decreased heart rate and contractility (β-adrenergic blockers) or to induce coronary vasodilation instead of vasoconstriction on exercise (calcium channel blockers and nitrates). Metabolic agents such as trimetazidine and ranolazine inhibit the oxidation of fatty acids and indirectly promote protective glycolysis. Currently very popular is the insertion

of a stent to keep open a stenotic artery that has been dilated. The problem of restenosis is greatly diminished by the local application of rapamycin, an antibiotic that blocks the protein kinase B growth path.

STUDENT QUESTIONS

1. What is meant by perfusion–contraction matching? Why is it important in ischemia?
2. In ischemia, anaerobic glycolysis is accelerated. Do you see this as a beneficial or harmful process? What are the reasons for your choice?
3. Trace the fate of $NADH_2$ (i.e., $NADH + H^+$) made by glycolysis during normal oxygenation and ischemia. What is the importance of these changes?
4. What are the changes in pathways of fatty acid metabolism found in ischemia? What is the potential significance in terms of the extent ischemic damage?
5. Intracellular acidosis develops during ischemia. Where do the protons come from and what is their significance?

CARDIOLOGIST-IN-TRAINING QUESTIONS

1. Soon after the onset of severe ischemia, there is myocardial contractile failure. What are the metabolic processes involved?
2. Describe the ischemic cascade.
3. During an attack of angina pectoris caused by pacing, there is an acute loss of potassium ions into the extracellular space. Why is this? What are the consequences?
4. Describe the changes in the cardiac action potential found in ischemia. How do these relate to the changes in the surface electrocardiogram found during a positive effort stress test?
5. What are the principles that explain the therapeutic steps that can be taken to reverse myocardial ischemia and angina pectoris?

REFERENCES

1. Erichsen JE. On the influence of the coronary circulation on the action of the heart. *Lond Med Gazette NS* 1842;2:361.
2. Virchow R. *Die Cellularpathologie in ihrer Begründung auf physiologische und pathologische Gewebelehre.* Berlin: Hischwald, 1858.
3. Burns A. *Observations on some of the most frequent and important diseases of the heart; on aneurysm of the thoracic aorta; on preternatural pulsation in the epigastric region; and on the unusual origin and distribution of some of the large arteries of the human body.* Edinburgh: Bryce, 1809.
4. Hochachka PW, Buck LT, Doll CJ, et al. Unifying theory of hypoxia tolerance: Molecular/metabolic defense and rescue mechanisms for surviving oxygen lack. *Proc Natl Acad Sci U S A* 1996;93: 9493–9498.
5. Heusch G, et al. Perfusion-contraction match and mismatch. *Basic Res Cardiol* 2001;96:1–10.

6. Kloner RA, et al. Consequences of brief ischemia: stunning, preconditioning, and their clinical implications. Part 1. *Circulation* 2001;104:2981–2989.
7. Rauch U, et al. Alteration of the cytosolic-mitochondrial distribution of high energy phosphates during global myocardial ischaemia may contribute to early contractile failure. *Circ Res* 1994;75: 760–769.
8. Owen P, et al. Glucose flux rate regulates onset of ischemic contracture in globally underperfused rat hearts. *Circ Res* 1990;66:344–354.
9. Cross HR, Opie LH, Radda GK, et al. Is a high glycogen content beneficial or detrimental to the ischemic rat heart? *Circ Res* 1996;78:482–491.
10. Tennant R. Factors concerned in the arrest of contraction in an ischemic myocardial area. *Am J Physiol* 1935;1935:677–682.
11. Katz AM, Hecht HH. The early "pump" failure of the ischemic heart. *Am J Med* 1969;47:497–502.
12. Jacobus WE, Pores IH, Lucas SK, et al. Intracellular acidosis and contractility in the normal and ischemic heart as examined by ^{31}p NMR. *J Mol Cell Cardiol* 1982;14(suppl 3):13–20.
13. Kubler W, Katz AM. Mechanism of early "pump" failure of the ischemic heart: possible role of adenosine triphosphate depletion and inorganic phosphate accumulation. *Am J Cardiol* 1977;40: 467–471.
14. Lee JA, et al. Mechanisms of acute ischemic contractile failure of the heart. Role of intracellular calcium. *J Clin Invest* 1991;88:361–367.
15. Guth BD, et al. Time course and mechanisms of contractile dysfunction during acute myocardial ischemia. *Circulation* 1993;87(suppl IV):35–42.
15a. Apstein CS, Varma N, Eberli FR. Ischemic diastolic dysfunction and postischemic diastolic stunning In: Yellon DM, Rahimtoola SH, Opie LH, eds. *New ischemic syndromes. Beyond angina and infarction*. Philadelphia: Lippincott–Raven, 1997:106–135.
15b. Serizawa T, Carabello BA, Grossman W. Effect of pacing-induced ischemia on left ventricular diastolic pressure-volume relations in dogs with coronary stenosis. *Circ Res* 1980;46:430–439.
16. Young LH, Renfu Y, Russell R, et al. Low-flow ischemia leads to translocation of canine heart GLUT-4 and GLUT-1 glucose transporters to the sarcolemma in vivo. *Circulation* 1997;95:415–422.
17. Steenbergen C, et al. Correlation between cytosolic free calcium, contracture, ATP, and irreversible ischemic injury in perfused rat heart. *Circ Res* 1990;66:135–146.
18. Marban E, et al. Quantification of (Ca^{2+})$_i$ in perfused hearts. Critical evaluation of the 5F-BAPTA and nuclear magnetic resonance method as applied to the study of ischemia and reperfusion. *Circ Res* 1990;66:1255–1267.
19. Leyssens A, et al. The relationship between mitochondrial state, ATP hydrolysis, (Mg^{2+})$_i$ and (Ca^{2+})$_i$ studied in isolated rat cardiomyocytes. *J Physiol* 1996;496:111–128.
20. Meissner A, et al. Contractile dysfunction and abnormal Ca^{2+} modulation during postischemic reperfusion in rat heart. *Am J Physiol* 1995;268:H100–H111.
21. Allen DG, et al. The effects of simulated ischaemia on intracellular calcium and tension in isolated ferret ventricular muscle. *J Physiol* 1988;396:91P.
22. Klein HH, et al. Na^+/H^+ Exchange inhibitor cariporide attenuates cell injury predominantly during ischemia and not at onset of reperfusion in porcine hearts with low residual blood flow. *Circulation* 2000;102:1977–1982.
23. Sawyer DB, et al. The sting of salt on an old, but open, wound—is Na^+ the cause of mitochondrial and myocardial injury during ischemia/reperfusion? *J Mol Cell Cardiol* 2002;34:699–701.
24. Williamson JR, et al. Effects of acidosis on myocardial contractility and metabolism. *Acta Med Scand* 1976;587:95–112.
25. Khuri SF, et al. The significance of the late fall in myocardial Pco_2 and its relationship to myocardial pH after regional coronary occlusion in the dog. *Circ Res* 1985;56:537–547.
26. Cross HR, et al. Is lactate-induced myocardial ischaemic injury mediated by decreased pH or increased intracellular lactate? *J Mol Cell Cardiol* 1995;27:1369–1381.
27. Guth BD, et al. Regional myocardial blood flow, function and metabolism using phosphorous-31 nuclear magnetic resonance spectroscopy during ischemia and reperfusion in dogs. *J Am Coll Cardiol* 1987;10:673–681.
28. Bak MI, et al. Acidosis during ischemia promotes adenosine triphosphate resynthesis in postischemic rat heart. *J Clin Invest* 1994;93:40–49.
29. Bing OHL, et al. Heart muscle viability following hypoxia: protective effect of acidosis. *Science* 1973;180:1297–1298.

30. Armiger LC, et al. Mitochondrial changes in dog myocardium induced by neutral lactate in vivo. *Lab Invest* 1974;31:29–33.
31. Wissner SB. The effect of excess lactate upon the excitability of the sheep Purkinje fiber. *J Electrocardiol* 1974;7:17–26.
32. Rovetto MJ, et al. Mechanisms of glycolytic inhibition in ischemic rat hearts. *Circ Res* 1975;37:742–751.
33. Cairns SP, Westerblad H. Allen DG. Changes in myoplasmic pH and calcium concentration during exposure to lactate in isolated rat ventricular myocytes. *J Physiol* 1993;464:561–574.
34. Lehninger AL, et al. Transport and accumulation of calcium in mitochondria. *Ann N Y Acad Sci* 1978;307:160–176.
34a. Maekawa K, Yokoyama M, Kaada Y, et al. A study on myocardial ischemia in the left ventricular wal with special reference to electrographic and metabolic changes. *Jpn Heart J* 1980;21:215–224.
34b. Neill WA, Ingwall JS, Andrews E, et al. Stabilization of a derangement in adenosine triphosphate metabolism during sustained, partial ischemia in the dog heart. *J Am Coll Cardiol* 1986;8:894–900.
34c. Watanabe I, Johnson TA, Buchanan J, et al. Effect of graded coronary flow reduction on ionic, electrical, and mechanical indexes of ischemia in the pig. *Circulation* 1987;76:1127–1134.
35. Hauser AM, et al. Sequence of mechanical electrocardiographic and clinical effects of repeated coronary artery occlusion in human beings: echocardiographic observations during coronary angioplasty. *J Am Coll Cardiol* 1985;5:193–197.
36. Nesto RW, et al. The ischemic cascade: temporal sequence of hemodynamic, electrocardiographic and symptomatic expressions of ischemia. *Am J Cardiol* 1987;57:23C–30C.
37. Gallagher KP, et al. Effect of exercise on the relationship between myocardial blood flow and systolic wall thickening in dogs with acute coronary stenosis. *Circ Res* 1983;52:716–729.
38. Matsuzaki M, et al. Effects of β-blockade on regional myocardial flow and function during exercise. *Am J Physiol* 1984;16:H52–H60.
39. Simonsen S, et al. The effect of free fatty acids on myocardial oxygen consumption during arterial pacing and catecholamine infusion in man. *Circulation* 1978;58:484–491.
40. Apstein CS, Grossman W. Opposite initial effects of supply and demand ischemia on left ventricular diastolic compliance: the ischemia-diastolic paradox. *J Mol Cell Cardiol* 1987;19:119–128.
41. De Bruyne B, et al. Comparative effects of ischemia and hypoxemia on left ventricular systolic and diastolic function in humans. *Circulation* 1993;88:461–471.
42. Rinaldi CA, et al. Randomized, double-blind crossover study to investigate the effects of amlodipine and isosorbide mononitrate on the time course and severity of exercise-induced myocardial stunning. *Circulation* 1998;98:749–756.
43. Ralevic V, et al. Substance P is released from the endothelium of normal and capsaicin-treated rat hind-limb vasculature, in vivo, by increased flow. *Circ Res* 1990;66:1178–1183.
44. Crea F, et al. Role of adenosine in pathogenesis of anginal pain. *Circulation* 1990;81:164–172.
45. Weiss JN, et al. Glycolysis preferentially inhibits ATP-sensitive K+ channels in isolated guinea pig cardiac myocytes. *Science* 1987;238:67–70.
46. Rodriguez B, et al. Mechanistic investigation of extracellular K^+ accumulation during acute myocardial ischemia: a simulation study. *Am J Physiol* 2002;283:H490–H500.
47. Holland RP, et al. TQ-ST segment mapping: critical review and analysis of current concepts. *Am J Cardiol* 1977;40:110–129.
48. Li RA, et al. Molecular basis of electrocardiographic ST-segment elevation. *Circ Res* 2000;87:837–839.
49. Cohen D, et al. Magnetic measurement of S-T and T-Q segment shifts in humans. Exercise-induced ST-segment depression. *Circ Res* 1983;53:274–279.
50. Ambrosio G, et al. Prolonged impairment of regional contractile function after resolution of exercise-induced angina. Evidence of myocardial stunning in patients with coronary artery disease. *Circulation* 1996;94:2455–2464.
51. Camici P, et al. Increased uptake of ^{18}F-fluorodeoxyglucose in postischemic myocardium of patients with exercise-induced angina. *Circulation* 1986;74:81–88.
52. Liu B, et al. Cardiac efficiency is improved after ischemia by altering both the source and fate of protons. *Circ Res* 1996;79:940–948.
53. Vandenberg JI, et al. Mechanisms of pHi recovery after global ischemia in the perfused heart. *Circ Res* 1993;72:993–1003.
54. Lopaschuk GD, et al. Glucose metabolism in the ischemic heart. *Circulation* 1997;95:313–315.

55. Heyndrickx GR, et al. Recovery of regional contractile function and oxidative metabolism in stunned myocardium induced by 1-hour circumflex coronary artery stenosis in clinically instrumented dogs. *Circ Res* 1993;72:901–913.
56. Jeremy RW, et al. Relation between glycolysis and calcium homeostasis in postischemic myocardium. *Circ Res* 1992;70:1180–1190.
57. Heusch G, et al. Endogenous nitric oxide and myocardial adaptation to ischemia. *Circ Res* 2000;146:146–152.
58. Erbel R, et al. Coronary microembolization. *J Am Coll Cardiol* 2000;36:22–24.
59. Opie LH. Myocardial ischemia—metabolic pathways and implications of increased glycolysis. *Cardiovasc Drugs Ther* 1990;4:777–790.

18

Acute Coronary Syndromes: Cell Death

"Atherosclerosis is an inflammatory disease."
Ross (1)

Acute coronary syndrome is the modern term for a group of clinical conditions presenting with acute chest pain, electrocardiographic changes in the ST segment, and enzyme release from the heart. The primary event is acute partial or complete obstruction to coronary flow, typically with a thrombus (clot) forming on severe preexisting atherosclerotic coronary artery disease. Our understanding of this spectrum of clinical conditions and its clinical management has advanced considerably since the previous edition of this book. Concepts of the basic chronic disease, coronary atherosclerosis, have shifted to emphasize the etiologic role not only of cholesterol disorders but also of the associated inflammatory reaction. When coronary occlusion is superimposed, the risk is a clinical diagnosis of acute myocardial infarction (AMI). The corresponding animal model is coronary artery ligation.

The clinical onset of AMI is characterized by severe, persisting, angina-like chest pain. If left untreated, the severity and duration of ischemia are sufficient to allow progression to ultimate cell necrosis (Fig. 18-1). The term infarction literally means "stuffed in" and refers to the swollen appearance of totally dead cells. The time taken for the whole sequence to develop will be only 20 to 60 minutes when there is little or no collateral flow and the myocardial oxygen uptake is relatively high. In contrast, the time is extended to 2 to 6 hours when the collateral flow is high and the myocardial oxygen uptake low (2). A crucial event in triggering this whole sequence is rupture of the atherosclerotic plaque (Fig. 18-2). When the coronary occlusion is incomplete, the clinical correlate is unstable angina, a condition in which AMI is threatened without actually occurring.

The best treatment for AMI is reperfusion as soon as possible, by either a pharmacologic agent breaking down the thrombus (thrombolytic) or physically opening the blocked artery by balloon angioplasty or urgent coronary bypass

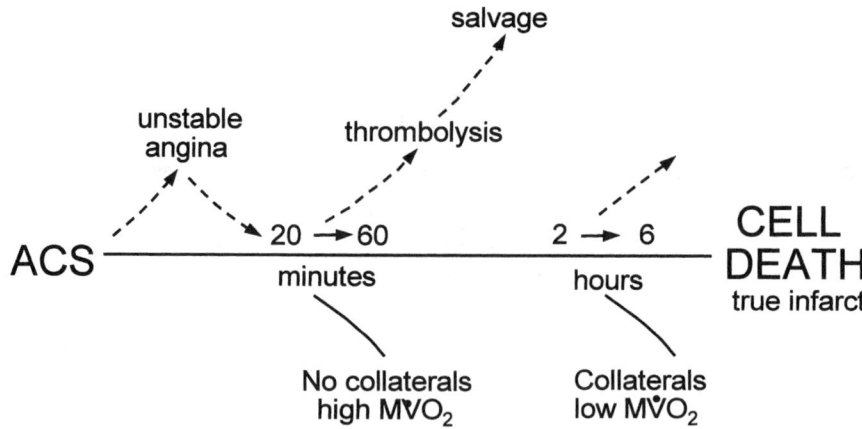

FIG. 18-1. Acute coronary syndrome (ACS) is a clinical syndrome in which a significant number of ischemic cardiac cells may eventually die. Although in the early stages, the condition is reversible and constitutes ischemia and not necrosis, clinicians include such reversible early ischemia in the overall syndrome of acute myocardial infarction. If the thrombus is broken down by therapeutic thrombolysis, the threatened myocardium can be salvaged. The therapeutic window is that time between the onset of chest pain and irreversible ischemia. In the presence of collateral flow and a low myocardial oxygen uptake (MVO_2), animal data suggest an interval of 2 to 6 hours, whereas in the presence of no collateral flow and a high oxygen uptake, the interval is 20 to 60 minutes.

surgery. The corresponding animal model is reperfusion by release of the coronary artery ligature. Although reperfusion saves many cells from dying, it also introduces the risk of reperfusion injury (see next chapter).

How does sustained ischemia progress to cell death? It can spread through the myocardial wall, often starting in the subendocardium, which is the most vulnerable for several reasons. This zone lies farthest from the source of the coronary blood supply via the epicardial arteries; there is more wall stress in the subendocardial zone after an increase in ventricular pressure that results from ischemic contractile failure, and there are transmural metabolic differences that render the subendocardium more susceptible to ischemic damage (Fig. 10-13). When developed, subendocardial ischemia spreads toward the subepicardium, a process that constitutes an advancing wave front (3).

The mechanism of the *wave front phenomenon* includes a progressively increasing intraluminal ventricular pressure as the left ventricle progressively fails, transmitted through the flaccid ischemic myocardium to more subepicardial layers. The larger the zone of initial ischemic damage is, the more rapid and severe the extent of contractile failure is and the faster the wave front advances. Thus, it is not possible to set exact limits for the time that divides reversible and

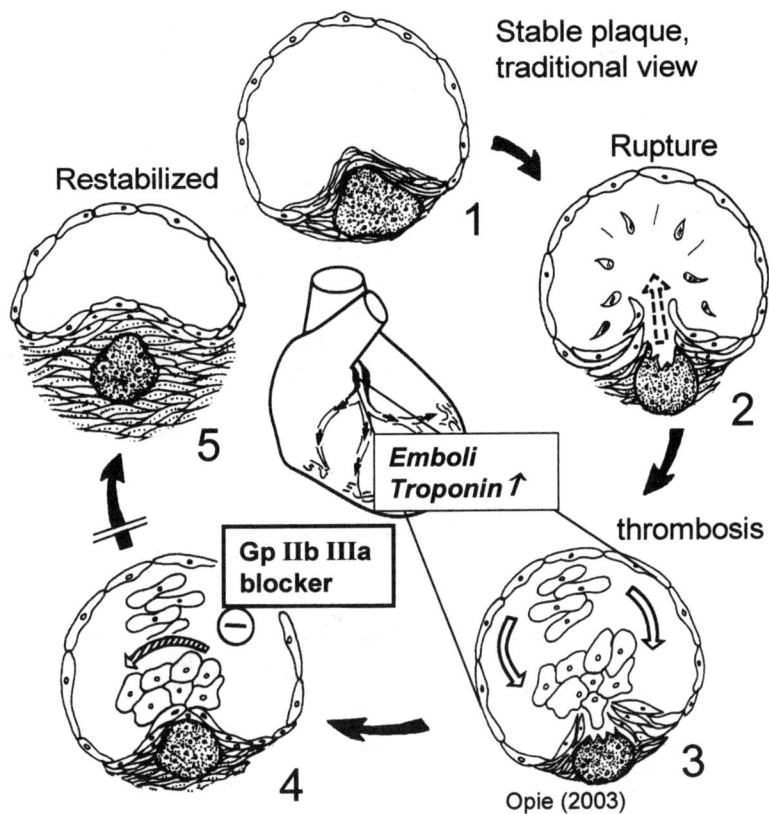

FIG. 18-2. Acute plaque rupture. A simplified schema based on traditional views stressing the internal growth of plaque rather than the updated concept of eccentric growth (Fig. 18-5). When plaque ruptures, there is local thrombosis with lumen occlusion, inhibited by drugs of the class that block the glycoprotein platelet receptor IIb-IIIa. Additionally, parts of the local thrombus are thought to break off and to travel downstream as emboli, thereby blocking off very small arterioles and causing microscopic areas of cell death and elevation of blood cardiac enzymes such as troponin.

irreversible ischemic damage. Nonetheless, it is clear that the earlier that reperfusion takes place, the better.

THE ATHEROSCLEROTIC PROCESS

The following brief summary of this complex process should be complemented by reference to the excellent review of Ross (1). The new concept is that atherosclerosis is an inflammatory response to endothelial dysfunction. This explains why it is not only the blood cholesterol level that is a marker of coronary disease but also C-reactive protein, a circulating indicator of the inflammatory process. Normally, intact vascular endothelium prevents the entry of lipoprotein molecules and protects the intima from invasion by cells such as macrophages. Endothelial dysfunction is the crucial initiating event (Fig. 18-3). Each of the primary risk factors for coronary artery disease (hypercholesterolemia, hypertension, and cigarette smoking) leads through different events to endothelial injury and dysfunction and hence to the atherosclerotic lesion. For example, in patients with hypercholesterolemia, the normal vasodilator responses to acetylcholine are changed into pathologic vasoconstriction (4). In hypertension, exercise causes coronary vasoconstriction rather than normal vasodilation, a change that is thought to reflect endothelial dysfunction (5).

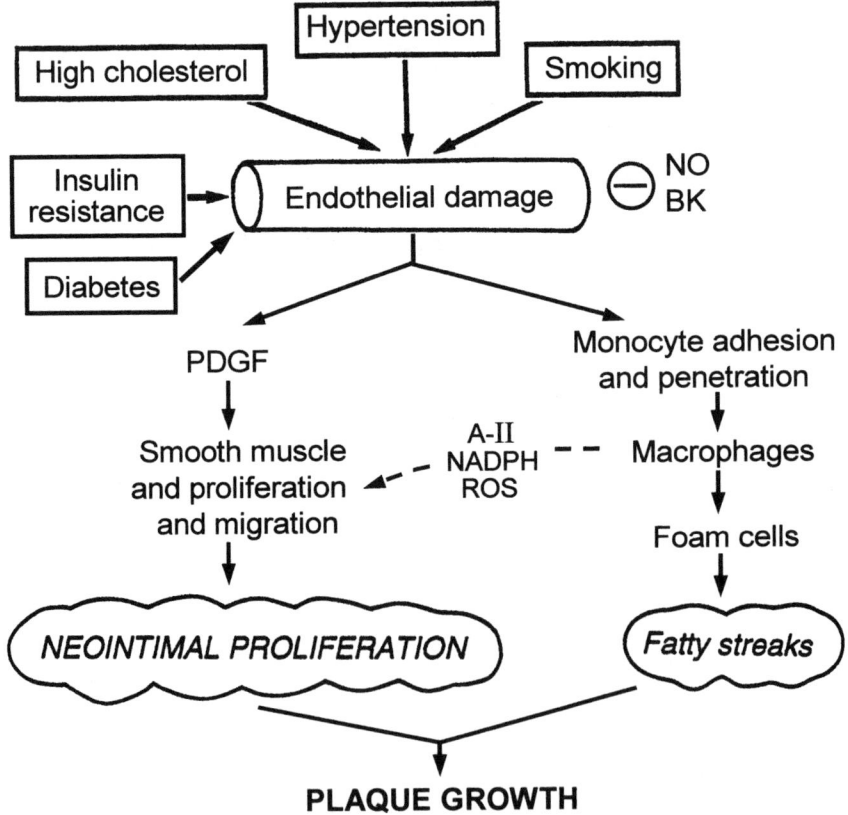

FIG. 18-3. Progression from endothelial damage to plaque. Note the multiple events occurring simultaneously but triggered by endothelial dysfunction as the focal point of primary risk factors for coronary disease. *NO*, nitric oxide; *BK*, bradykinin; *PDGF*, platelet-derived growth factor; *ROS*, reactive oxygen species.

Smoking produces free radicals and acts synergistically with hypercholesterolemia to promote endothelial dysfunction (6). Other risk factors, such as diabetes mellitus, insulin resistance, and increased blood levels of homocysteine, as well as some infectious agents, promote endothelial damage. Of these, diabetes is potentially the most serious, in that a person with diabetes without a history of a myocardial infarction (MI) has as severe a prognosis as a person without diabetes who has already had an MI. Endothelial permeability is increased by endothelial dysfunction to allow entry not only of macrophages and other leukocytes but also of harmful low-density cholesterol so that the developing lesion is a mixture of fat and inflammation.

Inflammatory Response

This response aims to neutralize the effects of endothelial dysfunction that promotes adhesion of leukocytes and platelets to the endothelium, with increased permeability that allows the passage of macrophages that in turn produce growth factors such as angiotensin II and adverse cytokines such as tumor necrosis factor-α (TNF-α). Growth factors are also released from the platelets adhering to the dysfunctional endothelium. Thus, the inflammatory response stimulates migration and proliferation of smooth muscle cells that mix with the area of inflammation to form an intermediate lesion that is the beginning of the atherosclerotic plaque. The inflammatory response, although potentially protective, also promotes progression to the atherosclerotic lesion by promoting infiltration of macrophages and lymphocytes into the advancing lesion, with consequent release of cytokines and several growth factors that can cause focal arterial necrosis (1). Angiotensin II, produced from macrophages, promotes formation of free radicals and stimulates fibroblasts to form fibrous tissue. Angiotensin II also stimulates apoptosis (7). The eventual result is the *vulnerable plaque* with a fibrous cap, ready to rupture and precipitate a potentially fatal thrombus.

Role of Macrophages

These scavenger cells are derived from circulating monocytes that have penetrated the endothelium to participate in the atherosclerotic process (Fig. 18-4). Macrophages attempt to remove noxious molecules such as oxidized low-density lipoprotein (LDL) in the process being transformed into foam cells. Macrophages may accumulate large amounts of lipid. This collection of foam cells and the increased growth of vascular smooth muscle cells and macrophages set the scene for the atherosclerotic fibrous plaque. Hemodynamic shear forces are thought to trigger plaque rupture, the usual antecedent event leading to an occlusive thrombus and total coronary occlusion (Fig. 18-5). Just which fibrous plaques rupture is not clearly defined, but considerable effort is now being put into detection of the highly vulnerable plaque. Some evidence suggests that the arteries that are not too severely narrowed are at most risk of rupture, presum-

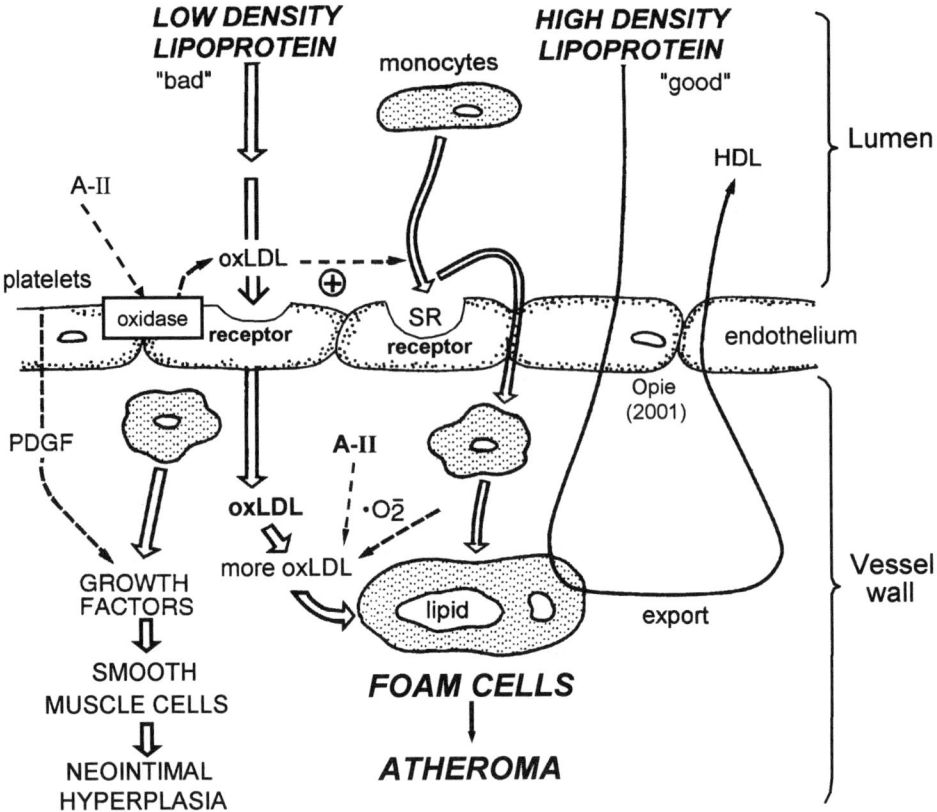

FIG. 18-4. Role of lipoproteins in atherosclerosis. When low-density lipoproteins become oxidized (*oxLDL*), they are trapped in the intima of the arterial wall to enter macrophages and to become foam cells. High-density ("good") lipoproteins (*HDL*) can reexport nonoxidized LDL. *PDFG*, platelet-derived growth factor.

ably because severe occlusion limits coronary perfusion and the hemodynamic stress required to precipitate the rupture.

Dietary Factors

Several of the important steps in atherogenesis are susceptible to dietary changes. The influence of a cholesterol-reducing diet on the blood levels of LDL is well known. More recently, the benefits of a Mediterranean-type diet have come into prominence, but the role of dietary antioxidants and especially vitamin E remains unproven (8).

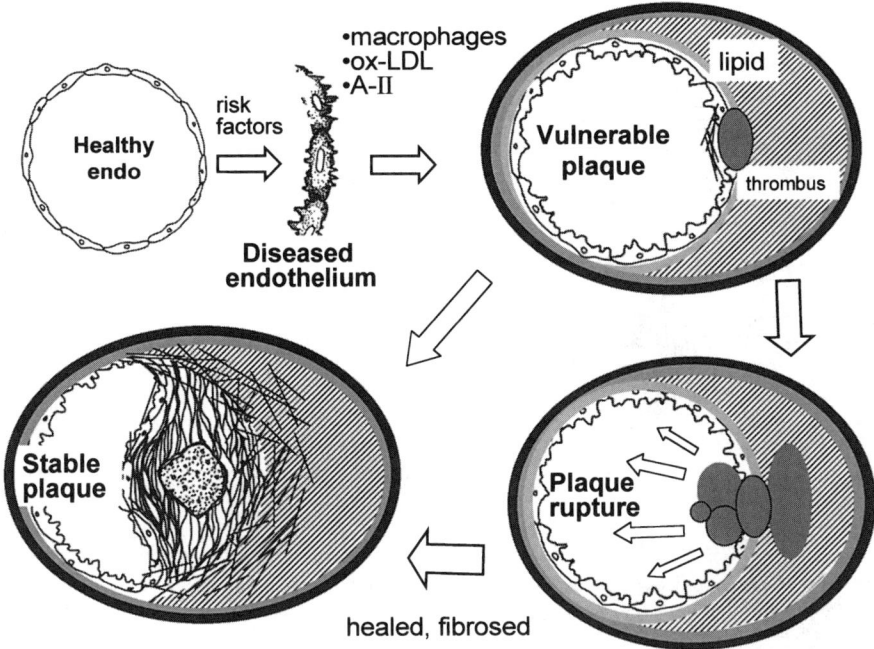

FIG. 18-5. **Current concepts of the atherosclerotic process** and production of the vulnerable plaque. The major difference from the traditional model (Fig. 18-2) is that the early plaque is unstable (top right), at a stage when the disease has grown eccentrically so that the lumen diameter is virtually unchanged. By the time the lumen diameter is much narrowed (bottom left), the plaque is relatively stable. Thus, "severe" coronary disease seen on a coronary angiogram might paradoxically be safer than an apparently normal lumen. For details, see Libby, *Circulation* 2001;104:365.

NECROSIS (ONCOSIS) VERSUS APOPTOSIS

The struggle for survival of the ischemic myocardium is governed by both the severity and duration of ischemia. Undoubtedly, prolonged severe ischemia leads to cardiac cell death. Previously, necrosis was regarded as the only mode of cell death, whereas currently it is known that some cells also die by apoptosis (Fig. 18-6). The term *necrosis* (Greek, *nekros*, dead) is now being replaced by oncosis (which means caused by swelling), the logic being that the crucial event in this mode of cell death is cell swelling and membrane rupture (Fig. 18-6). Nonetheless, the nonspecific term necrosis remains more widely used. The dead cells act as a stimulus to inflammation with macrophage infiltration, fibroblast activation, and ultimately scar formation (7). Contraction band necrosis is a different process, found near the border of the infarct. A proposed mechanism is

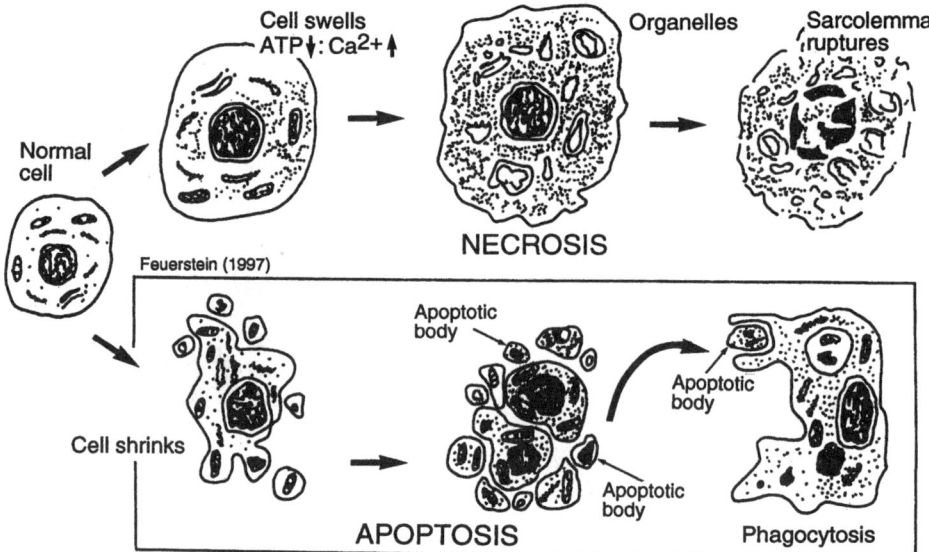

FIG. 18-6. **Contrasts between necrosis and apoptosis.** Note the current trend to replace the term necrosis with oncosis, the latter meaning cell death by oncotic pressure and rupture. (Courtesy of Dr. G. Feuerstein, Merck, New Jersey.)

that partially perfused cells take up a large amount of calcium ions, causing hypercontracture.

Apoptosis (Greek, *apo*, separation from) progresses to cell death by a different route: a genetically programmed series of biochemical events (Fig. 9-8) leads to shrinkage of the cell with intracellular degeneration yet with maintained sarcolemmal integrity (Fig. 18-6). Mitochondria are relatively spared, whereas the entire nucleus is cleaved into two or more portions with the microscopic appearance of DNA fragmentation and formation of DNA ladders. There are no residual fibrosis and scar formation as with necrosis. Rather, the neighboring cells cleanly remove the apoptotic bodies, leaving no trace behind (7).

Autophagic cell death is a third mode, known for a long time but now appreciated as a major cause of cell death in heart failure and infarction (9). Autophagic means self-eating in Greek, and the process depends on lysosomal activation and proteolysis (Fig. 18-7).

The overall evidence shows that cell death in ischemia and reperfusion is caused by both necrosis and apoptosis, but the relative proportion of each is still open to debate. One view is that apoptosis precedes necrosis after coronary artery occlusion until, with time, more necrosis occurs so that ischemic cell death is owing to both apoptosis and necrosis (7). Another view is that apoptosis is of prime importance during reperfusion (10). Because necrosis, apoptosis, and autophagic cell death all have different underlying mechanisms, they could hypothetically respond to different therapeutic approaches.

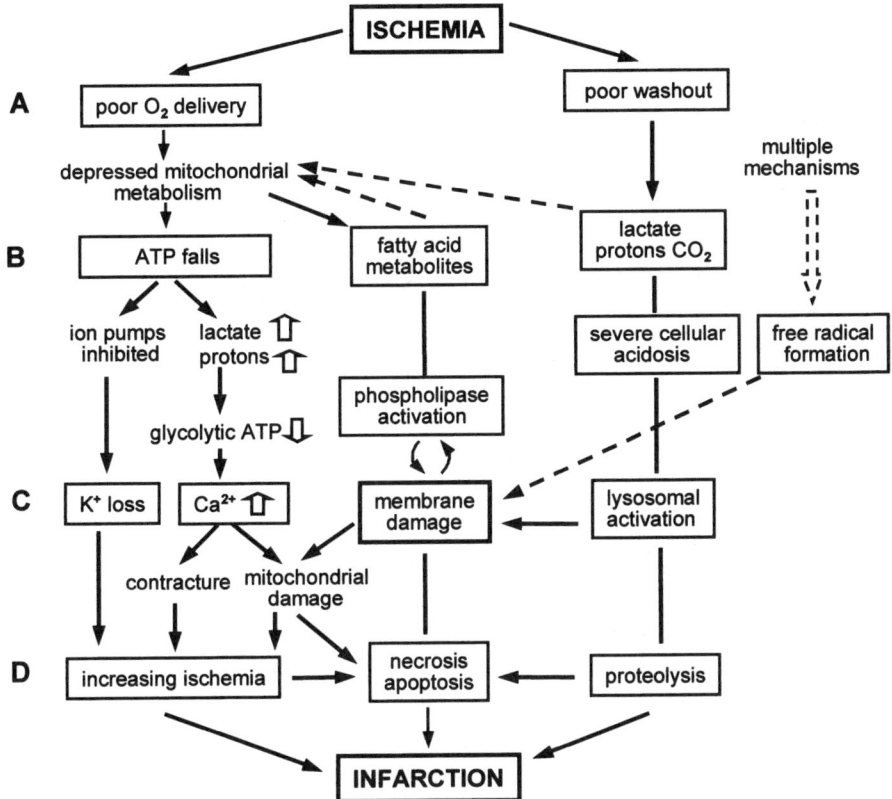

FIG. 18-7. Mechanisms of infarction. Proposed metabolic mechanisms by which ischemia can produce infarction. **A:** The two major effects of ischemia: poor oxygen delivery (hypoxia) and poor washout of metabolites. **B:** Depressed mitochondrial metabolism results in decreased production of adenosine 5′-triphosphate (*ATP*) and accumulation of fatty acid metabolites, which are normally metabolized in the mitochondria. Anaerobic metabolism causes accumulation of lactate and protons (the latter from breakdown of ATP), and continued residual respiration causes accumulation of CO_2. **C:** Decreased production of glycolytic ATP (a result of accumulation of lactate and/or protons) results in calcium accumulation. Inhibition of ion pumps by lack of ATP and by inhibition of fatty acid metabolites results in potassium loss as well as sodium and water retention with cell swelling (shown at right). Fatty acid metabolites also cause membrane damage, which may also result from lysosomal activation by severe cellular acidosis. **D:** The final events leading to infarction may be increasing ischemia caused by ischemic contracture, mitochondrial damage, enzyme loss as a result of membrane damage, and cell death by necrosis, apoptosis, or autophagic cell dell resulting from lysosomal activation.

Mechanisms of Apoptosis

Two different, although interacting, paths lead to apoptosis: one initiated by a surface receptor that responds to TNF-α and the other initiated by mitochondrial damage (Fig. 9-9). Specific factors that link ischemia to apoptosis include all those that damage the mitochondria such as acidosis, calcium overload (7), and the formation of excess reactive oxygen species in response to β-adrenergic stimulation (11). Apoptosis, although undesirable in the adult heart, can crucially lessen the risks of neoplastic disease. Tumor suppressor genes promote apoptosis in a variety of tissues. Such genes include p53, which is rapidly expressed in the reperfused myocardium to up-regulate another gene called Bax, which in turn mediates apoptosis (12). Conversely, the bcl-2 protein inhibits apoptosis, and the Bax-to-bcl-2 ratio is increased in cells destined to die by apoptosis (13).

INITIAL EVENTS IN ACUTE MYOCARDIAL INFARCTION

Animal models of AMI have generally used either acute occlusion by ligature of otherwise healthy coronary arteries or massive injections of catecholamines. The former procedure produces transmural MI, and the latter procedure causes subendocardial infarction. The ideal model would be spontaneously occurring severe coronary atherosclerosis. Superimposed thereon would be the triggering event, which is now known to be an occlusive thrombus (Fig. 18-5), frequently associated with platelet/fibrin microemboli (14).

Triggers of Myocardial Infarction

Emotional and physical stress may be identified as triggering factors in as many as one-half of cases of AMI in humans. Probably closely related is the increased onset of AMI and sudden death soon after awakening (15). Increased adrenergic activation is probably involved in both situations, originating from either intense central arousal or severe physical exercise. The mechanisms for the adverse adrenergic effects may include a series of events that may precipitate plaque rupture with superimposed thrombosis in those with preexisting coronary disease: (a) increased heart rate and contractility increase the oxygen demand (MVO_2) and precipitate ischemia, (b) increased arterial blood pressure associated with increased cardiac output and increased α-adrenergic–mediated peripheral vascular resistance exaggerate ischemia and damage the vascular endothelium, and (c) increased circulating free fatty acids have harmful effects on membranes and promote platelet aggregation. In addition, in high concentrations used experimentally, catecholamines may directly increase sarcolemmal permeability to cause the egress of intracellular enzymes. Although all these links to the onset of AMI are still speculative, they provide a challenging hypothesis. Even when AMI is not triggered by excess catecholamines, there is a very early increase in circulating catecholamine levels, especially in patients with large infarcts, and much evidence supports the concept that β-adrenergic activation can exaggerate the degree of myocardial ischemia.

MECHANISMS OF IRREVERSIBLE ISCHEMIC DAMAGE

The exact mechanism by which reversible ischemia finally evolves into irreversible infarction is still controversial. The consequences of both poor oxygen delivery and poor washout of metabolites may play a role, with the former probably being the predominant factor (Fig. 18-7). Because irreversibility is a consequence of either necrosis or apoptosis, each having a different etiology, simplification is difficult. Five current theories for the development of irreversible ischemic damage in the form of necrosis are (a) loss of a critical amount of adenosine 5′-triphosphate (ATP), (b) membrane damage induced metabolically or mechanically, (c) formation of free radicals, (d) calcium overload, and (e) sodium pump inhibition.

A critical level of ATP, although still often proposed, can be excluded as the sole cause of irreversibility because of the very different values for the critical level given by different authors and because of the now established concept of ATP compartmentation (mitochondrial versus cytoplasmic). It is impossible to say which compartment is depleted by measurements of overall ATP. However, the ATP theory is being revived and extended with the recent evidence that ATP produced by glycolysis may have a specific role in the prevention of membrane-related ischemic events, such as calcium influx (16) and potassium loss (17). Inhibition of glycolysis markedly accelerates cell death in dogs with coronary occlusion (18). Thus, inhibition of glycolysis with calcium overload is postulated to be one of the crucial events in the progression to ischemic cell necrosis (Fig. 18-8).

Inhibition of the sodium pump may precipitate an excess of internal sodium, which is turn leads to the increased osmotic pressure that helps to "pop" the cell membrane and cause irreversible damage (19). The proposed cause of the pump failure is inadequate synthesis of glycolytic ATP for the pump (20).

Membrane damage is, however, multifactorial in origin, including accumulation of free fatty acids inside and outside the ischemic cells and increased amounts of acyl-CoA and acylcarnitine (Fig. 18-9). There may be a self-perpetuating cycle whereby part of the membrane damage results from the action of phospholipases that break down membrane lipids, with formation of lysophosphoglycerides, which further promote membrane damage.

Oxygen free radicals may also contribute to membrane damage by lipid peroxide formation and are part of the signaling sequence leading to apoptosis (11). Free radicals are derived in part from neutrophils, particularly during the reperfusion phase of ischemic damage, and in part from damaged myocyte mitochondria (Fig. 19-4).

Calcium overload is a major component of irreversibility in response to catecholamine stimulation (21), severe reperfusion damage, or prolonged ischemia

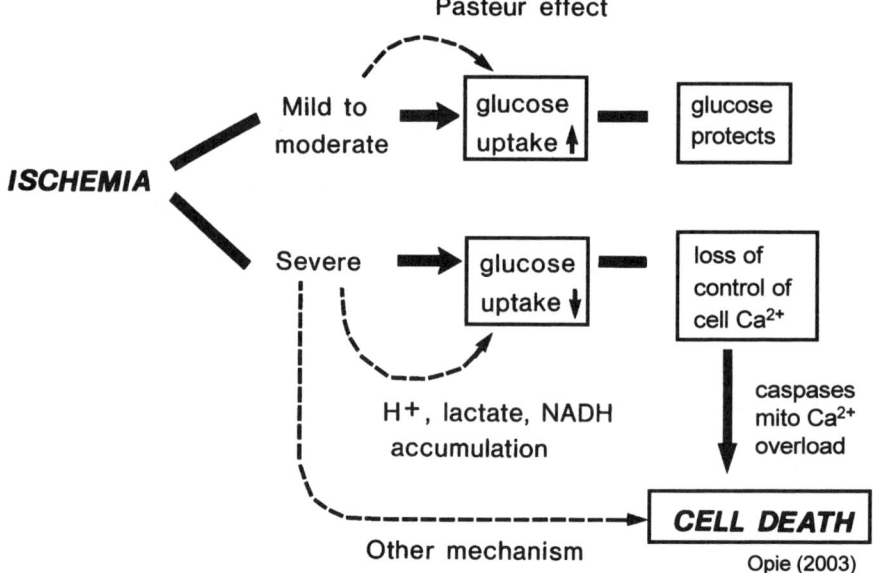

FIG. 18-8. Hypothesis relating the rate of glycolysis to cell death. During mild to moderate ischemia, glucose uptake is increased, providing the benefit of increased glycolytic adenosine 5′-triphosphate. During severe ischemia, the rate of glucose delivery becomes limiting (35). In addition, the accumulation of protons, lactate, and nicotinamide adenine dinucleotide (reduced form) (*NADH*) inhibits glycolysis and glucose uptake. Consequently, there is a loss of control of intracellular calcium with mitochondrial calcium overload and activation of caspases (Fig. 9-8).

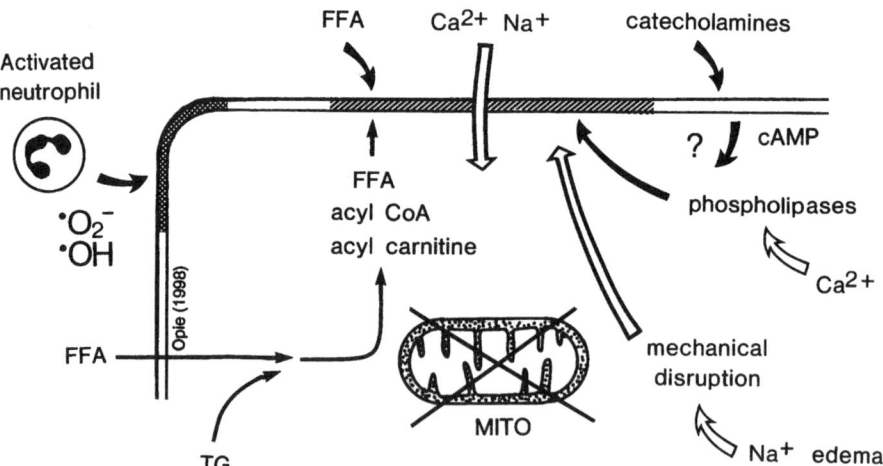

FIG. 18-9. Membrane damage in ischemia. Note the multiple mechanisms involved. *FFA*, free fatty acids; *TG*, triglyceride; *MITO*, inhibited mitochondrial metabolism; $\cdot O_2^-$ and $\cdot OH$, oxygen-derived free radicals; *cAMP*, cyclic adenosine 3′,5′-monophosphate.

(Fig. 18-7). The basic concept of calcium overload is that the mitochondria initially act as a buffer to take up calcium from the cytosol, which requires considerable energy. As a consequence, generalized cellular energy depletion is enhanced, the energy required for maintenance of ionic gradients becomes inadequate, and membrane integrity is lost. A modified form of this hypothesis is as follows. In ischemia, cytosolic calcium levels increase (Fig. 19-3), possibly as a result of a lack of ATP to regulate calcium uptake by the sarcoplasmic reticulum (21). Such increases in cytosolic calcium can activate phospholipases, increase resting tension, and provoke fatal arrhythmias (Fig. 20-8).

The mitochondrial permeability transition pore is a nonspecific pore located in and between the mitochondrial membrane that opens during ischemia and especially during early reperfusion in response to increased cytosolic calcium and other metabolic changes (22). This promotes mitochondrial damage by permitting major influx of electrolytes and water into the mitochondrial matrix, with risk of both necrosis and apoptosis.

CLINICAL DIAGNOSIS OF IRREVERSIBILITY

It is often important to distinguish patients with true AMI from those with other sources of chest pain such as unstable angina and among those with true AMI to diagnose irreversible damage. It is also important to know whether thrombolytic reperfusion has taken place. The release of intracellular enzymes and contractile proteins into the circulation is helpful (Fig. 18-10) in conjunction with the electrocardiogram (next section).

Release of Creatine Kinase

Creatine kinase of cardiac origin [CK-MB (myocardial bound)] is specific to the heart and can be detected within hours of the onset of AMI, but increased sensitivity and specificity are obtained by the assay of isoforms of CK-MB. There is only one form of CK-MB in the heart, $CK-MB_2$, but this is converted in the blood to $CK-MB_1$, which can be detected within 6 hours of the onset of symptoms (23).

Troponin T and Other Intracellular Proteins

Increases in blood levels of CK-MB isoform, myoglobin, and troponin T or I are indicators of the early diagnosis of AMI. For the purposes of ruling out AMI (often very important to cardiologists), release of myoglobin is earlier than that of troponin or CK (24). Nonetheless, in practice, the release of troponin is now standard practice in the assessment of acute chest pain. This is because bedside tests are now available that provide qualitative results (positive or negative) within 15 to 20 minutes, thus leading to rapid decision making in the emergency department assessment of acute coronary syndrome (25). The release of enzymes such as troponin is now regarded as diagnostic of MI.

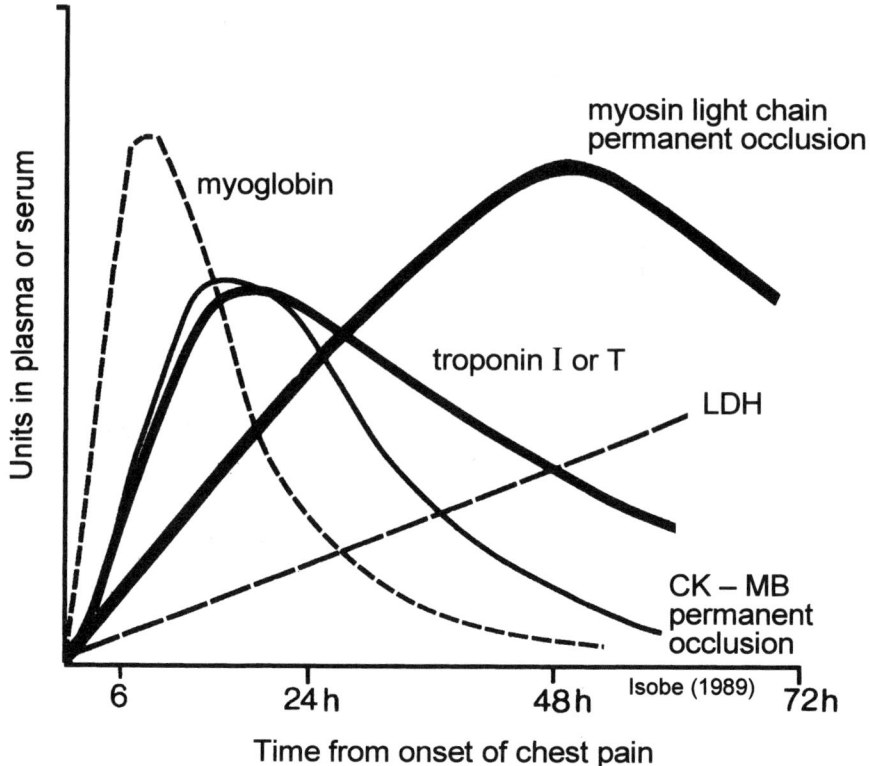

FIG. 18-10. Blood biochemical changes in acute myocardial infarction. Note the early increase in myoglobin and slightly later increase in troponin I or T and creatine kinase, myocardial bound (*CK-MB*) with later but more sustained increase in myosin light chain. Serum myosin light chain increases much later to attain a peak at approximately 48 hours. Reperfusion increases blood levels of troponin or CK-MB but not myosin light chain.

Magnetic Resonance Imaging

This modern technique can greatly assist in the correct diagnosis of acute coronary syndrome—if there is MI or not. It can diagnose regional ventricular wall abnormalities, myocardial perfusion, and myocardial viability (26). However, it is expensive and not widely available, and some patients cannot tolerate the tightly enclosed coffin-like conditions imposed by the magnetic resonance imaging machine.

Diagnosis of Patency after Reperfusion

After reperfusion, an important question is whether adequate patency has been achieved. The gold standard in invasive angiography and the degree of patency are arbitrarily classified according to the criteria in the Thrombolysis in

Myocardial Infarction study series. Grades 1 to 3 in this study reflect lesser to complete patency. Clearly, noninvasive indices are preferable. Early resolution of the ST abnormalities is one indirect method of assessing reperfusion.

Electrocardiographic Irreversibility

As ischemia is prolonged and irreversibility develops, there is a new series of electrocardiographic changes, characterized by Q waves and an acute infarction pattern (Fig. 18-11). The very early electrocardiographic changes of hyperacute infarction during the stage of myocardial ischemia are those of ST segment deviation (Fig. 5-27). The ST changes are those of depolarization caused by ischemic potassium ion shifts. Next, as the tissue undergoes necrosis, a Q wave develops (Fig. 5-29). Theoretically, the efficacy of an intervention to reduce experimental infarct size can be tested in humans by its capacity to lessen the development of electrocardiographic signs of necrosis, such as loss of frontal forces (decrease in R waves) and formation of Q waves, which occur over approximately 4 to 12 hours. Using this approach, early intravenous β-blockade diminishes the electrocardiographic features of infarction (27). The major factors preventing widespread use of

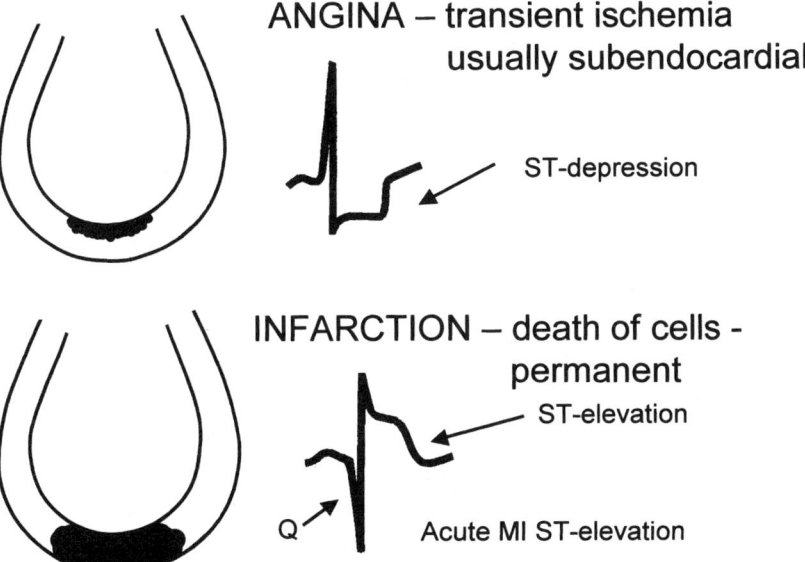

FIG. 18-11. Electrocardiographic changes of the clinical syndromes of angina and acute infarction. In angina, which is usually subendocardial, there is transient ST segment depression during the attack (Fig. 17-5). In acute infarction, necrosis causes Q wave formation, whereas ST elevation reflects ongoing ischemia (Fig. 5-29).

568   18. ACUTE CORONARY SYNDROMES: CELL DEATH

this electrocardiographic technique are the great individual variation in the evolution of the typical infarction pattern and the difficulty of following the changes in inferior infarction, which requires special sites for the precordial electrodes.

INFARCT SIZE

The infarct size is the amount of tissue irreversibly damaged by the infarction process. The larger the infarct is, the worse the prognosis. However, this crucial measurement is not easy to undertake in humans. Enzymatic estimation of the infarct size depends on many assumptions. The extent of electrocardiographic changes is only indirectly correlated with the infarct size. Probably the new technique of magnetic resonance imaging (26) will turn out to be the best imaging technique.

Infarct Size and Area at Risk

When there is occlusion of a major coronary artery, the whole territory supplied by that vessel becomes the area at risk of infarction (Fig. 18-12). Of this

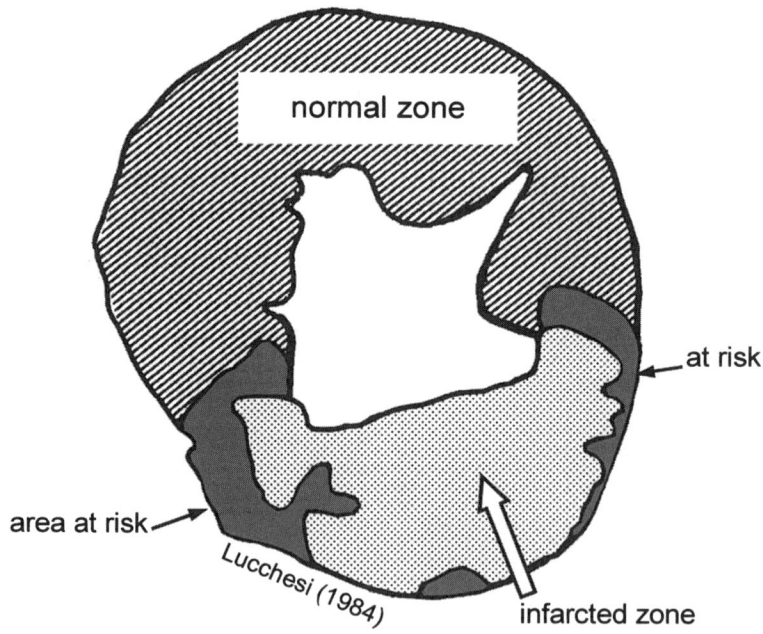

FIG. 18-12. Area at risk. The lateral and epicardial areas at risk can be saved from myocardial necrosis by appropriate intervention such as thrombolytic reperfusion. (Modified from Lucchesi BR, Romson, JL, Jolly SR. Do leukocytes influence infarct size? In: Hearse DJ, Yellon DM, eds. *Therapeutic approaches to myocardial infarct size limitation.* New York: Raven Press, 1984: 219–248.)

18. ACUTE CORONARY SYNDROMES: CELL DEATH

area, approximately 60% may undergo infarction in a typical rabbit heart experiment. Interventions that limit the infarct size include preconditioning, which reduces the infarct size to approximately 20% or even less of the area at risk (Chapter 19). A large number of other experimental procedures will reduce the infarct size less strikingly. The principles are that either the blood supply to the infarcted tissue is improved or the oxygen supply is conserved, for example, by decreasing the heart rate. However, there are reservations about applying these therapeutic principles to humans. First, it is still difficult to measure the infarct size and especially to continuously monitor the evolution of the infarction process. Second, clinicians are increasingly demanding that new therapies be designed to be additive in effect to those of urgent revascularization and that the end points of such studies should be mortality in megatrials, which are extremely expensive. Of the many agents tested experimentally, only early β-blockade and angiotensin-converting enzyme inhibition are currently in widespread use.

POSTINFARCTION REMODELING

After the onset of AMI, some patients undergo a progressive increase in left ventricular (LV) size manifest by a long-term increase in the end-diastolic and end-systolic volumes (Fig. 18-13). The increase in LV volume is particularly found in patients with large infarcts and clinical manifestations of heart failure. The process by which the left ventricle progressively enlarges is called remodeling. Strictly speaking, remodeling applies to other situations in which the myocardial structure is altered, including hypertrophy and cardiomyopathy. Furthermore, remodeling can be either beneficial (as found in some models of hypertrophy) or adverse. Generally, postinfarction remodeling refers to an adverse process occurring in the surviving, noninfarcted myocardium. One proposal is that increased wall stress, resulting from LV damage and fewer contractile cells, stimulates cardiac hypertrophy via the cardiac renin–angiotensin system (7), as in the case of myocardial stretch caused by a pressure load (Chapter 13). If left unchecked, this process will lead to apoptosis, with side-to-side slippage of cells giving rise to LV dilation (7).

Because *angiotensin II stimulates fibroblasts* (via transforming growth factor β) to promote the formation of cardiac fibrosis (Fig. 16-8), it would need the activity of the matrix metalloproteinases to split the collagen and hence to allow the ventricle to enlarge. This is where TNF-α is involved (28). TNF-α is synthesized in response to angiotensin II (29) and released from myocytes by stretch (30). TNF-α in turn stimulates the metalloproteinases that break down collagen and thereby allows the heart to dilate further (Fig. 16-8). Experimentally, inhibiting the metalloproteinases attenuates postinfarction LV dilation and infarct expansion (31). Established clinical therapy is with angiotensin-converting enzyme inhibition (Fig. 18-13), which beneficially alters remodeling, acting in a combination of preload and afterload reduction and inhibition of the cardiac renin–angiotensin system.

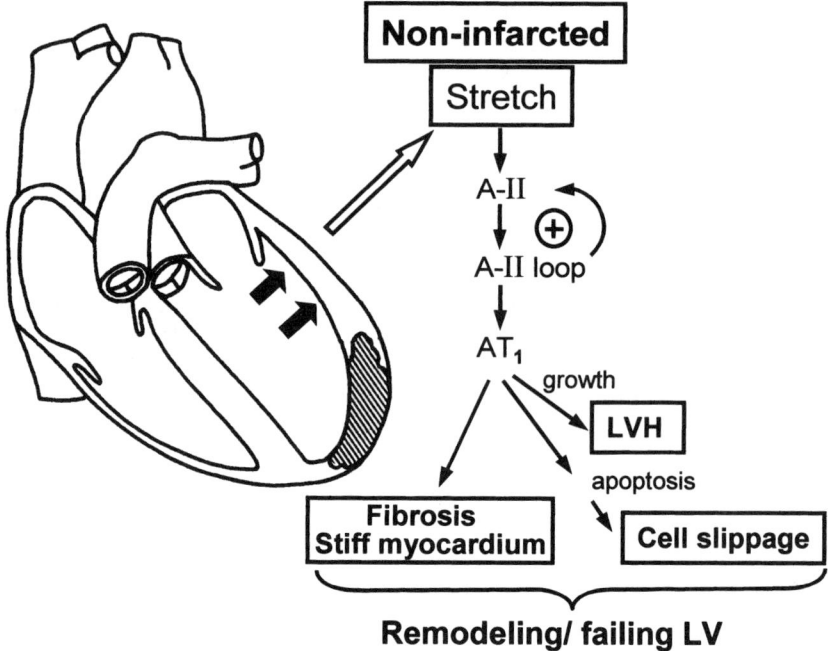

FIG. 18-13. Postinfarction remodeling. Role of large infarct in precipitation of left ventricular dilation by provoking increased wall stress in noninfarcted zone as a result of fewer contractile cells. The result is that there is increased stretch on these cells, with activation of the angiotensin II paths (including the angiotensin II loop shown in Figure 13-3), acting on the angiotensin II, subtype 1 receptor (AT_1) with multiple cellular consequences that lead to a remodeled dilated left ventricle. *LVH*, left ventricular hypertrophy.

STEM-CELL THERAPY

A new hypothesis is that not all adult cardiac cells are terminally differentiated but that there is a small and active population of resident primitive cells with the potential for continuous renewal of cardiomyocytes and coronary vascular cells as older cells die off (7). The further hypothesis is that stem cells from autologous bone marrow can adhere to the damaged myocardium and differentiate into myocardial cells (Fig. 18-14). Furthermore, if injected into an animal with experimental MI, the stem cells seem preferentially to "settle" in the zones of myocardial damage and to adopt some of the proprieties of cardiomyocytes. Why such cells should "home" in on the damaged tissue is totally unknown. Supposedly, a strong chemotactic agent forms in the ischemic tissue to attract the bone marrow cells "home" (7) where these cells can produce cardiac-specific proteins, including myosin and connexin 43 (32). Hence, cells originating from the bone marrow have *plasticity* and become *transdifferentiated* into cardiac myocytes, at least in part. Furthermore, skeletal myoblasts when implanted into a scar area can develop slow twitch characteristics, corresponding more to the

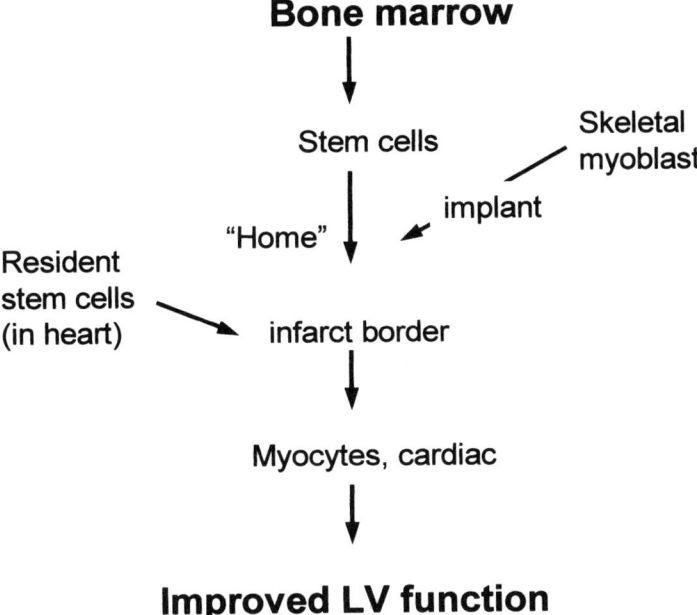

FIG. 18-14. **Proposed role of bone marrow and stem cells** in improving left ventricular function. How injected stem cells "home" on the infarct border is still unknown.

pattern of contraction in the myocardium (33). Although the clinical application of these studies may still only be on the horizon and the interpretation of the data remains controversial, such novel research has given rise to new hopes for "rebuilding a damaged heart" (34).

THE AGING HEART

Elderly patients with MI have a worse prognosis than younger patients. This may in part be because of the inevitable advance of atherosclerosis with age. A more interesting possibility is that the enlarged, aged cells have lost their capacity to adapt either by hypertrophy or cell division (7).

SUMMARY

1. *The mechanism of irreversible cell death* by necrosis is not simple and appears to be multifactorial. Although energy depletion, monitored by the level of total ATP, cannot be related directly to outcome because of ATP compartmentation and multiple modes of generation of ATP, energy depletion is crucial. Lack of energy leads to early redistribution of calcium ions in the cell, which activate phospholipases to damage the sarcolemma. Lack

of oxygen leads to accumulation of unmetabolized lipid products, such as acyl-CoA and acylcarnitine as well as reactive oxygen species. These processes increase sarcolemmal damage, as does intracellular edema fluid formation resulting from sodium pump failure and increased internal sodium. When membrane disruption occurs beyond a specific point, calcium ions will enter from outside, and such net gain of cellular calcium is associated with irreversible damage, large-scale release of enzymes, and the clinical "point of no return."

2. *Three modes of cell death.* These are necrosis (more correctly called oncosis), apoptosis, and autophagic cell death. In necrosis, there is eventual rupture of the cell membranes. In apoptosis, or programmed cell death, the cells eventually vanish without trace, making their quantification difficult. In autophagic cell death, the basic process is self-digestion by lysosomes. Each process contributes to irreversible ischemic damage, but how much is still under debate.

3. *The time scale for irreversible damage* is highly variable. Whereas severely or totally ischemic cells probably die after 20 to 60 minutes, in the presence of collateral flow and a low oxygen requirement, the point of no return can be delayed for as long as 2 to 6 hours.

4. *The ultimate extent of tissue death* is important and highly variable from patient to patient, depending on the extent and number of sites of coronary artery occlusion, the degree of spontaneous reperfusion, the overall metabolic state of the patient including circulating catecholamines and free fatty acids, and, above all, the pattern of preexisting collateral flow. The infarct size is difficult to quantify, although modern imaging techniques such as magnetic resonance imaging may attain this goal in the near future. Infarct size limitation involves either relief of the coronary occlusion by, for example, thrombolysis, or conservation of the oxygen supply, for example, reduction of heart rate by β-adrenergic blockade.

5. *Stem-cell therapy* is currently under vigorous assessment. The proposal is that stem cells derived from bone marrow or residing in the heart can transdifferentiate into myocytes resembling those found in the adult heart and thereby lessen the damage caused by prior MI.

REFERENCES

1. Ross R. Atherosclerosis—an inflammatory disease. *N Engl J Med* 1999;340:115–126.
2. Schaper W, et al. Influence of collateral blood flow and of variations in MVO2 on tissue-ATP content in ischemic and infarcted myocardium. *J Mol Cell Cardiol* 1987;19:19–37.
3. Reimer KA, et al. The wavefront phenomenon of ischemic cell death. I. Myocardial infarct size vs duration of coronary occlusion in dogs. *Circulation* 1977;56:786–794.
4. Zeiher AM, et al. Endothelial dysfunction of the coronary microvasculature is associated with impaired coronary blood flow regulation in patients with early atherosclerosis. *Circulation* 1991;84:1984–1992.
5. Frielingsdorf J, et al. Normalization of abnormal coronary vasomotion by calcium antagonists in patients with hypertension. *Circulation* 1996;93:1380–1387.
6. Heitzer T, et al. Antioxidant vitamin C improves endothelial dysfunction in chronic smokers. *Circulation* 1996;94:6–9.

7. Nadal-Ginard B, et al. Myocyte death, growth and regeneration in cardiac hypertrophy and failure. *Circ Res* 2003;92:139–150.
8. Gotto Jr AM. Antioxidants, statins and atherosclerosis. *J Am Coll Cardiol* 2003;41:1205–1210.
9. Hein S, et al. Progression from compensated hypertrophy to failure in the pressure-overloaded human heart. Structural deterioration and compensatory mechanisms. *Circulation* 2003;107:984–991.
10. Vanden Hoek T, et al. Reperfusion, not simulated ischemia, initiates intrinsic apoptosis injury in chick cardiomyocytes. *Am J Physiol* 2003;254:H141–H150.
11. Remondino A, et al. β-Adrenergic receptor-stimulated apoptosis in cardiac myocytes is mediated by reactive oxygen species/c-Jun NH_2-terminal kinase-dependent activation of the mitochondrial pathway. *Circ Res* 2003; 92:136–138.
12. Hayashida W, et al. Expression of p53 and Bax genes are induced in the ischemia-reperfused rat ventricle: Potential roles in myocardial apoptosis. *Circulation* 1996;94(suppl I):1–225.
13. Misao J, et al. Expression of bcl-2 protein, an inhibitor of apoptosis and Bax, an accelerator of apoptosis, in ventricular myocytes of human hearts with myocardial infarction. *Circulation* 1996;94: 1506–1512.
14. Erbel R, et al. Coronary microembolization. *J Am Coll Cardiol* 2000;36:22–24.
15. Kloner RA, et al. Natural disaster plus wake-up time: a deadly combination of triggers. *Am Heart J* 1999;137: 830–837.
16. Owen P, et al. Glucose flux rate regulates onset of ischemic contracture in globally underperfused rat hearts. *Circ Res* 1990;66:344–354.
17. Weiss J, et al. Functional compartmentation of glycolytic versus oxidative metabolism in isolated rabbit heart. *J Clin Invest* 1985;75:436–447.
18. Sebbag L, et al. Elimination of glycolytically-derived ATP markedly accelerates the onset of transmural cell death during myocardial ischemia in vivo in dogs. *Circulation* 1996;94(suppl I): 1–367(abst).
19. Jennings RB, et al. Myocardial ischemia revisited. The osmolar load, membrane damage, and reperfusion. *J Mol Cell Cardiol* 1986;18:769–780.
20. Cross HR, et al. The role of Na^+/K^+ ATPase activity during low flow ischemia in preventing myocardial injury: A ^{31}P, ^{23}Na and ^{87}Rb NMR spectroscopic study. *Magn Reson Med* 1995;34:673–685.
21. Marks AR. Calcium and the heart, a question of life and death. *J Clin Invest* 2003;111:597–600.
22. Hausenloy DJ, Yellon DM. The mitochondrial permeability transition pore: its fundamental role in mediating cell death during ischaemia and reperfusion. *J Mol Cell Cardiol* 2003;35:339–341.
23. Puleo PR, et al. Use of a rapid assay of subforms of creatine kinase MB to diagnose or rule out acute myocardial infarction. *N Engl J Med* 1994;331:561–566.
24. de Winter RJ, et al. Value of myoglobin, troponin T and CK-MB_{mass} in ruling out an acute myocardial infarction in the emergency room. *Circulation* 1995;92:3401–3407.
25. Hamm C, et al. Emergency room triage of patients with acute chest pain by means of rapid testing for cardiac troponin or troponin I. *N Engl J Med* 1997;337:1648–1653.
26. Kwong RY, et al. Detecting acute coronary syndrome in the emergency department with cardiac magnetic resonance imaging. *Circulation* 2003;107:531–537.
27. Yusuf S, et al. Early intravenous atenolol treatment in suspected acute myocardial infarction: preliminary report of a randomized trial. *Lancet* 1980;2:273–276.
28. Bradham WS, et al. Tumor necrosis factor-alpha and myocardial remodeling in progression of heart failure: a current perspective. *Cardiovasc Res* 2002;53:822–830.
29. Kalra D, et al. Angiotensin II induces tumour necrosis factor biosynthesis in the adult mammalian heart through a protein kinase C-dependent pathway. *Circulation* 2002;105:2198–2205.
30. Wachtell K, et al. Change in diastolic left ventricular filling after one year of antihypertensive treatment. The Losartan Intervention for Endpoint Reduction in Hypertension (LIFE) Study. *Circulation* 2002;105:1071–1076.
31. Mukherjee R, et al. Myocardial infarct expansion and matrix metalloproteinase inhibition. *Circulation* 2003;107:618–625.
32. Orlic D, et al. Stem cells for myocardial regeneration. *Circ Res* 2002;91:1092–1102.
33. Hagège AA, et al. Viability and differentiation of autologous skeletal myoblast grafts in ischemic cardiomyopathy. *Lancet* 2003;361:491–492.
34. Müller-Ehmsen J, et al. Rebuilding a damaged heart. Long-term survival of transplanted neonatal rat cardiomyocytes after myocardial infarction and effect on cardiac function. *Circulation* 2002;105: 1720–1726.
35. King LM, et al. Coronary flow and glucose delivery as determinants of contracture in the ischemic myocardium. *J Mol Cell Cardiol* 1995;27:701–720.

19

Myocardial Reperfusion: Stunning, Hibernation, and Preconditioning

Lionel H. Opie and Gerd Heusch

"Brief periods of coronary occlusion result in prolonged depression of myocardial function in the ischemic zone."

Heyndrickx et al. (1)

Myocardial reperfusion is no longer a laboratory event. Practicing cardiologists are now able to induce myocardial reperfusion after the onset of coronary thrombosis with thrombolytic agents, such as streptokinase or tissue plasminogen activator. Increasingly, mechanical reperfusion by angioplasty or urgent coronary bypass is seen as ideal reperfusion therapy. Despite very promising findings with reperfusion, clinicians have noted that the results are not always as positive as expected. Thus, sometimes even early restitution of blood flow leaves the function of the myocardium temporarily depressed, which has been termed the stunned myocardium (2). Experimentalists have long been impressed by the finding that restitution of coronary flow to the ischemic myocardium may precipitate an adverse sequence of events (3). This spectrum of events, including reperfusion arrhythmias, stunning, microvascular damage, and accelerated death of the more severely damaged cells despite reperfusion, is termed *reperfusion injury* (4).

These novel aspects of ischemia, such as stunning, hibernation, and preconditioning (Table 19-1), stand in contrast to the "classic" conditions, such as effort angina, and acute coronary syndromes, such as unstable angina and infarction. *Stunning* refers to postischemic impairment of myocardial function (Fig. 19-1). *Hibernation* is when the ventricle contracts poorly in the presence of severe coronary artery disease but "wakes up" after revascularization by coronary artery surgery. *Preconditioning* is the protective state that lessens the severity of ischemia/reperfusion injury when it follows one or more brief episodes of preceding ischemia, each such episode being followed by reperfusion. Although the vast body of evidence favoring the entity of preconditioning has been found in experimental animals, current studies strongly suggest that it also occurs in humans (5).

TABLE 19-1. Proposed characteristics of conventional ischemia, stunning, hibernation and preconditioning

Parameter	Conventional ischemia	Stunning	Hibernation	Preconditioning Early phase	Preconditioning Late phase
Myocardial function	Reduced	Reduced	Reduced	Protected for hours by prior ischemia	Protected for days by prior ischemia
Coronary blood flow	Severely reduced	Postischemic; fully restored	Modestly reduced or possibly normal at rest and repetitively reduced during exercise	Brief ischemia: →Fully referfused →Index ischemia →Reperfused →Protection	Brief ischemia: →Fully reperfused →Index ischemia →Reperfused →Protection
Myocardial energy metabolism	Reduced: increasingly severe as ischemia proceeds	Normal or excessive	Reduced in relation to contractile decrease	Reduced ATP demand in index ischemic period	
Duration	Minutes to hours	Hours to days, possibly longer	Days to months, possibly longer	Protection lasts up to 3 hr	Protected for 1–3 days; "second window"
Outcome	Infarction if severe ischemia persists	Full recovery	Recovery if revascularization	Decreased postischemic infarct size; decreased surrogate damage	Decreased postischemic infarct size; decreased surrogate damage
Proposed mechanism	Insufficient glycolytic ATP to control cell calcium and to prevent irreversibility	Interaction between cystolic calcium overload and excess formation of ROS	Increased uptake of FDG reflects increased glycolytic ATP	Signal system from adenosine receptor to PKC to opening of mitochondrial K-ATP channel	Nuclear synthesis of protective proteins (COX-2, iNOS) in response to JAK-STAT and NF-κB

ATP, adenosine 5′-triphosphate; ROS, reactive oxygen species; FDG, fluorodeoxyglucose; PKC, protein kinase C; K, potassium; COX-2, cyclooxygenase 2; iNOS, inducible nitric oxide synthase; JAK-STAT, Janus kinase–signal transducer and activator of transcription; NF-κB, nuclear factor κB.

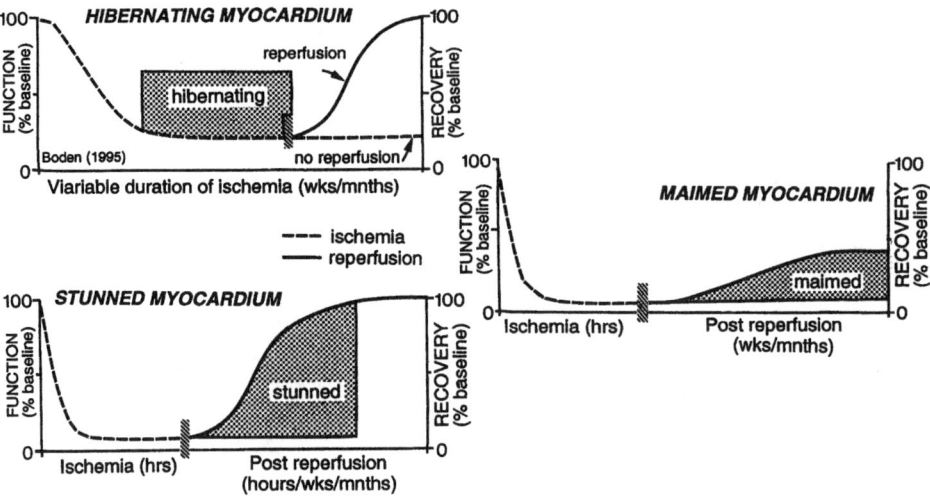

FIG. 19-1. **Hibernation, stunning, and maiming.** In the hibernating heart, chronic depression of function is relieved by revascularization. In the stunned heart, mechanical dysfunction results from reperfusion. In the maimed myocardium, there is some permanent damage resulting from prolonged ischemia, so that recovery is never complete. (Modified from Boden WE, et al. Incomplete, delayed functional recovery late after reperfusion following acute myocardial infarction: "maimed myocardium." Am Heart J 1995;130:922–932.)

STUNNED MYOCARDIUM

Not all the mechanical recovery occurs rapidly after reperfusion; full recovery may be delayed by hours, days, or even weeks. Because myocardial function eventually recovers fully, it is stunned during the phase of delayed recovery (2). In 1975, Heyndrickx et al. (1) made the seminal discovery that regional ischemia in the dog heart when induced for only 5 minutes was followed by depressed mechanical function lasting more than 3 hours. Furthermore, 15 minutes of coronary occlusion resulted in more than 6 hours of left ventricular (LV) dysfunction. Of considerable importance was the point that such short periods of ischemia did not result in any residual necrosis. The impaired postischemic function could not be accounted for by any impairment of blood flow in the previously occluded vessel. Thus, as Braunwald and Kloner (2) state, transient ischemia may interfere with normal myocardial function, biochemical processes, and ultrastructure for prolonged periods.

Duration of Ischemia and Stunning

If the absence of necrosis is an essential part of the definition, as required by Bolli, then it becomes clear that the longer and more severe the period of ischemia is, the less the contribution of true stunning is and the greater the contribution of permanent damage to postinfarction dysfunction. The typical duration of total ischemia that is soon followed by completely reversible stunning is 5 to 20 minutes (1). Increasing the duration of severe ischemia from 30 to 90 minutes results in adverse events such as further increase in postischemic diastolic pressure, with a marked gain in total tissue and mitochondrial calcium. These observations explain why 1 hour of coronary artery occlusion in the dog followed by 4 weeks of reperfusion does not yield complete recovery (6). When this type of gradual and incomplete recovery over several days and even weeks results from a mixture of chronic stunning and irreversible damage, there never will be full functional recovery. This condition is sometimes called the *maimed myocardium* (7). Chronic stunning, with greatly delayed but eventual full recovery, and the maimed myocardium probably merge.

Mechanism of Stunning

Of the many theories to explain the development of stunning, the most plausible involve the formation of oxygen-derived free radicals and cytosolic calcium overload (Fig. 19-2) (8). Most logically, the delayed resynthesis of adenosine 5'-triphosphate (ATP), probably the consequence of the loss of adenosine and related compounds during the ischemic period, could be blamed. Nonetheless, even when there are no decrease in ATP and a rapid recovery of creatine phosphate after short periods of ischemia, there is already stunning (Fig. 17-3).

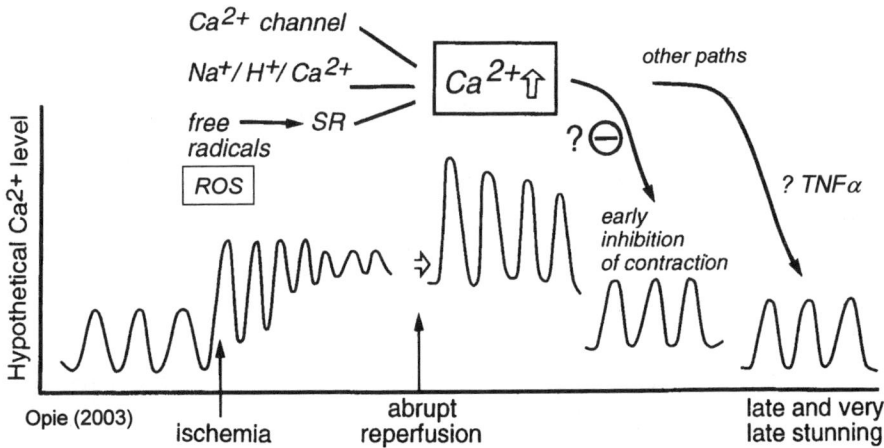

FIG. 19-2. Hypothetical cytosolic calcium levels. Note the proposed role of increased cytosolic calcium in causing early stunning after reperfusion and in hypothetically playing a role in late remodeling by stimulation of protein synthesis, possibly at the level of mitogen-activated protein kinase (*MAPK*). $Na^+/H^+/Ca^2$, sodium–proton and sodium–calcium exchange mechanisms; *SR*, sarcoplasmic reticulum; *ROS*, reactive oxygen species; *TNF*, tumor necrosis factor.

Calcium Overload

The mechanism of the contractile failure in stunning has not been finalized, but "alterations in calcium homeostasis seem to be a likely cause" (3). The fact that the stunned myocardium can respond well to inotropic stimulation by the catecholamines (9), calcium infusion (10), or postextrasystolic potentiation (9) suggests that stunning results from calcium abnormalities. There could be a lack of available intracellular calcium, a failure of uptake of calcium by the sarcoplasmic reticulum, or a failure of the contractile proteins to respond to normal calcium concentrations (11). Measurements of cytosolic calcium during early postischemic reperfusion show increased calcium levels and oscillations (Fig. 19-3) (12–14). The concept could be that internal cytosolic calcium overload damages the contractile apparatus to impair the normal physiologic response to calcium so that there is mechanical stunning (Fig. 19-2). The temporary cytosolic calcium overload during reperfusion has different possible sources, including decreased uptake into the sarcoplasmic reticulum (failure of availability of ATP), decreased extrusion from the cell (again failure of ATP), entry through the voltage-sensitive calcium channel (explaining inhibition of stunning by calcium channel blockers at the time of reperfusion), and activity of the sodium–calcium exchanger. All procedures leading to excess cytosolic calcium, including formation of free radicals, should be harmful and the use of various agents including

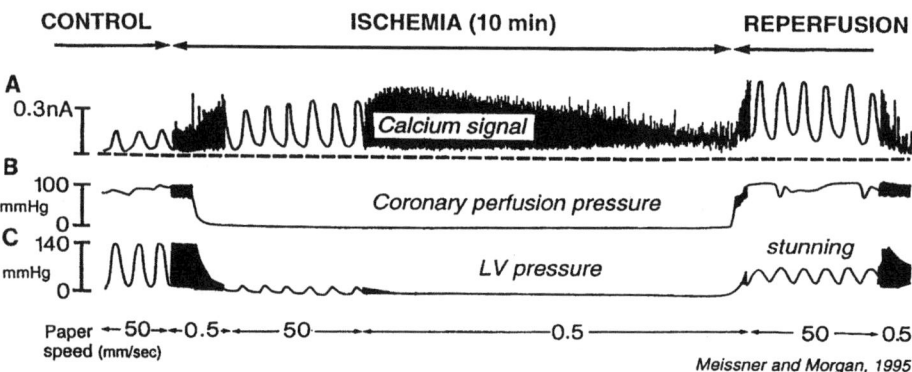

FIG. 19-3. Measured cytosolic calcium levels. Can left ventricular (*LV*) mechanical failure during and after severe ischemia be explained by changes in the cytosolic calcium? These data show that when there is abrupt ischemic LV failure [LV pressure decreases to zero (**C**)], then the calcium signal (**A**) increases before it decreases. Ischemia is designated by the abrupt decrease in coronary perfusion pressure to zero in this isolated rat heart preparation. During reperfusion, there is also a dissociation between the cytosolic calcium oscillations, which are increased (on right in **A**) in contrast to LV contraction that is decreased (on right in **B**), so that there is mechanical stunning. Hypothetically, excess calcium oscillations damage the contractile proteins. (From Meissner A, et al. Contractile dysfunction and abnormal Ca^{2+} modulation during postischemic reperfusion in rat heart. *Am J Physiol* 1995;268:H100–H111, with permission.)

the calcium channel blockers as well as Na^+-H^+ exchange inhibitors should be beneficial.

REACTIVE OXYGEN SPECIES AND OXIDATIVE STRESS

Free radicals are highly reactive chemical species that differ from standard compounds in having unpaired electrons in their outer orbitals. Oxygen-derived free radicals are biologically the most important and are often called reactive oxygen species (ROS). They include the superoxide radical $\cdot O_2^-$ (Fig. 19-4), in which the dot indicates the free radical and the negative charge indicates the electron gained (superoxide anion). There is danger that the superoxide anion can react with hydrogen peroxide to form the even more highly reactive hydroxyl ion ($\cdot OH$) in which there is no charge because normally the hydroxyl group carries the negative charge and gaining an electron confers a neutral compound. Nonetheless, this compound is "one of the most aggressive species of oxygen free radicals" (15). Singlet oxygen (Table 19-2) is not, strictly speaking, a free

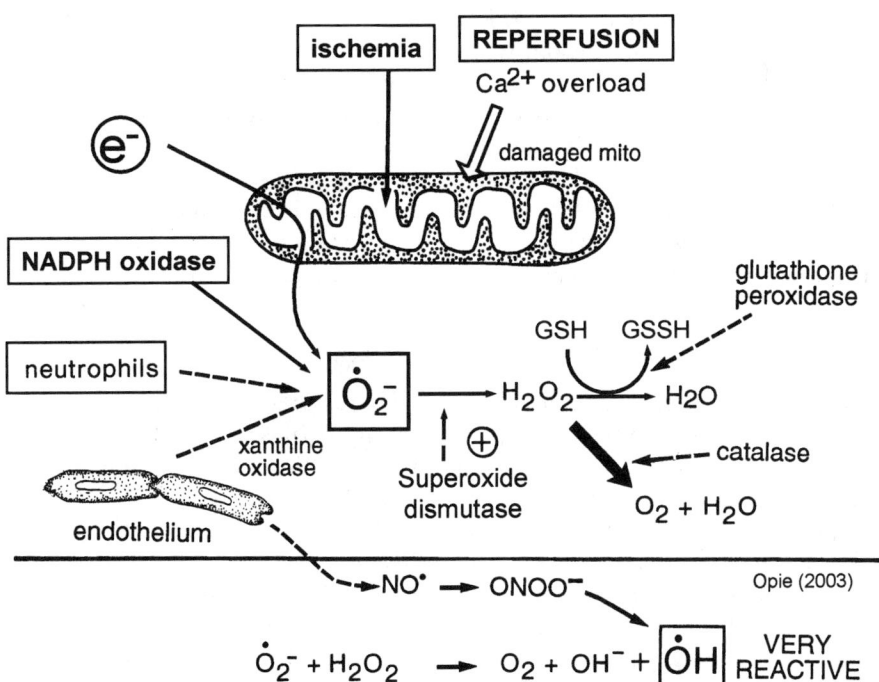

FIG. 19-4. Pathways for generation of oxygen free radicals with superoxide ($\cdot O_2^-$) and hydroxyl ($\cdot OH$) ions. *GSH*, reduced glutathione; *GSSG*, oxidized glutathione. Note the formation of peroxynitrite from nitric oxide ($\cdot NO$). For nicotinamide adenine dinucleotide phosphate (reduced form), see Figure 9-12.

TABLE 19-2. *Potentially cytotoxic oxygen-derived species*

·O_2^-	Superoxide anion radical
H_2O_2	Hydrogen peroxide (not a free radical)
·OH	Hydroxyl radical
ROO·	Lipid peroxide radical (R = lipid chain)
$^1O_2$	Singlet oxygen[a]
$ONOO^-$	Peroxynitrite

[a]In singlet oxygen, the two outer electrons occupy the same orbital and spin in opposite directions, hence being unstable. One mechanism for formation of singlet oxygen is by light activation of molecular oxygen in the presence of a photosensitizer, such as rose bengal. Another proposed mechanism is during superoxide dismutation.

radical but has two outer electrons spinning in opposite directions, which accounts for its instability.

Major Sources of Reactive Oxygen Species

First, mitochondria are physiologic sources of ROS, mostly made at complex 3 in the electron transport chain (Fig. 11-13), where some of the electrons form superoxide. During reperfusion, when mitochondria are damaged by lipid peroxides (next section), ROS are more likely to form (16). Another source of ROS is the nicotinamide adenine dinucleotide phosphate (reduced form) oxidase system, especially important in mediating the effects of angiotensin in vascular smooth muscle cells but also found in ventricular myocytes where they contribute to growth signaling (16). Third, nitric oxide, itself a free radical and normally a "good guy" causing vasodilation and protecting the endothelium, can, when in excess, form the "bad guy" peroxynitrite (Table 19-3).

Role of Reactive Oxygen Species in Stunning

In a classic paper, Hearse et al. showed that restoration of oxygen to the previously anoxic heart was accompanied by signs of severe cell injury (16a). That led to the later hypothesis that a burst of ROS production on reperfusion was a major cause of reperfusion injury, including stunning (3). ROS have complex roles in the heart (Figs. 9-9 and 9-11), varying from physiologic participation in the angiotensin signaling system that promotes cell growth to apoptosis and even cell necrosis at higher and more cytotoxic levels of ROS (16). Currently, there is good evidence that the hydroxyl radical is the key mediator of stunning (17). One early and still valid proposal was that *peroxidation* of polyunsaturated lipids of the membranes could be caused by ROS and specifically by the hydroxyl radical (Table 19-2) to contribute to reperfusion injury. When membranes are damaged by lipid peroxidation, increased permeability to calcium follows.

TABLE 19-3. *Free radical generation: some essential equations*

Reduction of O_2 to H_2O
$O_2 + e^- \rightarrow \cdot O_2^-$ (superoxide radical)
$\cdot O_2 + e^- + 2H^+ \rightarrow H_2O_2$ (hydrogen peroxide)
$\cdot O_2^- + H_2O_2 + H^+ \rightarrow O_2 + H_2O + \cdot OH$ ($\cdot OH$ = hydroxyl radical)
$\cdot OH + e^- + H^+ \rightarrow H_2O$
Iron-related reactions
$Fe^{2+} + H_2O_2 \rightarrow Fe^{3+} + \cdot OH + OH^-$ (Fenton reaction)
$Fe^{3+} + \cdot O_2^- \rightarrow Fe^{2+} + O_2$
$\cdot O_2^- + H_2O_2 \rightarrow O_2 + \cdot OH + OH^-$ (Haber–Weiss reaction)
Lipid peroxidation
   Initiation   Lipid-H + $\cdot OH \rightarrow H_2O$ + lipid$\cdot$
                         Lipid$\cdot$ + $O_2 \rightarrow$ lipid OO$\cdot$
   Propagation   Lipid OO$\cdot$ + lipid-H $\rightarrow$ lipid – OOH + lipid$\cdot$
   Termination   Lipid$\cdot$ + lipid$\cdot$ $\rightarrow$ lipid – lipid
Xanthine oxidase reaction[a]
ATP $\rightarrow$ adenosine $\rightarrow$ xanthine
Xanthine + H_2O + $2O_2 \rightarrow$ uric acid + $2 \cdot O_2^-$ + $2H^+$
NADPH oxidase
NADPH + $2O_2 \rightarrow NAD(P)^+ + H^+ + 2\cdot O_2^-$
Peroxynitrite
$\cdot NO + \cdot O_2^- \rightarrow ONOO^-$

[a]Xanthine oxidase is not found in the human myocardium, although it may be present in vascular endothelial cells.
ATP, adenosine 5′-triphosphate; NADPH, nicotinamide adenine dinucleotide (reduced form).

Antioxidant Defense Mechanisms

These occur naturally and protect against the formation of free radicals (Fig. 19-4, Table 19-4). Thus, the key enzyme protecting against lipid peroxidation is glutathione reductase, which uses reduced glutathione for hydrogen donation to the membrane lipids, thereby keeping them reduced. It is when such defense mechanisms are overcome that the harmful effects of ROS become evident, in which case a logical therapy is to remove excess free radicals by compounds that

TABLE 19-4. *Naturally occurring defence systems against free radicals*

Superoxide dismutase
   $2 \cdot O_2^- + 2H^+ \rightarrow H_2O_2 + O_2$
Catalase (peroxisome bound)
   $2 H_2O_2 \rightarrow O_2 + 2H_2O$
Glutathione peroxidase
   2 GSH + lipid-OOH $\rightarrow$ GSSG + lipid-OH + H_2O
   2 GSH + $H_2O_2 \rightarrow$ GSSG + $2H_2O$
Nonenzymatic scavengers
   α-Tocopherol
   β-Carotene
   Vitamin A
   Ascorbate
   Sulfhydryl group
   Thioether compounds

act as radical scavengers (Table 19-4). This proposal is supported by strong experimental data (3). Thus far, however, no clinical tests with such drugs have been successful in modifying reperfusion injury, which has somewhat dampened the interests of cardiologists in free radicals.

Interaction of Calcium and Reactive Oxygen Species

Calcium-mediated and ROS-mediated components to reperfusion damage may be interactive (Fig. 19-5) (8). Thus formation of ROS increases cytosolic calcium by a variety of mechanisms: an effect on membrane phospholipids with an increase in cytosolic calcium, mitochondrial production of free radicals with mitochondrial injury, additive or parallel effects of calcium overload on ATP

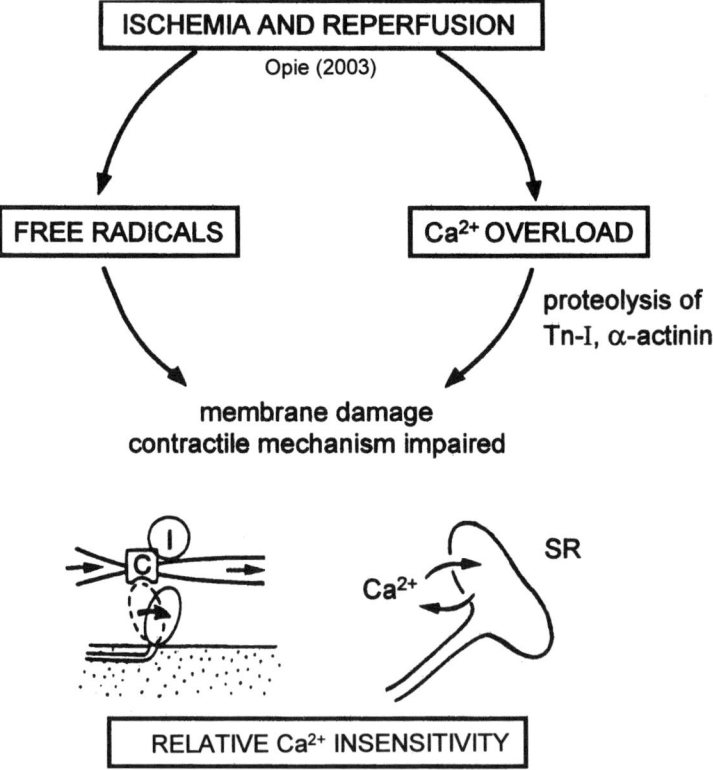

FIG. 19-5. Two major mechanisms for reperfusion injury: formation of free radicals and calcium overload. This scheme reconciles these apparently conflicting hypotheses, showing their combined role in causing membrane damage and relative calcium insensitivity of contractile mechanism (actin–myosin interaction on the left and sarcoplasmic reticulum on the right). (From Opie LH. Reperfusion injury and its pharmacologic modification. *Circulation* 1989;80: 1049–1062, with permission.)

depletion, and activation of the calcium release channel of the ryanodine receptor of the sarcoplasmic reticulum with enhanced release of calcium. ROS, especially hydroxyl radicals, stimulate sodium–calcium exchange in the reverse mode (Fig. 6-7) to cause calcium overload and acute diastolic dysfunction (15).

Stunning in the Clinical Setting

After Balloon Angioplasty

These observations have been made in conditions most closely mimicking the original animal experiments and particularly emphasize diastolic contractile abnormalities (3).

Postanginal and Postthrombolytic Stunning

Although the recovery from angina by cessation of exertion has been known from the early descriptions centuries ago, more recent work has shown that myocardial mechanical recovery is also delayed (Fig. 17-11). Thus, regional wall motion abnormalities persist for at least 30 minutes after treadmill exercise testing (18). Unstable angina is also followed by echocardiographic changes (3). In postthrombolytic patients, there is the delayed recovery, over days and weeks, of function. Such chronic dysfunction may be a complex mixture of prolonged stunning, ventricular remodeling, and myocyte damage. In a few clinical studies, calcium channel blockers have reduced postthrombolytic or postanginal stunning.

Bypass Surgery

Bypass surgery involves myocardial ischemic arrest and reperfusion. Diastolic dysfunction is associated with an increase in LV diastolic chamber stiffness. The impairment in ventricular function may also, in more severe cases, be systolic with clinical heart failure that requires inotropic stimulation. As much as 24 to 48 hours may be required for complete recovery (3). All these clinical observations tie in well with the now established concept that "ischemia does something" that impairs mechanical activity even after the actual ischemic event is over.

OTHER ASPECTS OF REPERFUSION INJURY

Reperfusion Arrhythmias

Experimentally, reperfusion arrhythmias can occur within seconds of the onset of reperfusion. As in the case of stunning, there are two main theories for arrhythmias: excess cytosolic calcium and formation of free radicals. During prolonged periods (30 minutes) of severe hypoxia in guinea pig papillary muscle, there is a slow, steady increase in diastolic tension, i.e., hypoxic contracture, followed by automaticity on reoxygenation (4). Direct measurements show large cytosolic calcium oscillations during early reperfusion (14). Restoration of ATP with reperfusion must provide the energy for the excess recycling of calcium. The result is the specific electrophysiologic phenomenon of delayed afterdepolarizations, which probably explains at least some types of reperfusion arrhythmias. Calcium overcycling repetitively evokes the transient inward current that predisposes to ventricular automaticity. Of note, inhibitors of calcium movement in or out of the sarcoplasmic reticulum are able to decrease reperfusion arrhythmias.

Duration of Ischemia and Arrhythmias

There is a relationship between the incidence of reperfusion arrhythmias and the degree of reversibility of ischemia. No reperfusion arrhythmias arise in dead cells. This postulate is compatible with the idea that energy in the form of ATP is required for the cytosolic recycling of calcium that underlies at least some types of reperfusion arrhythmias. There is a bell-shaped curve of incidence of reperfusion arrhythmias with a peak incidence when the ischemia lasts between 5 and 20 minutes. Thereafter, the incidence decreases, presumably as the ATP stores are depleted and calcium ions cannot recycle.

Severity of Ischemia

Relatively little is known about the influence of the severity of ischemic injury on subsequent reperfusion injury. Increased heart rate increases the severity of ischemic injury and also increases the incidence of reperfusion arrhythmias. Two agents known to reduce heart rate, the beta-blocker propranolol and the calcium antagonist diltiazem, decrease reperfusion calcium uptake and reperfusion arrhythmias, respectively. Hence, it is probable that the severity of ischemia is a factor determining the severity of reperfusion arrhythmias and probably other aspects of reperfusion injury.

Speed of Reperfusion

Experimentally, sudden rather than gradual reperfusion is associated with a greater degree of reperfusion injury. In patients, reperfusion by thrombolysis is slow, over many minutes, and not abrupt, in seconds, as it is in many animal experiments. This difference may explain why some aspects of reperfusion injury, such as arrhythmias, are less common in humans than in animals. In cases of transient severe coronary spasm, rapid relief of spasm is much faster and may precipitate reperfusion ventricular arrhythmias.

Microvascular Damage and No Reflow

No reflow is the multifactorial phenomenon occurring when removal of coronary occlusion does not lead to full restoration of coronary flow (19) or when early complete reperfusion is followed by a later close down (20). Clearly, the benefits of reperfusion are lessened by no reflow. There is probably a combination of endothelial swelling and edema of the microvessels, with added plugging by neutrophils and/or platelets and fibrin (19). The postulated role of the neutrophils that accumulate during reperfusion is similar to that in postpump syndrome (next section). Microvascular damage also can decrease formation of vasodilatory substances, such as nitric oxide, from the endothelium and promote formation of vasoconstrictors. At least some of the microvascular damage is caused by ROS and is decreased by free radical scavengers. A proposed mechanism for the formation of ROS is the reintroduction of neutrophils into the ischemic zone with damage to the endothelium. The result could be platelet activation, which could explain or contribute to no reflow.

Postpump Syndrome, Cytokines, and Neutrophils

Although most patients recover well from cardiopulmonary bypass, in some, there is a widespread inflammatory response, caused by activation of a variety of cells including monocytes, macrophages, endothelial cells, and T cells. These cells liberate cytokines such as tumor necrosis factor-α (TNF-α) and the interleukins. Interleukin-8 is also known as the neutrophil-activating factor, and its messenger RNA is induced in the myocardium during cardiopulmonary bypass. Neutrophils are attracted to any area of injury, "roll on" and adhere to the endothelium, and then either return to the bloodstream or undergo transendothelial migration, the whole process known as *neutrophil trafficking*. Neutrophil adhesion is promoted by endothelial surface receptors such as the selectins and intercellular adhesion molecules, which interact with the neutrophil surface. When inside the vascular interstitial space, the neutrophils are activated and thought to liberate damaging free radicals and leukotrienes. The proposal is that such neutrophil trafficking promotes postsurgery myocardial and even whole body damage.

Postreperfusion Accelerated Cell Death

The prototype experiments on reperfusion damage and cell death were performed by Jennings et al. (21). They found that on reperfusion of a coronary artery, there was a massive increase in the tissue level of calcium, with the appearance of contraction bands and intramitochondrial dense bodies (probably deposits of calcium phosphate). Such changes were greatly delayed when coronary occlusion was maintained. They proposed that reperfusion led to excess uptake of calcium into the cytosol through a sarcolemma damaged during the ischemic period, with the cytosolic overloading followed by subsequent mitochondrial calcium excess and impaired ability of mitochondrial manufacture of ATP. This sequence could explain accelerated reperfusion-related cell death. Since then, necrosis and apoptosis have been differentiated (Chapter 18), with recent studies focusing on apoptosis (Fig. 9-9).

Reperfusion has a protective effect in decreasing the extent of ischemic apoptosis, yet provoking a paradoxical acceleration of apoptosis in other cells, which may be those previously destined to die (22). Apoptosis in reperfusion is mediated by caspases and initiated by a variety of death-inducing ligands, including TNF-α (23). If ischemic necrosis and apoptosis are two different processes and if apoptosis is more specifically associated with reperfusion, then it is difficult to avoid the conclusion that reperfusion causes some cells to die that would otherwise have lived. Supporting evidence is that administration of insulin and other growth factors at the time of reperfusion decreases infarct size, probably at least in part by an antiapoptotic mechanism (24).

HIBERNATION AND CHRONIC LEFT VENTRICULAR DYSFUNCTION

Whereas stunning is caused by reperfusion, hibernation is cured by revascularization. Hibernation is a chronic clinical condition in which part of the myocardium does not contract normally (systolic dysfunction) in the presence of severe coronary artery disease without another obvious cause, such as concurrent angina or myocardial infarction, and responds to revascularization by improved mechanical function (Fig. 19-6). The original description of Rahimtoola (25) was "a state of persistently impaired myocardial and left ventricular

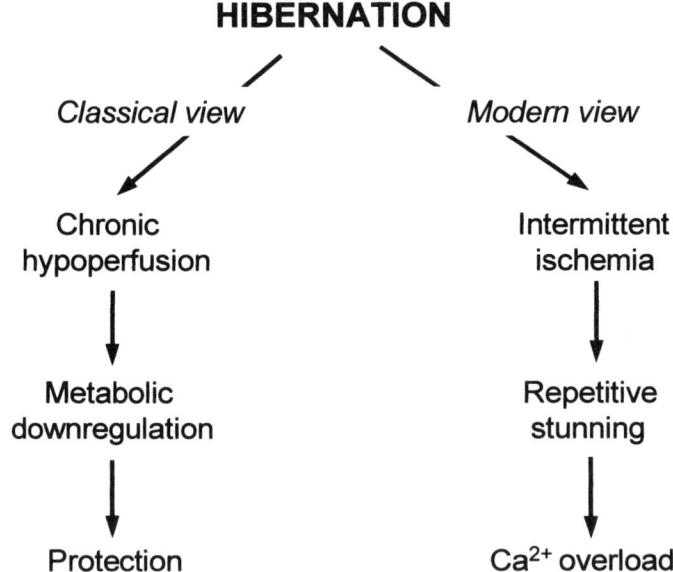

FIG. 19-6. Two views on hibernation. The classic view is that hibernation is associated with chronic hypoperfusion of the hibernating myocardium. The current and revised view is that intermittent ischemia causes repetitive stunning with similar consequences.

function at rest due to reduced coronary blood flow that can be partially or completely restored to normal if the myocardial oxygen supply/demand relationship is favorably altered, either by improving blood flow and/or by reducing demand." A challenging finding is that the resting blood flow may only be modestly or marginally reduced despite severe coronary artery disease. In any case, the flow reduction is not severe enough to damage the myocardium permanently, which would preclude recovery of function after revascularization.

Mechanism of Hibernation

A critical stenosis that limits coronary flow reserve is a "mandatory prerequisite" for hibernation (26). The initial hypothesis was that decreased coronary flow gave rise to metabolic down-regulation, the major change being inhibited contractile activity. This concept was supported by models of short-term hibernation in which flow reduction was matched by contraction decrease. Complexity was introduced by the finding that coronary flow in humans with hibernation was only modestly reduced, not enough to account for the degree of decline in contractile function (27). The updated proposal is that severe coronary artery disease is associated with repetitive, intermittent and often silent ischemia (Fig. 19-7), giving rise to repetitive episodes of stunning, which, when summated, translate into chronic impairment of LV function.

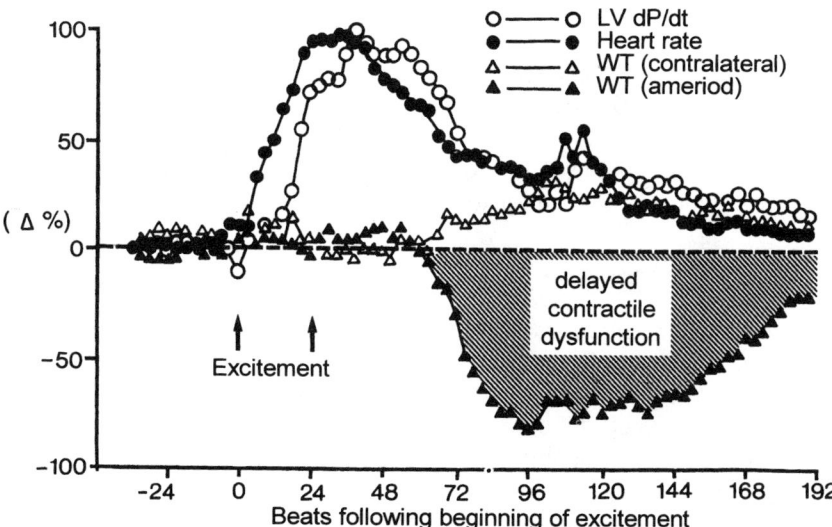

FIG. 19-7. Transient ischemia and contraction. Brief excitement in the presence of coronary stenosis in a pig model causes tachycardia, transiently increased contractility followed by delayed contractile dysfunction. (From Shen et al. Mechanism of impaired myocardial function during progressive coronary stenosis in conscious pigs. *Circ Res* 1995;76:479–488, with permission.)

New Animal Models

These are becoming more and more sophisticated. Partial coronary occlusion with reperfusion through a critical stenosis in a pig model within 2 weeks reproduces hibernation with matched decreases in coronary flow and function (28) in contrast to the perfusion–contraction mismatch in the stunned myocardium. When this model is studied after 3 months, the hearts become tolerant of attempts to aggravate ischemia by epinephrine infusion (29). Thus, there have been cellular adaptations that resemble the "rescue mechanism" for surviving hypoxia (30). When so adapted, the hibernating myocardium could theoretically go on surviving for a very long, in accord with some clinical observations. However, the mechanism of the impaired contraction requires further investigation.

Signaling in Hibernation

Heusch et al. (31) and others (32) have proposed that inflammatory processes such as those involving TNF-α could be important in the development of the hibernating myocardium. The basis of these observations is the increased gene expression of TNF-α in the hibernating human myocardium (32), the contractile depression induced by TNF-α, and the close similarity of the signaling systems to those induced by microembolization (31). Speculatively, showers of emboli from thrombi on coronary stenoses could be causing progressive loss of contractile function in hibernation.

Disuse Atrophy

Ventricular unloading can cause shrinkage of myocardial cells and accumulation of collagen and fibroblasts. Some changes, such as the loss of myofibrils, are common to the histology of some of the hibernating segments and to disuse atrophy. A simple hypothesis would therefore be that during sustained hibernation, lack of contraction would lead to disuse atrophy.

Clinical Significance of Hibernation

If hypocontractile myocardium is still viable and can respond to revascularization, then it is possible to improve LV function in patients with severe coronary disease, thereby easing symptoms and improving prognosis—hence, the active search for viable hibernating myocardium. Of the various radionuclide methods for assessing viability (Fig. 19-8), positron emission tomography is often regarded as the metabolic gold standard for preoperative detection of hibernation. Viability is indicated by a "mismatch" pattern whereby the tissue signal of labeled deoxyglucose is increased relative to the myocardial blood flow, which is either decreased, low normal, or even normal at rest (Fig. 11-21). Other methods for detection of viability include a positive inotropic response to dobu-

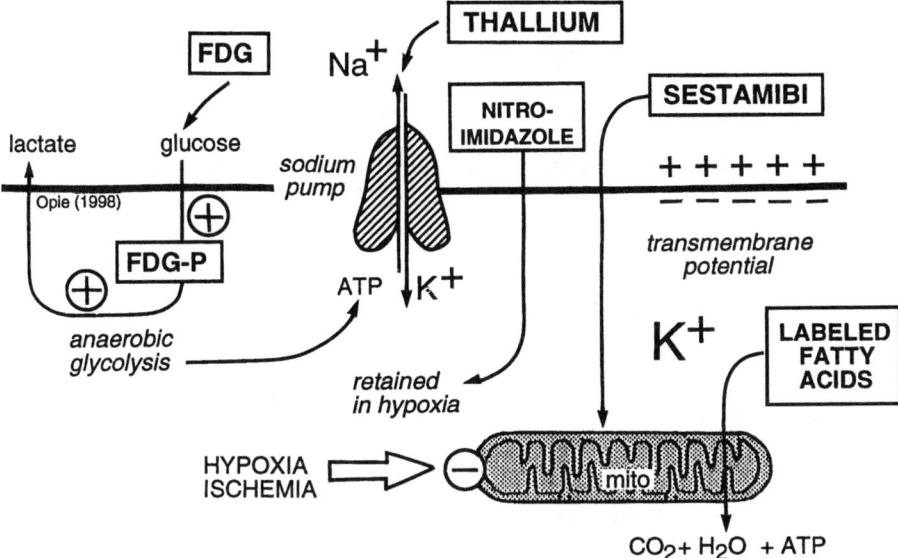

FIG. 19-8. Myocardial viability and tracers. Different radionuclide tracers are able to track different aspects of ischemic metabolism. Thallium indicates here either redistribution or reinjection techniques. *FDG*, fluorodeoxyglucose; *FDG-P*, phosphorylated fluorodeoxyglucose.

tamine as shown on the echocardiogram and/or a positive redistribution thallium scan. Thallium is taken up into viable cells by the sodium pump. Positron emission tomography, thallium single-photon emission computed tomography, and dobutamine echocardiography, when compared, give somewhat similar results with thallium being the least sensitive.

Spectrum of Changes in Hibernation

Clinical hibernation extends from one condition in which regional function returns promptly on the operating table on revascularization to another condition recognized by a much delayed mechanical recovery and overt histologic changes. Different observers using different techniques are likely to describe different entities under the term of hibernation, which in reality is not a uniform condition but rather a spectrum of conditions. It must also be considered that in humans, there would probably be multiple coronary stenoses of varying degrees of severity and varying consequences, extending from transient ischemia and stunning to reversible hibernation and irreversible cell death. Thus, the overall picture in human disease is much more complex than that found even in sophisticated animal models.

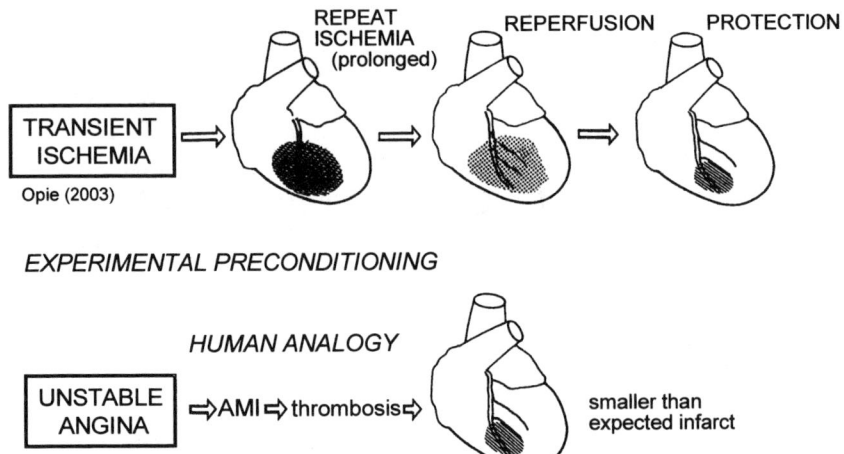

FIG. 19-9. Preconditioning. Top: Experimental protocol. Bottom: Proposed application in patients. For review, see Yellon and Downey (43).

PRECONDITIONING: THE POTENTIAL MODIFIER OF ISCHEMIC STATES

Whereas many repetitive episodes of ischemia should produce cumulative damage, one or more bursts of short-lived severe ischemia followed by complete reperfusion cause preconditioning, first described by Jennings' group (21,33). Preconditioning is one of the most powerful and consistent protectors against severe ischemia, found across a wide range of species, organs, and tissues. When preconditioned, the myocardium is protected against a greater subsequent ischemic insult, with less threat of infarction (Fig. 19-9). In addition, there are other surrogates of successful preconditioning such as decreased postischemic stunning, fewer reperfusion arrhythmias, or less apoptosis (34).

Variations on the Theme

Although preconditioning is classically initiated by one or more periods of total ischemia, each followed by reperfusion, nonetheless, there are variants. First, ischemic preconditioning can be achieved by partial coronary occlusion (rather than total) and without intermittent reperfusion. Thus, myocardial infarction with a "stuttering" pattern of onset may be less severe than expected. Another deviation from the classic pattern of preconditioning is *intraischemic preconditioning*, whereby an initial brief period of no-flow ischemia increases myocardial tolerance to subsequent low-flow ischemia without any intervening reperfusion period (Fig. 19-10) (35). Other variations are that preconditioning can follow transient vigorous β-adrenergic stimulation, cycles of calcium depletion and repletion, or rapid cardiac pacing, hypoxia, or stretch (34). Precondi-

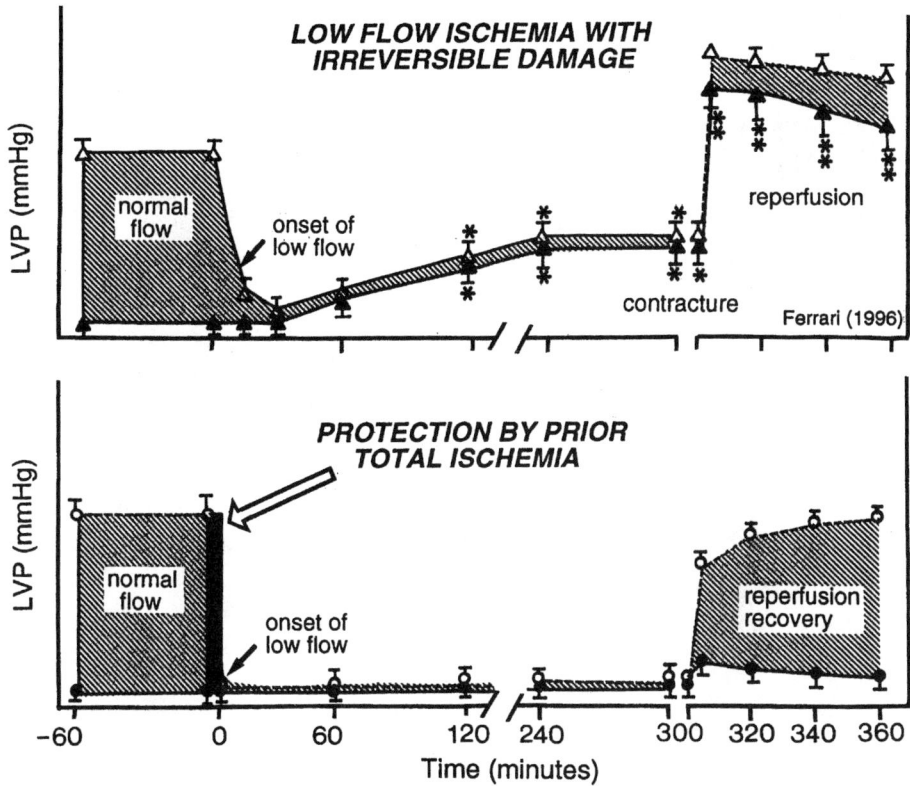

FIG. 19-10. Intraischemic preconditioning. This condition describes "increased tolerance to sustained low-flow ischemia by a brief episode of no-flow ischemia without intermittent reperfusion" (35). From data of Ferrari et al., 1996.

tioning is thus invoked by many more stimuli than previously appreciated. Furthermore, although the protective effect of preconditioning against subsequent ischemia is generally limited to 2 to 3 hours, Yellon's group (36) described a second window of protection occurring approximately 24 to 96 hours after the initial preconditioning episode (Fig. 19-11).

Classic or Early Preconditioning

The first or "classic" phase of preconditioning is hypothesized to involve a trigger molecule released by the short preconditioning phase or cycles of ischemia. As a simplification, the following may represent one of the cascades involved in the genesis of classic preconditioning (Fig. 19-12). One of several possible triggers is adenosine, which stimulates its G_i-coupled receptor protein to transmit the signal to protein kinase C, which then leads to activation of the

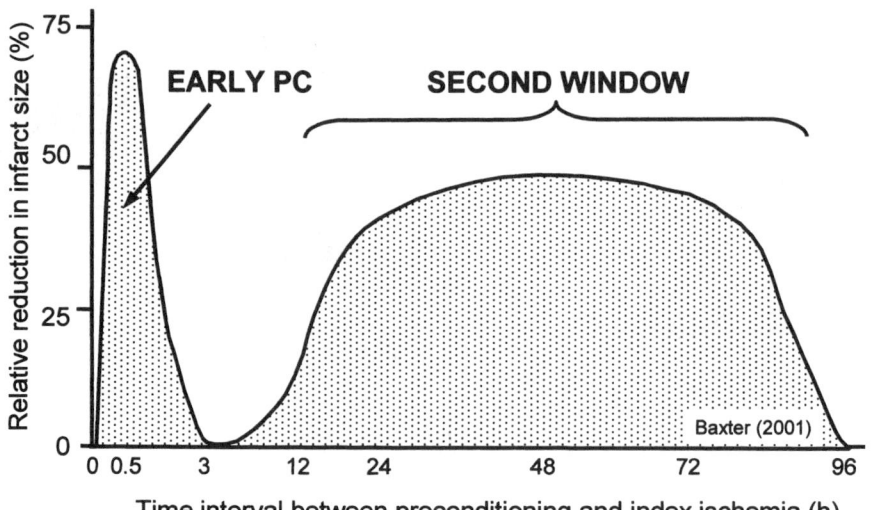

FIG. 19-11. Two phases of preconditioning (PC), early and late. (From Baxter GF, Ferdinandy P. Delayed preconditioning of myocardium: current perspectives. *Basic Res Cardiol* 2001;96:329–344, with permission.)

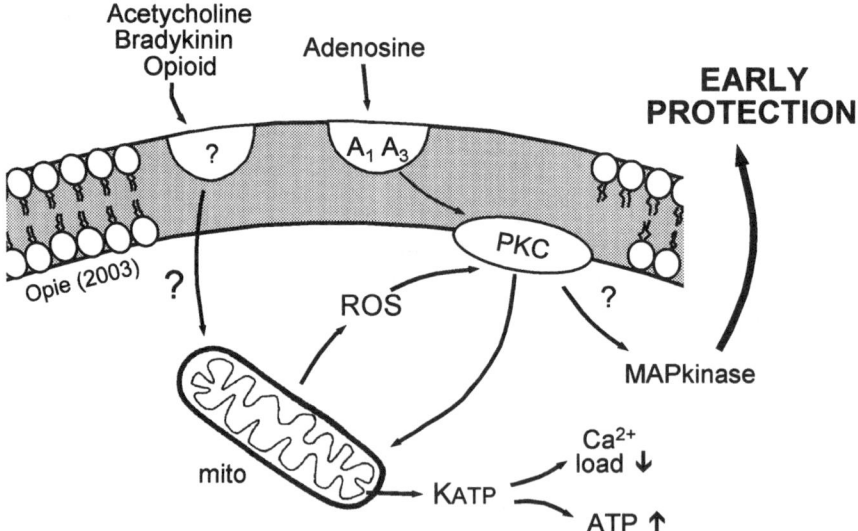

FIG. 19-12. Early phase preconditioning. Adenosine, acting mainly by A_1 and A_3 receptors, is thought to play a crucial role and acts by activation of protein kinase C and particularly the ε-isoform. Further steps leading to opening of the mitochondrial adenosine 5′-triphosphate–sensitive potassium channel (K_{ATP}) are not clear. Other effects could be via the inhibitory protein G_i or the mitogen-activated protein kinase cascade (Fig. 9-3). *ROS*, reactive oxygen species.

mitochondrial ATP-sensitive potassium channel (K_{ATP}). First, it was thought that the sarcolemmal K_{ATP} channel was involved, and by its opening, it shortened the action potential duration, thus limiting the entry of potentially noxious calcium ions. Later, emphasis shifted to the role of the mitochondrial K_{ATP} channel (17), the opening of which was proposed to protect the mitochondria from calcium overload (37). Even more recently, modest mitochondrial uncoupling has been invoked, meaning that paradoxically a process that dissociates mitochondrial oxygen consumption from ATP production is protective, perhaps by limiting the excess production of ROS (38).

Other paths or zigzags between paths may be involved. For example, Cohen et al. (39) found that in contrast to that of adenosine, the signaling system for acetylcholine, bradykinin, and opioids travels "directly" to the mitochondria, which generate a burst of ROS production that sets in motion further signals including activation of protein kinase C. What is clear is that the paths leading from brief ischemia to protection against subsequent ischemia are still not fully elucidated. Speculatively, some mild mitochondrial damage with modest uncoupling of respiration may be protective (Fig. 19-13).

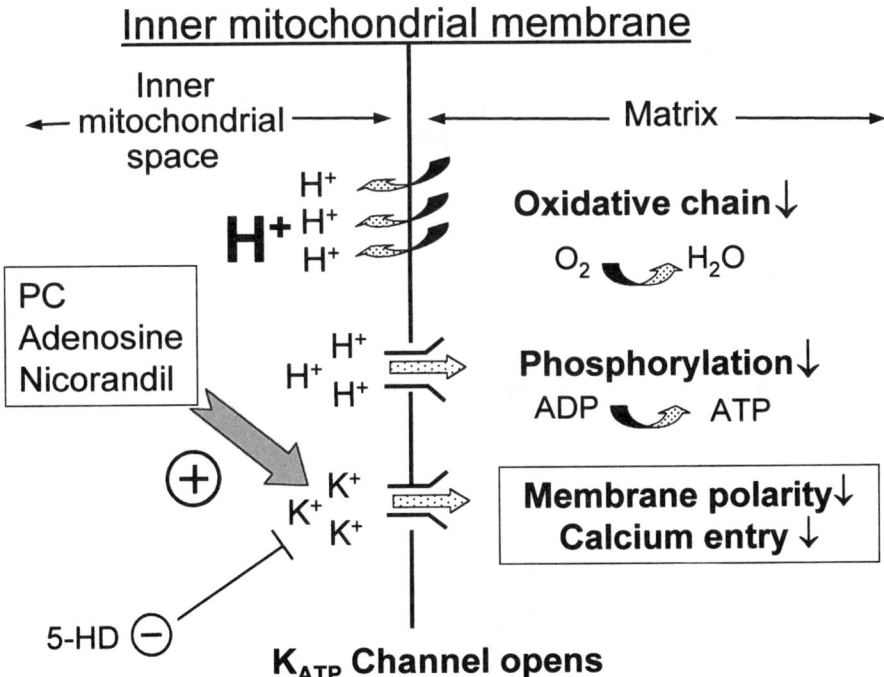

FIG. 19-13. **The mitochondrial hypothesis for preconditioning.** Opening of the mitochondrial K channel leads to depolarization of the inner mitochondrial membrane and mild uncoupling. Calcium entry is decreased. *5HD*, 5-hydroxydecanoate, an inhibitor of this K channel; *PC*, preconditioning. Based on the data of Minners et al. (44).

Delayed or "Second Window" Ischemic Preconditioning

This phase is even more complex in its genesis. "Late preconditioning is a polygenic phenomenon that requires the activation of multiple stress-responsive genes" (40). Some of the triggers released by the initial transient ischemia, such as nitric oxide, adenosine, and ROS, set in motion a series of signals that lead to synthesis of new cardioprotective proteins such as nitric oxide synthase, cyclooxygenase-2, superoxide dismutase, and others (40). Besides brief ischemia, preconditioning stimuli include heat stress, severe exercise, cytokines, and "stress in general" (40). There are two major paths involved (41). One leads via protein kinase C to activation of the nuclear factor κB and the other via JAK-STAT (Janus kinase–signal transducer and activator of transcription) to nuclear promoters and nuclear synthesis (Fig. 19-14). Again, the complete story is far from being told.

Does delayed preconditioning merely delay the onset of myocardial infarction, or does it permanently reduce infarction size? Bolli's group settled this point by studying rabbits 28 days after 30 minutes of coronary occlusion followed by reperfusion (42). Not only was infarct size reduced but recovery of LV mechan-

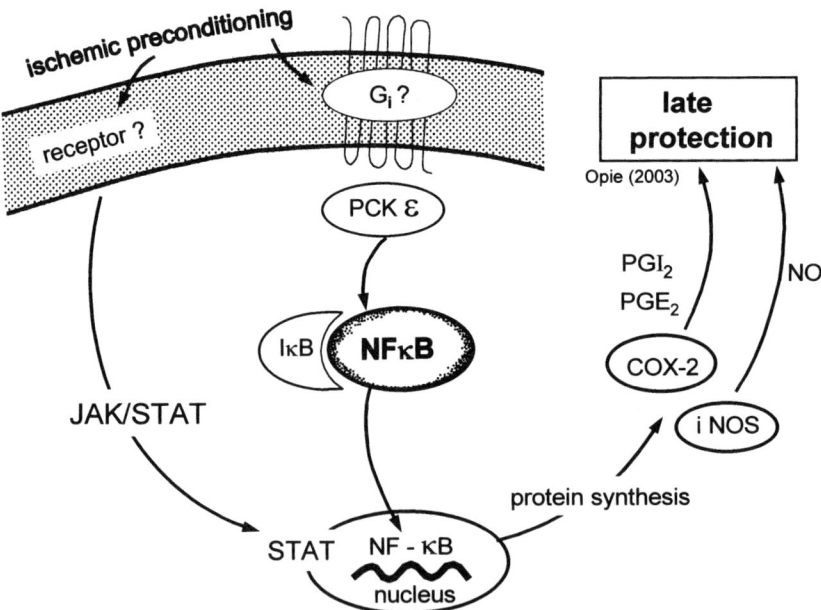

FIG. 19-14. Late phase preconditioning. Note that preconditioning occurs in two phases, early and late (second window of protection, *SWOP*, see Figure 19-11), the latter probably involving nuclear protein synthesis. Figure based on the concepts of Bolli et al. (41). For Janus kinase–signal transducer and activator of transcription (JAK-STAT), see Figure 9-10. For nuclear factor κB, see Figure 9-11. *COX-2*, cyclooxygenase-2; *NO*, nitric oxide; *iNOS*, inducible nitric oxide synthase; *PG*, prostaglandin.

ical function, measured by wall thickening, was more rapid. Thus, late preconditioning does reduce myocardial cell death.

Preconditioning in Patients

Preconditioning is, therefore, an important phenomenon of major clinical relevance because it potentially protects against myocardial infarction. Although the clinical evidence of preconditioning is not yet fully firm, there is increasing evidence that it occurs in humans (5,43). Patients with effort angina having one attack may be protected from subsequent attacks as in "warm-up" angina. Those undergoing coronary angioplasty have more severe features of ischemia, such a potassium release and ST segment elevation on the electrocardiogram, on the first when compared with subsequent balloon inflations. Patients with preinfarction angina may experience a less severe infarction than those thought to undergo sudden coronary occlusion without the opportunity for preconditioning. Thus, not only are there many stimuli to the preconditioned state, but there are also several potential mechanisms, and the consequences are multiple. Hence, the possibility must be considered that preconditioning occurs in any state of repetitive ischemia and also in patients.

Ischemia, stunning, hibernation, necrosis, and normal myocardium may coexist (2). Furthermore, there may be variations in the myocardial response to ischemia and in the coronary blood supply as well as the possibility of repetitive ischemic episodes each followed by reperfusion and stunning and/or by early or late preconditioning. Several or even all components of this multifarious spectrum of conditions could coexist in the same patient (Table 19-5).

TABLE 19-5. *The mixed cardiac response to ischemia*

Variations in myocardial response to ischemia
    Transient anaerobic metabolism
    Anaerobic metabolism plus serious ionic imbalance (Na/Ca/H) with threatened necrosis
    Tissue necrosis and eventual fibrosis, including inflammatory response and cytokine production
    Tissue repair including activation of protein synthesis and remodeling/hypertrophy
Variations in coronary blood supply
    Coronary artery disease with one or more of the following:
        Endothelial damage with impaired production of nitric oxide
        Increased vascular smooth muscle tone (vasoconstriction) or if severe and localized, vasospasm
        Platelet thrombi
        Plaque rupture
        Occluding thrombus with or without recanalization
        Inadequate blood supply from increased oxygen demand and restricted supply (exercise, emotion, acute hypertension)
Response to ischemia/reperfusion
    Repetitive stunning including maiming
    Hibernation (may include above)
    Repetitive preconditioning

SUMMARY

1. *Reperfusion injury* refers to a syndrome of related conditions that may follow reperfusion of the ischemic myocardium. For example, thrombolytic reperfusion may cause arrhythmias, stunning, and no reflow. Whether reperfusion can actually accelerate cell death remains controversial, but solid evidence points to reperfusion-induced apoptosis.
2. *There are at least two mechanisms for reperfusion damage:* cytosolic calcium overload and formation of ROS. Other important events include reintroduction of neutrophils into the ischemic area, microvascular damage, and no reflow.
3. *Stunning* is the delayed but full recovery of mechanical function after reperfusion. It varies in duration from minutes to hours to days and can experimentally be lessened by a number of interventions including sodium–calcium exchange inhibition and calcium channel blockers as well as by a variety of free radical scavengers.
4. *Hibernation* is the state of myocardial dormancy in the presence of severe coronary artery disease that can be revived by revascularization. Two current hypotheses are perfusion–contraction matching with downgraded myocardial energy requirements and repetitive cumulative stunning.
5. *Preconditioning* is the increased myocardial resistance to ischemia–reperfusion damage that is evoked by one or more prior episodes of transient ischemia followed by reperfusion. There is an early transient phase (classic preconditioning) lasting hours and a late phase lasting 1 to 3 days. The signaling paths involved are not well understood. One hypothesis for the early phase is that adenosine or other trigger substances released during the period of the transient and protective ischemia activates protein kinase C, which in turn promotes opening of the mitochondrial ATP-sensitive potassium channel, the later being the protective event. Such a sequence remains controversial.
6. *Late-phase or "second window" preconditioning.* Two main paths may be involved, that leading via protein kinase C to nuclear factor κB and that leading via JAK-STAT to nuclear activation. The result is formation of protective proteins such as nitric oxide synthase, cyclooxygenase-2, and superoxide dismutase.
7. *Clinical implications.* The recognition that stunning and especially hibernation can occur in patients with coronary artery disease and that preconditioning can also modify the severity of subsequent ischemia means that the clinical manifestations of ischemia and reperfusion in humans have become very complex. Stunning may explain much delayed mechanical recovery after thrombolytic therapy of acute myocardial infarction. Hibernation is now being actively searched for and diagnosed in efforts to improve LV function by revascularization. Preconditioning gives powerful protection against myocardial infarction and may be the basis of future therapeutic agents.

REFERENCES

1. Heyndrickx GR, et al. Regional myocardial functional and electrophysiological alterations after brief coronary artery occlusion in conscious dogs. *J Clin Invest* 1975;56:978–985.
2. Braunwald E, Kloner RA. The stunned myocardium: prolonged, postischemic ventricular dysfunction. *Circulation* 1982;66:1146–1149.
3. Kloner RA, Jennings RB. Consequences of brief ischemia: stunning, preconditioning, and their clinical implications. Part 1. *Circulation* 2001;104:2981–2989.
4. Opie LH. Reperfusion injury and its pharmacologic modification. *Circulation* 1989;80:1049–1062.
5. Heusch G. Nitroglycerin and delayed preconditioning in humans: yet another new mechanism for an old drug? *Circulation* 2001;103:2876–2878.
6. Lavallee M, et al. Salvage of myocardial function by coronary artery reperfusion 1, 2 and 3 hours after occlusion in conscious dogs. *Circ Res* 1983;53:235–247.
7. Boden WE, et al. Incomplete, delayed functional recovery late after reperfusion following acute myocardial infarction: "maimed myocardium." *Am Heart J* 1995;130:922–932.
8. Bolli R, et al. Molecular and cellular mechanisms of myocardial stunning. *Physiol Rev* 1999;79:609–634.
9. Becker LC, et al. Reversal of dysfunction in postischemic stunned myocardium by epinephrine and postextrasystolic potentiation. *J Am Coll Cardiol* 1986;7:580–589.
10. Ito BR, et al. Reversibly injured, postischemic canine myocardium retains normal contractile reserve. *Circ Res* 1987;61:834–846.
11. Heusch G, et al. Calcium responsiveness is regional myocardial short-term hibernation and stunning in the in situ porcine heart—inotropic responses to postextrasystolic potentiation and intracoronary calcium. *Circulation* 1996;93:1556–1566.
12. Brooks WW, et al. Reperfusion induced arrhythmias following ischemia in intact rat heart: role of intracellular calcium. *Cardiovasc Res* 1995;29:536–542.
13. Gao WD, et al. Relationship between intracellular calcium and contractile force in stunned myocardium. Direct evidence for decreased myofilament responsiveness and altered diastolic function in intact ventricular muscle. *Circ Res* 1995;76:1036–1048.
14. Meissner A, et al. Contractile dysfunction and abnormal Ca^{2+} modulation during postischemic reperfusion in rat heart. *Am J Physiol* 1995;268:H100–H111.
15. Zeitz O, et al. Hydoxyl radical-induced acute diastolic dysfunction is due to calcium overload via reverse-mode Na^+-Ca^{2+} exchange. *Circ Res* 2002;90:988–995.
16. Sawyer DB, et al. Role of oxidative stress in myocardial hypertrophy and failure. *J Mol Cell Cardiol* 2002;34:379–388.
16a. Hearse DJ, Humphrey SM, Nayler WG. Ultrastructural damage associated with reoxygenation of the anoxic myocardium. *J Mol Cell Cardiol* 1975;7:315–324
17. Kloner RA, et al. Consequences of brief ischemia: stunning, preconditioning, and their clinical implications. Part 2. *Circulation* 2001;104:3158–3167.
18. Kloner RA, et al. Stunned left ventricular myocardium after exercise treadmill testing in coronary artery disease. *Am J Cardiol* 1991;68:329–334.
19. Rezkalla SH, et al. No-reflow phenomenon. *Circulation* 2002;105:656–662.
20. Maes A, et al. Impaired myocardial tissue perfusion early after successful thrombolysis. Impact on myocardial flow, metabolism and function at late follow-up. *Circulation* 1995;92:2072–2078.
21. Jennings RB, et al. Myocardial necrosis induced by temporary occlusion of a coronary artery in the dog. *Arch Pathol* 1960;70:82–92.
22. Fliss H, et al. Apoptosis in ischemic and reperfused rat myocardium. *Circ Res* 1996;79:949–956.
23. Jeremias I, et al. Involvement of CD95/Apo1/Fas in cell death after myocardial ischemia. *Circulation* 2000;102:915–920.
24. Jonassen AK, et al. Myocardial protection by insulin at reperfusion requires early administration and is mediated via Akt and a p70s6 kinase cell-survival signaling. *Circ Res* 2001;89:1191–1198.
25. Rahimtoola SH. The hibernating myocardium. *Am Heart J* 1989;117:211–221.
26. Heusch G. Hibernating myocardium. *Physiol Rev* 1998;78:1055–1085.
27. Camici PG, et al. Pathophysiological mechanisms of chronic reversible left ventricular dysfunction due to coronary artery disease (hibernating myocardium). *Circulation* 1997;96:3205–3214.
28. Thomas SA, et al. Dissociation of regional adaptations to ischemia and global myolysis in an accelerated swine model of chronic hibernating myocardium. *Circ Res* 2002;91:970–977.
29. Fallavollita JA, et al. Hibernating myocardium retains metabolic and contractile reserve despite regional reductions in flow, function and oxygen consumption at rest. *Circ Res* 2003;92:48–55.

30. Hochacka PW, et al. Unifying theory of hypoxia tolerance: Molecular/metabolic defense and rescue mechanisms for surviving oxygen lack. *Proc Natl Acad Sci U S A* 1996;93:9493–9498.
31. Heusch G, Schulz R. Hibernating myocardium. New answers, still more questions! *Circ Res* 2002; 91:863–865.
32. Kalra DK, et al. Increased myocardial gene expression of tumour necrosis factor-alpha and nitric oxide synthase-2: a potential mechanism for depressed myocardial function in hibernating myocardium in humans. *Circulation* 2002;105:1537–1540.
33. Murry CE, et al. Preconditioning with ischemia: a delay of lethal cell injury in ischemic myocardium. *Circulation* 1986;74:1124–1136.
34. Schulz R, et al. Signal transduction of ischemic preconditioning. *Cardiovasc Res* 2001;52:181–189.
35. Schulz R, et al. Intraischemic preconditioning. Increased tolerance to sustained low-flow ischemia by a brief episode of no-flow ischaemia without intermittent reperfusion. *Circ Res* 1995;76:942–950.
36. Baxter GF, Ferdinandy P. Delayed preconditioning of myocardium: current perspectives. *Basic Res Cardiol* 2001;96:329–344.
37. Murata M, et al. Mitochondrial ATP-sensitive potassium channels attenuate matrix Ca^{2+} overload during simulated ischemia and reperfusion. *Circ Res* 2001;89:891–898.
38. Minners J, et al. Ischemic and pharmacological preconditioning in Girardi cells and C2C12 myotubes induce mitochondrial uncoupling. *Circ Res* 2001;89:787–792.
39. Cohen MV, et al. Acetylcholine, bradykinin, opioids, and phenylephrine, but not adenosine, trigger preconditioning by generating free radicals and opening mitochondrial K(ATP) channels. *Circ Res* 2001;89:273–278.
40. Bolli R. The late phase of preconditioning. *Circ Res* 2000;87:972–983.
41. Bolli R, Shinmura K, Tang XL, et al. Discovery of a new function of cyclooxygenase (COX)-2: COX-2 is a cardioprotective protein that alleviates ischemia/reperfusion injury and mediates the late phase of preconditioning. *Cardiovasc Res* 2002;55:506–519.
42. Takano H, et al. Late preconditioning enhances recovery of myocardial function after infarction in conscious rabbits. *Am J Physiol* 2000;279:H2372–H2381.
43. Yellon DM, Downey . Preconditioning the myocardium: from cellular physiology to clinical cardiology. *Physiol Rev* 2003 *(in press)*.
44. Minners J, van den Bos EJ, Yellon DM, et al. Dinitrophenol, cyclosporin A, and trimetazidine modulate preconditioning in the isolated rat heart: support for a mitochondrial role in cardioprotection. *Cardiovasc Res* 2000;47:68–73.

20

Electricity Out of Control: Arrhythmias

"The pain in his arm seizing him, he fell down dead, without the least motion of any limb."
The mode of death of the Chancellor of the University of Oxford, 1674 (1)

A useful, practical classification of arrhythmias (abnormal heart rhythms, also called dysrhythmias) is according to their origin, i.e., supraventricular or ventricular. Supraventricular arrhythmias may, in turn, be divided into supraventricular tachycardias or bradyarrhythmias. Ventricular arrhythmias frequently are ischemic in origin. This chapter first concentrates on supraventricular and then on ventricular tachyarrhythmias. There are three main proposals for the mechanisms underlying the development of such arrhythmias. First, automaticity may develop in otherwise nonautomatic tissue (Fig. 20-1). Second, there may be a reentry circuit. Third, afterdepolarizations may give rise to triggered activity or atypical ventricular tachycardia. Note that sinus arrhythmias, including sinus tachycardia and bradycardia as well as heart block are discussed with the conduction system in Chapter 5.

BASIC ARRHYTHMOGENIC MECHANISMS

There are three basic arrhythmogenic mechanisms common to both atrial and ventricular arrhythmias: ectopic automaticity (Greek, *ectopic*, out of place), afterdepolarizations, and reentry circuits (1). *Automaticity* is the development of a new site of depolarization in nonnodal tissue at the site of an ectopic focus (Fig. 20-1). Hence, they are often called ectopic beats, even though the ectopic depolarization may not progress to a ventricular beat. An entirely healthy cell would not depolarize except in response to the wave of depolarization, so that an ectopic depolarization represents either a site of cell damage or abnormal excitation. Automaticity varies in its implications all the way from relatively harmless ectopic beats to those that occur so rapidly as to impair the filling function of the heart (2). *Reentry circuits* occur between different conduction paths, one slow and

600   20. ELECTRICITY OUT OF CONTROL: ARRHYTHMIAS

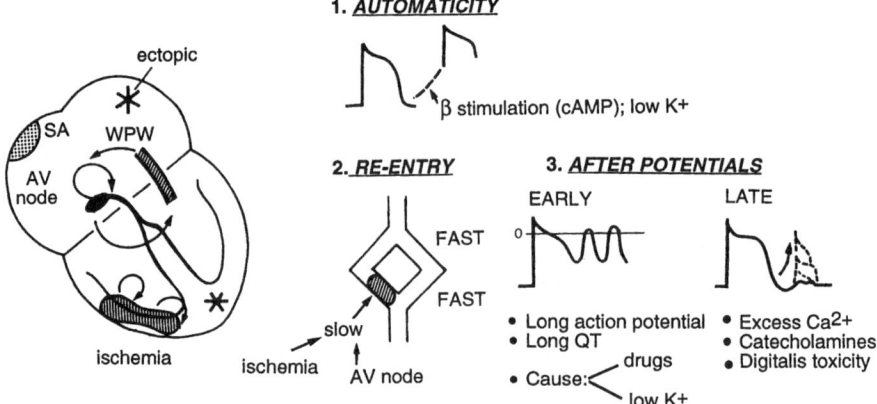

FIG. 20-1. Basic arrhythmogenic mechanisms: *1*, automaticity with ectopic depolarizations ("ectopic beats"); *2*, reentry paths; and *3*, afterpotentials. On the left, atrial ectopic beats may provoke supraventricular tachycardias that usually involve reentry through the atrioventricular (*AV*) node or the existence of a Wolff–Parkinson–White (*WPW*) bypass tract with rapid conduction through the AV node to the ventricles. Ventricular ectopic beats may likewise provoke ventricular tachycardias especially in the presence of an infarcted or ischemic zone. For cellular mechanisms, see text. For reentry circuits, see Figure 20-2.

the other fast (Fig. 20-2). A discharging automatic focus generated in the slow branch may not be able to conduct past the slow and still depolarized zone, so it travels "backward" and around the fast circuit to reenter the slow branch, a unidirectional block which is now past its refractory period. Thus, the impulse can travel from the slow to the fast branch and, by repeating the travel path, can indefinitely continue to cause a sustained reentry arrhythmia (3). *Afterdepolarizations*, also called afterpotentials, are probably caused by large inward sodium currents generated in conditions of calcium overload, as calcium ions move out and sodium ions move in by the electrogenic sodium–calcium exchanger (Fig. 4-4). These inappropriate inward currents cause depolarizations occurring shortly after repolarization or even during the repolarizing process. Afterdepolarizations are more much likely to give rise to serious arrhythmias if the individual has a genetic predisposition to an abnormally prolonged QT interval on electrocardiography [long QT syndrome (LQTS)]. Much current research focuses on the genetic factors that act on ion channels to increase the susceptibility to arrhythmias (2).

SUPRAVENTRICULAR ARRHYTHMIAS

Atrial Ectopic Depolarizations

The most common atrial arrhythmia is the ectopic depolarization, which is almost a physiologic event (Fig. 20-3). Normally harmless, such ectopic depolarizations may initiate supraventricular tachycardias in those predisposed by physiologic or anatomic pathways for reentry circuits. The mechanisms whereby

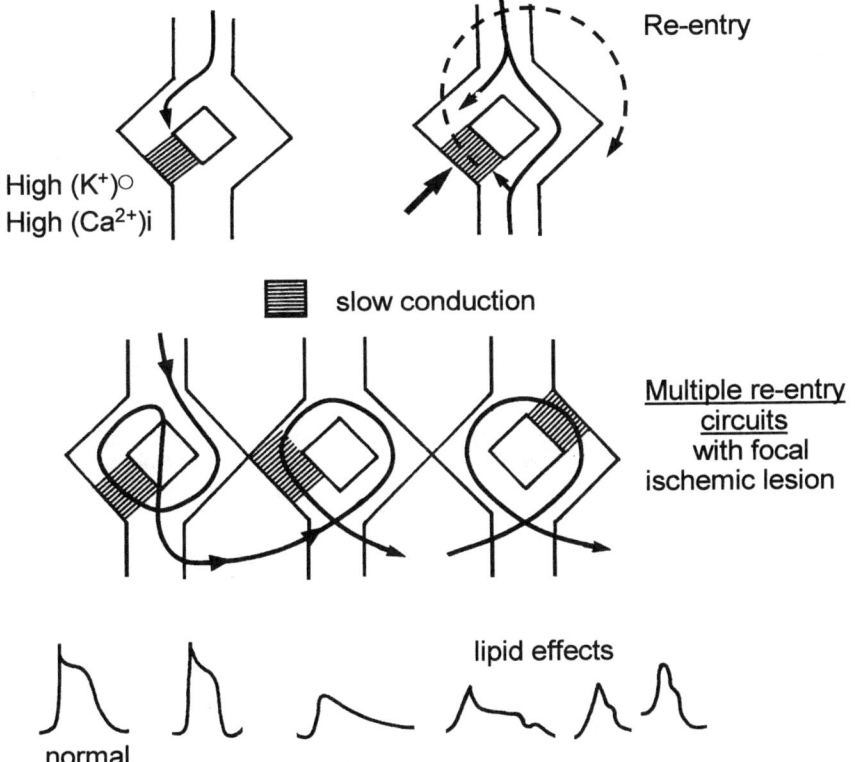

FIG. 20-2. Model for formation of the reentry circuit. The model postulates that the impulse can bifurcate into two paths, which then rejoin. When the electrical impulse reaches the zone of slow conduction, the impulse is blocked at that site (at top on left). That allows the normal impulse arriving from the other path of the bifurcation to penetrate the slow conduction zone from the other side and hence to create reentry (at top on right). The cause of the slow conduction may either be the existence of functional slow pathways as postulated in the AV node or focal ischemia with abnormal action potentials. How multiple reentry circuits could form from focal ischemic injuries with abnormal action potentials is shown at bottom. The electrical heterogeneity predisposes to reentry circuits.

ectopic depolarizations develop are still not fully understood; they probably originate when potentially automatic tissue, normally suppressed by the sinus node, is provoked into firing by a combination of factors including β-adrenergic stimulation and local disease such as fibrosis or ischemia.

Refractory Period

Ectopic beats can only develop when the sodium channel opens in response to the initiating stimulus. During the *absolute refractory period* (Fig. 20-4), an early electrical stimulus cannot evoke any response because repolarization is not

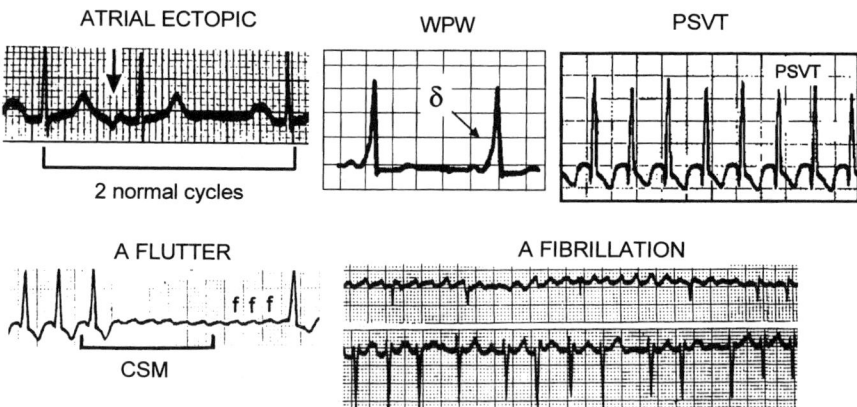

FIG. 20-3. Supraventricular arrhythmias. The most common and least serious is the atrial ectopic depolarization (or "beat"), which may, however, trigger paroxysmal supraventricular tachycardia (*PSVT*), especially in those with a bypass tract [Wolff–Parkinson–White syndrome (*WPW*), recognized by the delta wave]. In atrial flutter, the characteristic f (flutter) waves may only be revealed by carotid sinus massage (*CSM*). In atrial fibrillation, there are no P waves and a totally irregular ventricular response (Fig. 20-6).

sufficiently far advanced to regain the voltage range in which the sodium channel can operate. In the *relative refractory period*, toward the end of the action potential, the voltage is sufficiently negative to allow some sodium channels to open in response to an appropriate voltage stimulus. The rate of depolarization of such an ectopic focus is slower than normal because only some of the sodium channels open. As a result, fewer calcium channels open and the action potential

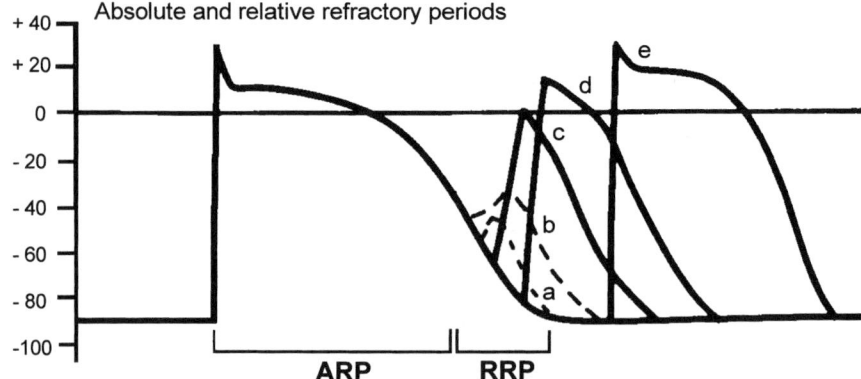

FIG. 20-4. Refractory periods. In normal heart tissue, an added stimulus during the action potential fails to elicit any response, the voltage being far from that required to open the sodium channels. This is the absolute or effective refractory period (*ARP, ERP*). During the relative refractory period (*RRP*), successively later stimuli, *a* to *e*, evoke a progressively greater and a more complete action potential. Even later, when the repolarization has decreased the voltage to less than that required to open sodium channels, there is a full response.

duration is decreased. When the ectopic beat develops during electrical diastole, full sodium channel opening is possible with a normal action potential. However, the ectopic beat brings with it its own refractory period, which prevents what would have been the next normal beat from developing. The ectopic beat is followed by a post-ectopic pause, longer than the interval between two normal cycles (Fig. 20-3). Thus, the heart "skips a beat" as in response to excitement.

Supraventricular Paroxysmal Tachycardias

Supraventricular arrhythmias are those originating in the atria, including the atrioventricular node. By definition, those with ventricular response rates greater than 100 beats per minute are tachycardias. A common variety occurring particularly in the younger age groups is *paroxysmal supraventricular tachycardia* (PSVT) (Fig. 20-3). There is a reentry circuit involving the atrioventricular (AV) node (Fig. 20-5). Strictly, these are called *AV nodal reentry tachycardias*. The

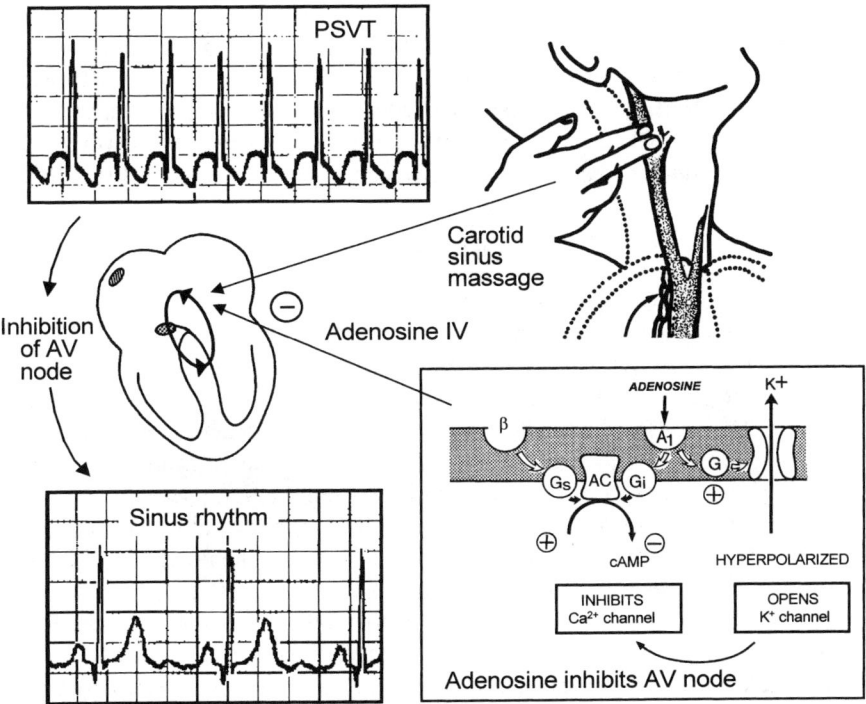

FIG. 20-5. Carotid sinus massage to inhibit reentry through the atrioventricular (*AV*) node and to stop paroxysmal supraventricular tachycardia (*PSVT*). Failing this physiologic mode of therapy, adenosine can be given intravenously; note the mode of action on adenosine receptor subtype 1 (A_1) via inhibitory G protein (G_i) to oppose stimulatory effects of cyclic adenosine 3',5'-monophosphate (*cAMP*). Additionally, adenosine "opens" the potassium channel of the nodal tissue to hyperpolarize nodal cells and to inhibit the reentry circuit.

result is that the atria and ventricles beat very rapidly and regularly (150 to 250 beats/min) so that ventricular filling may become impaired. At the higher atrial rates, AV block may develop as the capacity of the slow fibers of the AV node to conduct the rapid impulses to the ventricles is exceeded. Usually there is no background or organic heart disease in PSVT. Therapeutically, increased inhibition of the AV node can cut the reentry circuit by *carotid sinus massage* that reflexively stimulates the vagal system, or by intravenous adenosine that inhibits the AV node by a dual mechanism (Fig. 20-5).

Bypass Tract and Wolff–Parkinson–White Syndrome

When there is an anatomic bypass tract, another type of reentry circuit is possible (Fig. 20-1). In this condition, called Wolff–Parkinson–White syndrome after the three cardiologists who described the condition, an atrial ectopic impulse can travel in and out of the anatomic tract that bypasses the AV node to cause a tachycardia very similar to PSVT. The major difference is that because the AV node is completely bypassed, very rapid atrial arrhythmias can travel down the bypass tract to reach the ventricles to cause potentially fatal ventricular tachycardia. The resting electrocardiogram is also different from that found in PSVT in which in between attacks, the pattern is normal. In Wolff–Parkinson–White syndrome, when in sinus rhythm, the atrial impulse arrives more rapidly than normal at the ventricles by the bypass tract, thereby causing a characteristic hump on the upstroke of the QRS complex (delta wave, Fig. 20-3).

Atrial Flutter

The name refers to the *flutter waves* or f atrial waves that replace the normal P waves and are clearly visible on the electrocardiogram when there is AV block (Fig. 20-3). The mechanism of atrial flutter, previously controversial, involves a reentry circuit in the right atrium revolving around the tricuspid annulus, forming the anterior border (3). The left atrium, although passively activated from the right by an interatrial anatomic path called the Bachman bundle, is not needed to maintain the tachycardia. Electrocardiographically, the f waves reflect the atrial reentry circuit at rates of approximately 250 to 350 beats per minute, usually close to 300. Only some of these impulses reach the ventricles. The normal AV node cannot conduct impulses much faster than an atrial rate of 200 beats per minute, so that block results. Thus, an atrial rate of approximately 300 beats per minute gives a ventricular rate of approximately 150 beats per minute (2:1 block). Usually atrial flutter occurs with organic heart disease, and the fast ventricular rate may cause symptoms such as angina or syncope. With a 2:1 block, one of the atrial complexes may decrease on the QRS complex so that the diagnosis is in doubt until carotid sinus stimulation increases the degree of block by enhancing vagal tone (Fig. 20-3). When AV nodal disease is also present, the degree of block may be higher (4:1 or even 8:1; note the usual progression in multiples of two).

Atrial Fibrillation

This is the most common of all serious arrhythmias. Frequently, there is a chronic predisposing condition damaging the atria, such as left ventricular failure, hypertension, mitral stenosis, thyrotoxicosis, or increased fibrosis with old age. The word fibrillation is derived from the Latin (*fibril*, a small fiber). The contractions of the atria are no longer coordinated. Rather, it seems as if many small fibers are contracting separately. Only some of these numerous atrial beats are transmitted at irregular intervals through the filter of the AV node to the ventricles, which characteristically have a "chaotic" rhythm response (Fig. 20-6). The initial event is either an early atrial beat in the atrial vulnerable period or an increased rate of atrial flutter. For more than 50 years, there have been two leading theories to explain the mechanism of atrial fibrillation (AF). First, the abnormal beats could arise from one or more ectopic foci spreading through the atria irregularly as a result of the disease-induced inhomogeneities of conduction. Second, and more favored now, there is multicircuit reentry, facilitated by shortening of the action potential duration and reduction of the effective refractory

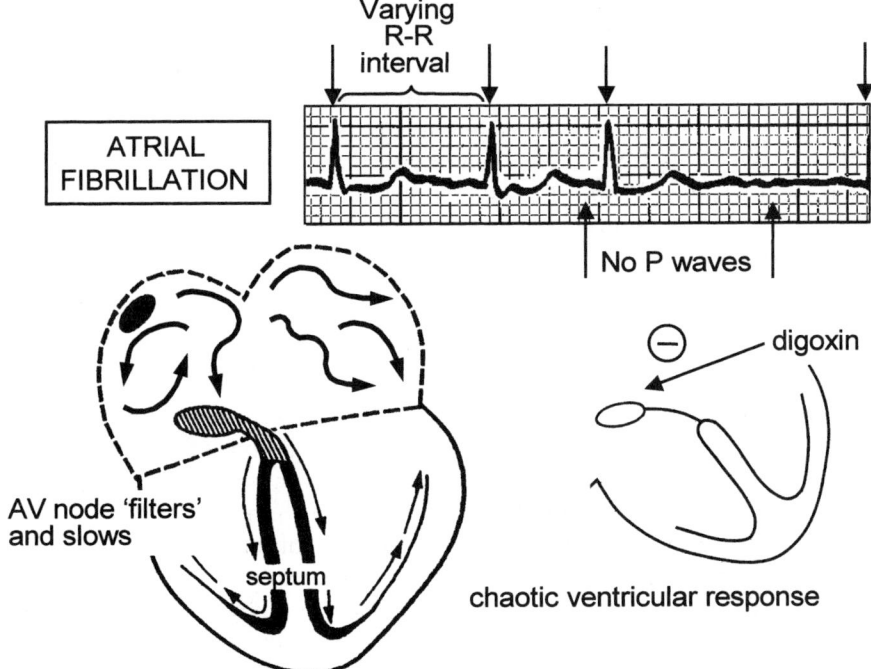

FIG. 20-6. Atrial fibrillation with macroreentry circuits. The atrioventricular (*AV*) node "filters" these many stimuli to let through only some to the ventricles; hence, the ventricular response is chaotic and irregular. The characteristic electrocardiogram shows varying R-R intervals and total absence of P waves. Digoxin may be used in chronic cases to slow the ventricular response rate, especially when there is also left ventricular failure.

period. For example, the action potential duration is reduced by vagal cholinergic activity, so that, paradoxically, highly trained athletes with their increased vagal tone are more prone to AF. In AF, the wave front of depolarization undergoes fractionation because of numerous inhomogeneities, so that multiple wave fronts form with the characteristic loss of P wave on the electrocardiogram.

Additional effects of AF, other than those on the heart rhythm, have only recently been recognized. First, the "atrial booster" effect of atrial contraction is lost, which itself may contribute to decreased ventricular function. Second, there are several remodeling processes. AF, a form of contractile dysfunction, can worsen itself metabolically by *metabolic remodeling*, with increased oxidative stress and decreased energy production via creatine kinase (4). The proposal is that the additional atrial metabolic demands lead to atrial ischemia and fibrosis, thereby further damaging the atria and converting episodes of AF into chronically sustained AF. *Electrical remodeling* refers to the progressively adverse effects of AF on the atria, whereby marked reduction in the density of the L-type calcium current decreases the action potential duration and shortens the refractory period (5). This means a greater chance of more AF attacks and increasingly poor atrial function in between attacks, with a greater risk of sustained chronic AF. The ideal therapy for sustained AF is early electrical defibrillation.

Atrial stunning is another recently recognized problem. Reversion to sinus rhythm may be followed by a prolonged period of poor atrial contraction, which in turn predisposes to atrial thrombosis formation and hence to embolization and cerebral stroke. As in ventricular stunning, excess accumulation of calcium ions and/or formation of free radicals may be responsible. In chronic sustained or intermittent AF, the AV node can be inhibited and the ventricular rate slowed by the calcium antagonist drugs verapamil and diltiazem or by the digitalis compound digoxin. Carotid sinus massage will not work because there are no reentry circuits traveling through the AV node.

VENTRICULAR ARRHYTHMIAS

Ventricular ectopic depolarizations are potentially serious, such as the R-on-T configuration that threatens the potentially lethal conditions of ventricular tachycardia and fibrillation (Fig. 20-7). The basic mechanisms involved are similar to those already described for atrial ectopic beats. When three or more ventricular ectopic depolarizations occur in rapid succession, ventricular tachycardia results. Now there is insufficient time for diastolic filling, so that cardiac output may decrease with risk of acute myocardial ischemia, especially when there is associated coronary artery disease. By a variety of mechanisms, still to be discussed, such ischemia predisposes to the development of a totally disorganized ventricular rhythm called *ventricular fibrillation* (fibrillate, movement of small fibers) in which regular cardiac pumping activity ceases and sudden cardiac death will develop unless a strong external electrical current is applied by an external defibrillator. Ventricular automaticity arises especially in Purkinje fibers.

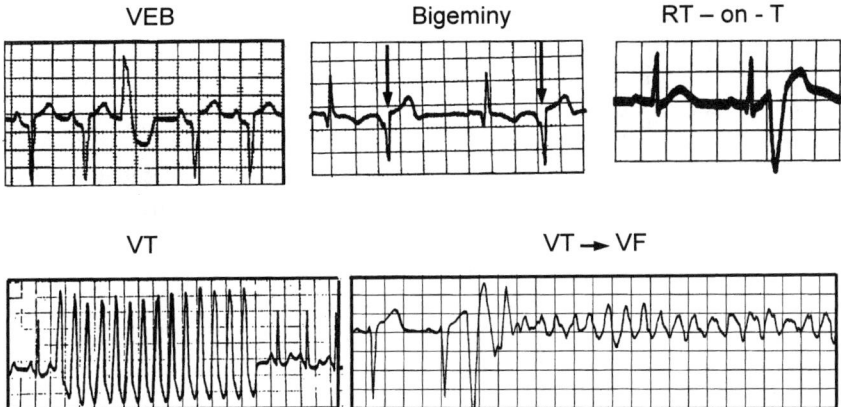

FIG. 20-7. Examples of ventricular arrhythmias. Single ventricular ectopic beats (*VEB*) (top left) may be of no consequence or may indicate heart disease. Paired beats (Latin, *bigeminy*, twins) point to digoxin poisoning. An early ectopic beat, the R-on-T phenomenon, is particularly prone to evoke ventricular tachycardia (*VT*) that in turn may degenerate into ventricular fibrillation (*VF*).

Purkinje fibers, normally quiescent, can develop phase 4 depolarization (as in ischemia) when partially depolarized, so that the threshold for firing is more easily reached. The pacemaker current I_f can operate at voltages between −90 and −60 mV, explaining why partial depolarization caused by ischemia predisposes to automaticity in these fibers.

Hypokalemia (e.g., K^+ = 2.7 mmol/L) increases phase 4 depolarization, whereas a high normal level (5.4 mmol/L) decreases phase 4 depolarization. If the potassium level is sufficiently high, catecholamine stimulation, which normally also evokes phase 4 depolarization in Purkinje fibers, becomes ineffective. When cyclic adenosine 3′,5′-monophosphate (cAMP) is introduced by iontophoresis into spontaneously active cardiac Purkinje fibers, there is a shortened action potential and a steeper rate of phase 4 depolarization, in keeping with catecholamine effects. Catecholamine stimulation and a low external level of potassium should be a potent arrhythmogenic combination. Acute myocardial infarction (AMI) in humans is characterized by acute liberation of catecholamines, which are known to decrease arterial blood potassium. In addition, some patients with acute infarction will have been given diuretic therapy, a frequent cause of hypokalemia that in turn predisposes to ventricular arrhythmias, including ventricular fibrillation.

Ventricular Reentry Circuits

Ventricular reentry circuits may develop whenever there is electrical inhomogeneity of the myocardium, which in turn reflects the focal ionic and metabolic abnormalities that cause slow conduction in one limb of a reentry circuit (Fig. 20-

2). Slow conduction is achieved by inhibition of the fast channel with residual slow channel activity, resulting from ischemic or other injury to the conduction tissue. These conditions predispose to the development of reentry, which when rapid and regular is one cause of ventricular tachycardia (the other being a rapidly firing automatic focus). After myocardial infarction, chronic focal scarring seems to be the basis for the reentry circuits, which cause sustained ventricular tachycardias, again with risk of ventricular fibrillation. In acute ischemic damage, heterogeneous areas of slow conduction can cause *microreentry circuits* that are thought to underlie the development of ventricular fibrillation. The five major theories to explain slow conduction in ischemic tissue are as follows. The first is the effect of localized hyperkalemia and partial depolarization. Second, the development of slow responses in completely depolarized tissue may occur when the tissue content of cAMP increases. Third, residual fast channel activity may explain why some apparently slow responses are sensitive to fast channel inhibitors. Fourth, disturbed metabolism of lipids and calcium may directly affect the action potential. Fifth, electrical coupling between cells may be disrupted.

Potassium and Depolarization

In the early 1950s, Harris et al. (6) found increasing coronary venous potassium values during the onset of arrhythmias after coronary arterial ligation. Since then, there has been increasing evidence of links between potassium and arrhythmogenesis. The mechanism whereby potassium loss promotes very early arrhythmias after coronary ligation cannot be merely depletion of cell potassium, which requires 2 to 4 hours to become evident. *Hyperkalemia*, found in coronary venous blood very early after coronary occlusion as potassium ions leave ischemic cells, may play a more important role. As ischemic cells are depolarized to values less negative than -50 mV, the rapid inward current is inactivated, and the resting potential approaches the threshold potential for the inward calcium current. The intravenous or intraarterial infusion of potassium salts rapidly produces ectopic activity, possibly by promoting electrical inhomogenity. Eventually ventricular fibrillation develops, even in otherwise normal hearts.

Metabolic Shortening and Lengthening of Action Potential Duration

Variations in the action potential duration between ischemic and nonischemic cells, between sites with different severities of ischemia, and between the shortened action potential of ischemia and the prolonged potential of hypertrophic cells produce the critical differences in the refractory state of the myocardium that explain dispersion of refractoriness and of electrical homogeneity. The metabolic causes of such differences include, first, accumulation of lipid breakdown products such as lysophosphoglycerides that induce narrowing of the action potential in some cells and lengthening in others (7). Second, these membrane-active agents may also predispose to slow conduction by depressing most of the components of the membrane currents (8). Third, the action potential duration is shortened by ischemic inhibition of glycolysis (9). Conversely, adenosine 5'-triphosphate (ATP) made by glycolysis has a special role in the maintenance of the action potential duration, as supported by the effects of direct intracellular injection of ATP (10).

Cytosolic Calcium and Electrical Alternans

Electrical alternans is a condition in which there are alternating beat-to-beat variations in the action potential duration and in the force of contraction. The cause may be insufficient glycolytically produced ATP to control calcium entry and release from the sarcoplasmic reticulum (11). The alternation of the action potential duration is matched by corresponding variations in the amplitude of the intracellular calcium transient (12). Local abnormalities of cytosolic calcium, as found in ischemia, can contribute to nonuniformity of the action potential duration across the ventricular surface. This process leads to a dispersion of refractoriness throughout the ventricles, which is an essential precondition for ventricular fibrillation.

Impaired Intercellular Conduction

Conduction between cells normally proceeds by the gap or nexus junctions (Fig. 3-8). Two changes found in ischemia, increased intracellular calcium ion activity and decreased pH (acidosis), can uncouple intercellular conduction to block conduction and to predispose to arrhythmias. Anatomically, gap junction defects induced by postinfarction remodeling help to define the reentry paths that underlie some types of ventricular tachycardia (13).

Delayed Afterdepolarizations or Afterpotentials

Ventricular myocardium can develop automatic activity in specified experimental conditions that cause *delayed afterdepolarizations* (DADs) or afterpotentials. Normally, ventricular cells have a flat phase 4 with no spontaneous depolarization. Delayed depolarizations are abnormal oscillations found in ventricular or Purkinje cells in some abnormal circumstances, including digitalis poisoning and microinjection of cAMP into the cell. The factor common to these two stimuli is the increase in cytosolic calcium ion concentration, which induces a transient diastolic inward current (I_{ti}), probably by promoting sodium–calcium exchange (Fig. 20-8). DAD tends to be a cyclical event with a series of ever-smaller waves, which probably reflect calcium ion oscillations in the cytosol because there are accompanying aftercontractions. When reperfusion restores ATP, the conditions are right for oscillatory movements of calcium ions. Depletion of calcium from the sarcoplasmic reticulum can stop the development of the afterdepolarizations. The current causing the repetitive afterdepolarizations is

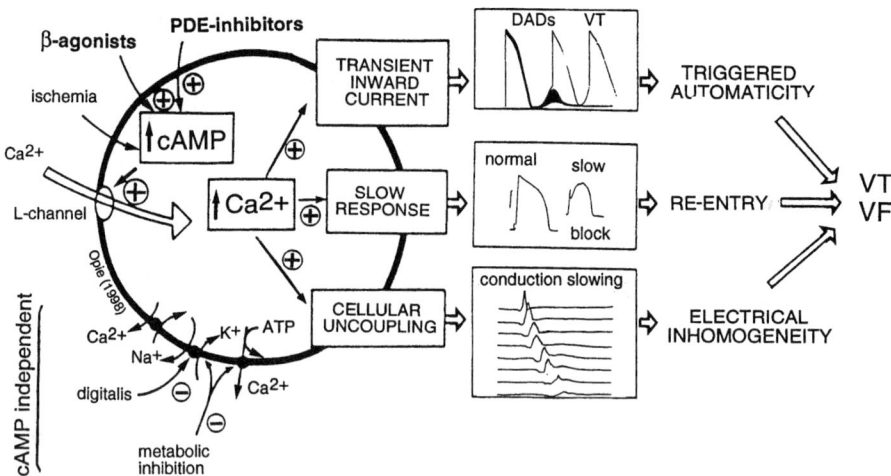

FIG. 20-8. Calcium-dependent ventricular arrhythmias. Links between cyclic adenosine 3′,5′-monophosphate (*cAMP*), cytosolic calcium, and specific calcium–mediated electrophysiologic abnormalities thought to predispose to ventricular tachycardia (*VT*) and ventricular fibrillation (*VF*).

activated (switched on) by increased intracellular calcium. Therefore, the calcium antagonist verapamil and low external calcium both inhibit the phenomenon. DADs are thought to underlie the development of ventricular automaticity during digitalis poisoning.

Triggered automaticity may result from repetitive afterdepolarizations in ventricular muscle and can convert a focus of automaticity into a sustained ventricular arrhythmia. This sequence seems most likely to occur when there is prior inhibition of the sodium pump by digoxin or a low external potassium concentration. In Purkinje fibers, DADs can develop, even at normal external potassium levels and theoretically be a cause of automaticity even in the absence of excess digitalis. Afterdepolarizations are suspected of contributing to some of the ventricular arrhythmias of AMI (14) and in the remodeled postinfarction myocardium (15).

Early Afterdepolarizations

There are several differences between early afterdepolarizations (EADs) and DADs. First, the EADs occur before the end of complete repolarization, whereas the DADs occur well thereafter (Fig. 20-1). Second, the EADs disappear as the heart rate increases, explaining why bradycardia predisposes to the development of torsade de pointes and why tachycardia induced by pacing or isoproterenol is effective in the therapy of that condition. In contrast, tachycardia exaggerates true DADs, perhaps because the rapid repetitive opening of the calcium channel overloads the cell with calcium. A similarity is that both EADs and DADs may develop the same type of triggered activity and ventricular tachycardia in the postinfarction heart (15). There is a wide spectrum of cellular mechanisms causing the EADs. An important predisposing condition is cytosolic calcium overload as may occur in heart failure with excess β-adrenergic stimulation, which in turn provokes increased inward current by the sodium–calcium exchange mechanism (16). Besides inducing phase 4 depolarization, hypokalemia can prolong the QT interval by interfering with the repolarizing potassium current with risk of arrhythmia development. Especially dangerous is the combination of diuretic-induced hypokalemia with antiarrhythmic drugs that may also prolong the QT interval, such as quinidine, disopyramide, amiodarone, and sotalol. Equally dangerous is the combination of diuretic hypokalemia with heart failure, now recognized as an acquired form of the LQTS (17).

The type of ventricular arrhythmia resulting from EADs characteristically has QRS complexes that rhythmically increase and decrease in amplitude called torsade de pointes (twisting of the points) or atypical ventricular tachycardia (see next section). The danger is ventricular fibrillation. The mechanism is complex and may include differential changes in refractoriness in different parts of the myocardium and development of EADs as recorded by suction electrodes in patients. It is very likely that such EADs could contribute to triggered activity (15).

ARRHYTHMIAS OF CHANNELOPATHIES

Inherited Versus Acquired Long QT Syndrome

The channelopathies are disorders of ion channels predisposing to potentially lethal cardiac arrhythmias and caused by genetic variations (17). As the genes become identified that are responsible for each of the major ion channels (Fig. 20-9), there are potentially more and more channelopathies. Examples are the three major genetic causes of LQTS now named LQT1, LQT2, and LQT3 (2,18). To prolong the action potential duration and hence the QT interval, either the repolarizing potassium currents must be inhibited or the inward currents prolonged. The abnormal genes that cause three molecular abnormalities have been identified (Fig. 20-10). In LCT1, there is a defect in the slow component of the repolarizing potassium current I_{Ks}. In LQT2, the gene HERG (human ether-a-go-go related gene) that expresses the rapid repolarizing current I_{kr} is defective. Specifically, resultant mutations in the pore-forming region of the corresponding K channel markedly increase the risk of arrhythmias (19). LQT3 results from abnormalities of a sodium channel, SCN5A, thereby allowing increased inward sodium currents. The latest addition is LQT4, a rare condition with a defect in the anchoring protein ankyrin-B that normally ensures that some key proteins governing ion transport are correctly inserted into the cell membranes (20). Each type can predispose to sudden cardiac death, presumably by precipitating torsade

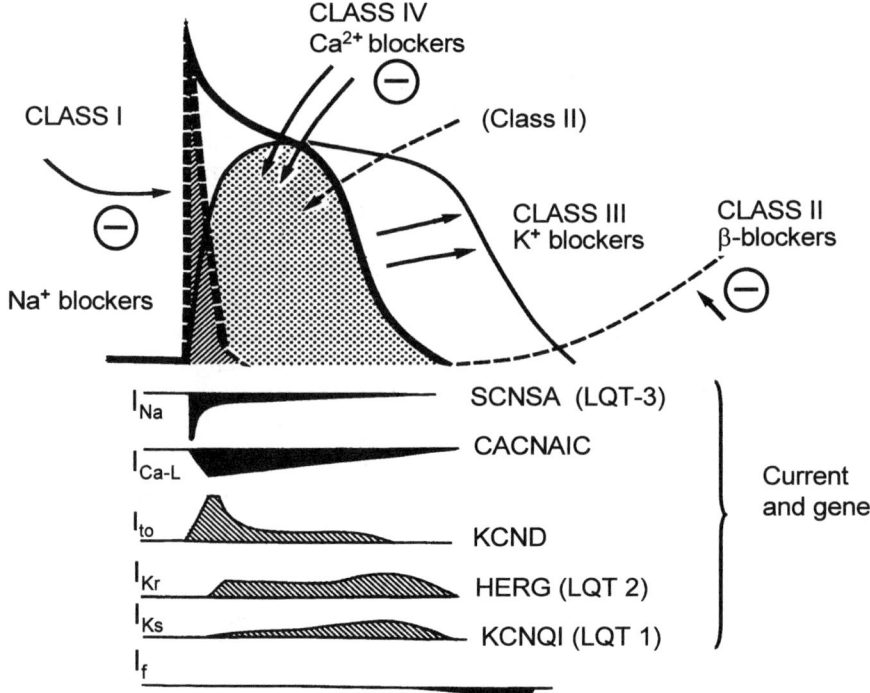

FIG. 20-9. The classic four types of antiarrhythmic agents and genetic basis of normal ion channels. Top: Class I agents decrease phase 0 of the rapid depolarization of the action potential (rapid sodium channel). Class II agents, β-blocking drugs, have complex actions including inhibition of spontaneous depolarization (phase 4) and indirect closure of calcium channels, which are less likely to be open when not phosphorylated by cyclic adenosine 3′,5′-monophosphate. Class III agents block outward potassium channels to prolong the action potential duration and hence refractoriness. The class IV agents verapamil and diltiazem and the indirect calcium antagonist adenosine all inhibit the inward calcium channel, which is most prominent in nodal tissue, particularly the atrioventricular node. Most antiarrhythmic drugs have more than one action. **Bottom:** The normal currents of the cardiac action potential and the genes that encode them. (LQT1 to 3, represent long QT syndrome, forms 1 to 3; see Figure 20-10.)

de pointes; there are somewhat differing clinical pictures. For example, LQT1 has malfunctioning I_{Ks} channels that do not shorten the action potential as they should during catecholamine release as in exercise, risking EADs and arrhythmias during exercise (21). Mutations in LQTS genes are closely linked to sudden infant death syndrome (22).

In acquired LQTS, now increasingly being reported, several drugs, such as the class III antiarrhythmics and the newer antihistaminics such as terfenadine, may block an amino acid subunit of the HERG channel that contains a genetic mutant (23). The result is a prolonged QT interval with risk of torsade de pointes (Fig. 20-11). "A drug concentration, which may slightly prolong the action potential

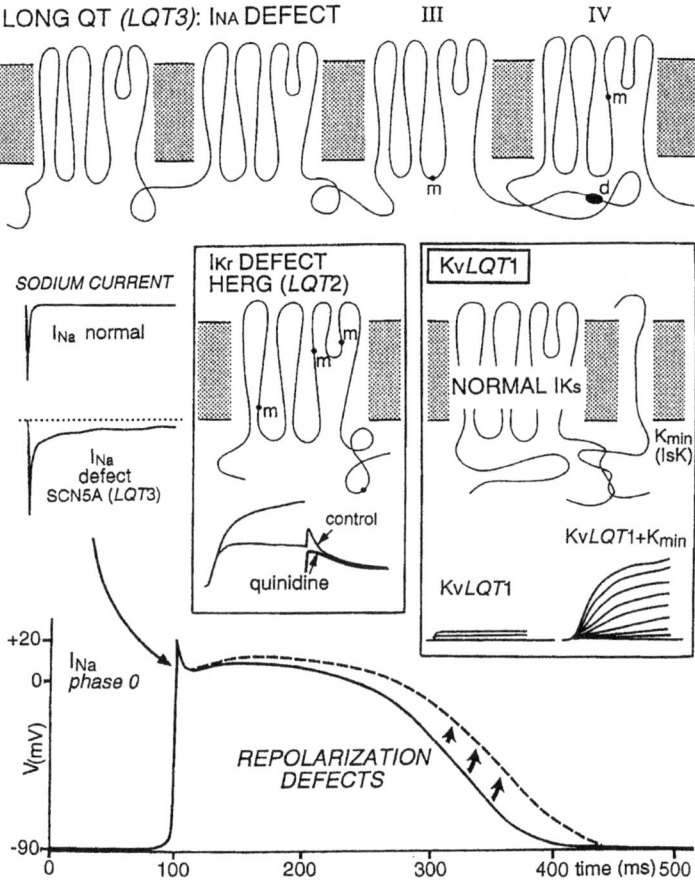

FIG. 20-10. **Inherited long QT abnormalities.** For details, see Attali (35) and Schwartz et al. (21).

plateau and actually be antiarrhythmic in some patients may produce excessive prolongation in others," thereby becoming proarrhythmic (23).

Gain-of-Function Mutations

There are at least two examples. The first, already mentioned, is when increased sodium channel activity results in QT prolongation. The second is in familial AF (24). The causative mutation lies in the KCNQ1 (KvLQT1) gene that encodes the pore-forming subunit of the cardiac potassium channel K_s. The gain of function means that the cardiac action potential in the atria is shortened (increased repolarizing current K_s) thereby predisposing to AF.

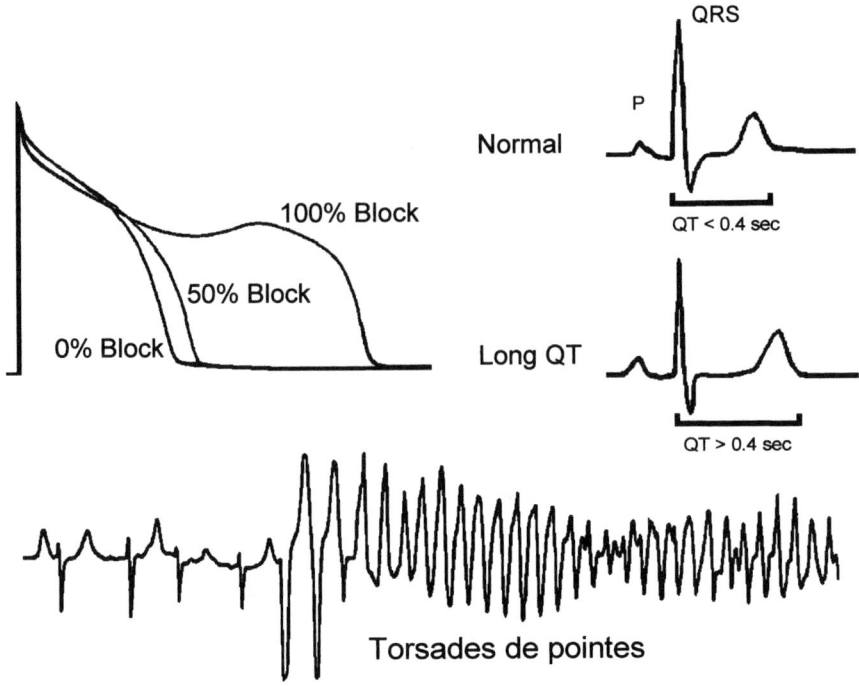

FIG. 20-11. Evolution of torsade de pointes based on QT prolongation. Note the effect of the progressive block of repolarizing potassium currents (see class III antiarrhythmics, Fig. 20-9) with prolongation of the QT interval. Note the risk of ventricular fibrillation, a fatal arrhythmia unless abruptly treated.

VENTRICULAR ARRHYTHMIAS IN ACUTE MYOCARDIAL INFARCTION

In AMI, ventricular arrhythmias vary from ectopic beats to ventricular tachycardia and fibrillation, indicating an increasing degree of severity because ventricular fibrillation is fatal if untreated. In general, AMI is characterized by an increased sympathetic activity that is proarrhythmic by promotion of calcium overload (Fig. 20-8). Four processes currently are thought to be basic to the genesis of such cardiac arrhythmias: (a) increased automaticity, (b) slowing of conduction in specific areas of the heart with resultant reentry and reexcitation, (c) variable shortening or lengthening of the refractory period with increased dispersion of refractoriness between the ischemic and nonischemic zones, and (d) EADs or DADs (as possible causes of automaticity). Increased dispersion of refractoriness to conduction between the ischemic and nonischemic zones sets the stage for reentrant arrhythmias. Unidirectional abnormalities of conduction between ischemic and nonischemic zones have been recorded, as have areas of localized fibrillation that can, it is thought, spread from the ischemic to nonischemic zone.

Localized hyperkalemia and consequent depolarization allow a current of injury to flow from the nonischemic to the ischemic zone, an example of the *current of injury* (Fig. 20-12). The current leaving the nonischemic zone will tend to depolarize the nonischemic side of the border zone and, as such, may actually trigger arrhythmias (particularly in Purkinje fibers). Purkinje fibers can be the site of origin of both slowly conducted normal impulses and ectopic foci.

Heterogeneity, both metabolic and histologic, is proarrhythmic. Apart from the differential duration of the action potential in epicardium and endocardium (Fig. 4-22) and the superior survival of Purkinje fibers, the persistence of a variable collateral circulation increases heterogeneity. Complex and multiple metabolic lesions induce numerous and varying changes in the action potential pat-

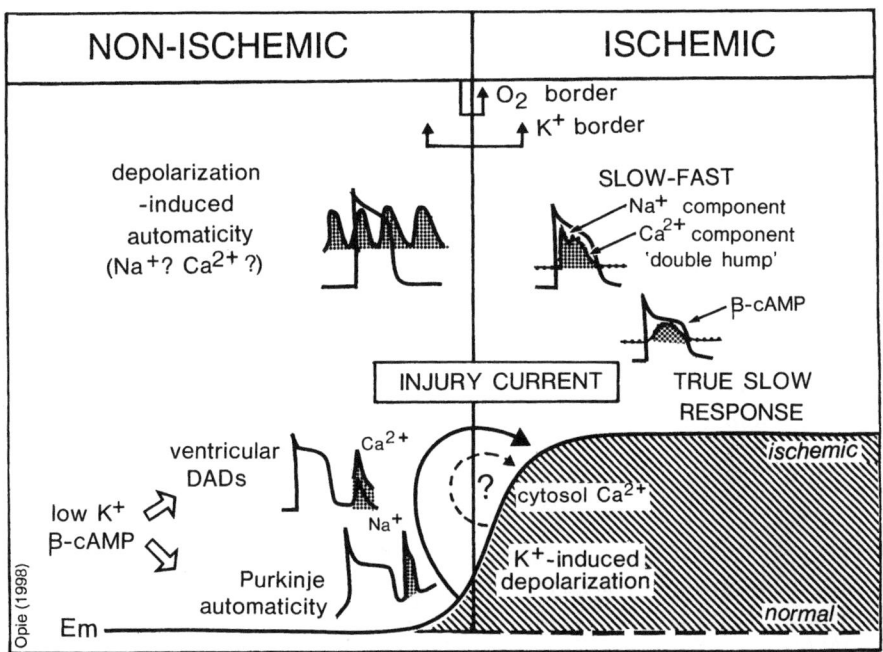

FIG. 20-12. Injury current. Metabolic differences between ischemic and nonischemic tissue that underlie the development of ventricular arrhythmias of early-phase acute myocardial infarction. Points of emphasis are the current of injury between ischemic and nonischemic zones, the development of Purkinje fiber automaticity especially when arterial potassium is low and there is β-adrenergic stimulation (*β-cAMP*), and delayed afterdepolarizations (*DADs*), which can give rise to triggered ventricular automaticity. Note also the formation of abnormal action potentials in the ischemic zone that predispose to abnormalities of impulse conduction and hence to reentry (Fig. 20-2). Slow-fast action potentials have the fast sodium component inhibited by ischemic depolarization, which tends to close the sodium channel and allow the calcium channel to become more dominant, giving the action potential a double-hump appearance. The true slow response is also found in totally depolarized fibers stimulated by cyclic adenosine 3′,5′-monophosphate. Such action potentials also predispose to conduction abnormalities. *Em*, resting membrane potential.

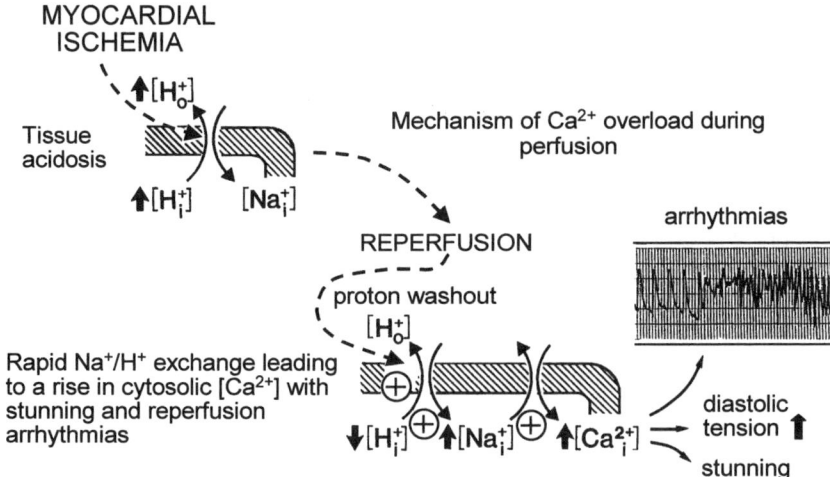

FIG. 20-13. **Reperfusion arrhythmias.** Rapid sodium–proton (H^+) exchange leading to an increase in cytosolic calcium ion concentrations with reperfusion arrhythmias.

tern (Fig. 20-12). Changes in receptor density (such as increased numbers of β-adrenergic receptors), hypokalemia, and other general metabolic disturbances may all play a role. It seems likely that there is no unique causal event to link metabolic changes and ischemic arrhythmias but rather that a variety of factors, each arrhythmogenic in some specific experimental conditions, could be interacting in the very complex situation in patients with AMI. Such multiple mechanisms may explain the difficulties frequently encountered in treating the ventricular arrhythmias of acute infarction.

Reperfusion Arrhythmias

These ventricular arrhythmias, occurring predictably and very soon after the start of experimental reperfusion, are specific to the reperfusion process and a manifestation of reperfusion injury (25). In patients undergoing reperfusion by thrombolytic therapy, reperfusion arrhythmias are much less common for complex reasons, probably including a much slower rate of reperfusion. The two main theories for the development of these arrhythmias are excess intracellular calcium cycling (Fig. 20-13) and formation of free radicals. In sufficiently high concentrations, free radicals can damage the sarcoplasmic reticulum (26) to cause calcium overload, thereby promoting calcium-dependent arrhythmias.

ANTIARRHYTHMIC DRUGS

Antiarrhythmic agents, currently divided into four classes (Table 20-1), should be active on two of the major factors provoking arrhythmias: automatic-

TABLE 20-1. *Classification of antiarrhythmic agents*

Class	Drugs
Sodium channel blockers	Quinidine and quinidine-like agents (major effect: inhibition of fast Na⁺ channel; action potential duration lengthened)
	Lidocaine and lidocaine-like agents (major effect: fast channel inhibition; action potential duration shortening)
	Sodium channel blocking agents with powerful inhibitory effects on the conduction system: encainide, flecainide, and others
Beta-blocking agents (cAMP inhibitors)	Propranolol and all other beta-blockers
Potassium channel inhibitors (repolarizing K⁺ current); agents widening action potential duration as their major effect	Amiodarone and others
Calcium channel antagonist agents active on the atrioventricular node	Verapamil and diltiazem; adenosine and other potassium channel openers (acting indirectly to inhibit calcium channel)

cAMP, cyclic adenosine 3′,5′-monophosphate.

ity and reentry circuits. The development of ectopic beats depends on the opening of the fast channel even if it does not open as rapidly as normal.

Class I antiarrhythmic agents preferentially inhibit abnormal depolarizations (Fig. 20-9). As a class, these drugs exert use-dependent block, so that their effect is greater at high heart rates (27). However, it must not be supposed that class I drug action is simple or well understood. For example, the drug lidocaine acts in part by termination of reentry circuits, a property linked to the rapid rate of recovery from use-dependent block (27) and in part by block of the ATP-dependent potassium channel K_{ATP} (28) so that ischemic potassium loss and regional inhomogeneity are decreased. Lidocaine also inhibits DADs, probably by a reduction of internal calcium as the internal sodium decreases.

Class II antiarrhythmic agents are the β-adrenergic blocking agents. β-Adrenergic stimulation enhances automaticity by several mechanisms. First, phase 4 depolarization in Purkinje fibers is stimulated. Second, DADs are provoked. Third, the slow response may develop in depolarized cells (Fig. 20-12).

Class III antiarrhythmic agents prolong the duration of the refractory period, thereby slowing or stopping conduction through one limb of the reentry circuit besides lessening ectopic formation. These agents generally inhibit the rapid component of the delayed rectifier repolarizing current (I_{Kr}). Not only do they prolong the action potential duration, but they all have torsade de pointes as an inevitable potential side effect (Fig. 20-11).

Class IV antiarrhythmic agents inhibit the calcium channel of the AV node or part of it, acting on the same circuit as adenosine to inhibit supraventricular reentry arrhythmias (Fig. 20-5).

Proarrhythmic Effect of Antiarrhythmic Agents

Postinfarction patients have a risk of sudden death, and the mechanism is thought to be at least in part the development of ventricular tachycardia or fibrillation. A simple hypothesis is that postinfarction ventricular arrhythmias predispose to potentially fatal arrhythmias. Therefore, it has seemed logical to test the effect of ventricular antiarrhythmics on postinfarction arrhythmias. Unexpectedly, some class I antiarrhythmic agents increased the risk of death or nonfatal cardiac arrest by more than threefold (29). These agents (encainide and flecainide) powerfully inhibit the conduction system and hence predispose to electrical heterogeneity and to reentry arrhythmias. In addition, class III agents and some class I agents (those that are quinidine-like) prolong the action potential duration and may predispose to EADs, triggered ventricular activity, and the ventricular arrhythmia called torsade de pointes. Thus, routine prophylactic postinfarction antiarrhythmic drug therapy cannot be justified, with the exception of the proven beneficial effects of β-blockade, which decreases postinfarction mortality.

ARRHYTHMIAS IN HEART FAILURE

Congestive heart failure is a serious condition, often still fatal, and lethal arrhythmias are thought to be a common mode of exit. The dilated left ventricle may activate stretch receptors that in turn directly or indirectly increase cell calcium (Fig. 20-14). Increased circulating concentrations of catecholamines and angiotensin II will also tend to increase cell calcium. An increased cytosolic calcium level increases release of calcium from the sarcoplasmic reticulum. Thereby, electrogenic sodium–calcium exchange (Fig. 4-4) is enhanced, and the transient inward current I_{ti} is evoked with risk of DADs (30). In heart failure, the cardiac action potential is prolonged, in part because of reduced expression of the repolarizing potassium channels. Furthermore, smaller calcium transients (Fig. 16-9) lead to less rapid inactivation of the inward calcium current. Thus, there is more opportunity for the late opening of the L channels with a late inward current that is the likely cause of EADs (31). Increased catecholamine stimulation also contributes to reactivation of L-type calcium currents (30). Failing myocytes have additional abnormal electrophysiologic properties, such as the emergence in ventricular myocytes of I_f, the hyperpolarization-activated current (32), and prolonged action potentials resulting from prior hypertrophy.

Therapeutic agents used in the treatment of heart failure may also promote arrhythmias (Fig. 20-15). For example, diuretic drugs may cause hypokalemia as a side effect, thereby predisposing to afterpotentials. The potassium-retaining diuretic spironolactone, known to reduce mortality in heart failure, may act (at least in part) by inhibiting the HERG repolarizing potassium current to prolong the action potential duration with a class III type antiarrhythmic effect (33). Positive inotropes increase cell calcium and are potentially arrhythmogenic.

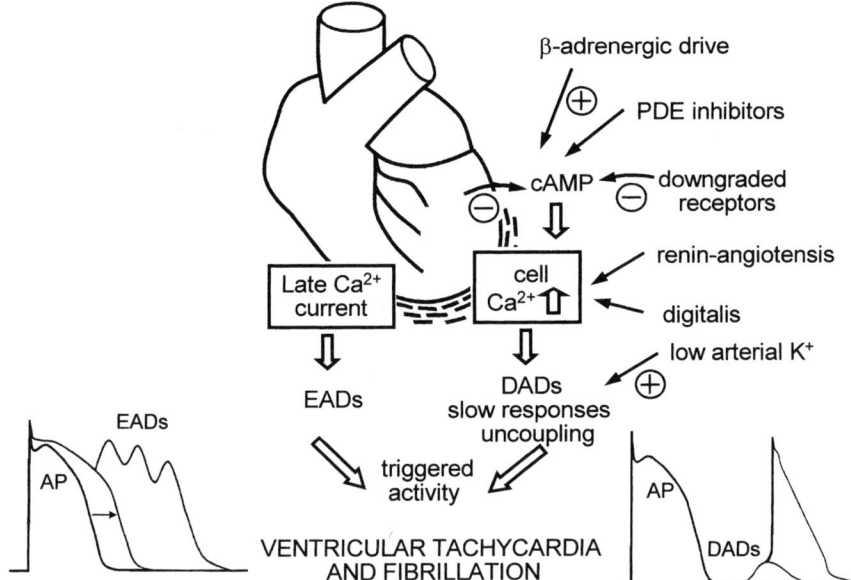

FIG. 20-14. **Arrhythmias of heart failure.** Proposed proarrhythmic mechanisms in left ventricular (*LV*) failure and arrhythmias, most of which are thought to implicate calcium ions and to arise from early afterdepolarizations (*EADs*) or delayed afterdepolarizations (*DADs*) (Fig. 20-1). The EADs reflect late calcium currents, whereas DADs reflect cytosolic calcium overload with compensatory overaction of sodium–calcium exchange with electrogenic sodium ion entry. Impaired function of the sarcoplasmic reticulum contributes to the prolonged calcium transients. In left ventricular failure, formation of cyclic adenosine 3′,5′-monophosphate is impaired and myocardial function can be improved by the combined administration of both phosphodiesterase (*PDE*) inhibitors and β-adrenergic stimulation with, however, risks of ventricular arrhythmias (Fig. 20-15). *AP*, action potential.

Cardiac Memory

The heart responds to some repetitive events such as serious arrhythmias, by evoking a "memory" response (34). The pathways concerned are remarkably similar to those concerned with cerebral memory, also involving angiotensin II. Hypothetically, altered myocardial ventricular stress–strain relationship induces angiotensin II that in turn evokes a nuclear response and synthesis of memory proteins. A specific example lies in the action potential pattern. The action potential duration is prolonged because the memory process down-regulates the repolarizing current I_{to}. Therefore, the memory process has an effect similar to that of class III antiarrhythmic drugs.

Proarrhythmic Risks of Positive Inotropic Agents

Digitalis agents, besides being positively inotropic by inhibition of the sodium–potassium pump, are potentially arrhythmogenic at toxic blood levels. DADs,

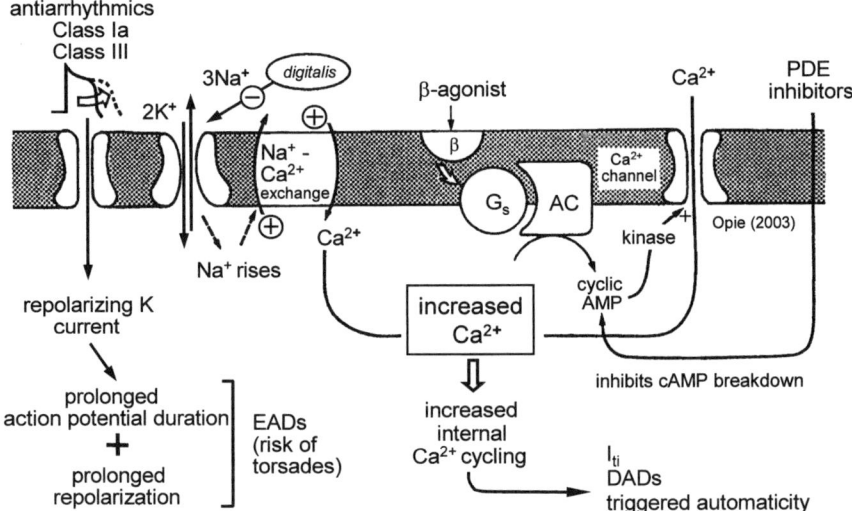

FIG. 20-15. Drug-induced arrhythmias resulting from abnormalities of calcium ions. On the left is shown the proposed mechanism whereby agents prolonging the action potential duration (*APD*) enable late calcium currents to flow, with development of early afterdepolarizations (*EADs*) and risk of torsade de pointes. On the right are the effects of agents that increase cytosolic Ca^{2+}, with risk of excess internal recycling of Ca^{2+} in and out of the sarcoplasmic reticulum and formation of delayed afterdepolarizations (*DADs*). See also Figure 20-14. PDE, phosphodiesterase.

resulting from cytosolic calcium overload and excess calcium recycling, are thought to underlie the development of ventricular automaticity during digitalis poisoning. β-Agonists and phosphodiesterase inhibitors produce a positive inotropic effect by elevating cellular cAMP and hence the cytosolic calcium level (Fig. 20-15). Because excess cytosolic calcium is potentially arrhythmogenic (Fig. 20-8), such positive inotropes have an implicit risk of arrhythmia development. The risk is increased when there is hypokalemia, frequently found in patients with severe heart failure treated by excess diuretics.

SUMMARY

1. *Mechanisms for ventricular arrhythmias.* The major three are the development of automaticity, reentry circuits, and abnormalities of repolarization, such as EADs and DADs. Automaticity in Purkinje fibers is particularly predisposed to by hypokalemia or catecholamine stimulation. Ventricular reentry circuits presuppose electrical heterogeneity, such as localized depolarization. Focal changes in extracellular potassium and intracellular calcium could contribute significantly. For example, differing intracellular calcium concentrations in various sites in ischemic tissue are thought to predispose to electrical alternans, which is a risk factor for ventricular fibrillation.

2. *Afterdepolarizations.* DADs particularly occur in conditions of cytosolic calcium overload, such as heart failure, early reperfusion, digitalis intoxication, or excess therapy with some inotropic agents. EADs are associated with congenital or drug-acquired prolongation of the QT interval. Afterdepolarizations predispose to torsade de pointes, a potentially lethal arrhythmia.
3. *Congenital LQTS.* The genes responsible for the abnormalities of the repolarizing potassium currents (in particular HERG) and the inward sodium current have been identified.
4. *Ventricular arrhythmias of AMI.* The initiating ectopic beat, which may trigger micro- and macroreentry circuits, is thought to be in the nonischemic zone. The current flowing from the nonischemic to the ischemic zone is the current of injury. Reperfusion arrhythmias have two main origins: cytosolic calcium overload with DADs and formation of free radicals in the form of reactive oxygen species.
5. *Arrhythmias of heart failure* may be caused by EADs or DADs, both related to abnormalities of calcium ion movements. Some therapeutic drugs, such as those stimulating contraction (positive inotropes), may also induce arrhythmias.
6. *Antiarrhythmic drugs may paradoxically promote arrhythmias* (proarrhythmic effect) and should, therefore, be used with care and only for specific indications.

STUDENT QUESTIONS

1. For which conditions is carotid sinus massage used, and how does it work?
2. What is AF, and how is it diagnosed by electrocardiography?
3. Hypokalemia predisposes to arrhythmias; however, regional loss of potassium with local venous hyperkalemia is arrhythmogenic. Explain this apparent contradiction.
4. Describe how abnormalities of internal calcium could be arrhythmogenic in ischemia and in heart failure.
5. What are the differences between EADs and DADs?

CARDIOLOGIST-IN-TRAINING QUESTIONS

1. Adenosine is given intravenously for some types of supraventricular arrhythmias. Describe its mechanism of action. Which arrhythmias respond best and which do not respond at all?
2. What is a reentry circuit? When might it be arrhythmogenic?
3. What is HERG? Describe the genetic abnormalities of the LQTS.
4. What are the cellular and electrophysiologic origins of the current of injury?
5. Why are patients with congestive heart failure prone to ventricular arrhythmias?
6. How can drugs cause arrhythmias?

ACKNOWLEDGMENT

Professor P. J. Schwartz, Pavia, Italy, critically reviewed the section on channelopathies.

REFERENCES

1. Major RH. *Classic descriptions of disease.* Springfield, IL: Charles C Thomas, 1945.
2. Keating MT, et al. Molecular and cellular mechanisms of cardiac arrhythmias. *Cell* 2001;104: 569–580.
3. Marine JE, et al. Different patterns of interatrial conduction in clockwise and counterclockwise atrial flutter. *Circulation* 2001;104:1153–1157.
4. Mihm MJ, et al. Impaired myofibrillar energetics and oxidative injury during human atrial fibrillation. *Circulation* 2001;104:174–180.
5. Van Wagoner DR, et al. Molecular basis of electrical remodeling in atrial fibrillation. *J Mol Cell Cardiol* 2000;32:101–117.
6. Harris AS, et al. Excitatory factors in ventricular tachycardia resulting from myocardial ischemia: potassium a major excitant. *Science* 1954;119:200–203.
7. Corr PB, et al. Arrhythmogenic amphiphilic lipids and the myocardial cell membrane [Editorial]. *J Mol Cell Cardiol* 1982;14:619–626.
8. Clarkson CW, et al. On the mechanism of lysophosphatidylcholine-induced depolarization of cat ventricular myocardium. *Circ Res* 1983;52:543–556.
9. Opie LH, et al. Biochemical aspects of arrhythmogenesis and ventricular fibrillation. *Am J Cardiol* 1979;43:131–148.
10. Taniguchi J, et al. Modification of the cardiac action potential by intracellular injection of adenosine triphosphate and related substances in guinea pigs single ventricular cells. *Circ Res* 1983;53: 131–139.
11. Huser J, et al. Functional coupling between glycolysis and excitation-contraction coupling underlies alternans in cat heart cells. *J Physiol* 2000;524:795–806.
12. Lee H-C, et al. Effect of ischemia on calcium-dependent fluorescence transients in rabbit hearts containing indo 1. Correlation with monophasic action potentials and contraction. *Circulation* 1988;78: 1047–1059.
13. Peters NS, et al. Disturbed connexin-43 gap junction distribution correlates with the location of reentrant circuits in the epicardial border zone of healing canine infarcts that cause ventricular tachycardia. *Circulation* 1997; 95:988–996.
14. Opie LH, Clusin WT. Cellular mechanism for ischemic ventricular arrhythmias. *Annu Rev Med* 1990; 41:231–238.
15. Qin D, et al. Cellular and ionic basis of arrhythmias in postinfarction remodeled ventricular myocardium. *Circ Res* 1996;79:461–473.
16. Volders PGA, et al. Progress in the understanding of cardiac early afterdepolarization and torsade de pointes: time to revise current concepts. *Cardiovasc Res* 2000;46:376–392.
17. Marban E. Cardiac channelopathies. *Nature* 2002;415:213–218.
18. Priori SG, et al. Risk stratification in the long-QT syndrome. *N Engl J Med* 2003;348:1866–1874.
19. Moss AJ, et al. Increased risk of arrhythmic events in long-QT syndrome with mutations in the pore region of the human ether-a-go-go related gene potassium channel. *Circulation* 2002;105:794–799.
20. Mohler PJ, et al. Ankyrin-B mutation causes type 4 long-QT cardiac arrhythmia and sudden cardiac death. *Nature* 2003;421:634.
21. Schwartz PJ, et al. Genotype-phenotype correlation in the long-WT syndrome. Gene-specific triggers for life-threatening arrhythmias. *Circulation* 2001;103:89–95.
22. Schwartz PJ, et al. Molecular diagnosis in a child with sudden infant death syndrome. *Lancet* 2001; 358:1342–1343.
23. Kass RS, et al. Channel structure and drug-induced cardiac arrhythmias. *Proc Natl Acad Sci U S A* 2000;97:11683–11684.
24. Chen Y-H, et al. KCNQ1 Gain-of-function mutation in familial atrial fibrillation. *Science* 2003;299: 251–253.
25. Opie LH. Reperfusion injury and its pharmacologic modification. *Circulation* 1989;80:1049–1062.

26. Xu KY, et al. Hydroxyl radical inhibits sarcoplasmic reticulum Ca^{2+}-ATPase function by direct attack on the ATP binding site. *Circ Res* 1997;80:76–81.
27. Fei H, et al. Termination of reentry by lidocaine in the tricuspid ring in vitro. Role of cycle-length oscillation, fast use-dependent kinetics, and fixed block. *Circ Res* 1997;80:242–252.
28. Olschewski A, et al. ATP-dependent potassium channel in rat cardiomyocytes is blocked by lidocaine. Possible impact on the antiarrhythmic action of lidocaine. *Circulation* 1996;93:656–659.
29. Cardiac Arrhythmia Suppression Trial. (CAST). Preliminary report: effect of encainide and flecainide on mortality in a randomized trial of arrhythmia suppression after myocardial infarction. *N Engl J Med* 1989;321:406–412.
30. Verkerk AO, et al. Ionic mechanism of delayed afterdepolarization in ventricular cells from human end-stage failing hearts. *Circulation* 2001;104:2728–2733.
31. Bers DM. Calcium and cardiac rhythms. Physiological and pathophysiological. *Circ Res* 2002;90: 14–17.
32. Cerbai E, et al. Characterization of the hyperpolarization-activated current, I_f, in ventricular myocytes from human failing heart. *Circulation* 1997;95:568–571.
33. Caballero R, et al. Spironolactone and its main metabolite, canrenoic acid, block human ether-a-go-go related gene channels. *Circulation* 2003;107:889–895.
34. Rosen MR. The heart remembers: clinical implications. *Lancet* 2001;357:468–471.
35. Attali B. A new wave for heart rhythms. *Nature* 1996;384:24–25.

Subject Index

Page numbers followed by f indicate figures; those followed by t indicate tables; and those followed by CP indicates color plate.

A

A band, 45, 46f
Abnormal coronary vasomotion, 300
ACE. See Angiotensin-converting enzyme
Acetyl-CoA, 322, 324
Acetylcholine
  parasympathetic nervous system, 16
  receptors. See Cholinergic receptors
  vasodilation, 284t
Acetylcholine-regulated potassium
    channel, 125
Actin
  cytoplasmic, 11CP
  filaments, 44–45
  isoforms, 238t
  myosin interactions, 223–224, 223f,
    7CP
α-Actinin, 59t, 11CP
Action potential
  cardiac currents, 94t
  cardiomyocytes, 50, 75f, 105f
  ionic conductances, 87f
  ischemic changes, 539–540
  metabolic effects on duration, 608–609
  overload hypertrophy changes, 417,
    418f
  phases, 73–74, 75f, 104–106
  plateau-terminating currents, 106t
  Purkinje cells, 73–74, 75f, 105f
  smooth muscle cells, 65–66
  sodium–calcium exchanger, 106, 107f,
    108
Activation threshold, 85
Acute coronary syndromes. See
    Myocardial infarction
Acylcarnitine carrier, 323f

Adenosine
  antiarrhythmic activity, 617t
  atrioventricular node inhibition, 132
  cardioprotective effects, 339–340
  cyclic AMP response, 203t
  heart rate effects, 204
  interactions with nitric oxide and K_{ATP}
    channel, 288
  preconditioning role, 591, 592f, 593
  production, 286, 287f
  receptors. See Purinergic receptors
  signaling, 339–340, 340f
  vasodilation, 24, 29, 279, 286, 287f
Adenosine deaminase, 286, 287f
Adenosine diphosphate (ADP)
  cardiac concentration, 338
  metabolic pathway regulation, 334t
Adenosine monophosphate (AMP),
    metabolic pathway regulation, 334t,
    340
Adenosine triphosphate (ATP)
  breakdown, 337–338, 339f
  cardiac consumption, 306
  cardiac content, 222
  cardiac uses, 334, 334t
  creatine phosphate synthesis, 335
  hydrolysis, 222
  ion flux requirements, 114–115, 114t,
    163
  ischemic metabolism
    requirements, 343–344, 343f,
      529–530, 534
    breakdown, 344
  magnesium affinity, 534
  metabolic pathway regulation, 334t
  mitochondrial production, 47, 49

Adenosine triphosphate (ATP) (contd.)
  pools and compartments, 336f, 337
  synthesis. See Oxidative
    phosphorylation
  transfer in circulation, 37, 38f
Adenylate cyclase
  heart failure effects, 511t
  hormone and drug effects, 203–205
  signaling, 198, 201, 202f
Adenylate kinase, 338
ADH. See Antidiuretic hormone
ADP. See Adenosine diphosphate
Adrenaline. See Epinephrine
Adrenergic nervous system. See
  Sympathetic nervous system
α-Adrenergic receptors
  activation effects on circulation, 17, 18t, 285, 289–290
  β-adrenergic receptor comparison, 210t
  classification, 210, 290
  functions, 210
  G protein coupling, 210
  positive inotropic effect, 211
  postsynaptic receptors, 26
  presynaptic receptors, 26
  signal transduction, 188, 210–211, 285
  vascular tone modulation, 26–27, 285, 289–290
  vasoconstriction, 24, 439f, 440t
β-Adrenergic receptors
  activation effects on circulation, 17, 18t, 19–21, 23f, 291
  α-adrenergic receptor comparison, 210t
  β_1-adrenergic receptors
    agonists, 193
    antagonists, 192
    chronotropic effect, 209
    density in heart, 192
    down-regulation in heart failure, 510–511
    dromotropic effect, 209
    inhibition in heart failure, 509f
    inotropic effect, 208–209
    lusitropic effect, 209
    tissue distribution, 191
  β_2-adrenergic receptors
    compensatory role in heart failure, 511–512
    physiologic effects, 209
    signaling, 193
    tissue distribution, 191
  β_3-adrenergic receptors in heart failure
    anchoring proteins, 197–198, 197f
    blockers. See Beta-blockers
    calcium transients in heart failure, 500f
    classification, 19, 291
    contractility effects, 369
    contraction–relaxation cycle effects, 231–232, 232f
    desensitization, 195–196, 195f, 508–509, 509f
    drug therapy effects, 196–197
    G protein coupling, 198–200
    heart failure response, 216, 508–512, 509f, 510f
    internalization, 195f, 196
    ischemia response, 215–216
    positive inotropic and relaxant effects stimulation, 177–178, 178f
    resensitization, 196
    sarcolemmal membrane density, 77t
    signal transduction, 21–22, 186, 187f, 193, 198–207
    sinoatrial node pacemaker activity regulation, 24
    structure, 193, 194f
    vascular tone modulation, 26–27, 291
    vasodilation role, 24, 25f, 29, 291
Adrenomedullin, heart failure response, 516
Afterdepolarization, 599–600, 600f, 609–611
Afterload
  aortic impedance, 450
  blood pressure relationship, 364, 364f, 449–450
  cardiac output contribution, 465–467
  definition, 359, 461t
  heart failure increase, 513f
  measurement, 363–364
  preload relationship, 364–365, 369–370
Aging
  blood pressure effects, 431, 446–447, 448f, 449f
  cardiomyocyte apoptosis, 404–405
  cardiomyopathy of the elderly, 491
  exercise capacity, 478
  myocardial infarction prognosis, 571

β-Agonist receptor kinase (β-ARK)
  β-adrenergic receptor desensitization, 195
  heart failure response, 216
  ischemia response, 216
  regulation of expression, 196
  therapeutic targeting, 197
AKAP. *See* A kinase anchoring protein
A kinase anchoring protein (AKAP), 198
Akt
  activation in disease, 257
  growth signaling, 188, 206
  restenosis role, 547
  substrates, 257
Aldosterone
  blood volume control, 31f
  heart failure role, 495–496, 507
Allopurinol, congestive heart failure management, 517
Ambulatory monitoring, blood pressure, 443–444
Amiodarone, 611, 617t
Amlodipine, mechanism of action, 92
AMP. *See* Adenosine monophosphate
AMP-activated protein kinase, 325, 338–339, 342
Anaerobic glycolysis, 341, 342f
Angina pectoris
  electrocardiography, 154–155
  pain mechanisms, 538–539
  Prinzmetal angina, 299
Angiography
  cardiac output measurement, 467
  coronary blood flow measurement, 302
Angiotensin II
  atherosclerosis role, 557
  blood pressure regulation, 437–438, 438t, 439f
  heart failure role, 495–496, 504, 505f, 512–513
  inhibition for left ventricular hypertrophy regression, 421–423
  norepinephrine release modulation, 26
  overload hypertrophy role, 406–407, 406f, 410–411, 411f, 413–414
  pathology, 249–250, 253
  processing, 31, 249–250, 250f
  vasoconstriction, 31, 250, 253, 286
Angiotensin II receptors
  AT-I, 251, 406

AT-II, 251, 407, 422
  G protein coupling, 251–252
  signaling, 251–253, 251f, 406
Angiotensin-converting enzyme (ACE)
  function, 249–250
  growth response, 412f
  inhibitors
    congestive heart failure management, 517
    ischemia treatment, 546
    remodeling promotion, 569
ANP. *See* Atrial natriuretic peptide
Anrep effect, 450
Antiarrhythmic drugs. *See* Arrhythmia
Antidiuretic hormone (ADH)
  blood pressure regulation, 438, 440
  heart failure response, 513
Aorta
  arterial pressure pattern, 12f
  pressure buffering function, 12, 13f
Aortic compliance, 364
  wall stress relationship, 372
Aortic impedance, 364, 450
Aortic regurgitation
  contractility dysfunction, 397
  hemodynamics, 493–494, 493f
Aortic stenosis, 492–493, 492f
Aortic valve, anatomy, 7
Apoptosis
  aging cardiomyocytes, 404–405
  heart failure, 496–497
  mechanisms, 562
  necrosis comparison, 559–560, 560f
  reperfusion injury, 586
  signaling
    caspases, 262f, 263
    death receptor pathway, 262
    mitochondrial pathway, 262–263
    overview, 248f, 261, 262f
β-ARK. *See* β-Agonist receptor kinase
Arrestin
  β-adrenergic receptor desensitization, 195
  scaffolding function, 197–198
Arrhythmia. *See also specific arrhythmias*
  antiarrhythmic drugs
    class I, 617
    class II, 617
    class III, 617
    class IV, 617

Arrhythmia, antiarrhythmic drugs (contd.)
  proarrhythmic effects, 618
  types, 616–617, 617t
calcium overload
  diastolic calcium overload, 79–180
  overview, 178–179
electrocardiography, 141–142, 142f
exercise induction, 478
heart failure arrhythmias, 618–620
mechanisms, 599–600, 600f
myocardial infarction arrhythmias, 614–616
reentry circuits
  atrial, 599–600, 600f, 601f, 604–605
  ventricular, 607–608
  refractory period, 601–603, 602f, 605–606
reperfusion injury, 583–584, 616, 616f
sodium–calcium exchanger role, 108
supraventricular arrhythmias, 600–606
ventricular arrhythmias, 606–616
Arterial blood pressure, 12–13, 431
Arteriole
  anatomy, 11–12, 282
  arterial pressure patterns, 12f
  neurotransmitter regulation, 24, 25f
  peripheral vascular resistance. *See* Peripheral vascular resistance
  resistance, 11–12, 33–34, 284
Artery, definition, 10
Atherosclerosis. *See also* Coronary artery disease; Ischemia; Myocardial infarction
  angiotensin II role, 253
  dietary factors, 558
  endothelial dysfunction, 556
  inflammatory response, 557
  macrophage role, 557–558
  plaque rupture, 553, 555f, 557
  progression from endothelial damage to plaque, 555–558, 556f, 559f
  risk factors, 556–557
  vulnerable plaques, 557, 559f
Athlete heart characteristics, 476f, 477
ATP. *See* Adenosine triphosphate
ATP-sensitive potassium channel, 101–102, 101f, 288, 295, 539, 593
Atrial cell
  function, 65
  morphology, 65
Atrial conduction, internodal tracts, 129–130
Atrial ectopic depolarizations
  electrocardiography, 602f
  mechanisms, 602
  refractory period, 601–603, 602f
Atrial fibrillation
  electrocardiography, 605, 605f
  familial mutations, 613
  reentry circuits, 605
  remodeling, 606
  stunning after cardioversion, 606
Atrial flutter
  electrocardiography, 602f
  reentry circuit, 604
Atrial natriuretic peptide (ANP)
  blood pressure regulation, 440
  heart failure response, 515–516, 516f
  overload hypertrophy expression, 417
  vasodilation, 289
Atrial systole, 357–358
Atrioventricular (AV) node
  autonomic control, 131–132
  definition, 10
  delay. *See* Heart block
  electrocardiography, 144, 145f
  electrophysiology, 131
  impulse propagation from sinoatrial node, 127–129, 128f, 129f
  inhibitors
    adenosine, 132
    calcium channel blockers, 132
  nodal rhythm, 146
  refractory period, 131
  regions, 131
  slow calcium channel, 130f
Atrioventricular nodal reentry tachycardia, 603–604
Atrium. *See also* Left atrium
  function, 390
  left ventricle comparison, 390–391, 391t
Automaticity
  sinoatrial node, 119–120
  triggered, 610
Autonomic nervous system. *See* Parasympathetic nervous system; Sympathetic nervous system
AV node. *See* Atrioventricular node

SUBJECT INDEX 629

B
BAD, 263
Bainbridge reflex, 435–435, 435f, 464
Balloon angioplasty, 547, 583
Baroreceptors
  definition, 20
  distribution, 27–28
  exercise effects, 433–434, 433f
  medullary autonomic control, 28f
  reflex bradycardia, 28
  reflex tachycardia, 28
Baroreflex response, 433–435, 433f, 434
Bax, 562
Bcl-2, 263, 562
Beta-adrenergic receptor kinase, 509f
Beta-blockers
  β-adrenergic receptor downregulation, 196–197
  antiarrhythmic activity, 617, 617t
  congestive heart failure management, 517
  cyclic AMP response, 203t
  effects on cardiac output with exercise, 473
  heart failure management, 512
  ischemia management, 537, 546
  ryanodine receptor effects, 510f
  toxicity, 190
Bifascicular block, 149
Blood pressure. *See also* Hypertension
  afterload relationship, 364, 364f, 449–450
  aging effects, 431, 446–447, 448f, 449f
  ambulatory measurement, 443–444
  autonomic control
    Bainbridge reflex, 435–435, 435f
    baroreceptors, 433–434, 433f
    baroreflex response, 433–435, 433f, 434
    flow-pressure receptors, 435, 435f
    integrated control, 436–437, 436f
    nucleus solitarius, 433
    vasomotor center, 433
  diastolic blood pressure, 431
  diurnal changes, 13, 14f
  diurnal variation, 431, 443
  epinephrine response, 19f
  exercise effects, 446, 447f
  mental stress response, 443–444, 444f
  neurohormonal control

angiotensin-II, 437–438, 438t, 439f
antidiuretic hormone, 438, 440
atrial natriuretic peptide, 440
epinephrine, 437
norepinephrine, 437
renin–angiotensin system, 436–438
  orthostatic stress response, 445–446, 446f
  peripheral vascular resistance control. *See* Peripheral vascular resistance
  systolic blood pressure, 431
  white-coat syndrome, 444
BNP. *See* Brain natriuretic peptide
Bowditch staircase effect, 365, 366f, 396, 465
Bradycardia
  athletes, 477
  electrocardiography, 143f
  inducers, 142, 144t
Bradykinin system, 250f
Brain natriuretic peptide (BNP), heart failure response, 515–516, 516f
Bypass surgery, postoperative stunning, 583

C
Caffeine, sarcoplasmic reticulum calcium effects, 170–171, 170t
Calcineurin
  growth regulation, 176–177
  nuclear factor-κB interactions, 265f
  overload hypertrophy role, 405, 406, 414f
Calcitonin gene related peptide (CGRP)
  cyclic AMP response, 204–205
  vasodilation, 284t
Calcium
  actin–myosin interaction mediation, 223–224, 223f
  concentrations in heart ventricles, 78t
  contraction–relaxation cycle regulation
    β-adrenergic effects, 231–232, 232f
    mechanism of control, 231
    overview, 229–230, 230f
    sensitivity modulation, 241t
    troponin C binding, 229–231
  cycling in heart failure, 508f
  cytosolic level reduction mechanisms, 163t
  electrical alternans role, 609

Calcium (*contd.*)
  flux. *See* Calcium channels; Excitation–contraction coupling; Ryanodine receptor; Sarcoplasmic reticulum
  free concentration relationship to tension development, 159, 161f, 164f
  growth regulation, 176–177, 177f
  heart failure abnormalities, 498, 500f, 508f, 511t
  ischemia abnormalities, 533
  Krebs cycle regulation, 329
  mitochondrial uptake and release, 329–330
  overload
    arrhythmias, 178–180
    diastolic calcium overload, 179–180
    irreversible ischemic damage, 563, 565
    stunning, 578–579, 578f
  reactive oxygen species interactions, 582–583, 582f
Calcium-activated potassium channel, 101
Calcium channels
  action potential, 50, 73–74, 75f, 105
  blockers, 88, 92–93, 132, 546, 617t
  gating mechanisms, 83, 85
  L-type channels, 91–92, 91f, 92t, 94t, 105
  regulation
    inhibition, 88, 90
    phosphorylation, 90–91
  sarcolemmal membrane density, 77t
  sodium channel comparison, 86t
  states, 90f
  structure, 88, 89f
  T-type channels, 91–92, 91f, 92t, 94t, 105
Calcium pumps
  regulation, 112–113
  sarcolemma
  sarcoplasmic reticulum, 163
Calmodulin
  calcium binding effects, 176
  glycogenolysis role, 321
Calreticulin, 175
Calsequestrin, 175
cAMP. *See* Cyclic adenosine monophosphate
Capillaries
  anatomy, 34, 35f, 282–283, 282t
  exchange mechanisms, 34–35

peripheral circulation, 8, 9f, 11
recruitment, 283t
Starling hypothesis for fluid exchange, 35f, 36
Carbon dioxide tension (pCO_2)
  ischemia, 534
  vasodilation, 289
Cardiac cycle
  heart sound origins, 358t
  overview, 355, 356f, 356t
  systole, 355–357
  ventricular filling, 357–358
  ventricular relaxation, 357
Cardiac output
  afterload contribution, 465–467
  beta-blockade effects in exercise, 473
  contractility contribution, 467
  definition, 373, 460
  determinants, 460, 461f, 461t
  distinguishing from work, 460–461
  dynamic versus static exercise
    central integration and reflexes, 467–468, 470f
    hemodynamic response, 467–468, 471f
    posture effects, 472–473
    pressure–volume loops, 471–472, 472f, 473f
  emotional stress effects, 479–480
  epinephrine response, 19f, 20f
  heart rate contribution
    adrenergic outflow and heart transplants, 464
    force–frequency relationship, 465
    overview, 460, 461f, 462, 463f, 464
    tachycardia of exercise, 464
  measurement, 467
  preload contribution, 465
Cardiomyocyte
  action potential, 50, 75f, 105f
  contraction–relaxation cycle. *See* Contraction–relaxation cycle
  cytoskeleton
    definition, 44
    proteins, 59t
  cytosol, 44
  extracellular matrix, 62–65
  glycocalyx, 49–50

intercellular communication, 54–57
ion channels, 50
ionic balance, 73, 74f
mitochondria, 44, 47, 48f, 49
morphology, 43t
myofibers, 43
myofibrils, 43
nuclei, 44, 53–54
polarization, 44
sarcolemma, 43–44, 49–50
sarcoplasmic reticulum, 52–53
species comparison of number and size, 404–405
T tubules. See T tubule
volume in heart, 42–43
Cardiomyopathy
cardiomyopathy of the elderly, 491
dilated cardiomyopathy, 490–491, 491f
hypertrophic cardiomyopathy, 489–490, 490f, 491f, 9CP, 10CP
tachycardiomyopathy, 491
Cardioplegia, 345
Cardiopulmonary bypass, postpump syndrome, 585
Cardiotrophin-1 (CT-1), 264f, 265
Carnitine palmityltransferase, 324
Carotid sinus massage, 28–29, 603f, 604, 606
Caspases, 262f, 263
Catalase, antioxidant defense, 581t
Catecholamines. See Epinephrine; Norepinephrine
Catenin, 59t
Caveolae, 52
Cesalpino, 5
c-fos, overload hypertrophy expression, 415, 415t
cGMP. See Cyclic guanosine monophosphate
CGRP. See Calcitonin gene related peptide
Chloride channels, 103–104, 104f
Cholinergic nervous system. See Parasympathetic nervous system
Cholinergic receptors
activation effects on circulation, 17, 18t, 19, 285, 291
negative inotropic effect, 213
parasympathetic vagal stimulation, 212–213

sarcolemmal membrane density, 77t
signal transduction, 22, 187f, 201f, 212–215
sinoatrial node pacemaker activity regulation, 24
Chordae tendinae, function, 6–7
Citrate cycle. See Krebs cycle
c-jun, overload hypertrophy expression, 415, 415t
c-myc, overload hypertrophy expression, 415, 415t
CK. See Creatine kinase
Collagen
heart failure role, 419–420, 496, 497f
matrix, 62–63, 63t, 64f
Collagenases, 64–65
Collateral flow, 297–298, 298f
Concentric remodeling, 488, 489f
Conducting system, anatomy, 10f
Congestive heart failure
definition, 504
diastolic failure, 504–506, 506f
neurohormonal vicious circle, 504, 505f
pathophysiologic mechanisms, 499t
receptors and signling systems, 511t
signs and symptoms, 507t
systolic failure, 504–506, 507f
treatment
allopurinol, 517
angiotensin-converting enzyme inhibitors, 517
beta-blockers, 517
digitalis, 517
gene therapy, 517
principles, 517
surgery, 517–518
vasodilators, 517
Connexins, 56, 59t
Connexon, 56
Contractility
β-adrenergic effects, 369. See also frontispiece
cardiac output contribution, 467
change effects on pressure–volume loops, 378, 378f
clinical indices, 382t
echocardiography, 384
ejection phase indices, 383–384
left ventricular function curves, 381

Contractility, clinical indices (contd.)
  maximal rate of left ventricular pressure generation, 381, 383, 383f
  pressure–volume loops, 385
  conceptual problems, 369
  definition, 367, 461t
  dysfunction in disease, 396–397, 508f
  force–velocity relationship and idealized contractility, 367–368, 368f
  ischemic impairment, 528–529, 528t
  isotonic contraction, 368–369
  perfusion–contraction match, 526, 527f
  perfusion–contraction mismatch, 526, 527f
Contraction–relaxation cycle
  calcium regulation
    β-adrenergic effects, 231–232, 232f
    mechanism of control, 231
    overview, 229–230, 230f
    sensitivity modulation, 241t
    troponin C binding, 229–231
  cross-bridge cycle, 45, 46f, 47, 221, 226–227, 2CP, 5CP, 6CP
  cross-bridge states, 227, 228f
  cycling rate, 227–228
  energetics, 221–222
  inotropic versus length effects on contractile apparatus, 239f
  ischemia and myofilaments
    creatine kinase, 242
    myosin ATPase, 242
    rigor state and ischemic contracture, 241–242
    troponin release in myocardial infarction, 242
  microanatomy, 223–226
  myofibrils, 44–45, 46f, 47
  phosphorylation of contractile proteins
    myosin binding protein C, 234
    myosin light chain, 233–234, 233f
    troponin I, 232–233
    troponin T, 234
  Rayment five-step molecular model, 228–229
  sarcomere gene mutations in cardiomyopathy
    dilated cardiomyopathy, 240

  heart failure, 241
  hypertrophic cardiomyopathy, 239–240
  restrictive cardiomyopathy, 240
  sarcomere length and Starling law
    ascending limb of Starling curve, 234, 235f, 236
    descending limb of Starling curve, 236
Cornell voltage-duration product, 150
Coronary artery disease. See also Atherosclerosis; Ischemia
  collateral flow, 297–298, 298f
  hemodynamic effects, 295
  stenosis and vascular resistance, 295–297, 296f
Coronary autoregulation, 292–293, 294f
Coronary circulation. See also Coronary artery disease; Ischemia
  abnormal coronary vasomotion, 300
  anatomy, 37–38, 279, 280f, 281
  autonomic control, 289–291
  metabolic vasodilation, 286–289, 299t
  measurement of blood flow, 300–302
  neuromodulation, 279, 280f, 281f, 284–286, 290f
  variations in flow
    coronary autoregulation, 292–293, 294f
    erectile effect, 295
    exercise effects, 294–295
    myogenic control, 293–294
    phasic coronary flow, 292, 293f
    reactive hyperemia, 291
Coronary spasm, 299–300
Coronary vascular reserve, 302, 495
Coronary vascular resistance (CVR), 282
Costamere, 58, 60–62, 11CP
CP. See Creatine phosphate
Creatine kinase (CK)
  contraction role, 242
  functions, 335–336
  MB isozymes, 335–336, 565
  myocardial infarction diagnosis, 336
Creatine phosphate (CP)
  ATP formation, 335
  cardiac functions, 334–335
  metabolic pathway regulation, 334t
Cristae, 47

Cromakalim, ATP-sensitive potassium channel activation, 102
Cross-bridge cycle. *See* Contraction–relaxation cycle
Cross-talk, receptors, 215, 257
αβ-Crystallin, 240
CT-1. *See* Cardiotrophin-1
Current, definition, 79
Current of injury, 540–541, 615, 615f
CVR, *See* Coronary vascular resistance
Cyclic adeneosine monophosphate (cAMP)
  cardiac effects, 202t
  compartmentation, 203
  drug response, 203t
  heart failure effects, 511t, 512
  hormone receptor signaling, 203–205, 204f
  organelle effects, 205–206
  protein kinase A activation, 205–206, 205f
  signal transduction, 186, 201
  synthesis, 198, 202f
  vascular smooth muscle cell effects, 203
Cyclic guanosine monophosphate (cGMP)
  cyclic nucleotide vasodiltory system, 441
  signal transduction, 188, 201, 213
Cyclopiazonic acid, sarcoplasmic reticulum calcium effects, 170t
Cytoskeleton
  mechanotransduction, 266–267
  overload hypertrophy
    biomechanical strain, 409
    load transduction, 407, 407f
    stretch-induced changes, 409, 410f

D

DADs. *See* Delayed afterdepolarizations
DAG. *See* Diacylglycerol
Debranching enzyme, 321
Delayed afterdepolarizations (DADs), 609–610, 614, 617–618
Depolarization, 73, 85, 104, 106, 539, 608
Desmin, 58, 59t, 60, 240, 11CP
Desmosome, 57, 58f
Diacylglycerol (DAG), signal transduction, 188, 210–211
Diastole

cellular factors influencing relaxation, 385–387, 387f
  definition, 6f, 358–359, 358t, 12CP
  dysfunction diagnosis, 395t
  early diastolic velocity, 388–389
  functional indices, 388t
  isovolumic relaxation, 387–388
  left ventricle sucking, 389–390
  left ventricular dysfunction, 390
  phases, 385, 386f
Diastolic distensibility, 391, 393f
Diastolic failure, 504–506, 506f
Diastolic filling, 12CP
Diazoxide, ATP-sensitive potassium channel activation, 102
Digitalis
  atrial stunning management, 606
  congestive heart failure management, 517
  contraction–relaxation cycle effects, 235f
  mechanism of action, 112
  proarrhythmic activity, 619–620
Dilated cardiomyopathy, 490–491, 491f
Diltiazem, 606, 617t
Dipyridamole, adenosine deaminase inhibition, 286
Disopyramide, 611
Distensibility, 496
Disuse atrophy, 588
DNA
  structure, 258
  transcription, 256–257, 257f
Dobutamine, inotropic effects, 193
Dopamine, cardiac response, 205
Doppler, tissue, 384
Dynamic coronary stenosis, 296, 299
Dyskinesia, 529
Dystroglycans, 11CP
Dystrophin, 59t, 62, 240, 491, 11CP

E

EADs. *See* Early afterdepolarizations
Early afterdepolarizations (EADs), 610–611, 614, 618
ECG. *See* Electrocardiogram
Echocardiography
  cardiac output measurement, 467
  contractility measurement, 384
  diastolic function, 388–390

ECM. *See* Extracellular matrix
EGF. *See* Epidermal growth factor
Ejection fraction
  contractility measurement, 383–384
  definition, 373
Elastin, 63, 63t
Electrical alternans, 609
Electrocardiogram (ECG)
  atrial ectopic depolarization, 602f
  atrial fibrillation, 605, 605f
  atrial flutter, 602f
  bundle branch block, 147–149
  electrical axis, 140
  f wave, 602f, 604
  historical perspective, 137–138, 137f
  ischemia
    angina, 154–155
    current of injury, 540–541
    epicardial versus endocardial electrocardiogram, 542
    faction potential changes, 539–540
    potassium loss and depolarization, 539, 541
    ST segment changes, 541–543, 543f, 544
    T-wave inversion, 543–544
  leads
    bipolar standard leads, 138
    limb leads, 138–139, 138f, 139f
    unipolar precordial chest leads, 139, 140f
  left ventricular hypertrophy, 136f, 150, 151f
  myocardial infarction, 150–154
  PR interval, 134, 135f, 144, 145f
  P wave, 134, 135f
  QRS complex, 134–135, 135f, 136f
  Q wave, 134, 135f, 153–154, 153f
  right ventricular hypertrophy, 150, 151f
  R wave, 134–135, 135f
  signal sources, 133, 134f, 139, 141f
  sinoatrial rate
    arrhythmia, 141–142, 142f
    bradycardia, 142–144
    heart rate determination, 141
    tachycardia, 142–144
  ST segment, 134–135, 135f, 150–153
  S wave, 135, 135f
  T wave, 134–135, 135f, 136f, 137

ventricular arrhythmias, 607f
Wolff–Parkinson–White syndrome, 602f
Emotional stress
  blood pressure effects, 443–444, 444f
  heart rate effects, 443–444, 444f
  hemodynamic response, 479–480, 479f, 480t
  sudden cardiac death, 480
Encainide, 617t
Endocardium, anatomy, 8–9
Endothelial dysfunction
  hypertension, 454–455, 454f, 455f
  hypertrophy progression to heart failure, 495
  plaque progression, 555–558, 556f, 559f
Endothelin
  heart failure role, 514
  hypertension role, 454f
  overload hypertrophy role, 411–413
  peripheral vascular resistance control, 441
  vasoconstriction, 286, 299–300
Epidermal growth factor (EGF), overload hypertrophy role, 413
Epinephrine
  blood pressure regulation, 19f, 437
  cardiac output response, 19f, 20f
  cyclic AMP response, 203t
  sympathetic activation, 16, 17f
  vascular tone effects, 26–27
  vasodilation, 24, 25f, 29, 284t
ERK. *See* Extracellular-regulated kinase
Excitation–contraction coupling
  calcium
    efflux from cells, 176
    influx via sodium–calcium exchanger, 167, 167f
    ion movements, 160f, 162–163
    sparks, 168
    storage and control, 175
  local control theory, 168
  overview, 159, 160f
  positive inotropic and relaxant effects of β-adrenergic stimulation, 177–178, 178f
  sarcoplasmic reticulum
    calcium release, 164–166
    calcium transients, 163–164, 164f
    calcium uptake, 163, 166

cessation of calcium release, 168–169
inositol 1,4,5-triphosphate induction of calcium release, 171, 172f
timing of events, 166–167
Exercise
abnormal coronary vasomotion, 300
aging and capacity, 478
arrhythmia induction, 478
autonomic stimulation, 474–475
beta-blockade effects on cardiac output, 473
blood pressure effects, 446, 447f
blood redistribution, 32
cardiac energy metabolism, 475
central cardiovascular control centers, 474
coronary flow effects, 294–295
dynamic versus static exercise
central integration and reflexes, 467–468, 470f, 474–475
hemodynamic response, 467–468, 471f
posture effects on cardiac output, 472–473
pressure–volume loops, 471–472, 472f, 473f
ergoreflexes, 474
myocardial oxygen demand effects, 467, 468f, 526f
sudden cardiac death, 481
tachycardia induction mechanism, 464
training
athlete heart characteristics, 476f, 477
cardiac protection mechanisms, 477–478
exercise phenotype, 476–477
transplanted heart response, 216–217
vasodilation, 442
Extracellular matrix (ECM)
collagen, 62–63, 64f
fibroblasts, 62
matrix metalloproteinases, 64–65
proteins, 62, 63t
remodeling in heart failure, 496, 497f
Extracellular-regulated kinase (ERK), 255–256, 408–409

F

Fascia adherens junction, 57
Fatty acids

fasted state metabolism, 307, 309, 309f
ischemia metabolism, 533
metabolism
beta-oxidation, 325
glucose–fatty acid cycle, 309, 311
insulin effects, 313, 314f
malonyl-CoA inhibition of oxidation, 324–325
overview, 306, 307f
mitochondrial transfer, 323–324, 324f
regulation of metabolic genes, 271–272
uptake, 322, 322f, 324t
Fetal phenotype, overload hypertrophy, 415–416, 415t
FGF. *See* Fibroblast growth factor
Fibroblast growth factor (FGF), overload hypertrophy role, 411, 413
Fibroblast, cardiac, 62, 64
Fibronectin, 63–64, 63t
Fibrosis, 62, 419–420, 422, 422f
Fick principle, 467
Fixed coronary stenosis, 296
Flecainide, 617t
Foam cell, 557
Focal adhesion complex, 61, 11CP
Focal adhesion kinase, 61
Force
conceptual model, 374–375, 374f
definition, 373–374
Force–frequency relationship, 365–367, 366f, 465
Force–velocity relationship, 367–368, 368f
Forskolin, cyclic AMP response, 203t, 205
Frank–Starling law, 362–363, 363f, 503, 503f
Free radicals. *See* Reactive oxygen species; Peroxynitrite
Futile cycle, 333
f wave, 602f, 604

G

Galen, 3
Gap junction, 16, 54, 56, 609
GATA-4, 256
Glucagon, cyclic AMP response, 203
Glucose
exercise-induced uptake, 475

Glucose (contd.)
  metabolism. See also Glycogen;
      Glycolysis
    energy balance during oxidative
        metabolism, 318f
    fed state metabolism, 309, 310f
    overview, 306, 307f
    positron emission tomography,
        346–347, 347f
    oxygen extraction ratio, 308t, 310t
    regulation of metabolic genes, 271–272
    transporters, 311–312
Glucose–fatty acid cycle, 309, 311
Glutathione peroxidase, antioxidant
    defense, 581t
Glyceraldehyde 3-phosphate
    dehydrogenase, 342
Glycocalyx, structure and function, 49
Glycogen
  breakdown, 320–321, 320f
  cardiac functions, 321
  storage diseases, 321
  synthesis, 319–320, 320f
Glycogenin, 321
Glycogen synthase kinase, 415
Glycolysis
  anaerobic, 308f, 341, 342f, 343
  enzymes, 314–315
  ischemic metabolism, 341–343, 342f, 533
  overview, 306, 308f, 314–315, 314f
  regulation, 315, 315t
G protein-coupled receptors. See also
    specific receptors
  anchoring proteins, 197–198, 197f
  G protein cycle, 198, 199f
  signal transduction, 21–22, 186, 188,
      193, 198–207
  structure, 193, 194f
Growth factors. See specific factors

H

Harvey, circulation concepts, 5f, 6
Heart block
  first-degree block, 145, 146f
  second-degree block, 145, 146f
  third-degree block, 145, 146f
Heart cells, types, 42t
Heart failure. See also Overload
    hypertrophy

β-adrenergic receptor response, 216,
    508–512, 509f
adrenomedullin response, 516
antidiuretic hormone response, 513
arrhythmias
  cardiac memory, 619
  drug induction, 618–620, 620f
  mechanisms, 618, 619f, 620f
atrial natriuretic peptide response,
    515–516, 516f
beta-blocker therapy, 510f, 512
brain natriuretic peptide response,
    515–516, 516f
calcium cycling, 508f
cardiac performance enhancers, 397t
cardiomyocyte hypertrophy versus
    hyperplasia, 260–261
causes, 485, 486t
circulation control, 37
clinical syndrome. See Congestive heart
    failure
contractility dysfunction, 396–397, 386t
cyclic AMP generation, 511t, 512
diastolic distensibility, 391, 393f
efficiency of work, 379, 380f
endothelin role, 514
hypertrophy progression to failure
  aldosterone role, 495–496
  angiotensin II role, 495–496
  apoptosis, 496–497
  calcium flux abnormalities, 498,
      500f
  collagen deposition, 496
  compensation loss, 494–495
  coronary vascular reserve
      impairment, 495
  endothelial defects, 495
  extracellular matrix remodeling, 496,
      497f
  metabolic defects, 497–498, 500, 501f
  myocardial outstripping of blood
      supply, 495
  myosin isoforms, 502
  sarcomere overstretching, 502–503
  Swan–Ganz catheterization studies,
      503, 503f
metabolic defects, 347
nitric oxide in dilated cardiomyopathy,
    216

primary myocardial failure. *See*
    Cardiomyopathy
sarcoplasmic reticulum role
    heart rate pacing, 181–182
    ryanodine receptor
        hyperphosphorylation, 180–181,
        181f
    SERCA deficiency and inhibition, 180
sodium retention and edema, 514
tumor necrosis factor-α role, 515
wall stress, 371–372
Heart rate
    adenosine effects, 204
    Bowditch staircase effect, 365
    cardiac output component, 460, 461f,
        462, 463f, 464
    definition, 141, 461t
    determination, 141, 143f
    diurnal changes, 13, 14f
    exercise induction mechanism, 464
    force–frequency relationship, 365–367,
        366f, 465
    intrinsic heart rate, 126–127
    maximal rate calculation by age, 462
    mental stress response, 443–444, 444f
    sarcoplasmic reticulum role in pacing in
        heart failure, 181–182
    stimulators, 462, 463t
    transplanted hearts, 465
Heart sounds, origins, 358t
Heparin, sarcoplasmic reticulum calcium
    effects, 170t
Hering–Breuer reflex, 141–142
Hexokinase, 314–315
Hibernation
    animal models, 588
    characteristics, 575t, 576f
    clinical significance, 588–589, 589f
    definition, 574
    disuse atrophy, 588
    mechanisms, 586–587, 586f, 587f
    signaling, 588
His bundle
    blood supply, 133
    function, 10, 130, 132
    idioventricular rhythm, 146
    Purkinje cells, 132–133
Hodgkin–Huxley hypothesis, 81–83
Hydralazine, 517

Hyperkalemia, 87, 608
Hyperplasia
    definition, 260–261, 402, 403f
    developmental changes in
        cardiomyocytes, 404
Hyperpolarization, 125–126
Hypertension
    cardiac complications, 451, 456
    definition, 431, 450–451
    endothelial dysfunction, 454–455, 454f,
        455f
    insulin resistance association, 453–454,
        453f
    lifestyle factors, 455–456
    low renin hypertension, 454
    mechanisms, 432f, 451, 452f
    neurogenic theory, 451
    obesity association, 453
    patterns in hypertrophy, 488–489, 489f
    salt-sensitive hypertension, 452
    sodium handling abnormalities,
        451–452, 452f
Hypertrophic cardiomyopathy, 489–490,
    490f, 491f
Hypertrophy. *See* Left ventricular
    hypertrophy; Overload hypertrophy;
    Right ventricular hypertrophy
Hypokalemia, ventricular arrhythmias,
    607, 620
Hypotension, 434f
Hypoxia, vasodilation, 289
H zone, 45, 46f

I

I band, 45, 46f
Idioventricular rhythm, 146
IGF-I. *See* Insulin-like growth factor-I
Inferior vena cava, 8
Inositol 1,4,5-triphosphate (IP_3)
    calcium release induction, 171
    signal transduction, 188, 210–211
Inotropic state. *See* Contractility
Insulin
    metabolic actions, 312–313, 313f
    overload hypertrophy role, 413
    receptor autophosphorylation, 256, 313
Insulin resistance
    atherosclerosis risks, 557
    cardiac metabolism, 345

Insulin resistance (contd.)
  hypertension association, 453–454, 453f
Insulin-like growth factor-I (IGF-I),
  overload hypertrophy role, 413
Integrin, 59t, 60–61, 61f
Intercalated disk, 54, 55f, 57f, 59t
Intermediate filament, 58
Ion channels. See also specific channels
  driving forces for ions, 79
  evolution, 81f
  gating
    kinetics, 81–83
    ligand gating, 83
    molecular mechanisms, 83, 85
    voltage gating, 79, 82–83, 85
  ionophores, 87–88
  selectivity, 83
  stretch-activated channels, 113, 410
  structure, 79–81, 80f, 81f, 82f
IP_3. See Inositol 1,4,5-triphosphate
Ischemia. See also Atherosclerosis;
  Coronary artery disease
  acidosis effects, 534–535
  adaptation
    metabolic changes, 528
    perfusion–contraction match, 526, 527f
    perfusion–contraction mismatch, 526, 527f
  angina pectoris. See Angina pectoris
  ATP-sensitive potassium channel role, 539
  β-adrenergic receptors, 215–216
  calcium abnormalities, 533
  contractility impairment, 528–529, 528t
  current of injury, 540–541, 615, 615f
  definition, 341, 525
  irreversible ischemic damage
    mechanisms, 563, 564f, 565
  magnesium abnormalities, 534
  metabolic therapy
    fatty acid metabolism inhibition, 348–349
    gene therapy, 349
    glycolysis coupling to glucose oxidation, 348
    glycolysis-promoting agents, 348
    omega-3 fatty acids, 349–350
    post-reperfusion abnormalities, 349
    principles, 347–348, 546

  metabolic vasodilation, 299t
  metabolism
    ATP loss, 344, 529–530, 534
    ATP requirements, 343–344, 343f
    fatty acids, 533
    glycolysis, 341–343, 342f, 533
    lactate accumulation, 535
    lipid metabolites in injury, 345–346, 346f
    malate–aspartate cycle and NADH accumulation, 535–536
    metabolite accumulation effects, 534
  mild versus severe ischemia effects, 531t
  mixed cardiac response, 595t
  myofilament effects
    creatine kinase, 242
    myosin ATPase, 242
    rigor state and ischemic contracture, 241–242
    troponin release in myocardial infarction, 242
  oxygen balance in ischemic zone, 537–538
  potassium current flow induction, 102–103
  preconditioning. See Preconditioning
  proton sources in acidosis, 532t
  recovery
    ion normalization, 544–545
    metabolism, 545–546
    time, 544, 545f
  reperfusion injury, 344
  severity and clinical effects, 536t
  silent ischemia, 539
  sodium abnormalities, 534
  subendocardial ischemia, 298–299
  supply versus demand ischemia, 537–538
  treatment
    beta-blockers, 537, 546
    calcium channel blockers, 546
    heart size control, 546
    nitrates, 546
    revascularization, 546–548, 547f
  vasodilation mechanisms, 295
Ischemic cascade, 536–537, 537f
Isometric contraction, 365
Isometric shortening, 368
Isoproterenol, 190, 191f
Isotonic contraction, 368–369

Isovolumic contraction, 357, 362, 381, 12CP
Isovolumic relaxation, 357, 387–388, 12CP

J
JAK. *See* Janus kinase
Janus kinase (JAK), 264f, 265–266, 406f, 422f
JNK. *See* Jun N-terminal kinase
Jugular venous pressure, 12CP
Junctional escape rhythm, 146
Jun N-terminal kinase (JNK), 255–256
Juxtaglomerular cells, 436f, 514f

K
Krebs cycle
  ATP yield, 326, 328t
  calcium regulation, 329
  mechanical work induction, 326–328, 328f
  overview, 326, 327f

L
Lactate
  fate, 317
  ischemic accumulation, 535
  oxygen extraction ratio, 308t, 310t
  synthesis, 316–317
Lactate dehydrogenase, 317
Laminin, 64
Laplace law, 370f, 371–372, 402, 421
LDL. *See* Low-density lipoprotein
Left anterior hemiblock, 147, 149, 149f
Left atrium
  anatomy, 6
  arterial pressure pattern, 12f
Left bundle branch block, 147, 147f, 148f
Left coronary artery, 281
Left posterior hemiblock, 149
Left ventricle
  anatomy, 6
  arterial pressure pattern, 12f
  failure. *See* Heart failure
  transmural distribution of fibers, 7–8
Left ventricular compliance
  causes of loss, 392–393
  definition, 391, 392f
  elasticity, 391, 392f
  Starling curve effects, 393, 394f

Left ventricular hypertrophy (LVH). *See also* Overload hypertrophy
  diastolic failure, 487
  electrocardiogram, 136f, 150, 151f
  hypertensive patterns, 488–489, 489f
  overload mechanisms, 485, 486f, 487
  regression and angiotensin II inhibition, 421–423
  valve lesions
    aortic regurgitation, 493–494, 493f
    aortic stenosis, 492–493, 492f
    mitral regurgitation, 493–494, 493f
    mitral stenosis, 492, 494f
  volume overload and left ventricular function, 487–488
  volume versus pressure load, 488, 489f
Left ventricular strain, 150, 151f
Leptin, food intake regulation, 313–314, 453f
Leukotrienes, coronary spasm role, 299
Lidocaine, 86, 617, 617t
LIM protein, 60f
Lipid peroxidation, reperfusion injury, 580
Lipotoxicity, 346
Long QT syndrome (LQTS)
  acquired form, 611–612
  afterdepolarization, 600
  hereditary channelopathies, 611–612, 613f
Losartan, left ventricular hypertrophy regression, 422
Low-density lipoprotein (LDL), oxidation, 557, 558f
Low renin hypertension, 454
LQTS. *See* Long QT syndrome
LVH. *See* Left ventricular hypertrophy
Lysophosphoglycerides, 345–346

M
Macrophage, atherosclerosis role, 557–558
Magnesium
  concentrations in heart ventricles, 78t, 113
  functions, 113
  ischemia abnormalities, 534
  transport, 113
Magnetic resonance imaging (MRI), myocardial infarction diagnosis, 566, 568

Malate-aspartate shuttle, 317, 319f, 328, 344, 535–536
Malonyl-CoA, 324–325, 349
MAPK. *See* Mitogen-activated protein kinase
Matrix metalloproteinases (MMPs), 64–65, 496, 497f
Maximal velocity of contraction, 367–369
Meerson three-stage model of pressure-induced hypertrophy development, 404
Mental stress. *See* Emotional stress
Metabolic syndrome, 453
Metabolism, oxidative, 310t, 325
Metacrine signaling, 247
Microcirculation, anatomy, 11, 34f
Microspheres, coronary blood flow measurement, 301
Minoxidil, ATP-sensitive potassium channel activation, 102
Minute work, 373
Mitochondria. *See also* Oxidative phosphorylation
  calcium uptake and release, 329–330
  cardiomyocytes, 44, 47
  cristae, 47
  energy production, 47, 49
  fatty acid uptake, 322–323, 322f
  myocardial oxygen demand and metabolism dynamics, 467, 469f
  permeability transition pore, 565
  preconditioning hypothesis, 593, 593f
  respiratory control, 329
  structure and function, 47, 48f, 49
Mitogen-activated protein kinase (MAPK)
  angiotensin II receptor signaling, 253–255
  overload hypertrophy role, 408–409, 413–414
  types, 255–256
Mitral regurgitation, 493–494, 493f
Mitral stenosis, 492, 494f
Mitral valve, anatomy, 6
MLP protein, 60f, 240
MMPs. *See* Matrix metalloproteinases
Monensin, 87
MRI. *See* Magnetic resonance imaging
Muscarinic receptors. *See* Cholinergic receptors

Myocardial infarction. *See also* Atherosclerosis; Coronary artery disease
  arrhythmias, 614–616
  autophagic cell death, 559
  diagnosis of irreversible damage
    creatine kinase release, 565, 566f
    magnetic resonance imaging, 566
    troponin release, 565, 566f
  electrocardiography
    Q wave changes, 153–154, 153f, 567, 567f
    ST segment changes, 150, 152f, 153, 553, 567, 567f
  infarct size
    area at risk, 568–569, 568f
    imaging, 568
  irreversible ischemic damage mechanisms, 563, 564f, 565
  mechanisms of infarction, 559–560, 561f
  necrosis versus apoptosis, 559–560, 560f
  patency after reperfusion, 566–567
  plaque rupture, 553, 555f
  postinfarction remodeling, 569, 570f
  prognosis in the elderly, 571
  reperfusion therapy, 553–554
  stages, 553, 554f
  stem cell therapy, 570–571, 571f
  triggers, 562–563
  wave front phenomenon, 554–555
Myocardial ischemia. *See* Ischemia
Myocardial oxygen demand
  determinants, 373–379, 526f
  exercise effects, 467, 468f, 526f
  heart rate effects, 462
  indices, 467, 470t
  mitochondrial metabolism dynamics, 467, 469f
  wall stress relationship, 372–373
Myocyte slippage, 496
Myofiber, 43, 1CP
Myofibril
  contraction–relaxation cycle, 44–45, 46f, 47, 1CP
  definition, 43
  proteins, 222t
  ultrastructure, 46f
Myoglobin, oxygen transport, 283
Myosin

binding protein-C, 10CP
filament, 224
head, 224–225, 225t, 4CP, 10CP
heart failure isoforms, 502
heavy chains, 224
isoforms, 237, 238t
light chains, 225, 233–234, 233f
structure, 224, 4CP
Myosin ATPase
  ischemia effects, 242
  isozymes, 237, 238f, 239
  regulation by calcium, 237
Myosin binding protein C, 225–226, 234, 240
Myosin filaments, 44–45
Myosin light chain kinase, 233–234, 233f

N

NADH, accumulation in ischemia, 535–536
Necrosis, apoptosis comparison, 559–560, 560f
Neuropeptide Y (NPY), vasoconstriction, 290
Neutrophil trafficking, 585
Nexus junction, 54
NF-κB. *See* Nuclear factor-κB
NFAT. *See* Nuclear factor of activated T cells
Nicorandil, ATP-sensitive potassium channel activation, 102
Nifedipine, mechanism of action, 92
Nigericin, 87
Nitric oxide (NO)
  blood pressure control, 437
  cholinergic receptor signaling, 125, 125f, 213–215, 214f
  donors in ischemia management, 546
  excess in disease, 216
  exercise response, 294–295
  functions, 270
  interactions with adenosine and K_{ATP} channel, 288
  peripheral vascular resistance control, 441
  peroxynitrite formation, 270
  signal transduction, 188, 268–269, 268f
  synthase isoforms, 269
  synthesis, 29–30, 214, 268–269
  vasodilation, 24, 29, 30f, 269, 285–286, 288

NMR. *See* Nuclear magnetic resonance
NO. *See* Nitric oxide
Nodal rhythm, 146
No reflow, microvascular damage, 584–585
Norepinephrine
  angiotensin II modulation of release, 26
  blood pressure regulation, 437
  circulation response, 20, 21f, 22f
  contraction–relaxation cycle effects, 235f
  cyclic AMP response, 203t
  ischemia response, 215
  receptors. *See* α-Adrenergic receptors
  release, 24, 25f, 26
  sympathetic activation, 16, 17f
  vascular tone effects, 26–27
  vasoconstriction, 24, 25f, 284t
NPY. *See* Neuropeptide Y
Nuclear factor of activated T cells (NFAT), calcineurin interactions, 177, 177f
Nuclear factor-κB (NF-κB)
  growth regulation, 265f, 267, 422f
  inhibitory protein, 267
Nuclear magnetic resonance (NMR), phosphate studies of metabolism, 341, 347
Nucleus
  cardiomyocytes, 44, 53–54
  functions, 54
Nucleus solitarius, baroreflex control, 27–28, 433

O

Obesity, hypertension association, 453
OER. *See* Oxygen extraction ratio
Overload hypertrophy. *See also* Left ventricular hypertrophy
  action potential changes, 417, 418f
  altered gene expression
    atrial natriuretic peptide, 417
    c-fos, 415, 415t
    c-jun, 415, 415t
    c-myc, 415, 415t
    contractile protein isoforms, 415–416, 416f, 417
    fetal phenotype, 415–416, 415t
    growth factor activation, 415
  cytoskeleton
    biomechanical strain, 409
    load transduction, 407, 407f

Overload hypertrophy, cytoskeleton (*contd.*)
stretch-induced changes, 409, 410f
estrogen protection, 417
hyperplasia comparison with
hypertrophy, 260–261, 402, 403f
Meerson three-stage model of
development, 404
molecular regulation
adrenergic stimulation, 413
angiotensin II, 406–407, 406f,
410–411, 411f, 413–414
calcineurin, 405, 406, 414f
endothelin, 411–413
epidermal growth factor, 413
fibroblast growth factor, 411, 413
insulin, 413
insulin-like growth factor-I, 413
mitogen-activated protein kinase,
408–409, 413–414
overview, 405, 405f
platelet-derived growth factor, 413
shared signaling systems, 414
systolic versus diastolic signaling,
60f, 408–409
transforming growth factor-β, 411, 431
tumor necrosis factor-α, 407–408
nonmyocardial cell effects, 410–411, 411f
physiologic hypertrophy in athletes, 477
pressure load, 402–404, 403f
ultrastructural changes
collagen accumulation, 419–420
fibrosis, 419–420
overview, 418–419, 419f, 420f
vascular remodeling, 420–421
volume load, 402–404, 403f
Oxidative phosphorylation
ATP production, 330
electron transport through respiratory
chain, 331–332, 332f
overview, 330, 331f
oxygen wasting and uncoupling, 333
proton pumping, 332f, 333
shuttling, 335–336
Oxidative stress. *See* Reactive oxygen
species
Oxygen demand. *See* Myocardial oxygen
demand
Oxygen extraction ratio (OER), 308t,
310t

Oxygen tension, tissues, 283–284

P

p38 mitogen-activated protein kinase,
255–256
Pacemaker cells, 119–120, 120f
Papaverine, 291
Papillary muscles, anatomy, 7
Parasympathetic nervous system
circulation regulation, 16, 18f, 23f
sinoatrial node regulation, 124–125, 124f
Paroxysmal supraventricular tachycardia
(PSVT), 603–604
pCO_2. *See* Carbon dioxide tension
Perfusion–contraction match, 526, 527f
Perfusion–contraction mismatch, 526, 527f
Pericardium
anatomy, 8
diastole effects, 395
Peripheral vascular resistance (PVR), 32f
arteriolar resistance, 11–12, 33–34,
432f, 452f
calculation, 32, 432
control
acute regulation, 432
autoregulation in regional
circulations, 442–443
cyclic nucleotide vasodilatory system,
441
endothelin, 441
integrated control, 436–437, 436f
myogenic properties, 442
nitric oxide, 441
temperature, 442
vasoconstrictor receptors, 440–441
factors affecting, 32–33
neurotransmitter regulation, 24
Poiseuille law, 33f, 34, 440
Peroxisome proliferator-activated receptor
(PPAR)
gene therapy targeting, 349
metabolic regulation of genes, 247,
270–272, 271f
Peroxynitrite, 270, 455, 455f, 580, 581t
PET. *See* Positron emission tomography
PFK. *See* Phosphofructokinase
Phasic coronary flow, 292, 293f
Phosphatidylinositol-3-phosphate kinase,
256–257

Phosphofructokinase (PFK), 315, 342
Phospholamban, 113, 172, 173f, 174–175
Phospholipase C (PLC)
    angiotensin II receptor signaling, 252
    negative inotropic effects, 211–212
    signal transduction, 188, 210–211
Phospholipids, cardiac membranes, 325–326
Phosphorylase *a*, 321
Phosphorylation/oxidation ratio, 325
Phosphorylation potential, 340–341
Pinacidil, ATP-sensitive potassium channel activation, 102
PKA. *See* Protein kinase A
PKB. *See* Protein kinase B
PKC. *See* Protein kinase C
PKG. *See* Protein kinase G
Platelet-derived growth factor, overload hypertrophy role, 413
PLC. *See* Phospholipase C
Poiseuille law, 33f, 34, 282, 296, 440
Polysome, 259
Positron emission tomography (PET)
    coronary blood flow measurement, 301
    metabolic imaging, 346–347, 347f, 346–347
Postural hypotension, 446
Potassium
    concentrations in heart ventricles, 77, 78t
    equilibrium potential, 78
    internal potassium activity, 78
    loss and depolarization in ischemia, 539, 541f
    rectification of currents, 103
    resting membrane potential role, 77–78
    vasodilation, 289
    ventricular arrhythmia role, 608
Potassium channels
    action potential, 50, 93, 95f, 105
    ATP-sensitive channel, 101–102, 101f, 288, 295, 539, 593
    calcium-activated channel BK_{Ca}, 101
    cardiac function of different types, 93, 94t
    classification, 93, 94t
    delayed rectifier potassium current in pacemaker cells, 122
    HERG channel, 95–96
    inwardly-rectifying channels, 96–97, 97f
    inward versus outward rectification, 98f
    ischemia-induced potassium current flow, 102–103
    K_{min}, 100
    ligand-operated channels, 99–100, 99t, 100f, 102–103
    physiologic versus pathologic channels, 103f
    repolarization, 109
    sarcolemmal membrane density, 77t
    slowly repolarizing channel, 94t, 95
    structure, 96f
    transient outward current, 97, 99
    vasodilation interactions with adenosine, nitric oxide, and K_{ATP} channel, 288
    voltage-gated channels, 93, 94t, 95, 96f
Potential energy, 376
Power
    definition, 373
    kinetic power, 375
    pressure power, 375
Power stroke, 5CP, 6CP
PPAR. *See* Peroxisome proliferator-activated receptor
Preconditioning
    characteristics, 575t, 576f
    clinical relevance, 595
    definition, 574
    delayed preconditioning mechanisms, 594–595
    early preconditioning mechanisms, 591, 592f, 593
    intraischemic preconditioning, 590, 591f
    mitochondrial hypothesis, 593, 593f
    models, 590, 590f
    phases, 591, 592f
Preload
    afterload relationship, 364–365, 369–370
    cardiac output contribution, 465
    definition, 359, 359f, 461t
    wall stress relationship, 372
Pressure–volume loops, 378, 378f, 385, 471–472, 472f, 473f, 8CP
Prinzmetal angina, 299
Proglycogen, 321
Promoter, 257–258, 258f
Propranolol
    antiarrhythmic activity, 617
    ischemia management, 537
    toxicity, 190

Prostacyclin, cyclic AMP response, 204
Prostaglandins, vasodilation, 289, 299
Protein kinase A (PKA)
　β-adrenergic receptor desensitization, 195–196
　anchoring proteins, 198
　cyclic AMP activation, 186, 205–206, 205f
　sarcoplasmic reticulum calcium regulation, 170, 177–178
　substrates, 206
Protein kinase B. See Akt
Protein kinase C (PKC)
　angiotensin II receptor signaling, 252–253
　heart failure activation, 241
　isozymes, 252
　preconditioning role, 591, 593
　signaling, 206–207, 207f
Protein kinase G (PKG), signaling, 207
Protein phosphatases, signaling, 207, 255–256
Protein synthesis
　cardiomyocytes, 260–261
　elongation factors, 259
　initiation factors, 259
　patterns, 260f
　posttranslational events, 259–260
　transcription, 257–259
　translation, 259–260
Protodiastole, 358–359
PSVT. See Paroxysmal supraventricular tachycardia
Pulmonary circulation, anatomy, 10–11
Purinergic receptors
　types, 287
　vasodilation mechanisms, 287–288
Purkinje cells
　action potential, 73–74, 75f, 105f
　arborization of fibers, 133
　His bundle, 132–133
　pacemaker currents, 132–133
Purkinje fibers, depolarization, 607
PVR. See Peripheral vascular resistance
Pyruvate
　fates, 316–317, 316f
　formation, 316
　oxygen extraction ratio, 308t
Pyruvate dehydrogenase, 316–317

Q
QRS complex, 604
QT interval, 600, 611, 614f
Quinidine, 86, 611, 617t

R
Raf, angiotensin II receptor signaling, 255
Rapamycin, restenosis inhibition, 547, 547f
Ras, angiotensin II receptor signaling, 254–255
Reactive hyperemia, 291
Reactive oxygen species (ROS)
　antioxidant defenses, 581–582, 581t
　calcium interactions, 582–583, 582f
　endothelial dysfunction, 454f, 455f
　generation reactions, 581t
　irreversible ischemic damage, 563
　oxidative stress, 267
　signaling, 248–249, 267–268
　sources, 267, 579–580, 579f
　stunning role, 580
　types, 579, 580t
Receptors. See also specific receptors
　cardiac types, 189t
　cross-talk, 215, 257
　dose–response curves, 190–191, 191f
　general mechanism, 187f, 189–190
　history of study, 188–189
　lock-and-key model, 190
Reentry circuit
　atrial, 599–600, 600f, 601f, 604–605
　ventricular, 607–608
Reflex bradycardia, 28
Reflex tachycardia, 28
Refractory period, 601–603, 602f, 605–606
Remodeling
　atrial fibrillation, 606
　postinfarction, 569, 570f
Renin, 30, 436f, 514f
Renin–angiotensin system
　blood pressure control, 436–437, 436f
　blood pressure regulation, 436–438
　blood volume regulation, 30–31
　enzymes, 249–250, 255f
　evolution, 249
　pathology, 31
Reperfusion injury. See also Hibernation; Preconditioning; Stunning
　accelerated cell death, 585–586

arrhythmias, 583–584, 616, 616f
definition, 344, 574
ischemia severity effects, 584
lipid peroxidation, 580
mechanisms, 582f
speed of reperfusion effects, 584
Repolarization, 73, 109
Restenosis, 547
Resting membrane potential, 77–78
Ribosome, protein synthesis, 54, 259–260
Right bundle branch block, 147, 148f
Right ventricular hypertrophy. *See also* Overload hypertrophy
electrocardiogram, 150, 151f
RNA polymerase, 258
ROS. *See* Reactive oxygen species
R-R interval, 605f
Ruthenium red, sarcoplasmic reticulum calcium effects, 170t
Ryanodine receptor (RyR)
arrays, 166
beta-blocker effects, 510f
caffeine effects, 170–171, 170t
calcium
release role, 165–166, 165f
response, 169–170
sparks, 168
store-regulated release, 175
damage in hypertrophy, 417
drug effects, 169, 170t
hyperphosphorylation in heart failure, 180–181, 181f
regulation of calcium release, 168–171
structure, 169
Ryanodine, sarcoplasmic reticulum calcium effects, 169, 170t
RyR. *See* Ryanodine receptor

S

SA node. *See* Sinoatrial node
Salbutamol, 193
Salt-sensitive hypertension, 452
Sarcolemma
calcium regulation, 49, 159, 163
cardiomyocyte association, 43–44
caveolae, 52
density of receptors and ion channels/pumps, 77t
fuzzy zone, 167
ion transfer, 73–74, 76f
polarization, 73
T tubules. *See* T tubule
Sarcomere
costamere, 58, 60–61, 11CP
gene mutations in cardiomyopathy
dilated cardiomyopathy, 240
heart failure, 241
hypertrophic cardiomyopathy, 239–240
restrictive cardiomyopathy, 240
length and Starling law
ascending limb of Starling curve, 234, 235f, 236
descending limb of Starling curve, 236
pressure-volume relation, 8CP
skeletal muscle versus cardiac muscle, 361
tension relationship, 261–263, 262f
mechanical force transmission, 60f
overstretching in heart failure, 502–503
structure, 45, 46f
Sarcoplasmic reticulum
calcium regulation, 52, 53f, 159
calcium storage and control, 175
diads, 52
excitation–contraction coupling
calcium release, 164–166
calcium transients, 163–164, 164f
calcium uptake, 163, 166
cessation of calcium release, 168–169
inositol 1,4,5-triphosphate induction of calcium release, 171
timing of events, 166–167
foot structure, 52
heart failure role
heart rate pacing, 181–182
ryanodine receptor hyperphosphorylation, 180–181, 181f
SERCA deficiency and inhibition, 180
network, 53
SERCA calcium uptake pump. *See* SERCA
triads, 52
Septic shock, nitric oxide excess, 216

SERCA
  ATP requirement, 171–172
  calcium store-regulated uptake, 175
  heart failure, deficiency and inhibition, 180
  phospholambin regulation, 172, 173f, 174–175
  phosphorylative regulation, 170, 174–175
  sarcoplasmic reticulum calcium uptake pump, 163, 166
  structure, 171
Serotonin, vascular tone effects, 285
Servetus, 3, 5
Sick sinus syndrome, 127, 144
Signal transducer and activator of transcription (STAT), 264f, 265–266
Sinoatrial (SA) node
  arrhythmias, 141–142, 142f
  automaticity, 119–120
  autonomic control
    hyperpolarization effects, 125–126
    intrinsic heart rate, 126–127
    nitric oxide, 125, 125f
    overdrive suppression, 127
    overview, 124–125
    parasympathetic activity, 124–125, 124f
    sympathetic activity, 124–125, 124f, 126f
  definition, 10
  depolarizing currents in heartbeat initiation
    background inward current, 122
    delayed rectifier potassium current, 122
    inward current, 123
    overview, 120, 121f, 122
    safety factors, 123
    slow inward nodal calcium currents, 122–123
  impulse propagation, 127–129, 128f, 129f
  pacemaker currents, 133t
  signaling in pacemaker activity, 24
  structure, 119–120, 120f
Smoking, atherosclerosis risks, 556
Smooth muscle cell. *See* Vascular smooth muscle cell

SOCS. *See* Suppressor of cytokine signaling
Sodium
  concentrations in heart ventricles, 78t
  ischemia abnormalities, 534
  retention in heart failure, 514
Sodium channels
  action potential, 50, 73–74, 75f, 85, 104
  activation, 2, 84f, 85
  antiarrhythmic agent targeting, 86
  calcium channel comparison, 86t
  depolarization role, 85, 104
  gating mechanisms, 83, 85
  patch recording, 82, 83f
  sarcolemmal membrane density, 77t
  sodium conductance versus current, 85–86
  threshold of activation, 85
Sodium–calcium exchanger
  action potential, 106, 107f, 108
  arrhythmia role, 108
  driving force, 108
  functions, 106
  ionic balance restoration, 74, 76f, 108–109, 163
  reversal potential, 106
  reverse mode exchange, 167, 167f
  stoichiometry, 106
  structure, 106
Sodium–potassium pump
  activation by ions, 112
  ATP requirement, 110, 334
  digitalis inhibition, 112
  functions, 74, 76f, 110, 111f
  sarcolemmal membrane density, 77t
  stoichiometry, 110–111
  structure, 111f, 112
Sodium–proton exchanger
  acid–base homeostasis, 109, 110f
  acidosis effects, 534
Sotalol, 611
Spectrin, 59t, 62, 11CP
ST segment, 541–543, 543f, 544f
Starling
  hypothesis for fluid exchange, 35f, 36
  law of the heart, 36–37, 234, 360, 360f
  left ventricular compliance effects on curve, 393, 394f
  sarcomere length and Starling law

ascending limb of Starling curve, 234, 235f, 236
descending limb of Starling curve, 236
skeletal muscle versus cardiac muscle, 361
tension relationship, 261–263, 262f
Starling curve familes, 360, 361f
STAT. *See* Signal transducer and activator of transcription
Stem cell therapy
myocardial infarction, 570–571, 571f
plasticity, 570
Stokes–Adams syndrome, 146
Stress. *See* Emotional stress; Wall stress
Stretch, versus tension, 409
Stretch-activated channels, 113, 410
Stroke volume
cardiac output component, 460
definition, 373
Stroke work, 373
Stroke work index, 373
Stunning
calcium overload, 578–579, 578f
cardioversion, 606
characteristics, 575t, 576f
clinical causes
angina recovery, 583
balloon angioplasty, 583
bypass surgery, 583
thrombolytics, 583
definition, 574
duration of ischemia and stunning, 576–577
mechanism, 577–579, 577f
reactive oxygen species role, 580
Substance P, 538
Sudden cardiac death
emotional stress, 480
exercise, 481
Sulfonylureas, ATP-sensitive potassium channel inhibition, 102
Superior vena cava, 8
Superoxide dismutase, antioxidant defense, 581t
Suppressor of cytokine signaling (SOCS), 264f
Swan–Ganz catheterization
cardiac output measurement, 467
hemodynamic measurements, 360

load reduction in heart failure, 503, 503f
Sympathetic nervous system
sinoatrial node regulation, 124–125, 124f, 126
stimulation
circulation response, 16, 17f, 20–21, 23f
heart failure, 507–512
Systemic circulation, anatomy, 5f, 10
Systemic vascular resistance. *See* Peripheral vascular resistance
Systole
cardiac cycle, 355–357, 12CP
definition, 7f, 358–359, 358t
dysfunction diagnosis, 395t
Systolic failure, 504–506, 507f

T
Tachycardia
electrocardiography, 143f
inducers, 142, 143t
Tachycardiomyopathy, 491
Talin, 59t
TATA box, 256–257, 257f
Tension. *See* Wall stress
Terfenadine, 612
Tetrodotoxin, sodium channel inhibition, 86–87
TGF-β. *See* Transforming growth factor-β
Thallium-201 scintigraphy, coronary blood flow measurement, 301–302
Thapsigargin, sarcoplasmic reticulum calcium effects, 170t
Theophylline, 286
Thermodilution, cardiac output measurement, 467
Thin filament, 4CP
Thyroid hormone, cyclic AMP response, 204
Titin, 45, 221, 223, 226, 236, 410, 3CP
TNF-α. *See* Tumor necrosis factor-α
Torsade de pointes, 612, 614f, 617
Training. *See* Exercise
Transcription factors
kinase activation, 256
promoter binding, 256–257, 257f
Transforming growth factor-β (TGF-β)
mechanotransduction, 266–267
overload hypertrophy role, 411, 431

Transitional cells, 120, 120f
Treppe effect. *See* Bowditch staircase phenomenon
Tricuspid valve, anatomy, 8
Triggered automaticity, 610
Tropomudulin, 224
Tropomyosin, 222–223, 240
Troponin C, 162–163, 222–223, 229–231, 4CP
Troponin I, 206, 222–223, 229, 232–233, 238t, 242, 386, 387f, 565
Troponin T, 222–223, 234, 238t, 240, 242, 565
T tubule
　functions, 50–52
　structure, 43, 46f, 51f
Tumor necrosis factor-α (TNF-α)
　adaptive and protective paths, 264
　apoptosis signaling, 262, 265
　atherosclerosis role, 557
　functions, 247–248, 263–264
　heart failure role, 515
　mechanotransduction, 266
　overload hypertrophy role, 407–408
　postinfarction remodeling, 569
T wave, 543–544

U

Uncoupling proteins, 333

V

Vagal nervous system. *See* Parasympathetic nervous system
Vascular smooth muscle cell
　action potential, 65–66
　calcium release mechanism, 172f
　cyclic AMP response, 203
　function, 65
　myofilaments, 65
　pathology, 66
　postpump syndrome role, 585
　structure, 65, 66f
Vasopressin. *See* Antidiuretic hormone
Vein, definition, 10

Venous capacitance system, 11
Venous return, 11
Ventricular ectopic depolarization, 606
Ventricular fibrillation, 606, 607f, 610f
Ventricular interactions, 394–395, 503
Verapamil, 606, 617t
Vesalius, 3, 4f
Vesicles, neurotransmitter release, 24–25
Vinculin, 59t, 61

W

Wall stress
　afterload relationship, 372, 449–450
　conceptual model, 370, 370f
　exercise, 475
　heart failure, 371–372
　Laplace law, 370f, 371–372
　myocardial oxygen demand relationship, 372–373
　preload relationship, 372
　tension, 370
Wave front phenomenon, 554–555
Wenkebach phenomenon, 477
White-coat syndrome, 444
Wiggers cycle, 12 CP
Wolff–Parkinson–White syndrome, 602f, 604
Work
　definition, 373
　efficiency of work
　　definition, 379
　　heart failure, 379, 380f
　　heat production, 379
　kinetic versus pressure work, 375
　left ventricle work diagram, 375–376, 376f
　myocardial oxygen consumption relationship, 376
　pressure versus volume work, 377–378, 377f, 378f, 380f

Z

Z disk, 45, 46f, 410, 11CP
Z line, 45, 46f, 223